Sjögren's Syndrome

Robert I. Fox · Carla M. Fox
Editors

Sjögren's Syndrome

Practical Guidelines to Diagnosis and Therapy

Springer

Editors
Robert I. Fox, MD, Ph.D.
Scripps Memorial Hospital & Research Foundation
Rheumatology Clinic
La Jolla, CA 92037, USA

Carla M. Fox, RN
Scripps Memorial Hospital & Research Foundation
Rheumatology Clinic
La Jolla, CA 92037, USA

ISBN 978-1-60327-956-7 e-ISBN 978-1-60327-957-4
DOI 10.1007/978-1-60327-957-4
Springer New York Dordrecht Heidelberg London

Library of Congress Control Number: 2011932791

Printed on acid-free paper

Springer is part of Springer Science+Business Media (www.springer.com)

Preface

"He who studies medicine without books
sails an uncharted sea,
but he who studies medicine without patients
does not go to sea at all."
—Sir William Osler (1849–1916)

Symptoms of dry eyes and dry mouth negatively affect the "quality of life" of the patient with Sjögren's Syndrome (SS). Patients have equated the "impact of sicca symptoms" at a level of disability equal to moderate angina and would be willing to "trade two to four years of (their) life expectancy" to be free of these symptoms. For example, a dry mouth alters the types of foods a patient can eat and thus interferes with "eating together." Eating serves far more than nutrition needs and represents a major part of social interaction for women at home, business, and relaxation with friends. Dry eyes interfere with the ability to use a computer for prolonged periods at work or at home, since staring at a computer screen involves a markedly decreased blink rate and exacerbates symptoms of aqueous tear deficiency.

Extraglandular manifestations can range from vasculitis to lymphoproliferative infiltrates of many organs. SS patients have a markedly increased risk incidence of lymphoma. Many older patients diagnosed with systemic lupus erythematosus (SLE) actually have SS. Since the correct diagnosis is not made for many years in most patients, their symptoms and signs due to glandular involvement are not adequately recognized and treated. Even in rheumatology, SS is not listed in the "Primer of Rheumatic Diseases," a major teaching instrument for residents and fellows in training.

This volume differs from other recent review publications that have appeared in "current opinion journals" or review volumes largely written by specialists in a single medical specialty. We have included a distinguished panel of authors in a broad spectrum of basic science, clinical, and surgical disciplines. Further, we have included authors from multiple areas of the world where SS has been studied.

Pathogenic studies reviewed in this volume include genetics and proteomics as well as cytokines and lymphoid regulation. The authors also emphasize that SS represents the intersection of the immune, secretory, and neural regulatory axes. An understanding of pathogenesis provides the backbone for understanding current diagnostic and therapeutic approaches. Further, basic science and astute clinical observation are the routes to future improved therapies.

Since the SS patient sees a wide variety of clinical and surgery specialists, we have included authors from many of the relevant areas to review their specialty's approach to diagnosis and therapy. For example, the management of SS often involves Ophthalmology, Oral Medicine, Oral Surgery, Otolaryngology, Gastroenterology, Dermatology, Nephrology, Chest Medicine, Hematology and Oncology, Neurology, and Rheumatology. Each specialty has been given the task of providing useful clinical hints as well as their "pearls of wisdom." By integrating the expertise by these eminent scholars in their respective clinical fields, we try to accomplish the fundamental goal of this book—to present cutting-edge diagnosis and therapeutic approaches to SS in one authoritative source.

The collaborative efforts of contributors in this book geographically span Europe, the Middle East, Asia, India, Australia, as well as the USA. This collection of enlightening chapters not only reflects our goal to recognize the outstanding contributions of each of these groups located around the world, but also emphasizes that the "medical world" is increasingly a global community composed of patients and their physicians.

In different regions of the world, the disease may have subtly different presentations, and the available diagnostic and therapeutic resources are dramatically different. Our patients increasingly present to us from different parts of the world, and they also travel to different regions for work or holiday. The inclusion of authors from around the world renders this resource an interconnective conduit between US rheumatologists and our counterparts throughout the world, in order to provide a universal spectrum of educational and clinical resources for our SS patients as well as for ourselves.

It is our hope that the reader finds this book to be a useful "first stop on Osler's journey" toward the procurement and utilization of reputable information that promotes the superior medical and nursing care that our courageous Sjögren's patients deserve.

We also wish to express our profound gratitude to: (a) our esteemed Authors, (b) our developmental editor Judi Brown, and (c) Springer Science+Business Media, for the immense amount of time, effort, and vision dedicated to the inception and evolution of this volume—without this degree of synergistic collaboration, this book would not have been possible.

La Jolla, California

Robert I. Fox
Carla M. Fox

Contents

Contributors

Ilias Alevizos Sjögren's Syndrome Clinic, National Institute of Dental and Craniofacial Research, Bethesda, MD, USA, alvizosi@nidcr.nih.gov

Elaine Alexander Sjögren's Syndrome Foundation Medical and Scientific Advisory Board, San Diego, CA, USA, elaine@easandiego.com

Jacqui E. Allen Department of Otolaryngology, University of Auckland, Auckland, New Zealand, jacquieallen@yahoo.com

Chiara Baldini Rheumatology Unit, University of Pisa, Pisa, Italy, chiara.baldini@gmail.com

Peter C. Belafsky The Center for Voice and Swallowing, University of California at Davis, Davis, CA, USA, pbelafsky@sbcglobal.net

Julius Birnbaum Division of Rheumatology, The Jerome L. Greene Sjögren's Syndrome Center, Johns Hopkins Bayview Medical Center, Baltimore, MD, USA, jbirnba2@jhmi.edu

Stefano Bombardieri Rheumatology Unit, University of Pisa, Pisa, Italy, s.bombardieri@int.med.unipi.it

Hendrika Bootsma Department of Rheumatology and Clinical Immunology, University of Groningen, Groningen, The Netherlands; University Medical Center, Groningen, The Netherlands, h.bootsma@reuma.umcg.nl

Simon J. Bowman Department of Rheumatology, University Hospitals Birmingham, Birmingham, England, simon.bowman@uhb.nhs.uk

Steven E. Carsons SUNY at Stony Brook School of Medicine, Stony Brook, NY, USA; Division of Rheumatology, Allergy and Immunology, Winthrop-University Hospital, Mineola, NY, USA, Scarsons@winthrop.org

Seunghee Cha Department of Oral Surgery and Diagnostic Sciences, University of Florida College of Dentistry, Gainesville, FL, USA; Department of Oral Biology, University of Florida College of Dentistry, Gainesville, FL, USA, SCHA@dental.ufl.edu

Edward K.L. Chan Department of Oral Biology, University of Florida College of Dentistry, Gainesville, FL, USA, echan@ufl.edu

John A. Chiorini Department of Molecular Physiology and Therapeutics Branch, National Institute of Dental and Craniofacial Research, Bethesda, MD, USA, jchiorin@mail.nih.gov

Philip L. Cohen Section of Rheumatology, Department of Medicine, Temple University School of Medicine, Philadelphia, PA, USA, philco@temple.edu

Debashish Danda Department of Clinical Immunology and Rheumatology, Christian Medical College, Vellore, India, debashishdandacmc@hotmail.com

Nicolas Delaleu Broegelmann Research Laboratory, The Gade Institute, University of Bergen, Bergen, Norway; Rheumatology Clinic, Scripps Memorial Hospital and Research Foundation, La Jolla, CA, USA, nicolas.delaleu@gades.uib.no

Carla M. Fox Rheumatology Clinic, Scripps Memorial Hospital and Research Foundation, La Jolla, CA, USA, carlafoxrn@mac.com

Robert I. Fox Rheumatology Clinic, Scripps Memorial Hospital and Research Foundation, La Jolla, CA, USA, robertfoxmd@mac.com

Jonn Terje Geitung Haraldsplass Deaconess University Hospital, Bergen, Norway, jtgeit@online.no; jonn.terje.geitung@haraldsplass.no

Tom Gordon Department of Immunology, Flinders Medical Center, Flinders, Australia, t.gordon@flinders.edu.au

Jacques-Eric Gottenberg Centre de Recherche Biomédical Strasbourgeois (CRBS), Hôpitaux Universitaires de Strasbourg, Université de Strasbourg, Strasbourg, France, jacques-eric.gottenberg@chru-strasbourg.fr

Katherine Morland Hammitt Sjögren's Syndrome Foundation, Lynchburg, VA, USA, khammitt@sjogrens.org

John B. Harley Division of Rheumatology, Cincinnati Children's Hospital Medical Center, Cincinnati, OH, john.Harley@cchmc.org

Jing He Department of Rheumatology and Immunology, People's Hospital, Peking University Medical School, Beijing, China, hejing_1105@yahoo.com

Gustaaf W. van Imhoff Department of Hematology, University of Groningen, Groningen, The Netherlands; University Medical Center, Groningen, The Netherlands, g.w.van.imhoff@int.umcg.nl

Malin V. Jonsson Institute of Medicine - Section for Rheumatology, University of Bergen, Bergen, Norway, malin.jonsson@odont.uib.no

Roland Jonsson Broegelmann Research Laboratory, The Gade Institute, University of Bergen, Bergen, Norway; Department of Rheumatology, Haukeland University Hospital, Bergen, Norway, roland.jonsson@gades.uib.no

Yrjö T. Konttinen Department of Medicine, Biomedicum Helsinki, Helsinki University Central Hospital, Helsinki, Finland; ORTON Orthopaedic Hospital of the ORTON Foundation, Helsinki, Finland; COXA Hospital for the Joint Replacement, Tampere, Finland, yrjo.konttinen@helsinki.fi

Katja Koskenpato Department of Medicine, Biomedicum Helsinki, Helsinki University Central Hospital, Helsinki, Finland, katja.koskenpato@helsinki.fi

Chak-sing Lau Division of Rheumatology and Clinical Immunology, Li Ka Shing Faculty of Medicine, The University of Hong Kong, Hong Kong, China, cslau@hku.hk

Zhan-Guo Li Department of Rheumatology and Immunology, People's Hospital, Peking University Medical School, Beijing, China, zgli98@yahoo.com

Menelaos N. Manoussakis Department of Pathophysiology, School of Medicine, University of Athens, Athens, Greece, menman@med.uoa.gr

Xavier Mariette Assistance Publique-Hôpitaux de Paris (AP-HP), Hôpital Bicêtre, Institut Pour la Santé et la Recherche Médicale (INSERM) U 1012, Université Paris-Sud 11, Le Kremlin Bicêtre, France, xavier.mariette@bct.aphp.fr

Mihaela C. Marthinussen Section for Cariology, Department of Clinical Dentistry, Faculty of Medicine and Dentistry, Bergen, mihaela.cuida@iko.uib.no

Paul E. Michelson Eye Care of La Jolla, Scripps Memorial Hospital, La Jolla, CA, USA; UCSD School of Medicine, La Jolla, CA, USA, pmichel2@san.rr.com

Ramnath Misra Department of Immunology, Sanjay Gandhi Post Graduate Institute of Medical Sciences, Lucknow, India, rnmisra2000@gmail.com

Kathy L. Moser Arthritis and Immunology Program, Oklahoma Medical Research Foundation, Oklahoma City, OK, USA, moserk@omrf.org

Haralampos M. Moutsopoulos Department of Pathophysiology, School of Medicine, University of Athens, Athens, Greece, hmoutsop@med.uoa.gr

Yoichi Nakagawa Second Department of Oral and Maxillofacial Surgery, Tsurumi University School of Dental Medicine, Yokohama, Japan, nakagawa-y@tsurumi-u.ac.jp

Nikolay P. Nikolov Sjögren's Syndrome Clinic, National Institute of Dental and Craniofacial Research, Bethesda, MD, USA, nikolovn@mail.nih.gov

Kazuhisa Nozawa Department of Rheumatology and Internal Medicine, Urayasu Hospital Juntendo University, Chiba, Japan; Institute for

Environment and Gender Specific Medicine, Juntendo University Graduate School of Medicine, Chiba, Japan; Department of Rheumatology, Juntendo Urayasu Hospital, Chiba, Japan, k-nozawa@juntendo.ac.jp

Sapan Pandya Department of Rheumatology, Vedanta Institute of Medical Sciences, Ahmedabad, India, sapancpandya@yahoo.com

Stephen C. Pflugfelder Department of Ophthalmology, Baylor College of Medicine, Houston, TX, USA, stevenp@bcm.edu

Justin Pijpe Department of Oral and Maxillofacial Surgery, Catharina Hospital Eindhoven, Eindhoven, The Netherlands; University Medical Center, Groningen, The Netherlands, j.pijpe@gmail.com

Raimo Pöllänen Department of Medicine, Biomedicum Helsinki, Helsinki University Central Hospital, Helsinki, Finland, raimo.pollanen@helsinki.fi

Alberto Vivó Porcar Department of Medicine, Biomedicum Helsinki, Helsinki University Central Hospital, Helsinki, Finland, siralbertvivoporcar@gmail.com

Pauliina Porola Department of Medicine, Biomedicum Helsinki, Helsinki University Central Hospital, Helsinki, Finland, pauliina.porola@helsinki.fi

Beata D. Przybyla Department of Microbiology and Immunology, University of Arkansas for Medical Sciences, Little Rock, AK, USA, BDPrzybyla@uams.edu

Manuel Ramos-Casals Sjögren Syndrome Research Group (AGAUR), Hospital Clinic, Barcelona, Spain, mramos@clinic.ub.es

Philippe Ravaud Centre d'Epidomiologie Clinique, INSERM U738, Hôpital Hotel Dieu, Paris, France, philippe.ravaud@htd.aphp.fr

Maureen Rischmueller Department of Rheumatology, The Queen Elizabeth Hospital/University of Adelaide, Adelaide, South Australia, maureen.rischmueller@health.sa.gov.au

María Lorés Rodriguez Department of Medicine, Biomedicum Helsinki, Helsinki University Central Hospital, Helsinki, Finland, maria.lores.rodriguez@gmail.com

John G. Routsias Department of Pathophysiology, School of Medicine, University of Athens, Athens, Greece, jroutsias@med.uoa.gr

Ichiro Saito Department of Pathology, Tsurumi University School of Dental Medicine, Yokohama, Japan, saito-i@tsurumi-u.ac.jp

Minoru Satoh Division of Rheumatology and Clinical Immunology, Department of Medicine, University of Florida, Gainesville, FL, USA; Department of Pathology, Immunology, and Laboratory Medicine, University of Florida, Gainesville, FL, USA, Minoru.Satoh@medicine.ufl.edu

Raphaèle Seror Assistance Publique-Hopitaux de Paris, Hôpital Bicêtre, Department of Rheumatology, Institut Pour la Santé et la Recherche

Médicale (INSERM) U 802, Université Paris-Sud 11, Le Kremlin Bicêtre, France, raphaele.se@gmail.com

Yehuda Shoenfeld Department of Medicine "B" and Zabludowicz Center for Autoimmune Diseases, Sheba Medical Center, Tel-Hashomer, Israel, shoenfel@tau.ac.il

Kathrine Skarstein Broegelmann Research Laboratory, Department of Immunology, The Gade Institute, University of Bergen, Bergen, Norway, kathrine.skarstein@gades.uib.no

Michelle Spaan Department of Medicine, Biomedicum Helsinki, Helsinki University Central Hospital, Helsinki, Finland, michelle.spaan@hotmail.com

Vasily Stegaev Department of Medicine, Biomedicum Helsinki, Helsinki University Central Hospital, Helsinki, Finland, vasily.stegaev@helsinki.fi

Michael E. Stern Inflammation Research Program, Allergan, Inc., Irvine, CA, USA, stern_michael@allergan.com

John H. Stone Division of Rheumatology, Allergy, and Immunology, Massachusetts General Hospital, Boston, MA, USA, jhstone@partners.org

Yoshinari Takasaki Department of Internal Medicine and Rheumatology, Juntendo University School of Medicine, Tokyo, Japan, tyoshi@juntendo.ac.jp

Elke Theander Skane University Hospital Malmö, Malmö, Sweden, elke.theander@med.lu.se

Moshe Tishler Department of Medicine "B", Asaf Harofe Medical Center, Zerifin, Israel 70300, tishlerm@netvision.net.il

Pamela Traisak Section of Rheumatology, Department of Medicine, Temple University School of Medicine, Philadelphia, PA, USA, pammy1000@hotmail.com

Kazuo Tsubota Department of Ophthalmology, Keio University School of Medicine, Tokyo, Japan, tsubota@z3.keio.jp

Athanasios G. Tzioufas Department of Pathophysiology, School of Medicine, University of Athens, Athens, Greece, agtzi@med.uoa.gr

Liisa Virkki Department of Medicine, Biomedicum Helsinki, Helsinki University Central Hospital, Helsinki, Finland, liisa.m.virkki@helsinki.fi

Claudio Vitali Section of Rheumatology, Department of Internal Medicine, Villamarina Hospital, Piombino, Italy, c.vitali@yahoo.it

Frederick B. Vivino Division of Rheumatology, Penn Presbyterian Medical Center, University of Pennsylvania School of Medicine, Philadelphia, PA, USA, frederick.vivino@uphs.upenn.edu

Frank A. Wollheim Lund University Hospital SUS, Lund, Sweden, frank.wollheim@med.lu.se

Part I
Introduction

Introduction

1

Robert I. Fox and Carla M. Fox

Keywords
Sjogren's syndrome • Keratoconjunctivitis sicca • Ophthalmology • Otolaryngology • Oral medicine • Gastroenterology • Neurology • Pathogenesis • Europe • China • India • Israel • Internet

The care of the Sjogren's syndrome (SS) patient is often shared by many specialists due to the multi-system involvement of this disease. Each of these specialists reads different journals and rarely attends common educational meetings. Thus, each specialty has a slightly different view of the "elephant" in the room. The primary goal of this book is to bring together a series of experts in different disciplines to provide a common dialogue regarding diagnosis and therapy for SS. Each chapter is written in a manner that preserves the sophistication of their respective field but that employs terminology that will be clear to other specialtists.

Although the rheumatologist frequently becomes the central "quarterback" in the treatment of the SS patient, he/she must be familiar with the diagnostic procedures and therapeutic approaches of the other specialties to avoid medication interactions and coordination of care. An additional goal for this volume is to include contributors from around the world including Europe, the Middle East, South America, Australia, and Asia as well as the USA. Different medications (including herbal) and different diagnostic methods are used in various parts of the world, based on medical resources and technology available. These chapters provide examples about how to manage our patients in a cost-efficient manner and new approaches to therapy. Also, it is important for "western physicians" to recognize "centers of excellence" among the emerging nations of the world because our patients increasingly travel to these regions for business and pleasure. Our patients may require medical care either for a complication of their SS or for an infection that is endogenous to that region while travelling. It is worth noting that in many parts of the world (as well as certain regions of the USA) the "primary" care of rheumatology patients is under the direction of non-surgical orthopedic surgeons in part to the shortage of available rheumatologists. This volume also is directed to "non-rheumatologist" who is providing care to the SS patient.

We are fortunate to have contributions in clinical specialties from

- Ophthalmology
- Oral medicine

R.I. Fox (✉)
Rheumatology Clinic, Scripps Memorial Hospital and Research Foundation, La Jolla, CA, USA
e-mail: robertfoxmd@mac.com

R.I. Fox, C.M. Fox (eds.), *Sjögren's Syndrome*, DOI 10.1007/978-1-60327-957-4_1,

- Otolaryngology (ENT)
- Hematology/Oncology
- Neurology and psychology
- Dermatology
- Orthopedic surgery
- Gastroenterology
- Nephrology

This multitude of specialists also creates a situation where there may be disagreements about diagnosis, duplication of efforts, and conflicting therapies. In order to coordinate therapy between so many specialists and to avoid conflicting information/medications to the patient, we extensively use the Internet and transfer of files to participating physicians. The patient also needs to be part of the educational and therapeutic process.

Patients are increasingly computer literate and we encourage them to educate themselves regarding their disease and its therapy using resources including the Internet. However, we caution them to use the Internet wisely and use a search engine such as Google scholar (rather than simply Google) to find validated information rather than the often frightening and misleading information found in various chat groups that are found during general web.

1.1 Historical Background

The clinical features (both glandular and extraglandular) of the disease, as we currently recognize SS in its florid form, were largely outlined in 1956 by Bloch et al. [1]. This clinical report from Massachusetts General Hospital outlined the clinical features associated with a characteristic minor salivary gland pathology that had been recently reported by Morgan et al. in 1953 [2] of the same institution. This pathology report by Morgan et al. acknowledged that they had "rediscovered" the minor salivary gland pathology that "Mikulicz" initially reported in 1892 [3] and had been later reported by Sjogren in 1933 [4]. A simple Google scholar search since 1956 lists over 76,000 different articles. Yet the etiology remains largely unknown and the therapy unsatisfactory.

In SS patients with severe dryness, positive autoantibodies, and positive lip biopsies, the issue is the extent of extraglandular involvement and the approaches to therapy. However, many rheumatology consults are requested for evaluation of SS in the patient in whom a positive ANA is detected during the workup of myalgias, arthralgias, neuropathy, nephritis, or chronic fatigue. In these patients, there has been considerable debate about the classification criteria for patients and the role of the immune system in causing the clinical symptoms. The diagnosis may then have a significant impact on the types of therapy used. This clinical problem is particularly difficult in patients with sicca symptoms and "fibromyalgia" symptoms. The diagnostic criteria for SS (Table 1.1) are discussed in Chapter 5 by Vitali et al. and approaches to therapy of fibromyalgia in Chapter 21 by Bowman. The "disconnect" between "severity of clinical symptoms as judged by patient" and the objective measurements such as tear flow, saliva flow, or neurologic symptoms observed by the clinician is very high. This has led some experts such as Prof. Graham Hughes in London to joke that SS is actually a neurologic disease with peripheral manifestations [5].

Until 2003, there were multiple sets of diagnostic criteria for primary SS including those by American, European (Scandinavian, Italian, and Greek), and Japanese groups [6–9]. The inclusion criteria were so significantly different among these groups that the diagnoses of "SS" rendered by European physicians were almost 10-fold when utilizing the EEC criteria than in two different US criteria [10]. This discrepancy was largely due to inclusion in the original European criteria of patients with fibromyalgia, hepatitis C-related sicca or dryness in association with Alzheimer's, or demyelinating disorders. Of importance to current readers, the discrepancy in diagnostic criteria led to confusion in the research and clinical trial literature. Thus, readers may be confused by very discrepant results and need to very carefully check the criteria used for inclusion in published studies.

Primary SS using the current consensus criteria is a systemic autoimmune disorder with a

Table 1.1 Revised classification criteria for Sjogren's syndrome

Requirements for classification of patients with primary SS:
(a) the presence of either positive salivary gland biopsy (described below) or positive antibody to SS-A or SS-B; and
(b) the presence of any three objective clinical signs for oral and ocular dryness (described below); and
(c) the presence of at least four clinical symptoms for oral and ocular dryness (described below).
I. Clinical symptoms
A. Ocular symptoms: a positive response to at least one of the following questions:
1. Have you had daily, persistent, troublesome dry eyes for more than 3 months?
2. Do you have a recurrent sensation of sand or gravel in the eyes?
3. Do you use tear substitutes more than three times a day?
B. Oral symptoms: a positive response to at least one of the following questions:
1. Have you had a daily feeling of dry mouth for more than 3 months?
2. Have you had recurrently or persistently swollen salivary glands as an adult?
3. Do you frequently drink liquids to aid in swallowing dry food?
II. Objective clinical signs
A. Ocular signs, that is, objective evidence of ocular involvement defined as a positive result for at least one of the following two tests:
1. Schirmer's test, performed without anesthesia ($\leq$5 mm in 5 min)
2. Rose Bengal score or other ocular dye score ($\geq$4 according to van Bijsterveld's scoring system)
B. Minor salivary gland biopsy:
Histopathology: In minor salivary glands (obtained through normal appearing mucosa), focal lymphocytic sialadenitis, evaluated by an expert histopathologist, with a focus score $\geq$1, is defined as a number of lymphocytic foci (which are adjacent to normal appearing mucous acini and contain more than 50 lymphocytes) per 4 mm^2 of glandular tissue
C. Salivary gland involvement: objective evidence of salivary gland involvement defined by a positive result for at least one of the following diagnostic tests:
1. Unstimulated whole salivary flow ($\leq$1.5 ml in 15 min)
2. Parotid sialography showing the presence of diffuse sialectasias (punctate, cavitary, or destructive pattern), without evidence of obstruction in the major ducts.
3. Salivary scintigraphy showing delayed uptake, reduced concentration, and/or delayed excretion of tracer
D. Autoantibodies: presence in the serum of the following autoantibodies:
1. Antibodies to Ro(SS-A) or La(SS-B) antigens or both
III. Criteria for secondary SS
In patients with a potentially associated disease such as rheumatoid arthritis, systemic lupus, or progressive systemic sclerosis, together with a positive minor salivary gland biopsy or antibody to SS-A or SS-B
IV. Exclusion criteria
Past head and neck radiation treatment
Hepatitis C infection
Acquired immunodeficiency disease (AIDS)
Pre-existing lymphoma
Sarcoidosis
Graft-versus-host disease
Use of anticholinergic drugs at the time of measurements considered abnormal (all measurements used to fulfill criteria need to be performed at a time duration after stopping drug for four half-lives of the drug)

prevalence of about 0.5% in the general population, with a female preponderance of 9:1, which is roughly similar to SLE [11]. This would make *SS one of the three most frequent autoimmune disorders* [10], although it has received far less research and therapeutic attention than SLE or PSS.

There *are two major age peaks of primary SS*, with

- the *first peak* incidence *after menarche* during the twenties to thirties;
- the *second peak* incidence *after menopause* in the mid-50-year age range;
- SS also presenting in children, as part of the spectrum of juvenile arthritis.

The criteria in current use is the European-American Consensus Group Modification of the European Community Criteria for SS [12] and is described in Chapter 5 by Vitali et al. The key feature of the new criteria is the requirement for objective evidence of the immune system in causing the sicca symptoms, as demonstrated by the requirement for either a characteristic minor salivary gland biopsy or autoantibody against SS-A. Due to logistics of obtaining biopsies in clinical practice, the patients usually fulfill their diagnostic criteria based on their antibody status. Therefore, the methodologic pitfalls that influence diagnosis are briefly discussed below.

Diagnosis of secondary SS (2° SS) has not yet been addressed by the American European Consensus Group. However, in practice we usually require the patient to fulfill the criteria for 1° SS and to additionally fulfill American College of Rheumatology (ACR) criteria for an established connective tissue disease such as RA, SLE, dermatomyositis or myositis, PSS, or biliary cirrhosis. For ease of comparison, the diagnostic criteria for SLE and PSS are provided in Chapter 3.

Exclusions to the diagnosis of 1° SS include previous radiotherapy to the head and neck, lymphoma, sarcoidosis, graft-versus-host disease, infection with hepatitis C virus, human T-lymphotropic virus type I, or HIV. Measurements of tear and saliva flow must be made in the absence of drugs that have anticholinergic side effects.

Although 1° SS patients are at increased risk for lymphoma, patients with pre-existing lymphoma are typically excluded from studies to ensure entry of a relatively homogeneous group into studies of therapy and prognosis.

In contrast to the patients with florid SS, there are a large number of patients referred to rheumatology with

- a low titer ANA and vague symptoms of myalgia, trigger points, and fatigue or vague cognitive deficits, who are termed fibromyalgia;
- a positive ANA but who lack the sicca features of SS, particularly patients in whom the ANA is detected as part of the workup for other problems such as neuropathy, pneumonitis, or nephritis.

1.2 Pitfalls in Diagnosis and Methodology

There are two common areas of confusion in clinical diagnosis of SS: (a) the specificity/sensitivity of the ANA and (b) the evaluation of the minor salivary gland biopsy. These tests are generally considered our "gold standards" for diagnosis of SS and most physicians do not recognize the variability in the results of these tests. Thus, rheumatologists must interpret these results based on the method of laboratory analysis (i.e., IFA or ELISA) and the experience of the pathologist in evaluating minor salivary gland biopsies.

Both primary care physicians and other specialists frequently use the ANA as a "screening" test in patients with rheumatic disease symptoms. The diagnosis of SS is frequently made in a patient with vague symptoms and a positive ANA. However, Tan et al. [13] reported that the frequency in "normal individuals" of a positive ANA titer using Hep-2 cells at titer 1:40 was 31.7% of individual, at 1:80 was 13%, at 1:160 was 5%, and at 1:320 was 3.3%.

Using a Bayesian analysis, Lightfoot et al. found similar results in ANA testing and calculated that the risk of an individual with an ANA 1:320 developing SLE or SS during a 10-year follow-up period was less than 5% [14]. Thus, it is a common mistake for patients or their primary care MDs to make the diagnosis of SLE or SS based solely on the finding of an abnormal autoantibody test result. The correct role for an ANA is to confirm the clinical diagnosis.

The recent increased use of enzyme-linked assays (ELISA) to measure ANA has been driven by the lower cost of this method. However, the ELISA tests have a lower sensitivity. Rheumatologists and patients may be confronted with the same serum sample that exhibits a strongly positive ANA by IFA and negative result by ELISA assay. An example of the importance of this discrepancy in laboratory method was the delay in diagnosis reported in a New England Journal clinical case study until the "negative" ELISA test result was replaced by positive result obtained using the conventional IFA measurement [15].

The laboratory tests for antibody to SS-A and SS-B showed a higher level of specificity for SS diagnosis but significant variation in results were dependent on the "vendor" of the substrate used in the assay [16].

The pathologist may be asked to help confirm the diagnosis of SS with a *minor salivary gland biopsy* [17]. Jonsson et al. present examples of salivary gland biopsies from an SS patient in Chapter 14. *The key features in reading the minor salivary gland biopsy* include an adequate number of valuable lobules (at least four) and the determination of an average *focus score* (a "focus" refers to a cluster of at least 50 lymphocytes) based on a survey of at least four lobules. Lobules that have been ruptured due to non-immune mechanisms (called "sialadenitis" due to rupture of ducts that release mucus) need to be discarded from the quantization of the focus score [18, 19]. The biopsy should not be taken from a region of the buccal mucosa where there is inflammation, as this can give false-positive results [19]. The sensitivity and specificity of the focus scoring method may be improved by looking at serial sections of salivary gland [20].

Non-specific sialadenitis including focal infiltrates was a relatively frequent finding in minor salivary gland biopsies taken in a "control population" studied at the National Institutes of Health, particularly among older patients [21]. The finding of germinal centers in a minor salivary gland biopsy of an SS patient may be prognostically important [22]. However, most pathologists are not experienced in reading these samples and rarely report the "focus score" or germinal centers. In one recent report, almost 50% of biopsies obtained for entrance into a clinical study of SS were reclassified when examined by a pathologist experienced in SS [23, 24]. Biopsies previously read as positive were reclassified as not fulfilling criteria and an equal proportion of negative biopsies were felt to be positive for focal infiltrates.

1.3 Methods to Assess Disease Activity

The recent introduction of a "disease activity index" by Vitali et al. will facilitate the clinical course and therapeutic trials of SS patients. Also, a recently standardized Disease Damage Index scale (Chapter 5 by Vitali et al.) will allow comparison of different patient populations and therapeutic protocols. This will facilitate studies on disease frequency, extraglandular manifestations, prognosis, and diagnostic markers and provide a basis for therapeutic studies. Seror et al. review this important step in standardization of the nomenclature and collaboration among different cohorts of SS patients in Chapter 30.

1.4 Summary

This volume on Sjogren's syndrome is different from the reviews that have been published in recent years or as "seminars in rheumatology" or as "current opinion" articles.

We have included a group of world-renowned experts in the field of ophthalmology, oral medicine and pathology, neurology, otolaryngology, nephrology, oncology, and other disciplines to present their points of view on diagnosis and therapy. Since each group of medical and surgical specialists reads and writes in their different journals, as well as attends different meetings, this volume is intended to help each specialty understand the opinions and treatments of other specialties.

We have included experts from different parts of the world, since the health-care resources and systems of delivery of health care in the USA differ substantially from those in other parts of the world.

Finally, we have tried to move the information into the Internet age. We feel that "frequently asked questions" may be best answered by making validated information available to patients and other health-care specialists over the Internet. For a disease that largely is a "quality of life" disorder, in contrast to an acute vasculitis or a heart attack, the time available to provide instruction about treatment of "dryness" or "fatigue" or "cognitive" changes is increasingly limited by our time during patient revisits. Thus, we have provided a series of "frequently asked questions" as well as "myths and pearls" that can easily be modified by each clinician and placed on their web sites for patients or other clinicians to access.

References

1. Bloch KJ, Buchanan WW, Wohl MJ, Bunim JJ. Sjögren's syndrome: a clinical, pathological and serological study of 62 cases. Medicine (Baltimore). 1956;44:187–231.
2. Morgan W, Castleman B. A clinicopathologic study of Mikulicz's disease. Am J Pathol. 1953;29:471–503.
3. Mikulicz JH. Uber eine eigenartige symmetrische Erkrankung der Tranen- und Mundspeicheldrusen. In: Billroth GT, editor. Beitr. Chir. Fortschr. Stuttgart; 1892. pp. 610–30.
4. Sjögren HS. Zur kenntnis der keratoconjunctvitis sicca (Keratitis folliformis bei hypofunktion der tranendrusen). Acta Opthalmol (Copenh). 1933;2:1–151.
5. Cervera R, Khamashta MA, Font J, Sebastiani GD, Gil A, Lavilla P, Aydintug AO, Jedryka-Goral A, de Ramon E, Fernandez-Nebro A. Morbidity and mortality in systemic lupus erythematosus during a 5-year period: a multicenter prospective study of 1,000 patients. Medicine. 1999;78:167.
6. Vitali C. Criteria for the classification of Sjogren's syndrome. Primer Rheum Dis. 1998;11:458 (appendix).
7. Manthorpe R. New criteria for diagnosing Sjogren's syndrome: a step forward?–or. Scand J Rheumatol. 2001;Suppl:14–20; discussion-2.
8. Fox R. Classification criteria for Sjogren's syndrome. Rheum Dis Clin North Am: Curr Controversies Rheumatol. 1994;20:391–407.
9. Homma M, Tojo T, Akizuki M, Yamagata H. Criteria for Sjögren's syndrome in Japan. Scand J Rheumatol. 1986;Suppl 61:26.
10. Fox RI. Sjogren's syndrome. Lancet. 2005;366:321–31.
11. Vitali C. Classification criteria for Sjogren's syndrome. Ann Rheum Dis. 2003;62:94–5; author reply 5.
12. Vitali C, Bombardieri S, Jonsson R, Moutsopoulos H, Alexander E, Carson S, Daniels T, Fox P, Fox R, Kassan S. Classification criteria for Sjogren's syndrome: a revised version of the European criteria proposed by the American-European Consensus Group. Ann Rheum Dis. 2002;61:554–8.
13. Tan EM, Feltkamp TE, Smolen JS, Butcher B, Dawkins R, Fritzler MJ, Gordon T, Hardin JA, Kalden JR, Lahita RG, Maini RN, McDougal JS, Rothfield NF, Smeenk RJ, Takasaki Y, Wiik A, Wilson MR, Koziol JA. Range of antinuclear antibodies in "healthy" individuals. Arthritis Rheum. 1997;40:1601–11.
14. Lightfoot R. Cost effective use of laboratory tests in rheumatology. Bull Rheum Dis. 1997;46:1–3.
15. Infirmary E, Stone J, Caruso P, Deshpande V. Case 24-2009: a 26-year-old woman with painful swelling of the neck. N Engl J Med. 2009;361:511–8.
16. Tan EM, Smolen JS, McDougal JS, Butcher BT, Conn D, Dawkins R, Fritzler MJ, Gordon T, Hardin JA, Kalden JR, Lahita RG, Maini RN, Rothfield NF, Smeenk R, Takasaki Y, van Venrooij WJ, Wiik A, Wilson M, Koziol JA. A critical evaluation of enzyme immunoassays for detection of antinuclear autoantibodies of defined specificities. I. Precision, sensitivity, and specificity. Arthritis Rheum. 1999;42:455–64.
17. Daniels T, Fox P. Salivary and oral components of Sjögren's syndrome. Rheum Dis Clin North Am. 1992;18:571.
18. Daniels TE. Labial salivary gland biopsy in Sjögren's syndrome. Arthritis Rheum. 1984;27:147–56.
19. Daniels TE, Whitcher JP. Association of patterns of labial salivary gland inflammation with keratoconjunctivitis sicca. Analysis of 618 patients with suspected Sjogren's syndrome. Arthritis Rheum. 1994;37:869–77.
20. Morbini P, Manzo A, Caporali R, Epis O, Villa C, Tinelli C, Solcia E, Montecucco C. Multilevel examination of minor salivary gland biopsy for Sjogren's syndrome significantly improves diagnostic performance of AECG classification criteria. Arthritis Res Ther. 2005;7:R343–8.
21. Radfar L, Kleiner DE, Fox PC, Pillemer SR. Prevalence and clinical significance of lymphocytic

foci in minor salivary glands of healthy volunteers. Arthritis Care Res. 2002;47:520–4.

22. Salomonsson S, Jonsson MV, Skarstein K, Brokstad KA, Hjelmstrom P, Wahren-Herlenius M, Jonsson R. Cellular basis of ectopic germinal center formation and autoantibody production in the target organ of patients with Sjogren's syndrome. Arthritis Rheum. 2003;48:3187–201.
23. Brennan MT, Sankar V, Leakan RA, Kleiner D, Atkinson JC, Wilkinson WE, Baum BJ, Pillemer SR. Risk factors for positive minor salivary gland biopsy findings in Sjogren's syndrome and dry mouth patients. Arthritis Rheum. 2002;47:189–95.
24. Yamada H, Nakagawa Y, Wakamatsu E, Sumida T, Yamachika S, Nomura Y, Mishima K, Saito I. Efficacy prediction of cevimeline in patients with Sjogren's syndrome. Clin Rheumatol. 2007;26: 1320–7.

A Note from Sweden: Recollection of Henrik Sjögren

2

Elke Theander and Frank A. Wollheim

Abstract

In 1933 the Swedish ophthalmologist Henrik Sjögren defended his doctoral thesis at the Karolinska Institute in Stockholm. He obtained a mediocre evaluation for his thesis and had to leave academia, but continued to publish from his outpost in Jönköping. Ultimately he got well-deserved international recognition for his work, after a study on "Sjögren's syndrome" was subsequently published in 1954 by W. Morgan in *New England Journal of Medicine*.

Keywords

Sjögren's syndrome • Henrik Sjögren • Sweden • Recollection of Sjögren's original patients • Aerobic exercise and fatigue

2.1 Introduction

Henrik Sjögren was born in Köping in central Sweden in 1899 and died in Lund in September of 1986, only months after being honorary president together with Jan Waldenström at the First International Sjögren's Syndrome meeting held outside Copenhagen earlier that year. He was a soft-spoken almost shy gentleman who never advertised himself and never complained of the harsh and unjustified critique he received when defending his thesis in 1933. Figure 2.1 is based on his patient data and drawn by Frank A. Wollheim [1]. When interviewed in connection with the 1986 meeting, he regretted that due to illness he was unable to attend in person. He wished the participants a successful meeting and said that he was particularly thrilled that one had now created "Sjögren's mice." The opening of the meeting featured a valse for piano that he had composed for his fiancée, and later wife, Maria Hellgren, in the early 1920s. Although he was an ophthalmologist and not a rheumatologist, it is fair to state that he made Swedish rheumatology world famous. Henrik Sjögren was an honorary member of the American Rheumatism Association and of the Swedish Society for Rheumatology. Before the advent of the Nazi regime in Germany, a large proportion of academic papers in Sweden were published in German language. This was also true of Sjögren's thesis. In 1943 the Australian ophthalmologist Bruce Hamilton approached Sjögren and

F.A. Wollheim (✉)
Lund University Hospital SUS, Lund, Sweden
e-mail: frank.wollheim@med.lu.se

R.I. Fox, C.M. Fox (eds.), *Sjögren's Syndrome*, DOI 10.1007/978-1-60327-957-4_2,

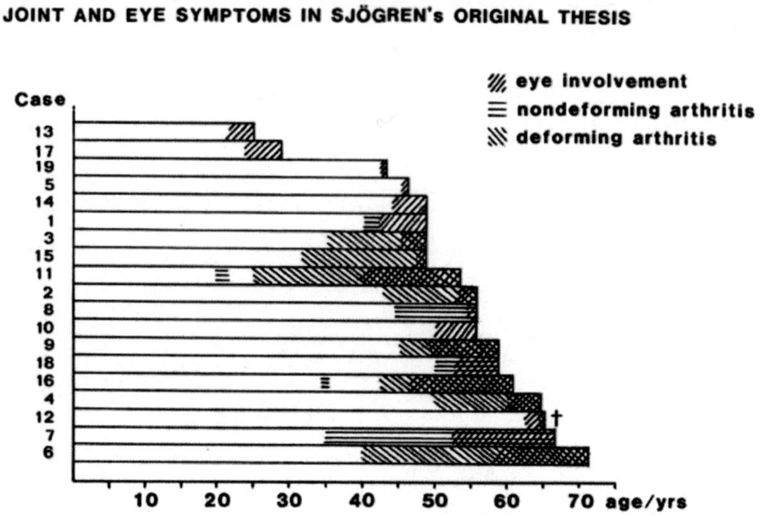

Fig. 2.1 Age, symptoms and disease course in the 19 first patients studied by Henrik Sjögren

obtained permission to translate it into English. This translation obtained much wider attention than the original German version and made Henrik Sjögren well-recognized internationally.

2.2 Prevalence and Incidence of Sjögren's Syndrome in Scandinavia

How prevalent is Sjögren's syndrome in Scandinavia? We have current data from two areas. One is the city of Malmö, with an adult population of approximately 200,000 inhabitants. Here we (ET) have identified 340 cases among individuals above the age of 18 years corresponding to a prevalence of 0.15% (E. Theander, unpublished personal communication). All these individuals have an established diagnosis based on the American–European Consensus Criteria from 2002 [1]. This would be similar to recently proposed prevalence estimates from Turkey [2], Greece [3], and Great Britain [4] using the same criteria set. The incidence is more difficult to estimate. We have encountered between four and seven new cases per year in the period starting in 2002. A rough estimate based on the Malmö experience would give an estimated average annual incidence of 2.5 new cases per 100,000 individuals per year or 1 in 40,000. It is likely that not all new cases come to our hospital unit; some may be cared for by their primary care physicians or escape health care or stay unsymptomatic. An earlier incidence estimate published for the population of Minnesota was 3.9 per 100,000 [5].

In Norway, a recent survey was performed in two health districts around the cities of Stavanger and Bergen. In this population of 852,342 individuals served by two university hospitals and one general rheumatism hospital, the Norwegian investigators found 431 patients with a diagnosis of primary Sjögren's syndrome registered at these hospitals, private rheumatologists, and in a salivary gland biopsy registry. This corresponds to an estimated prevalence of only 0.05%. There were no incidence data in this study [6].

The incidence and prevalence of secondary Sjögren's syndrome in Scandinavia has not been investigated to our knowledge and would be rather difficult to study.

2.3 Any Special Features in Swedish Patients with Sjögren's?

Several investigators in Spain and Greece have reported high prevalence of cryoglobulinemia in their patients. This has not been the experience in

Malmö, where only traces of cryoglobulin were found in a minority of 7% of patients, although active search and careful lege artis sampling was performed (E. Theander, unpublished personal communication). Neither have we found hepatitis C to be increased among the patients. It should be mentioned that the occurrence of hepatitis C is low in Sweden. With regard to the development of non-Hodgkin's lymphoma (NHL) in primary Sjögren's syndrome, we have detected differences in subtype of NHLs compared to other European countries. In Sweden we detect a high number of diffuse large B-cell lymphomas in addition to the commonly found MALT lymphomas [7, 8]. The difference may be mainly due to the assessment of risks by using health-care registries in contrast to cohort observations in some other studies. Otherwise we have not identified any special clinical features distinguishing Swedish patients.

2.4 Pearls of Wisdom

Fatigue and impaired physical capacity are common features in Sjögren's syndrome influencing an individual's quality of life. Therefore, we want to call attention to the successful application of intensive aerobic training reported from our unit in Malmö in 2007 [9]. We have recently performed a 4-year follow-up of the results of this controlled aerobic exercise program involving Nordic walking. The initial training consisted of 12 weeks of 45 min walking three times each week. Retesting at follow-up showed sustained higher physical activity and aerobic capacity in the treatment group and borderline less fatigue. Pain, anxiety, and depression did not differ between the groups [10]. The increased physical activity could have positive effects also on comorbidities such as cardiovascular health.

References

1. Wollheim FA. Henrik Sjögren and Sjögren's syndrome. Scand J Rheumatol Suppl. 1986;61: 11–6; Vitali C, Bombardieri S, Jonsson R, et al. Classification criteria for Sjögren's syndrome: a revised version of the European criteria proposed by the American–European Consensus Group. Ann Rheum Dis. 2002;61(6):554–8.
2. Birlik M, Akar S, Gurler O, et al. Prevalence of primary Sjogren's syndrome in Turkey: a population-based epidemiological study. Int J Clin Pract. 2009;63(6):954–61.
3. Trontzas PI, Andrianakos AA. Sjogren's syndrome: a population based study of prevalence in Greece. The ESORDIG study. Ann Rheum Dis. 2005;64(8): 1240–1.
4. Bowman SJ, Ibrahim GH, Holmes G, Hamburger J, Ainsworth JR. Estimating the prevalence among Caucasian women of primary Sjögren's syndrome in two general practices in Birmingham, UK. Scand J Rheumatol. 2004;33:39–43.
5. Pillemer SP, Mattesson EL, Jacobsson LTH, et al. Incidence of physician-diagnosed primary Sjögren's syndrome in residents of Olmsted County, Minnesota. Mayo Clinic Proc. 2001;76(6):593–9.
6. Göransson LG, Haldorsen K, Brun JG, Harboe E, Jonsson MV, Skarstein K, Time K, Omdal R. The point prevalence of clinically relevant primary Sjögren's syndrome in two Norwegian counties. Scand J Rheumatol 2011;First article:1–4.
7. Theander E, Henriksson G, Ljungberg O, Mandl T, Manthorpe R, Jacobsson LT. Lymphoma and other malignancies in primary Sjogren's syndrome. A cohort study on cancer incidence and lymphoma predictors. Ann Rheum Dis. 2006;65(6):796–803.
8. Smedby KE, Askling J, Mariette X, Baecklund E. Autoimmune and inflammatory disorders and risk of malignant lymphomas – an update. J Intern Med. 2008;264(6):514–27.
9. Strombeck BE, Theander E, Jacobsson LT. Effects of exercise on aerobic capacity and fatigue in women with primary Sjogren's syndrome. Rheumatology. 2007;46(5):567–71.
10. Theander E, Theander S, Karlelid L, Strömbeck B. Sustained effects of a supervised aerobic exercise program (Nordic walking) in women with primary Sjögren's syndrome. A 4-year follow-up. Abstract Book, 10th International Symposium on Sjögren's syndrome, Brest, France, October 1–3, 2009: p. 49.

Myths, Pearls, and Tips Regarding Sjögren's Syndrome

3

Robert I. Fox, Manuel Ramos-Casals, and John H. Stone

Abstract

Although SS is among the three most common rheumatologic disorders, there are few double-blind, placebo-controlled studies to rationally guide either topical or systemic therapy. Therefore, we wish to share some of the clinical "myths and pearls" that we have encountered, including the following:

(a) Although the diagnostic criteria of SS depend on a positive anti-SS-A/B antibody, there is significant variation among laboratories in the sensitivity and specificity of these tests. SS patients may have other autoantibodies (such as anti-centromere) antibodies and should not be excluded from diagnosis of SS.
(b) Many pathologists do not have experience in reading minor salivary gland biopsies. Outside review of biopsies at a center with expertise is frequently required.
(c) The severity of symptoms, as assessed by the patient, is strongly influenced by "fibromyalgia" (central pain sensitization), and this may partly explain the poor correlation between objective measurements of glandular (tear/mouth) and extraglandular (neuropathic) symptoms.
(d) The key extraglandular concerns among SS patients are lymphoma and central nervous system involvement. Development of cost-effective strategies to screen patients for these relatively uncommon complications is necessary.
(e) Oral dryness leads to change in socialization habits, when the patient can no longer eat with friends, family, or business colleagues. Ocular dryness interferes with work efficiently as patients increasingly sit in front of computer screens in low-humidity office buildings. Therapy must recognize that these problems not only are more than an "irritation" to the patient but also strongly influence their quality of life.

R.I. Fox (✉)
Rheumatology Clinic, Scripps Memorial Hospital
and Research Foundation, La Jolla, CA, USA
e-mail: robertfoxmd@mac.com

R.I. Fox, C.M. Fox (eds.), *Sjögren's Syndrome*, DOI 10.1007/978-1-60327-957-4_3,

Keywords
Sjögren's syndrome (SS)—[primary SS: 1 °SS/secondary SS: 2° SS] • Arthralgia • Antinuclear antibody (ANA) • Myalgia • Fibromyalgia • Central pain sensitization • Raynaud's phenomenon • Oral candidiasis • Dysphagia • Laryngotracheal reflux • Gastro-esophageal reflux disease (GERD) • Lymphadenopathy • Lymphoma • Vasculitic skin lesions • Pneumonitis • Neuropathy • Nephritis • Nonspecific interstitial pneumonitis (NSIP) • Erythrocyte sedimentation rate (ESR) • Sicca symptoms

3.1 Background: Overall Approach to Patient Care

In the era of increased demand on the time per patient for rheumatologists, SS patients represent the proverbial patient with a long list of questions regarding problems of topical therapy of dry eyes and mouth, most of which are not immediately life threatening. In addition to the limited time available, there is only a limited amount of information that a patient can retain during their visit.

3.1.1 Pearl

Use the Internet as a means to instruct the patient and help them become actively involved in the therapeutic process. Chapter 4 will contain a series of tables regarding choice of artificial tears, saliva, and topical therapy that will be included in the "Standards of Care" guidelines that are currently being formulated.

We have found that many of our patients have Internet addresses (or that their children or family members have computers). For those without computers, the local library offers access to the Internet, and instructions about simple Internet use are generally available there. Thus, during our patient visits, we attempt to provide the patient with a general overview of the treatment plan and then email them an "attachment" with more specific written instructions as needed.

Patients increasingly want to be an active partner in the treatment plan and we encourage this. However, we also warn them that the Internet can be a citadel of misinformation.

3.1.2 Pearl

A helpful hint (humorously referred to as a "pearl of wisdom") for the rheumatologist is to instruct patients *to restrict their Internet medical information searches to a much more reliable (albeit less well-known) search engine such as "Google Scholar"* (http://www.googlescholar.com).

The patient can be directed to the Internet to read available patient information on validated websites such as

- http://www.WebMD.com
- http://www.MedScape.com
- http://www.eMedicine.com
- http://www.sjogrens.org

3.2 Diagnosis Criteria and Laboratory Tests

3.2.1 Myth

There is now a validated diagnostic criteria structure for Sjögren's syndrome that has been adopted by the American College of Rheumatology (ACR).

Fact: Although rheumatologists are using the European–US consensus criteria described by Vitali et al. [1, 2], the ACR has *not* yet accepted these criteria. Although the criteria have been validated in a European cohort, it has not been systematically studied in any US cohort. The European criteria are listed in Table 3.1. An example of a salivary gland biopsy from an SS patient, characterized by focal lymphocytic infiltrates, is shown in Fig. 3.1.

Table 3.1 Consensus criteria for the diagnosis of primary and secondary Sjögren's syndrome. The diagnosis requires either a positive antibody to SS-A/SS-B or a characteristic minor salivary gland biopsy. Revised classification criteria for Sjögren's syndrome

I. Requirements for classification of patient with primary SS:
1. The presence of *either positive salivary gland biopsy* (described below) *or positive antibody to SS-A or SS-B*;
2. The presence of *any three objective clinical signs for oral and ocular dryness* (described below); and
3. The presence of *at least four clinical symptoms for oral and ocular dryness* (described below).
II. Clinical symptoms
A. Ocular symptoms: a positive response to *at least one* of the following questions:
1. Have you had *daily, persistent, troublesome dry eyes* for more than 3 months?
2. Do you have a *recurrent sensation of sand or gravel in the eyes*?
3. Do you use *tear substitutes* for more than three times a day?
B. Oral symptoms: a positive response to *at least one* of the following questions:
1. Have you had a *daily feeling of dry mouth* for more than 3 months?
2. Have you had *recurrently or persistently swollen salivary glands* as an adult?
3. Do you *frequently drink liquids to aid in swallowing* dry food?
III. Objective clinical signs
A. Ocular signs—that is, *objective evidence of ocular involvement* defined as a *positive result for at least one of the following* two tests:
1. *Shirmer's test*, performed without anesthesia (greater than 5 mm in 5 min)
2. *Rose Bengal* score or other ocular dye score (greater than 4 according to Van Bijsterveld's scoring system) B. Minor salivary gland biopsy
Histopathology: In minor salivary glands (obtained through normal-appearing mucosa): *focal lymphocytic sialadenitis*, evaluated by an expert histopathologist, *with a focus score greater than 1.*
• A *lymphocyte focus* is defined as a cluster of 50 or more lymphocytes—which are adjacent to normal-appearing mucous acini and not adjacent to areas where ruptured ducts have fibrotic regions.
C. Salivary gland involvement: objective evidence of salivary gland involvement defined by a positive result for at least one of the following diagnostic tests:
1. *Unstimulated whole salivary flow* (greater than 1.5 mL in 15 min)
2. *Parotid sialography* showing the presence of diffuse sialectasis (punctate, cavitary, or destructive pattern), without evidence of obstruction in the major ducts.
3. *Salivary scintigraphy* showing delayed uptake, reduced concentration, and/or delayed excretion of tracer.
D. Autoantibodies: presence in the serum of the following autoantibodies:
• antibodies to Ro (SSA) or
• La (SSB) antigens, or both
IV. Criteria for secondary SS
Patients who fulfill criteria for primary SS *and* with an associated well-defined rheumatologic disorder such as
• rheumatoid arthritis,
• systemic lupus, *or*
• progressive systemic sclerosis.
V. Exclusion criteria
1. Past head and neck radiation treatment
2. Hepatitis C infection
3. Acquired immunodeficiency disease syndrome (AIDS)

Table 3.1 (continued)

4. Pre-existing lymphoma
5. Sarcoidosis
6. Graft versus host disease
7. Use of anticholinergic drugs at the time of measurements considered abnormal (all measurements used to fulfill criteria need to be performed at a time duration after stopping drug for four-half lives of the drug) [1].

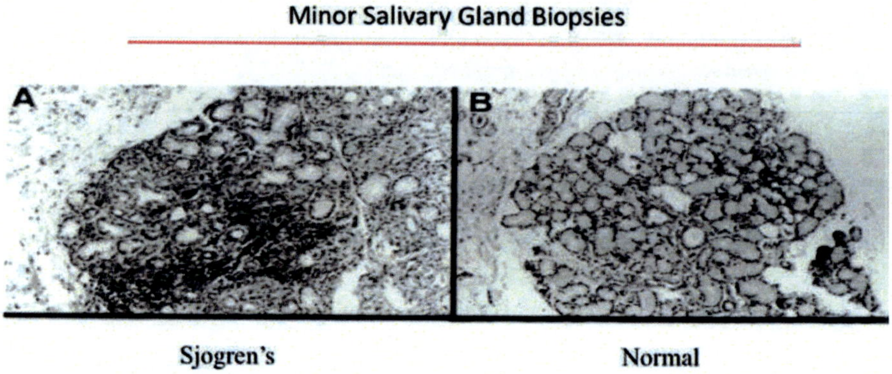

Fig. 3.1 Minor salivary gland biopsies. **a** Biopsy from a Sjögren's patient where clusters of lymphocytes (termed foci) can be seen. *Arrows* also denote regions of the glandular lobule where the acini and ducts remain intact but non-functioning. **b** Biopsy from a patient with symptoms of a dry burning mouth but that lacks focal lymphocytic infiltrates

3.2.2 Pearl

There are recent criteria for disease activity and disease damage indices.

Comments: The same EEC consortium (Vitali et al. (Vitali, 2007 #16385)) that spearheaded the new consensus criteria has recently presented an activity and disease damage index (Tables 3.1 and 3.2) that will serve as a starting point for a uniform database basis for clinical data collection and research studies. These indices will provide the same type of standardization that the ACR criteria provided for RA.

3.2.3 Myth

The antinuclear antibody (ANA) and anti-Sjögren's SS-A (Ro) antibody are specific for primary Sjögren's syndrome.

Comments: Patients commonly arrive in the rheumatologist's office after the primary care physician has ordered a battery of tests for vague symptoms and a positive ANA and/or a positive anti-SS-A (Ro) emerged.

ANA assays can be useful in recognizing certain disease conditions but can create misunderstanding when the limitations are not fully appreciated. The ANA has a higher sensitivity than specificity. Tan et al. [3] measured the range of antinuclear antibodies (ANAs) in "healthy" individuals.

- Fifteen international laboratories experienced in performing tests for ANA by indirect immunofluorescence participated in analyzing coded sera from healthy individuals.
- Except for the stipulation that HEp-2 cells should be used as substrate, each laboratory used its own in-house methodology so that the data might be expected to reflect the output of a cross-section of worldwide ANA reference laboratories.

Table 3.2 Distinct clinical features in patients with Sjögren's syndrome and systemic lupus erythematosus.

SS is not simply SLE with only four criteria

SS is characterized by infiltration of lymphocytes into ocular and salivary glands, so it is more lymphocyte aggressive, and may also include other systems such as:

- **parotid and lymph node swelling**
- **respiratory / lung (pneumonitis) rather than pleurisy**
- **renal / kidney (interstitial nephritis) rather than glomerulonephritis**
- **neurological (central and peripheral)**
- **skin (hyperglobulinemic purpura)**

So it is no surprise that SS patients have lymphoproliferative features such as lymphoma

Although patients with SS and SLE share many features in common, the distinguishing feature of SS is the infiltrative nature of lymphocytes into extranodal sites, including salivary and lacrimal glands, as well as into lungs, kidneys, and neural system. In some cases, the lympho-aggressive characteristic in SS is manifested by increase in frequency of non-Hodgkin's lymphoma. In comparison, SLE can be considered to largely mediate its tissue damage from autoantibody, immune complex, and complement-mediated damage.

- The sera were analyzed at four dilutions: 1:40, 1:80, 1:160, and 1:320.
- They found that in healthy individuals, the frequency of ANA did not differ significantly across the four age subgroups spanning 20–60 years of age.
- This putatively normal population was ANA positive in 31.7% of individuals at 1:40 serum dilution, 13.3% at 1:80, 5.0% at 1:160, and 3.3% at 1:320.

An interesting finding of this study was a remarkably higher incidence of "false"-positive ANAs in patients with either a monoclonal gammopathy or a myelodysplastic syndrome; this observation was attributed to the association of autoantibody with a "dysregulated" immune system at the bone marrow level.

The same consortia of research labs (led by Tan et al. (Tan, 1997 #6375; Tan, 1996 #5941; Tan, 1999 #99186629; Tan, 1973 #354)) also studied ELISA detection methods using normal and patent sera.

- Precision, based on evaluation of replicate samples, varied from very good to poor for particular antigens [4–6].
- Similar results were reported in more recent laboratory standardization reports [5–7].

Lightfoot has used Bayesian calculation to determine that an individual with an ANA of 1:320 (and lacking other clinical criteria to suggest either SS or SLE) has less than a 1:100 chance in developing SLE or SS during a 5-year follow-up interval.

In a more recent analysis, Lopez-Hoyos et al. [5–7] confirmed the complexity in the clinical laboratory of standardizing ANA testing. ANA testing by indirect immunofluorescence (IIF) assays is not an automated laboratory test. Efforts are being made to develop easy and semi or automated methods to screen for ANAs using microchip-binding technology. However, the affinity columns used to prepare the chips will be "as good as" the sera that are defined as definite SS—and previously we have noted the problems in diagnosis. Similarly, the "positive" sera that go with each assay kit will need to be carefully chosen for their sensitivity and specificity.

3.2.4 Myth

SS Patients with "atypical antibody profiles" such as an ANA with anticentromere pattern or

ANCA always represent overlap syndromes with other conditions such as progressive systemic sclerosis (PSS) or Wegener's granulomatosis [8].
Comments: Although patients may develop an overlap syndrome with other autoimmune disorders such as PSS, the pattern of autoantibodies in patients with SS correlates more closely with their HLA-DR than with their clinical presentation [9, 10].

Ramos-Casals et al. [5, 6] studied 402 patients diagnosed with primary SS.

- Eighty-two (20%) patients showed atypical autoantibodies (36 had antiphospholipid (aPL), 21 anti-DNA, 13 ANCA, 10 anti-RNP, 8 ACA, 6 anti-Sm, 2 anti-Scl70, and 1 anti-Jo-1 antibodies).
- Patients with atypical autoantibodies had no statistical differences in extraglandular manifestations (except for a higher prevalence of Raynaud's phenomenon, 28% vs 7%).

3.2.5 Pearl

MRI sialography can be used to visualize the ductal structure of the major salivary glands.
Comments: It is not necessary to perform a sialogram to assess the salivary status of SS patients or to visualize the ductal structures for punctual sialadenitis. This is important since most US academic centers do not have experience in retrograde sialography that is mentioned in consensus diagnostic criteria and this invasive method may have morbidity if done by inexperienced radiologists or ENT.

MRI of the parotid and submandibular glands has vastly improved. If an MRI of the soft tissues of the neck is required (for example, in a case of parotid gland swelling), then we ask for a gadolinium contrast study with "fat suppression" views that provides a nice evaluation of the glandular tissues [11, 12]. Although ultrasound of the glands has proven useful at certain research centers (particularly in Europe), a great deal of experience is required to obtain reproducible results. As a result of readily available MRI at most academic medical centers in the United States, experience with ultrasound imaging of the glands has not been fully developed.

3.2.6 Pearl

Salivary flow rates can be evaluated by non- or minimally invasive methods.
Comments: This is important to correlate measurements of patient's symptoms with objective signs of dryness. Technetium scans of salivary function are performed after coating the tongue with a lemon concentrate [13–15]. The uptake of contrast material and its rate of secretion into the gland can be quantitated.

Although the decreased flow rate is not specific to SS (i.e., many processes can contribute to decreased uptake or secretion), the method is useful in the evaluation of the patient who complains that "I don't feel any saliva in my mouth," but the oral mucosal tissues appear to be relatively intact. The finding of a normal technetium scan should point the rheumatologist toward other causes of the patient's severe mouth complaints.

3.2.7 Pearl

There is significant variation when collecting saliva by oral expectoration or "sponge" methods [16, 17].
Comments: Simple expectorated saliva can be collected on a preweighed sponge placed under the tongue (called the Saxon test) [18]. However, there is significant variability in these measurements in the same patient over the course of the day or when measurements are repeated [16]. The reasons for the variability include

- time since last meal
- last oral stimulation (including tooth brushing)
- history of smoking as well as
- medications taken for other medical problems [5, 6, 19]

Although the variability in flow rates in both normal and SS is noted above, it is worth pointing out that the "normal salivary flow rate" for unstipulated saliva from the parotid gland is 0.4–0.5 mL/min/gland. The normal flow rate for unstipulated, "resting," or "whole" saliva is 0.3–0.5 mol/min; for *stimulated* saliva, 1–2 mol/min. Values less than 0.1 mol/min are typically considered xerostomia, although reduced flow may not always be associated with complaints of dryness.

3.3 Myths and Pearls About Clinical Presentations

3.3.1 Pearl

Do not spend too much time worrying about the clinical extraglandular distinction between the diagnosis of SS and SLE.

We will discuss some important clinical and therapeutic distinctions between these entities below, but it is generally sufficient for the patient to understand that their SS can be considered an "SLE-like" condition. This is important when the patient goes to other specialists or to the emergency room, where the diagnostic entity of SS is less well recognized. Since SLE is much more widely recognized, the other physicians will not attribute important clinical presentations such as drug toxicities, a heart attack, or pulmonary emboli to the "mysterious" manifestations of SS.

Comments: *There is a close relationship between SS and a subset of patients with SLE* [5, 6, 20]. The genetics, antibody profiles, and therapy of the subset of SLE patients with SS-A antibodies closely resemble that subset of SLE patients [21]. It has been suggested that many older patients diagnosed with "mild" SLE actually better fulfill the diagnosis of SS [22]. This is shown schematically in Fig. 3.2, which shows the overlap of SS, SLE, and fibromyalgia patients with a positive ANA.

There are several "humorous" ways that our clinic has described SS. It has been suggested that SS is really an SLE with only four criteria, due to the close relationship in HLA-DR, autoantibodies, and response to therapies [20, 23–25]. However, there are distinct differences in the patterns of disease involvement.

It might be more accurate to describe SS as having similar features as SLE but with "homing receptors" that yield

1. *Interstitial infiltrates* in salivary and lacrimal glands (that normally lack infiltrates)
2. *Increased rates of lymphoma*

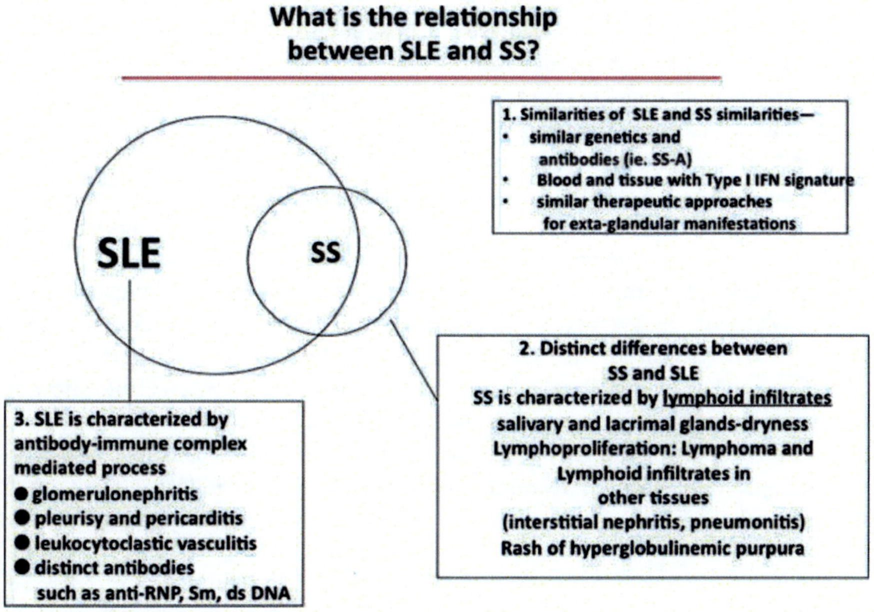

Fig. 3.2 Overlap of clinical features with Sjögren's syndrome, systemic lupus erythematosus, and fibromyalgia. There is significant clinical overlap between patients with primary Sjögren's syndrome (SS) and systemic lupus erythematosus (SLE). Both groups may possess a positive ANA and anti-SS-A antibody. One approach is to consider SLE as a group of disorders that are each characterized by their own profile of autoantibodies (and associated HLA-DR genes) and that one subset of SLE has close correspondence to SS. The SS patients have particular clinical features such as dry eyes and dry mouth as well as extraglandularmanifestations that include increased frequency of lymphoma

3. *Interstitial pneumonitis* (in contrast to pleurisy of SLE)
4. *Interstitial nephritis* (in contrast to glomerulonephritis)
5. *Slightly different types of rashes* (such as hyperglobulinemia purpura) [26].

Thus, SS patients can have the same autoantibody and immune complex-mediated complications as we find in SLE (i.e., ITP, hemolytic anemia, glomerulonephritis), but in the SS patient, our differential must include lymphocyte-aggressive processes such as lymphocytic interstitial pneumonitis, mixed cryoglobulinemia, or lymphoma (Table 3.2).

3.3.2 Myth

There is a close relationship between lacrimal gland flow rates as measured by Schirmer's test and patient's symptoms of ocular dryness [27, 28].

Comments: Tears do not only have an aqueous component, but also have proteins and *mucins that form a lubricating gel [29]. The tears have a different composition in terms of mucins, osmolality, and proteins than that found in saliva. Also, the lipid component of the tears (secreted by the meibomian glands, discussed below) is important in retarding evaporation [27, 32–36].

Thus, the volume of tears is determined by its aqueous content produced by the lacrimal gland as well as the mucins [37] (especially MUC4) produced by goblet cells of the ocular surface that contribute to the viscosity of the tear film [27, 33, 37]. The number of goblet cells can be ascertained by simple exfoliative cytology of the conjunctival surface or by conjunctival biopsy [38] (a method generally used in research or clinical trial settings).

3.3.3 Pearl

Patients may complain of dry eye, but their symptoms may also be due to increased evaporative loss associated with inflammation of the meibomian glands, a condition known as "blepharitis" [27, 33, 37].

Comments: Of importance in normal individuals, the tear film evaporation is retarded by a lipid layer produced by the meibomian glands (located at the edge of the eyelids). The rate of evaporative loss depends on

(a) *the lipid layer*,
(b) *the outside ambient humidity*, and
(c) *the blink rate* (discussed below), which determines the spreading.

Each of these factors may be important in treating the patient with dry or painful eyes.

The thickness of the lipid layer of the tear film in SS patients and the rate of evaporative loss of tears increased in SS patients [39].

3.3.4 Pearl

There is a poor correlation of measurement of saliva and patient's complaints of dry mouth.

Comments: Unfortunately, there is a poor correlation between patients' descriptions of oral comfort and observed salivary flow rates [40–42]. This may reflect the misconception that saliva is "water" rather than a complicated mixture of water–proteins–mucins. This lubricating film provides a decreased viscosity for the oral mucosa and allows the tongue to more easily function during deglutition and talking [43].

In a recent report (Alliende, 2007 #18598), reduced sulfating of mucin MUC5B was more closely linked to complaints of xerostomia in SS patients than aqueous water flow. Mucins are sulfated oligosaccharides that sequester water to provide lubrication and low viscosity of movement of the oral mucosa. They are familiar to many of us as the Lewis antigens that are secreted in saliva.

This defect in sulfating of MUC5B probably results from the inflammatory microenvironment due to release of cytokines and the disorganization of the basal lamina as a result of metalloproteinases that leads to dedifferentiation of acinar mucous cells (Alliende, 2007 #18598).

3.3.5 Pearl

A dry mouth is not necessarily a painful mouth.
Comments: The physician should look for signs of oral candidiasis such as angular cheilitis or erythematous changes of the hard palate as well as lichen planus-like changes in buccal recess [44].

Many patients have a dry mouth and this may be a normal part of the aging process [45, 46]. However, some event usually brings the patient to clinical attention. Frequently, *a dry mouth is converted to a painful mouth by the occurrence of oral yeast infections*, particularly in a patient who is on corticosteroids and has recently been taking antibiotics [47–49].

Alterations in the oral microbial flora as well as relative decreases in the salivary flow of naturally occurring antifungal agents such as transferrin or calprotectin [50], histatins [51], and other small molecules of the defensin family [52] may further predispose the SS patient to oral *Candida* [47–49]. A role for decreased level of antioxidants with these symptoms and the potential exacerbating role of medications with anticholinergic side effects must always be considered [46, 53].

Daniels et al. [44, 54, 55] have pointed out the importance of recognizing erythematous candidiasis, which presents as reddish petechiae frequently on the hard palate. It may be important for the patient to remove his/her denture in order to see the lesions. Also, lichen planus-like lesions on the buccal mucosa (especially in the buccal recesses).

Treatment of the oral candidiasis may require a rather prolonged treatment with topical antifungal drugs [43], using mouth rinses similar to those employed by the radiation therapists (often called XYZ mouth rinses) and topical application of nystatins [55].

3.3.6 Pearl

Burning mouth is a common complaint and may not be associated with a systemic autoimmune disorder such as SS.

Comments: Other causes of burning mouth syndrome must also be considered, including *nutritional deficiencies, hormonal changes associated with menopause, local oral infections, denture-related lesions, hypersensitivity reactions, medications, and systemic diseases including diabetes mellitus* [56]. In many cases, no clear cause can be found, and the dry mouth is attributed to a local neuropathy or to a manifestation of depression [46, 53].

Patton et al. [57] reported a series of 45 patients with burning mouth in whom a diagnosis of SS (or above causes) could not be established. They suggested a localized neuropathy or psychogenic causes in these patients and recommended a trial of topical clonazepam and antioxidants (alpha-lipoic acid) in some patients and systemic agents used in neuropathy (gabapentin, pregabalin) or antidepressants with benefit in neuropathy (SSRIs, SNSRIs, or NSRIs) in other patients. Agents with known anticholinergic side effects such as tricyclics were not tolerated.

3.3.7 Pearl

Suspect laryngotracheal reflux in the patient who exhibits repeated "throat clearing" during their visit to the rheumatologist.
This problem can present as hoarseness, coughing at night, and even as a "post-nasal drip." The imbalance is due to decreased saliva volume, and the content predisposes to dysfunction of the gastro-esophageal sphincter, gastro-esophageal reflux, and laryngotracheal reflux [58, 59]. The latter condition can be suspected when the patient engages in *repeated "throat clearing"* during the interview or has "unexplained" hoarseness. Of importance, the reflux of acid into the trachea can stimulate the vagus nerve and mucus secretions, thus emulating symptoms from panic attack (choking) to sinus infections [58, 59].

3.3.8 Pearl

SS patients have more difficulty swallowing certain types of tablets or capsules than do other patients.

Comments: SS patients have deglutition problems due to dryness and lack of viscosity (associated with altered mucin production). As a result, they have difficulty with both swallowing and esophageal transit of many medications.

When possible, smaller "polished" tablets are preferred. An example is "branded" hydroxychloroquine (Plaquenil) that is a polished tablet, in comparison to many of the generics that are larger in size and contain a residue with bitter taste on the unpolished surface. Also, certain capsules (particularly large capsules containing iron replacement) may become adherent to the dry esophageal mucosa where they may even cause erosion. For these reasons, "polished" (coated) tablets are preferred to "sticky" capsules.

3.3.9 Pearl

Thyroid disease is more frequent in SS patients.
Comments: The most common thyroid disorder found in association with SS was autoimmune thyroiditis, and the most common hormonal pattern was subclinical hypothyroidism [60]. pSS was *ten times more frequent* in patients with autoimmune thyroid disease, and autoimmune thyroiditis was *nine times more frequent* in pSS [60].
The co-existence of SS and thyroiditis is significantly more frequent and suggests a common genetic or environmental factor predisposition with similar pathogenic mechanisms [60, 61]. Therefore, SS should be studied in patients with thyroid disease and vice versa.

Antigens are shared by both thyroid and salivary glands, which could be responsible for the association between both the diseases. Immunogenetic studies have suggested that both diseases have a common genetic predisposition. SS and thyroid disease patients were mostly women with positive antithyroglobulin, antiparietal cell, and antithyroid peroxidase antibodies [60, 62].

3.3.10 Pearl

Autonomic neuropathy is more frequent in SS patients.
Comments: In one recent study, autonomic neuropathy was more common among both SS and SLE patients [63]. Vagal dysfunction was established by applying three tests:
1. valsalva maneuver,
2. deep breathing test, and
3. heart rate response to standing.

Sympathetic dysfunction was examined by applying two tests:
1. blood pressure response to standing and
2. handgrip test.

In all cardiovascular reflex tests, frequencies of abnormal results were significantly higher among the SS and SLE patients than among the controls [63].

In a separate recent study by Mandl et al. [64], orthostatic test [64], orthostatic systolic and diastolic blood pressure responses (lSBP ratio and lDBP ratio), and finger skin blood flow test [64] were reported.
- Orthostatic systolic and diastolic blood pressures were significantly decreased.
- The VAC score significantly increased in patients with pSS compared to controls, indicating both parasympathetic and sympathetic system dysfunction.

3.3.11 Pearl

When SS occurs in males, look for other clinical stigmata of Klinefelter syndrome.
Comments: In some studies, up to 10% of SS patients are male [65]. In general, the clinical presentation, laboratory findings, extraglandular manifestations, and minor salivary biopsies are similar to females, with slightly lower percent exhibiting a positive ANA and higher percent exhibiting hematologic abnormalities [65].

In one study, up to 15% of the male SS patients had symptoms of Klinefelter's syndrome (lack of reproductive capacity, low testosterone, and abnormal XXY karyotype).

These findings are interesting in view of the finding of translocation of a Toll receptor in the BXSB mouse involving a portion of the X chromosome to the Y chromosome, since this is the only male mouse model to develop SS-like or SLE-like features.

3.3.12 Pearl

Pulmonary hypertension may develop in SS patients.

Comments: Although dyspnea is most frequently associated with scleroderma, pulmonary hypertension needs to be considered in the SS patient.

A recent study reviewed an unexpected 9 cases of PAH [66] in a cohort of 500 SS patients. The rheumatologist should make sure that the cardiac echo is performed (i.e., valves imaged) and interpretation being specifically read for PAH since most technicians perform the study to evaluate left heart function rather than a detailed examination of the tricuspid valve and the estimated pulmonary pressure. Further, in the real world of the busy cardiologist, the echocardiograms are read as a "string" of different studies where the cardiologists are concentrating on left ventricular function (without recognizing that the ordering rheumatologist wanted information on PAH).

If PAH is detected, then the patient also needs to be evaluated for occult pulmonary emboli and the occurrence of circulating anticoagulants.

3.3.13 Myth

Cutaneous vasculitis in SS is usually a lymphocytic vasculitis.

Comment: In fact, cutaneous vasculitis in SS is usually a leukocytoclastic vasculitis, the most common feature of which is palpable purpura [67]. In up to 30% of cases of vasculitis associated with SS, cryoglobulinemia (occurring as part and parcel of the SS) is also present.

Other prominent features of vasculitis in SS are

- Urticarial lesions in approximately 25% of those with vasculitis
- Medium-vessel disease mimicking PAN in <5% (but bearing a bad prognosis when it presents) [67]

3.3.14 Pearl

More than 25% of patients with primary SS have sensorineural hearing loss.

Comment: Sensorineural hearing loss was detected in 38 (27%) of 140 patients with primary SS included in 4 studies [68–71]. An association with immunologic parameters such as aPL, ANA, Ro, or La has been suggested. Boki et al. [71] found that primary SS is associated with sensorineural hearing loss preferentially affecting the high frequencies, although clinically significant deficits are not common, with no evidence of retrocochlear disease or increased vestibular involvement [71, 72].

3.3.15 Pearl

Urinary tract symptoms and cystitis are underdiagnosed in primary SS.

Comment: Two recent studies have investigated lower urinary tract symptoms in primary SS. Walker et al. [73] found severe urological symptoms (increased frequency, urgency, and nocturia) in 61% of patients, with biopsy-proven interstitial cystitis being found in some cases [5, 6]. Similar results have recently found that 5% of Finnish SS patients fulfilled the criteria for interstitial cystitis [74]. Using a different approach, a high percentage of patients were identified as having a biomarker associated with interstitial cystitis (APF, antiproliferative factor made by bladder epithelial cells) and clinical features of SS among an Australian cohort [75].

3.3.16 Myth

Muscular biopsy is a key tool in the diagnosis of muscular involvement in SS.

Comment: Myalgias are found in nearly 30% of patients with primary SS, although the causes are diverse, including both non-inflammatory (mainly fibromyalgia) and inflammatory (mainly myositis) processes. The key study was performed by Lindvall et al. [76] and they found that analytical data and histological findings do not correlate with clinical myositis. Thus, one third of patients with clinical myositis have normal histology while nearly half of the patients with histologically confirmed myositis have no clinical features.

3.4 Myths and Pearls About Pathogenesis

3.4.1 Myth

Dryness in SS results from the total destruction of the gland.

Comments: In a lip biopsy from an SS patient with severe dryness, attention is usually focused on the dense lymphoid infiltrates (shown in Fig. 3.1, *frame A*). However, it should be noted that residual acinar units are still visible [77].

Indeed, morphometric analysis has shown that *only about 50% of the gland acinar or ductal tissue is replaced or destroyed* [26, 78]. This may seem somewhat surprising, since a kidney or liver continues to function until its functional units are over 90% destroyed.

The interesting question is "*why has the residual gland stopped functioning?*" Kontinnen et al. [79] have demonstrated that the glandular tissue (outside the lymphoid infiltrate) still has its neural innervation based on immunohistology. Studies in man and murine models have indicated the presence of receptors for acetylcholine and other critical neurotransmitters [80–82]. It has been shown in animal models that the release of and response to neurotransmitters are strongly influenced by inflammatory cytokines including TNF and IL-1 [83–85].

Further, the release of metalloproteinases in the inflammatory environment may interfere with the secretory gland's ability to maintain spatial orientation necessary for glandular function [86]. Recently, there has been increased interest in the potential role of antibodies directed against the muscarinic M3 receptor [87, 88].

3.4.2 Pearl

The environment plays a key role in exacerbating the patient's symptoms.

Comments: Although the patient has a *decreased* rate of aqueous tear formation and *increased* rate of evaporative loss due to the inflammatory process, each of these processes may be exacerbated by environmental factors.

Factors such as *low humidity* can be partially helped by humidifiers and the effect of dry winds by "wrap around" sunglasses or "side shields" on glasses. However, additional factors such as the *markedly decreased "blink rate" associated with the use of computer monitors* are not usually appreciated.

Wolf et al. [89] have pointed out that the modern work place environment is often an office with low humidity where individuals spend a great deal of the day staring at computer screens. Using cameras mounted on the computers, they could demonstrate a *90% decrease in the normal blink rate as the workers concentrated on their computer monitors*. Thus, concentration on the "screen" can override the normal corneal surface conditions that lead to blinking and spreading of the available tears [90, 91].

3.4.3 Pearl

Antibody SS-A may play an integral role in the induction of SS and the type I IFN gene signature in salivary gland biopsies.

Comments: Recent studies by Bave and others have demonstrated that anti-SS-A antibody complex to the ribonucleoprotein complex (SS-A bound to hYRNA) can bind to Fcj receptors on plasmacytic dendritic cells. The internalized immune complex can then gain access to Toll receptors located in cytoplasmic vacuoles and stimulate production of type I IFN. This model ties together the genetics (HLA-DR3 that is associated with production of anti-SS-A antibodies) and the finding of activated plasmacytic dendritic cells that produce interferon type I. Thus, the contribution of the innate (HLA-DR independent) and acquired (HLA-DR dependent) pathways can be appreciated as potential targets (alone or in synergy) for therapy.

3.4.4 Myth

The only problem with saliva is that the volume of flow is diminished.
Comments: Recent studies have compared the content of saliva in normals and in SS patients and have shown significant differences in the profile of proteins present as well as alteration in the post-translational processing of existing salivary proteins.

Normal saliva is the viscous, clear, watery fluid secreted from the parotid, submaxillary, sublingual, and smaller mucous glands of the mouth. Saliva contains *two major types* of protein secretions:

1. a serous secretion containing the digestive enzyme ptyalin and
2. a mucous secretion containing the lubricating aid *mucin*.

The pH of saliva falls between 6 and 7.4. Saliva also contains large amounts of potassium and bicarbonate ions and to a lesser extent sodium and chloride ions. In addition, saliva contains several antimicrobial constituents, including thiocyanate, lysozyme, immunoglobulins, lactoferrin, and transferrin.

Mass spectrometry and expression microarray profiling have been used to identify candidate protein and mRNA biomarkers of primary SS [5, 6, 92–94]. Sixteen WS proteins were found to be down-regulated and 25 WS proteins were found to be up-regulated in primary SS patients compared with matched healthy control subjects (Hu, 2007 #90) [5, 6].

In a separate study, SS saliva showed significant alterations in post-translational modification of carbonic anhydrase and the presence of proteins associated with oxidative stress injury [95].

Low salivary dehydroepiandrosterone and androgen-regulated cysteine-rich secretory protein 3 (crisp3) levels have recently been reported in saliva of SS patients [96]. This is important since it may help explain some of the hormonal influence on salivary function.

3.4.5 Pearl

The gene signature in the SS dry eye is associated with interferon gamma signature.
Comments: As a result of the dryness, the ocular surface develops a form of squamous metaplasia, and conjunctival biopsies have demonstrated an interferon gamma gene signature [33]. This points out the difference between the type I interferon signature in the gland (described above) and the chronic inflammatory reaction on the ocular surface as well as the potentially different requirements for therapy.

3.5 Myths and Pearls About Treatment

3.5.1 Myth

TNF inhibitors have been shown to be beneficial in Sjögren's syndrome.
Comments: Although an initial pilot study suggested the benefit of infliximab in SS [97], a larger multicenter study did not confirm this initial observation [98]. Two studies have examined etanercept (25 mg twice weekly) in SS [99, 100] for 12 weeks, and these pilot studies did not report reduction in sicca symptoms or signs in SS. Also, treatment with etanercept (25 mg twice weekly) did not affect minor salivary gland biopsy results.

3.5.2 Pearl

Salivary gland toxicity may accompany ^{131}I treatment of thyroid disease.
Comments: Although not commonly appreciated, salivary gland toxicity may be an adverse effect

of high-dose radioiodine (^{131}I) [101]. A recent study of 20 patients revealed that 11 (15%) had symptoms of xerostomia within the first 48 h, continuing for 12 months in 7 of these patients. The onset of toxicity in a further nine (12%) patients with persistent symptoms did not occur until 3 months after therapy [101].

3.5.3 Pearl

The salivary gland biopsy of SS patients exhibits a gene signature of type I interferon. This may play an important role in determining the therapeutic agents that are most likely to be successful in trial.

Comments: Among the candidates for therapy may be Toll receptors, whose stimulation led plasmacytic dendritic cells to release type I IFN. Expression of TLR2, TLR3, TLR4, and myeloid differentiation factor 88 (MyD88) in labial salivary glands has been demonstrated by immunohistochemistry [102].

Phosphorylation of extracellular signal-regulated kinase (ERK), c-Jun N-terminal kinase (JNK), p38 (map kinase), Akt, and activation of nuclear factor-kappaB (NF-kappaB) p65 have expressions that are markedly increased in the SS salivary gland. These activated genes were found in salivary-infiltrating mononuclear cells as well as in acinar cells and ductal epithelial cells. The results suggest that TLR-mediated immune response in SS acts through the mitogen-activated protein kinase pathway [102].

Recently, several groups [103–105] have demonstrated the increased migration of plasmacytic dendritic cells into the gland due to chemokines and their receptors, increased, production of cytokines that organize germinal centers and alter the ratio of T-regulatory cells. This inflammatory microenvironment promotes a cycle of continuing lymphoproliferation in both glandular and extraglandular sites in the SS patient [103–105]. The identification of these locally expressed cytokines, chemokines, and their receptors provide new therapeutic opportunities.

3.5.4 Pearl

Ask patients about their use of Chinese or other herbal medications.

Comments: Many patients do not inform their physicians about herbal drugs, as they consider them "nutritional" supplements (and are marketed as such). However, the agents may have significant direct toxicities on the SS patient, such as promoting profound hypokalemia in the SS patient with interstitial nephritis [5, 6, 106] or interaction with other "Western drugs" [107–111].

In our experience, the "herbal" medicines come in the form of "Chinese" herbs or "Indian ayurvedic medicine." In addition to the adverse effect of the herb itself, the preparations may be contaminated with heavy metals (especially common in ayurvedic medications) or pesticides that were used at the time of crop harvesting. Obviously, these candidates can vary from lot to lot of the preparation, even with "scrupulous" and even more unpredictably with material obtained from "street" venders.

3.5.5 Pearl

Cosmetic procedures around the eye can exacerbate SS.

Comments: Three types of procedures come to mind:

1. LASIK surgery for the eye
2. Blepharoplasty (eyelid "lift")
3. Botox® injection

Pre-existing SS is considered a contraindication to LASIK surgery, due to the increased dryness after the procedure [112]. This increased dryness presumably results from the "flap" cut by the microtome across the cornea, which would be expected to sever the nerve bodies from afferent sensory nerves innervating the cornea. The resulting "neuropathic" eye is more sensitive to abrasions as well as to the sensation of dryness (friction as the upper lid traverses the globe).

Blepharoplasty may interrupt the basal tearing that occurs in the lower lid by the glands of

Sherring. This is because the stretching of the lid may disrupt the delicate neural interconnections within the network of glands (these are the same glands that you stimulate when you massage your eyes). Another problem that we have encountered after blepharoplasty is increased zones of exposure keratitis. Particularly when sleeping, the lower lid may not make adequate contact with the upper lid, leading to a zone of increased evaporative loss and resulting desiccative injury.

Finally, a standard model for induction of keratoconjunctivitis sicca is Botox® [113].

3.5.6 Pearl

SS patients have unique and particular needs at the time of anesthesia and surgery.

Comments: *Operating rooms typically have low humidity and patients are at risk for flare of their KCS or corneal abrasions.* We have found this to be particularly true in the post-operative recovery room, where the patient is partially awake with fluttering eyelids, receiving direct flow of oxygen (usually not humidified) to the face, and not really aware of their eye symptoms as they awaken from anesthesia. Therefore, we recommend the use of ocular lubricants during surgery to prevent complications.

Also, the anesthesiologist must be careful with the amount of *anticholinergic agents* given during intubation, as the SS patient may be unduly sensitive and develop inspissated secretions that cannot easily be cleared in the post-operative period (i.e., after abdominal or chest surgery) when raising tenacious secretions is difficult.

Finally, the use of *oral saliva substitutes* should be encouraged. It is expected that patients will be "NPO" (nothing by mouth) prior to many surgeries. In the absence of normal saliva, they will have unnecessary discomfort if they are not allowed to have their artificial saliva. We have found this particularly true when the patient is a "late in the day" case for elective procedures such as joint replacement.

3.5.7 Pearl

A wide range of peripheral neuropathies may be present in SS and constitute one of the most difficult aspects to treat.

Comments: Early attention to peripheral neuropathies is extremely important. The types of neuropathy include sensory including pure sensory and ganglionic neuronopathy. Sural nerve biopsy [114] frequently shows vascular or perivascular inflammation of small epineurial vessels (both arterioles and venules) and in some cases necrotizing vasculitis. Loss of myelinated nerve fibers was relatively common and loss of small diameter type I nerve fibers occurs.

Pathology in cases of sensory (doral root ganglion) consists of loss of neuronal cell bodies and infiltration of T cells [114]. Also, peripheral motor neuropathies can include mononeuritis multiplex (that derives from vasculitis) and CIPD ("chronic idiopathic peripheral demyelination") associated with anti-MAG (myelin-associated glycoprotein) disease. In addition, patients may suffer from trigeminal and other cranial neuropathies, autonomic neuropathy, and mixed patterns of neuropathy [114].

Sural nerve biopsy may show vascular or perivascular inflammation of small epineurial vessels (both arterioles and venules) and in some cases necrotizing vasculitis [114]. Loss of myelinated nerve fibers is common and loss of small diameter nerve fibers occurs. Peripheral neuropathy in PSS often is refractory to treatment although newer biological agents may provide more effective treatment options.

References

1. Vitali C, Palombi G, Baldini C, Benucci M, Bombardieri S, Covelli M, Del Papa N, De Vita S, Epis O, Franceschini F, Gerli R, Govoni M, Bongi SM, Maglione W, Migliaresi S, Montecucco C, Orefice M, Priori R, Tavoni A, Valesini G. Sjogren's syndrome disease damage index and disease activity index: scoring systems for the assessment of disease damage and disease activity in Sjogren's syndrome, derived from an analysis of a cohort of Italian patients. Arthritis Rheum. 2007;56:2223–31.

2. Vitali C. Classification criteria for Sjogren's syndrome. Ann Rheum Dis. 2003;62:94–5; author reply 5.
3. Tan EM, Feltkamp TE, Smolen JS, Butcher B, Dawkins R, Fritzler MJ, Gordon T, Hardin JA, Kalden JR, Lahita RG, Maini RN, McDougal JS, Rothfield NF, Smeenk RJ, Takasaki Y, Wiik A, Wilson MR, Koziol JA. Range of antinuclear antibodies in "healthy" individuals. Arthritis Rheum. 1997;40:1601–11.
4. Tan EM, Smolen JS, McDougal JS, Butcher BT, Conn D, Dawkins R, Fritzler MJ, Gordon T, Hardin JA, Kalden JR, Lahita RG, Maini RN, Rothfield NF, Smeenk R, Takasaki Y, van Venrooij WJ, Wiik A, Wilson M, Koziol JA. A critical evaluation of enzyme immunoassays for detection of antinuclear autoantibodies of defined specificities. I. Precision, sensitivity, and specificity. Arthritis Rheum. 1999;42:455–64.
5. Ramos-Casals M, Nardi N, Brito-Zeron P, Aguilo S, Gil V, Delgado G, Bove A, Font J. Atypical autoantibodies in patients with primary Sjogren syndrome: clinical characteristics and follow-up of 82 cases. Semin Arthritis Rheum. 2006;35: 312–21.
6. Ramos-Casals M, Solans R, Rosas J, Camps MT, Gil A, Del Pino-Montes J, Calvo-Alen J, Jimenez-Alonso J, Mico ML, Beltran J, Belenguer R, Pallares L. Primary Sjogren syndrome in Spain: clinical and immunologic expression in 1010 patients. Medicine (Baltimore) 2008;87:210–19.
7. Lopez-Hoyos M, Rodriguez-Valverde V, Martinez-Taboada V. Performance of antinuclear antibody connective tissue disease screen. Ann NY Acad Sci. 2007;1109:322–9.
8. Liberatore G, Jackson-Lewis V, Vukosavic S, Mandir A, Vila M, McAuliffe W, Dawson V, Dawson T, Przedborski S. Inducible nitric oxide synthase stimulates dopaminergic neurodegeneration in the MPTP model of Parkinson disease. Nat Med. 1999;5:1403–9.
9. Arnett F. Histocompatibility typing in the rheumatic diseases: diagnostic and prognostic implications. Med Clin NA. 20:371–87.
10. Arnett FC, Hamilton RG, Reveille JD, Bias WB, Harley JB, Reichlin M. Genetic studies of Ro (SS-A) and La (SS-B) autoantibodies in families with systemic lupus erythematosus and primary Sjogren's syndrome. Arthritis Rheum. 1989;32:413–9.
11. Eracleous E, Kallis S, Tziakouri C, Blease S, Gourtsoyiannis N. Sonography, CT, CT sialography, MRI and MRI sialography in investigation of the facial nerve and the differentiation between deep and superficial parotid lesions. Neuroradiology 1997;39:506–11.
12. Makula E, Pokorny G, Kiss M, Voros E, Kovacs L, Kovacs A, Csernay L, Palko A. The place of magnetic resonance and ultrasonographic examinations of the parotid gland in the diagnosis and follow-up of primary Sjogren's syndrome. Rheumatology (Oxford) 2000;39:97–104.
13. Hakansson U, Jacobsson L, Lilja B, Manthorpe R, Henriksson V. Salivary gland scintigraphy in subjects with and without symptoms of dry mouth and/or eyes, and in patients with primary Sjogren's syndrome. Scand J Rheumatol. 1994;23:326–33.
14. Helman J, Turner RJ, Fox PC, Baum BJ. ^{99m}Tc-pertechnetate uptake in parotid acinar cells by the $Na^+/K^+/Cl^-$ co-transport system. J Clin Invest. 1987;79:1310–3.
15. Kohn WG, Ship JA, Atkinson JC, Patton LL, Fox PC. Salivary gland ^{99m}Tc-scintigraphy: a grading scale and correlation with major salivary gland flow rates. J Oral Pathol Med. 1992;21:70–4.
16. Burlage FR, Pijpe J, Coppes RP, Hemels ME, Meertens H, Canrinus A, Vissink A. Variability of flow rate when collecting stimulated human parotid saliva. Eur J Oral Sci. 2005;113:386–90.
17. Rosas J, Ramos-Casals M, Ena J, Garcia-Carrasco M, Verdu J, Cervera R, Font J, Caballero O, Ingelmo M, Pascual E. Usefulness of basal and pilocarpine-stimulated salivary flow in primary Sjogren's syndrome. Correlation with clinical, immunological and histological features. Rheumatology (Oxford) 2002;41:670–5.
18. Kohler PF, Winter ME. A quantitative test for xerostomia. The Saxon test, an oral equivalent of the Schirmer test. Arthritis Rheum. 1985;28: 1128–32.
19. Stevens WJ, Swartele FE, Empsten FA, De Clerck LS. Use of the Saxon test as a measure of saliva production in a reference population of schoolchildren. Am J Dis Child. 1990;144:570–1.
20. Isenberg DA. Systemic lupus erythematosus and Sjogren's syndrome: historical perspective and ongoing concerns. Arthritis Rheum. 2004;50: 681–3.
21. Diamond B. Systemic lupus erythematosus and Sjogren's syndrome. Curr Opin Rheumatol. 2007;19:405.
22. Garcia-Carrasco M, Cervera R, Rosas J, Ramos-Casals M, Morla RM, Siso A, Jimenez S, Pallares L, Font J, Ingelmo M. Primary Sjogren's syndrome in the elderly: clinical and immunological characteristics. Lupus 1999;8:20–3.
23. Isenberg D. Sjogren's syndrome – a house of cards. Clin Rheumatol. 1995;14 Suppl 1:8–10.
24. Moutsopoulos HM. Sjogren's syndrome or autoimmune epithelitis? Clin Rev Allergy Immunol. 2007;32:199–200.
25. Tsonis IA, Avrameas S, Moutsopoulos HM. Autoimmunity and pathophysiology. J Autoimmun. 2007;29:203–5.
26. Fox RI. Sjogren's syndrome. Lancet 2005;366: 321–31.
27. Macri A, Pflugfelder S. Correlation of the Schirmer 1 and fluorescein clearance tests with the

severity of corneal epithelial and eyelid disease. Arch Ophthalmol. 2000;118:1632–8.
28. Spiteri A, Mitra M, Menon G, Casini A, Adams D, Ricketts C, Hickling P, Fuller ET, Fuller JR. Tear lipid layer thickness and ocular comfort with a novel device in dry eye patients with and without Sjogren's syndrome. J Fr Ophtalmol. 2007;30:357–64.
29. Pflugfelder SC, Liu Z, Monroy D, Li DQ, Carvajal ME, Price-Schiavi SA, Idris N, Solomon A, Perez A, Carraway KL. Detection of sialomucin complex (MUC4) in human ocular surface epithelium and tear fluid. Invest Ophthalmol Vis Sci. 2000;41:1316–26.
30. Afonso AA, Monroy D, Stern ME, Feuer WJ, Tseng SC, Pflugfelder SC. Correlation of tear fluorescein clearance and Schirmer test scores with ocular irritation symptoms. Ophthalmology 1999;106:803–10.
31. Behrens A, Doyle JJ, Stern L, Chuck RS, McDonnell PJ, Azar DT, Dua HS, Hom M, Karpecki PM, Laibson PR, Lemp MA, Meisler DM, Castillo JM, O'Brien T P, Pflugfelder SC, Rolando M, Schein OD, Seitz B, Tseng SC, Setten GV, Wilson SE, Yiu SC. Dysfunctional tear syndrome: a Delphi approach to treatment recommendations. Cornea 2006;25:900–7.
32. de Paiva CS, Pflugfelder SC. Tear clearance implications for ocular surface health. Exp Eye Res. 2004;78:395–7.
33. De Paiva CS, Villarreal AL, Corrales RM, Rahman HT, Chang VY, Farley WJ, Stern ME, Niederkorn JY, Li DQ, Pflugfelder SC. Dry eye-induced conjunctival epithelial squamous metaplasia is modulated by interferon-gamma. Invest Ophthalmol Vis Sci. 2007;48:2553–60.
34. Luo L, Li DQ, Corrales RM, Pflugfelder SC. Hyperosmolar saline is a proinflammatory stress on the mouse ocular surface. Eye Contact Lens. 2005;31:186–93.
35. Pflugfelder SC, Huang AJ, Feuer W, Chuchovski PT, Pereira IC, Tseng SC. Conjunctival cytologic features of primary Sjogren's syndrome. Ophthalmology 1990;97:985–91.
36. Pflugfelder SC, Jones D, Ji Z, Afonso A, Monroy D. Altered cytokine balance in the tear fluid and conjunctiva of patients with Sjogren's syndrome keratoconjunctivitis sicca. Curr Eye Res. 1999;19:201–11.
37. Pflugfelder SC, Solomon A, Stern ME. The diagnosis and management of dry eye: a twenty-five-year review. Cornea 2000;19:644–9.
38. Yoon KC, Jeong IY, Park YG, Yang SY. Interleukin-6 and tumor necrosis factor-alpha levels in tears of patients with dry eye syndrome. Cornea 2007;26:431–7.
39. Goto E, Matsumoto Y, Kamoi M, Endo K, Ishida R, Dogru M, Kaido M, Kojima T, Tsubota K. Tear evaporation rates in Sjogren syndrome and non-Sjogren dry eye patients. Am J Ophthalmol. 2007;144:81–5.
40. Atkinson JC, Fox PC. Sjogren's syndrome: oral and dental considerations. J Am Dent Assoc. 1993;124:74–6.
41. Fox PC, Mandel ID. Effects of pilocarpine on salivary flow in patients with Sjogren's syndrome [letter; comment]. Oral Surg Oral Med Oral Pathol. 1992;74:315–8.
42. Wolff A, Fox PC, Ship JA, Atkinson JC, Macynski AA, Baum BJ. Oral mucosal status and major salivary gland function. Oral Surg Oral Med Oral Pathol. 1990;70:49–54.
43. Wu AJ, Fox PC. Sjogren's syndrome. Semin Dermatol. 1994;13:138–43.
44. Daniels S. We all need to know about Sjogren's syndrome. Nurs Times. 2007;103:15.
45. Hershkovich O, Shafat I, Nagler RM. Age-related changes in salivary antioxidant profile: possible implications for oral cancer. J Gerontol A Biol Sci Med Sci. 2007;62:361–6.
46. Nagler RM. Salivary glands and the aging process: mechanistic aspects, health-status and medicinal-efficacy monitoring. Biogerontology 2004;5:223–33.
47. Abraham CM, al-Hashimi I, Haghighat N. Evaluation of the levels of oral *Candida* in patients with Sjogren's syndrome. Oral Surg Oral Med Oral Pathol Oral Radiol Endod. 1998;86:65–8.
48. Almstahl A, Kroneld U, Tarkowski A, Wikstrom M. Oral microbial flora in Sjogren's syndrome. J Rheumatol. 1999;26:110–4.
49. Rhodus NL, Michalowicz BS. Periodontal status and sulcular *Candida albicans* colonization in patients with primary Sjogren's syndrome. Quintessence Int. 2005;36:228–33.
50. Sweet SP, Denbury AN, Challacombe SJ. Salivary calprotectin levels are raised in patients with oral candidiasis or Sjogren's syndrome but decreased by HIV infection. Oral Microbiol Immunol. 2001;16:119–23.
51. Tsai H, Bobek LA. Human salivary histatins: promising anti-fungal therapeutic agents. Crit Rev Oral Biol Med. 1998;9:480–97.
52. Peluso G, De Santis M, Inzitari R, Fanali C, Cabras T, Messana I, Castagnola M, Ferraccioli GF. Proteomic study of salivary peptides and proteins in patients with Sjogren's syndrome before and after pilocarpine treatment. Arthritis Rheum. 2007;56:2216–22.
53. Nagler RM, Hershkovich O. Relationships between age, drugs, oral sensorial complaints and salivary profile. Arch Oral Biol. 2005;50:7–16.
54. Daniels TE, Fox PC. Salivary and oral components of Sjogren's syndrome. Rheum Dis Clin North Am. 1992;18:571–89.
55. Daniels TE, Wu AJ. Xerostomia – clinical evaluation and treatment in general practice. J Calif Dent Assoc. 2000;28:933–41.

56. Maltsman-Tseikhin A, Moricca P, Niv D. Burning mouth syndrome: will better understanding yield better management? Pain Pract. 2007;7: 151–62.
57. Patton L, Siegel M, Benoliel R, De Laat A. Management of burning mouth syndrome: systematic review and management recommendations. Oral Surg Oral Med Oral Pathol Oral Radiol Endodontol. 2007;S39:1–13.
58. Belafsky PC, Postma GN. The laryngeal and esophageal manifestations of Sjogren's syndrome. Curr Rheumatol Rep. 2003;5:297–303.
59. Postma GN, Belafsky PC, Aviv JE, Koufman JA. Laryngopharyngeal reflux testing. Ear Nose Throat J. 2002;81:14–8.
60. Jara LJ, Navarro C, Brito-Zeron Mdel P, Garcia-Carrasco M, Escarcega RO, Ramos-Casals M. Thyroid disease in Sjogren's syndrome. Clin Rheumatol. 2007;26:1601–6.
61. D'Arbonneau F, Ansart S, Le Berre R, Dueymes M, Youinou P, Pennec YL. Thyroid dysfunction in primary Sjogren's syndrome: a long-term followup study. Arthritis Rheum. 2003;49:804–9.
62. Fox PC. An Autoimmune Exocrinopathy. Ann NY Acad Sci. 2007;1098:15–21.
63. Stojanovich L, Milovanovich B, de Luka SR, Popovich-Kuzmanovich D, Bisenich V, Djukanovich B, Randjelovich T, Krotin M. Cardiovascular autonomic dysfunction in systemic lupus, rheumatoid arthritis, primary Sjogren syndrome and other autoimmune diseases. Lupus. 2007;16:181–5.
64. Mandl T, Wollmer P, Manthorpe R, Jacobsson LT. Autonomic and orthostatic dysfunction in primary Sjogren's syndrome. J Rheumatol. 2007;34: 1869–74.
65. Cervera R, Font J, Ramos-Casals M, Garcia-Carrasco M, Rosas J, Morla RM, Munoz FJ, Artigues A, Pallares L, Ingelmo M. Primary Sjogren's syndrome in men: clinical and immunological characteristics. Lupus. 2000;9:61–4.
66. Launay D, Hachulla E, Hatron PY, Jais X, Simonneau G, Humbert M. Pulmonary arterial hypertension: a rare complication of primary Sjogren syndrome: report of 9 new cases and review of the literature. Medicine (Baltimore) 2007;86:299–315.
67. Ramos-Casals M, Anaya J, Garcla-Carrasco M, Rosas J, BovÈ A, Claver G, Diaz L, Herrero C, Font J. Cutaneous vasculitis in primary Sjogren syndrome: classification and clinical significance of 52 patients. Medicine 2004;83:96.
68. Ramos-Casals M, Font J. Extrahepatic manifestations in patients with chronic hepatitis C virus infection. Curr Opin Rheumatol. 2005;17: 447–55.
69. Ramos-Casals M, Font J. Primary Sjogren's syndrome: current and emergent aetiopathogenic concepts. Rheumatology (Oxford) 2005.
70. Ramos-Casals M, Jara LJ, Medina F, Rosas J, Calvo-Alen J, Mana J, Anaya JM, Font J. Systemic autoimmune diseases co-existing with chronic hepatitis C virus infection (the HISPAMEC Registry): patterns of clinical and immunological expression in 180 cases. J Intern Med. 2005;257:549–57.
71. Boki KA, Ioannidis JP, Segas JV, Maragkoudakis PV, Petrou D, Adamopoulos GK, Moutsopoulos HM. How significant is sensorineural hearing loss in primary Sjogren's syndrome? An individually matched case–control study. J Rheumatol. 2001;28:798–801.
72. Ramos-Casals M, Tzioufas A, Font J. Primary Sjogren's syndrome: new clinical and therapeutic concepts. Br Med J. 2005;64:347.
73. Walker J, Gordon T, Lester S, Downie-Doyle S, McEvoy D, Pile K, Waterman S, Rischmueller M. Increased severity of lower urinary tract symptoms and daytime somnolence in primary Sjögren's syndrome. J Rheumatol. 2003;30:2406.
74. Leppilahti M, Tammela TL, Huhtala H, Kiilholma P, Leppilahti K, Auvinen A. Interstitial cystitis-like urinary symptoms among patients with Sjogren's syndrome: a population-based study in Finland. Am J Med. 2003;115:62–5.
75. Rosamilia A. Painful bladder syndrome/interstitial cystitis. Best Pract Res Clin Obstet Gynaecol. 2005;19:843–59.
76. Lindvall B, Bengtsson A, Ernerudh J, Eriksson P. Subclinical myositis is common in primary Sjögren's syndrome and is not related to muscle pain. J Rheumatol. 2002;29:717.
77. Silverman B, Brown L, Bright R, Kaczmarek R, Arrowsmith-Lowe J, Kessler D. Reported complications of silicone gel breast implants: an epidemiologic review. Ann Int Med. 1996;124:744–56.
78. Fox RI, Stern M. Sjogren's syndrome: mechanisms of pathogenesis involve interaction of immune and neurosecretory systems. Scand J Rheumatol Suppl. 2002;3–13.
79. Konttinen YT, Hukkanen M, Kemppinen P, Segerberg M, et al. Peptide-containing nerves in labial salivary glands in Sjögren's syndrome. Arthritis Rheum. 1992;35:815–20.
80. Beroukas D, Goodfellow R, Hiscock J, Jonsson R, Gordon TP, Waterman SA. Up-regulation of M3-muscarinic receptors in labial salivary gland acini in primary Sjogren's syndrome. Lab Invest. 2002;82:203–10.
81. Beroukas D, Hiscock J, Gannon BJ, Jonsson R, Gordon TP, Waterman SA. Selective down-regulation of aquaporin-1 in salivary glands in primary Sjogren's syndrome. Lab Invest. 2002;82:1547–52.
82. Beroukas D, Hiscock J, Jonsson R, Waterman SA, Gordon TP. Subcellular distribution of aquaporin 5 in salivary glands in primary Sjogren's syndrome. Lancet 2001;358:1875–6.

83. Fox RI, Konttinen Y, Fisher A. Use of muscarinic agonists in the treatment of Sjogren's syndrome. Clin Immunol. 2001;101:249–63.
84. Hurst S, Collins S. Interleukin-1 beta modulation of norepinephrine release from rat myenteric nerves. Am J Physiol. 1993;264:G30–G5.
85. Hurst SM, Collins SM. Mechanism underlying tumor necrosis factor-alpha suppression of norepinephrine release from rat myenteric plexus. Am J Physiol. 1994;266:G1123–9.
86. Baum BJ, Dai Y, Hiramatsu Y, Horn VJ, Ambudkar IS. Signaling mechanisms that regulate saliva formation. Crit Rev Oral Biol Med. 1993;4:379–84.
87. Bacman S, Sterin-Borda L, Camusso JJ, Arana R, Hubscher O, Borda E. Circulating antibodies against rat parotid gland M3 muscarinic receptors in primary Sjogren's syndrome. Clin Exp Immunol. 1996;104:454–9.
88. Bacman SR, Berra A, Sterin-Borda L, Borda ES. Human primary Sjogren's syndrome autoantibodies as mediators of nitric oxide release coupled to lacrimal gland muscarinic acetylcholine receptors. Curr Eye Res. 1998;17:1135–42.
89. Wolkoff P, Nojgaard JK, Franck C, Skov P. The modern office environment desiccates the eyes? Indoor Air 2006;16:258–65.
90. Nakamori K, Odawara M, Nakajima T, Mizutani T, Tsubota K. Blinking is controlled primarily by ocular surface conditions. Am J Ophthalmol. 1997;124:24–30.
91. Tsubota K. Tear dynamics and dry eye. Prog Retin Eye Res. 1998;17:565–96.
92. Hu S, Loo JA, Wong DT. Human saliva proteome analysis and disease biomarker discovery. Expert Rev Proteomics. 2007;4:531–8.
93. Hu S, Loo JA, Wong DT. Human saliva proteome analysis. Ann NY Acad Sci. 2007;1098: 323–9.
94. Hu S, Wang J, Meijer J, Ieong S, Xie Y, Yu T, Zhou H, Henry S, Vissink A, Pijpe J, Kallenberg C, Elashoff D, Loo JA, Wong DT. Salivary proteomic and genomic biomarkers for primary Sjogren's syndrome. Arthritis Rheum. 2007;56: 3588–600.
95. Giusti L, Baldini C, Bazzichi L, Ciregia F, Tonazzini I, Mascia G, Giannaccini G, Bombardieri S, Lucacchini A. Proteome analysis of whole saliva: a new tool for rheumatic diseases – the example of Sjogren's syndrome. Proteomics 2007;7:1634–43.
96. Laine M, Porola P, Udby L, Kjeldsen L, Cowland JB, Borregaard N, Hietanen J, Stahle M, Pihakari A, Konttinen YT. Low salivary dehydroepiandrosterone and androgen-regulated cysteine-rich secretory protein 3 levels in Sjogren's syndrome. Arthritis Rheum. 2007;56:2575–84.
97. Steinfeld SD, Demols P, Salmon I, Kiss R, Appelboom T. Infliximab in patients with primary Sjogren's syndrome: a pilot study. Arthritis Rheum. 2001;44:2371–5.
98. Mariette X, Ravaud P, Steinfeld S, Baron G, Goetz J, Hachulla E, Combe B, Puechal X, Pennec Y, Sauvezie B, Perdriger A, Hayem G, Janin A, Sibilia J. Inefficacy of infliximab in primary Sjogren's syndrome: results of the randomized, controlled Trial of Remicade in Primary Sjogren's Syndrome (TRIPSS). Arthritis Rheum. 2004;50:1270–6.
99. Sankar V, Brennan MT, Kok MR, Leakan RA, Smith JA, Manny J, Baum BJ, Pillemer SR. Etanercept in Sjogren's syndrome: a twelve-week randomized, double-blind, placebo-controlled pilot clinical trial. Arthritis Rheum. 2004;50:2240–5.
100. Zandbelt MM, de Wilde P, van Damme P, Hoyng CB, van de Putte L, van den Hoogen F. Etanercept in the treatment of patients with primary Sjogren's syndrome: a pilot study. J Rheumatol. 2004;31: 96–101.
101. Hyer S, Kong A, Pratt B, Harmer C. Salivary gland toxicity after radioiodine therapy for thyroid cancer. Clin Oncol (R Coll Radiol). 2007;19:83–6.
102. Kawakami A, Nakashima K, Tamai M, Nakamura H, Iwanaga N, Fujikawa K, Aramaki T, Arima K, Iwamoto N, Ichinose K, Kamachi M, Ida H, Origuchi T, Eguchi K. Toll-like receptor in salivary glands from patients with Sjogren's syndrome: functional analysis by human salivary gland cell line. J Rheumatol. 2007;34:1019–26.
103. Mavragani CP, Moutsopoulos HM. The geoepidemiology of Sjogren's syndrome. Autoimmun Rev. 2010;9:A305–A10.
104. Theander E, Vasaitis L, Baecklund E, Nordmark G, Warfvinge G, Liedholm R, Brokstad K, Jonsson R, Jonsson MV. Lymphoid organisation in labial salivary gland biopsies is a possible predictor for the development of malignant lymphoma in primary Sjogren's syndrome. Ann Rheum Dis. 2011;70:1363–70.
105. Mariette X, Gottenberg JE. Pathogenesis of Sjogren's syndrome and therapeutic consequences. Curr Opin Rheumatol. 2010;22:471.
106. Atalar K, Afzali B, Lams B, Tungekar MF, Goldsmith DJ. Falls, hypokalaemia, and a dry mouth. Lancet 2007;370:192.
107. Chan K. Chinese medicinal materials and their interface with Western medical concepts. J Ethnopharmacol. 2005;96:1–18.
108. Chang YH, Lin HJ, Li WC. Clinical evaluation of the traditional Chinese prescription Chi-Ju-Di-Huang-Wan for dry eye. Phytother Res. 2005;19:349–54.
109. Ernst E. Harmless herbs? A review of the recent literature. Am J Med. 1998;104:170–8.
110. Ernst E. Herb–drug interactions: potentially important but woefully under-researched. Eur J Clin Pharmacol. 2000;56:523–4.

111. Nishimagi E, Kawaguchi Y, Terai C, Kajiyama H, Hara M, Kamatani N. Progressive interstitial renal fibrosis due to Chinese herbs in a patient with calcinosis Raynaud esophageal sclerodactyly telangiectasia (CREST) syndrome. Intern Med. 2001;40:1059–63.
112. Liang L, Zhang M, Zou W, Liu Z. Aggravated dry eye after laser in situ keratomileusis in patients with Sjogren syndrome. Cornea 2008;27:120–3.
113. Lekhanont K, Leyngold IM, Suwan-Apichon O, Rangsin R, Chuck RS. Comparison of topical dry eye medications for the treatment of keratoconjunctivitis sicca in a botulinum toxin B-induced mouse model. Cornea 2007;26: 84–9.
114. Mellgren SI, Goransson LG, Omdal R. Primary Sjogren's syndrome associated neuropathy. Can J Neurol Sci. 2007;34:280–7.

Providing Information to Referring Physicians and Patients

4

Robert I. Fox and Carla M. Fox

Abstract

Sjogren's syndrome (SS) contains both glandular (lacrimal and salivary gland) features and extraglandular manifestations that create multiple physical, emotional, occupational, and financial problems down the road. Although many physicians and medical centers are moving toward integrated electronic medical records, these systems will take years to develop for use within a given institution and more years for them to securely communicate with electronic systems outside their own institution. In general, these systems are not designed to communicate with patients due to issues of patient confidentiality. This chapter addresses an approach that we have been using to provide both referring physicians, members of the health care team, and patients with information.

Keywords

Information to patients • Internet • Criteria Sjogren's syndrome • Criteria systemic lupus erythematosus • Criteria systemic sclerosis • Criteria fibromyalgia • Blepharitis • Artificial tears • Artificial saliva • Sensitivity and specificity of ANA • Disease activity index • Disease damage index • Prevention dental caries

4.1 Background and Overview

4.1.1 Need for Written Information

In the limited time available for the rheumatology consult or follow-up visit, it is often not possible to address each of these areas that directly affects the patient's questions about diagnostic and therapeutic needs. Indeed, the "load of information" may too great to be absorbed by the patient during their increasingly mandated time-limited revisits. Also, physicians in other disciplines and oral health care professions need to receive copies of information as part of the "health care team" in order to provide an integrated program of care to their patients.

Although patient competence with computers will vary widely among patient groups, it is

R.I. Fox (✉)
Rheumatology Clinic, Scripps Memorial Hospital and Research Foundation, La Jolla, CA, USA
e-mail: robertfoxmd@mac.com

R.I. Fox, C.M. Fox (eds.), *Sjögren's Syndrome*, DOI 10.1007/978-1-60327-957-4_4,

surprising how quickly patients as "consumers" have learned how to access information over the Internet. However, with respect to medical issues, this ease of availability of information may have the problem of "information overload" or "misinformation" provided to the patient. Increasingly, physicians should assume that at least a proportion of their patients are going to search the Internet regarding diagnoses and therapies. Thus, we should take steps to guide their searches in positive, helpful, and productive directions.

In the time allowed for patient revisits, the SS patient has the most "vested interest" in understanding the details of therapy. They also have the most "time available" in optimizing their own care and understanding their medical tests and treatments. We have found that the most effective way to guide their efforts is to provide them a broad-stroke "overview" of the plan and then follow-up with accurate *written* information and instructions by email and links to proper websites.

Providing information that the patient can understand is the best approach to gaining compliance and patient education for these "quality of life" issues that is often not possible during their time in the rheumatologist's office. Thus, the physician must treat the patient as a partner in the therapy of their disease and present the information in a form that allows patient choices to be made on a rational basis. Providing them written information that they can read at their leisure will accomplish this.

We do not expect to change patients into "physicians" in terms of clinical decision-making, as it is our responsibility as physicians based on our training to make our best-informed judgments about diagnosis and therapy. However, patients are increasingly diligent and intelligent consumers, and they will pursue information.

It is our obligation to present that information and to inform the rest of the health care team of the status of the patient. In cases where patients may not feel computer competent or language presents a barrier, we have found that information sent to children or family members proves useful.

4.1.2 Use of Internet as a Method to Provide Information

(a) We *email* appropriate information to patients with our suggestions to avoid "information overload" at the time of office visit;
(b) We help *counter potential misinformation* that patients might receive from the Internet and "chat" groups regarding diagnosis and therapy;
(c) We *provide copies of information from the Internet* to other members of the health care team (i.e., referring physician, emergency room, and surgical colleagues and their nursing staff).

In doing so, we help spare a few trees that would provide the paper for the handouts by "going green" with electronically transmitted information.

4.1.3 Patient Access to Computers

We are aware that not all patients have a home computer, but a surprising number of patients, even older patients, have their own computer. In those patients who do not have one, their children, grandchildren, or close friends often have a computer, and other patients may have access to a public library where they can establish a free email account.

4.1.4 Types of Information Supplied to Patients and Referring Physicians

This chapter is a starting point for providing the informational content to patients and referring physicians on:

(a) *Diagnostic criteria* for SS and related diseases including SLE, scleroderma, and fibromyalgia; not every patient with a positive ANA or SS-A antibody has SS or SLE.
(b) *Pitfalls in interpretation of laboratory evaluations*; there is a difference between sensitivity and specificity of laboratory tests and significant variation between laboratories based on the method in which the test is performed.

(c) *Therapeutic hints* for glandular and extraglandular manifestations.
(d) *Informational resources* that might be mailed to the patient.

This information is in the "public domain" on the web but may be spread over many different websites. One of the current problems of the Internet/web is that a search for some topics such as "Sjogren's syndrome" currently brings up over 400,000 "hits," and the shear volume of data will overwhelm any patient in search of specific answers. Our goal is to make our patients' search for information more narrowly and better focused so they may more efficiently find validated information.

4.1.5 Future Guidelines of Diagnosis and Therapy Under Committee of the Sjogren's Syndrome Foundation

We are also working with the *Sjogren's Syndrome Foundation (SSF)* and the *American College of Rheumatology (ACR)* (see Chapter 13) to establish a standards of care and treatment guidelines website. Indeed, members of that collaborative committee provide many of the tables provided in this chapter. This website will initially be directed to physicians and include "standards of diagnosis and care" as well as a reference library and links to therapeutic studies.

4.2 Diagnostic Criteria for Sjogren's Syndrome (SS), Systemic Lupus Erythematosus (SLE), Scleroderma, and Fibromyalgia

4.2.1 Background: The Confusion Surrounding Criteria for Autoimmune Disorders

One of the initial problems encountered by the rheumatologist (and patient) is the distinction between Sjogren's syndrome (SS), systemic lupus erythematosus (SLE), scleroderma (PSS), and fibromyalgia (FM). The same patient with the same laboratory values may receive one or more of these diagnoses from their primary physician or specialist. Thus, it is worth providing the patient with the current criteria for diagnosis for each of these clinical entities, which has been diagnosed.

Although criteria for each of these diseases are available on the Internet, the shear volume of irrelevant and disconcerting information found on an Internet search for these topics is daunting. Thus, we have included these tables of diagnostic criteria as a "desktop" reference. It is worth noting that the diagnostic criteria for Sjogren's syndrome is the only one of these diagnostic categories NOT listed on the "American College of Rheumatology" website (http://www.rheumatology.org/practice/clinical/classification/index.asp).

This is because the SS criteria were developed in Europe and not independently validated in the American population. Nevertheless, these criteria for SS have been accepted as the entrance criteria for studies recognized by the US FDA for drug development.

4.2.2 Criteria for Sjogren's Syndrome

The question of whether a patient fulfills criteria for SS is a frequent source of referral to the rheumatologist as well as to ophthalmologist and oral medicine clinics.

In the patient with severe keratoconjunctivitis sicca, severe xerostomia, and characteristic autoantibodies, there is generally little debate over the diagnosis. However, a common scenario is the patient who presents with fatigue, vague myalgia, and cognitive symptoms and is found to have a positive anti-nuclear antibody (ANA) during evaluation. Indeed, the patient may get conflicting opinions about whether the diagnosis of SS is present or not.

The consensus criteria for SS were predominantly set up for research purposes, and they require both clinical and laboratory criteria. Thus, it is worth starting with the current European–American criteria for SS (Table 4.1). This provides a series of clinical questions and laboratory investigations that serve as a baseline.

Table 4.1 Revised classification criteria for Sjogren's syndrome

I. Requirements for classification of patient with primary SS:
1. The presence of *either positive salivary gland biopsy* (described below) *OR positive antibody to SS-A or SS-B*;
2. The presence of *any three objective clinical signs for oral and ocular dryness* (described below); *and*
3. The presence of *at least four clinical symptoms for oral and ocular dryness* (described below).
II. Clinical symptoms
A. *Ocular symptoms*: a positive response to *at least one* of the following questions:
1. Have you had *daily, persistent, troublesome dry eyes* for more than 3 months?
2. Do you have a *recurrent sensation of sand or gravel in the eyes*?
3. Do you use *tear substitutes* for more than three times a day?
B. *Oral symptoms*: a positive response to *at least one* of the following questions:
1. Have you had a *daily feeling of dry mouth* for more than 3 months?
2. Have you had *recurrently or persistently swollen salivary glands* as an adult?
3. Do you *frequently drink liquids to aid in swallowing* dry food?
III. Objective clinical signs
A. *Ocular signs*—that is, *objective evidence of ocular involvement* defined as a *positive result for at least one of the following* two tests:
1. *Schirmer's test*, performed without anesthesia (greater than 5 mm in 5 min)
2. *Rose Bengal* score or other ocular dye score (greater than 4 according to Van Bijsterveld's scoring system)
B. *Minor salivary gland biopsy*
Histopathology: In minor salivary glands (obtained through normal-appearing mucosa): *focal lymphocytic sialadenitis*, evaluated by an expert histopathologist, *with a focus score greater than 1.*
• A *lymphocyte focus* is defined as a cluster of 50 or more lymphocytes—which are adjacent to normal-appearing mucous acini and not adjacent to areas where ruptured ducts have fibrotic regions.
C. *Salivary gland involvement*: objective evidence of salivary gland involvement defined by a positive result for at least one of the following diagnostic tests:
1. *Unstimulated whole salivary flow* (greater than 1.5 ml in 15 min)
2. *Parotid sialography* showing the presence of diffuse sialectasis (punctate, cavitary, or destructive pattern), without evidence of obstruction in the major ducts
3. *Salivary scintigraphy* showing delayed uptake, reduced concentration, and/or delayed excretion of tracer
D. *Autoantibodies*: presence in the serum of the following autoantibodies:
• antibodies to Ro(SS-A) or
• La(SS-B) antigens, or both
IV. Criteria for secondary SS
Patients who fulfill criteria for primary SS *and* with an associated well-defined rheumatologic disorder such as:
• rheumatoid arthritis,
• systemic lupus, *or*
• progressive systemic sclerosis.
V. Exclusion criteria
1. Past head and neck radiation treatment
2. Hepatitis C infection
3. Acquired immunodeficiency disease syndrome (AIDS)

Table 4.1 (continued)

4. Pre-existing lymphoma
5. Sarcoidosis
6. Graft versus host disease
7. Use of anti-cholinergic drugs at the time of measurements considered abnormal (all measurements used to fulfill criteria need to be performed at a time duration after stopping drug for four-half lives of the drug).

Ref. [1].

It provides the patient and referring physician with the essential "data set" necessary.

Similarly, many SS patients have previously carried out the diagnosis of SLE (systemic lupus erythematosus), scleroderma (either limited or diffuse), or fibromyalgia. Therefore, these criteria are listed in Tables 4.2, 4.3, and 4.4; *classification criteria for Sjogren's syndrome: a revised version of the European criteria proposed by the American–European Consensus Group,* Table 4.1 [1].

Table 4.2 1988 revised criteria for diagnosis of systemic lupus erythematosus (SLE)[a]

I. Definite or probable systemic lupus
A. *Definite SLE*
• Five or more criteria (listed below), in general including a positive ANA
B. *Probable SLE*
• Four criteria, in general including a positive ANA
C. *Criteria*
1. *Malar rash: fixed erythema,* flat or raised, over the malar eminences, tending to spare the nasolabial folds
2. *Discoid rash erythematous*—raised patches with adherent keratotic scaling and follicular plugging; atrophic scarring may occur in older lesions
3. *Photosensitivity of skin*—rash as a result of unusual reaction to sunlight, by patient history or physician observation
4. *Oral ulcers; oral or nasopharyngeal ulceration,* usually painless, observed by physician
5. *Non-erosive arthritis*—involving two or more peripheral joints, characterized by tenderness, swelling, or effusion
6. Pleuritis or pericarditis
a. *Pleuritis*—convincing history of pleuritic pain or rubbing heard by a physician or evidence of pleural effusion
OR
b. *Pericarditis*—documented by electrocardiogram or rub or evidence of pericardial effusion
7. Renal disorder
a. *Persistent proteinuria* > 0.5 g/day or > than 3+ if quantitation not performed
OR
b. *Cellular casts*—may be red cell, hemoglobin, granular, tubular, or mixed
8. *Neurologic disorder*
a. *Seizures*—in the absence of offending drugs or known metabolic Derangements, e.g., uremia, ketoacidosis, or electrolyte imbalance
b. *Psychosis*—in the absence of offending drugs or known metabolic derangements, e.g., uremia, ketoacidosis, or electrolyte imbalance
9. *Hematologic disorder*
a. *Hemolytic anemia*—with reticulocytosis
OR
b. *Leukopenia*—$< 4{,}000/mm^3$ on $\geq$ two occasions
OR
c. *Lymphopenia*—$< 1{,}500/mm^3$ on $\geq$ two occasions

Table 4.2 (continued)

OR
d. *Thrombocytopenia*—$< 100{,}000/\text{mm}^3$ in the absence of offending drugs
10. *Immunologic disorder*
a. *Anti-DNA:* antibody to native DNA in abnormal titer
OR
b. *Anti-Sm:* presence of antibody to Sm nuclear antigen
OR
c. Positive finding of anti-phospholipid antibodies on:
1. *An abnormal serum level* of IgG or IgM anti-cardiolipin antibodies,
OR
2. *A positive test result for lupus anti-coagulant* using a standard method,
OR
3. *A false-positive test result* for at least 6 months confirmed by *Treponema pallidum* immobilization or fluorescent treponemal antibody absorption test
11. *Positive anti-nuclear antibody*—an abnormal titer of anti-nuclear antibody by immunofluorescence or an equivalent assay at any point in time and in the absence of drugs
II. Further points about diagnosis
A. When you get a positive ANA. . .order an ANA profile—which should include *anti-double-stranded DNA, anti-Smith, anti-SS-A and anti-SS-B, and anti-RNP*
B. Anti-dsDNA and anti-Sm antibodies
• These antibodies are virtually specific (96%) for SLE. However, their sensitivity is not as good
• 52% for *Crithidia* anti-dsDNA, 73% for Farr anti-dsDNA, and 18–31% for anti-Smith
C. If ANA is *negative* and clinical signs strongly suggest SLE, check for *anti-SS-A(Ro)* antibodies
• If this is positive, the patient probably has "*ANA-negative*" SLE (rare)
• As many as 62% of patients with "ANA-negative" SLE have anti-SS-A antibodies
D. Complement levels can also be helpful diagnostically—total serum hemolytic complement (*CH50*) and individual complement components (*C3 and C4*) may be low in patients with active SLE due to the presence of immune complexes;
Low sensitivity (40%) but high specificity (90%)

[a]See Refs. [2, 3] (http://www.rheumatology.org/practice/clinical/classification/index.asp).

Table 4.3 Criteria for the classification of systemic sclerosis (scleroderma)

A. The *American College of Rheumatology* (formerly American Rheumatism Association [ARA]) has defined criteria that are 97% sensitive and 98% specific for systemic sclerosis (SSc) as follows:
Major criterion:
• Proximal diffuse (truncal) sclerosis (skin tightness, thickening, non-pitting induration)
Minor criteria:
• Sclerodactyly (only fingers and/or toes)
• Digital pitting scars or loss of substance of the digital finger pads (pulp loss)
• Bilateral basilar pulmonary fibrosis
The patient should fulfill the major criterion or two of the three minor criteria. Raynaud's phenomenon is observed in 90–98% of SSc patients.

Table 4.3 (continued)

Subsets of systemic sclerosis

	Diffuse	Limited[a]
Skin involvement	Distal and proximal extremities, face, trunk	Distal to elbows, face
Raynaud's phenomenon	Onset within 1 year or at time of skin changes	May precede skin disease by years
Organ involvement	Pulmonary (interstitial fibrosis); renal (renovascular hypertensive crisis); gastrointestinal; cardiac	Gastrointestinal; pulmonary arterial hypertension after 10–15 years of disease in <10% of patients; biliary cirrhosis
Nailfold capillaries	Dilatation and dropout	Dilatation without significant dropout
Anti-nuclear antibodies	Anti-topoisomerase 1	Anti-centromere

[a] Also referred to as CREST (calcinosis, Raynaud's phenomenon, esophageal dysmotility, sclerodactyly, telangiectasia).

B. ABCD CREST criteria for the classification of systemic sclerosis

A classification of definite SSc requires *three or more* criteria.

1. *Autoantibodies*: autoantibodies to centromere proteins (CENPs) detected by indirect immunofluorescence; anti-Scl-70 (topoisomerase I) detected by double immunodiffusion; anti-fibrillarin (U3-RNP) detected by immunoprecipitation.

2. *Bibasilar pulmonary fibrosis* detected by chest radiograph: linear shadows or "honey-comb" reticular appearance most expressed at the periphery of the lungs and at the bases.

3. *Contracture of the joints* defined as permanent limitation of joint motion. The "prayer sign" is detected when a patient opposed the palmar surfaces of both hands with extended wrists. The sign is positive when the patient is unable to oppose the palms. This suggests joint or skin pathology or shortening of the forearm flexors.

4. *Dermal thickening* can be defined by the modified Rodnan skin score, which employs clinical palpation of the skin as described.

5. *Calcinosis cutis*, most often located on the fingers, is intra-cutaneous and/or subcutaneous deposits of hydroxyapatite that can ulcerate the skin; it can be detected by radiography, crystallographic, or chemical analysis.

6. *Raynaud's phenomenon* is a sudden pallor of an acral structure (e.g., fingers, whole hand, toes, tip of nose, earlobe, or tongue). The involved area may subsequently develop cyanosis and, with re-warming, becomes erythematous. Determination is by patient's history or physician's observation.

7. *Esophageal distal hypomotility* can be detected by cine/video barium esophagram, performed in the upright and supine positions. Reflux esophagitis can be detected by esophagogastroduodenoscopy in the forms of erosive esophagitis or Barret's esophagus.

8. *Sclerodactyly* is symmetric thickening and tightening of the skin on the digits. Before sclerodactyly develops, there could be a phase of non-pitting digital edema of varying duration. It is defined as non-pitting increase in soft tissue mass of the digits that extends beyond the normal confines of the joint capsules.

9. *Telangiectasias* are visible macular dilatations of superficial cutaneous blood vessels that collapse upon pressure and fill slowly when pressure is released. Common locations are the digits, face, lips, and tongue.

Refs. [4, 5]; http://www.rheumatology.org/practice/clinical/classification/index.asp

Table 4.4 1990 criteria for the classification of fibromyalgia

1. History of widespread pain

- *Definition*: Pain is considered widespread when *all* of the following are present:
  - o pain in the left side of the body,
  - o pain in the right side of the body,
  - o pain above the waist, and
  - o pain below the waist.
- In addition, axial skeletal pain (cervical spine or anterior chest or thoracic spine or low back) must be present.
- In this definition, shoulder and buttock pain is considered as pain for each involved side.

Table 4.4 (continued)

• "Low back" pain is considered lower segment pain.
2. Pain in 11 of 18 tender point sites on digital palpation
• *Definition:* Pain, on digital palpation, must be present in *at least 11* of the following 18 sites:
o *Occiput:* bilateral, at the suboccipital muscle insertions;
o *Low cervical:* bilateral, at the anterior aspects of the intertransverse spaces at C5–C7;
o *Trapezius:* bilateral, at the midpoint of the upper border;
o *Supraspinatus:* bilateral, at origins, above the scapula spine near the medial border;
o *Second rib:* bilateral, at the second costochondral junctions, just lateral to the junctions on upper surfaces;
o *Lateral epicondyle:* bilateral, 2 cm distal to the epicondyles;
o *Gluteal:* bilateral, in upper outer quadrants of buttocks in anterior fold of muscle;
o *Greater trochanter:* bilateral, posterior to the trochanteric prominence;
o *Knee:* bilateral, at the medial fat pad proximal to the joint line.
Digital palpation should be performed with an approximate force of 4 kg.
For a tender point to be considered "positive," the subject must state that the palpation was painful. "Tender" is not to be considered "painful."

*For classification purposes, patients will be said to have fibromyalgia if diagnostic criteria are satisfied. Widespread pain must have been present for at least 3 months. The presence of a second clinical disorder does not exclude the diagnosis of fibromyalgia (http://www.rheumatology.org/practice/clinical/classification/index.asp).

4.2.3 Initial (1982) and Revised 1997 Classification Criteria for Systemic Lupus Erythematosus (SLE)

The initial SLE criteria of the American College of Rheumatology classification criteria were devised in 1982 (Table 4.2) [2, 3]. In 1997, the immunologic disorder criteria were revised by a committee (without validation). All 11 criteria in the American College of Rheumatology criteria set have limitations. One of the most important laboratory tests, hypocomplementemia, was excluded entirely [3]. A subset of patients with SLE also fulfill criteria for SS and are termed "SLE with secondary SS."

4.2.4 Criteria for Systemic Sclerosis (SSc) (ACR and the ABCD CREST (Calcinosis, *R*aynaud's Phenomenon, *E*sophageal Dysmotility, *S*clerodactyly *T*elangiectasia Criteria)

Patients with early SSc may be difficult to distinguish from SS. Both groups of patients may have dry eyes/mouth, Raynaud's phenomena, and anti-centromere autoantibodies and/or typical capillaroscopic abnormalities (Table 4.3) [4–8]. Both groups may have heartburn and esophageal symptoms. However, SSc should be strongly considered if patients exhibit one of the following manifestations: digital ulcers/scars, puffy fingers, extensive telangiectasia, abnormal esophageal manometry, and shortness of breath with fibrotic lung disease on high-resolution chest CAT scan.

A subset of SSc patients have features suggestive of SS. Indeed, the salivary gland biopsies of some SSc patients show focal lymphocytic infiltrates, while others present with fibrosis of the glands in a pattern more consistent with the fibrotic pathology found in their other organs [9–13].

In comparison, undifferentiated connective tissue disease (UCTD) is a diagnosis applied to patients with a specific antibody (anti-RNP antibody) and capillaroscopic findings plus any disease manifestations listed above. With follow-up, many UCTD patients will subsequently fall into patterns more suggestive of SLE, SSc, or SS [14].

4.2.5 Criteria for Fibromyalgia

The American College of Rheumatology has established criteria for fibromyalgia—http://www.rheumatology.org/practice/clinical/classification/index.asp (Table 4.4).

Fibromyalgia is characterized by chronic widespread pain and allodynia—heightened and painful response to pressure. Fibromyalgia symptoms are not restricted to pain, leading to the use of the alternative term "central sensitization syndrome." Other symptoms include debilitating fatigue, sleep disturbance, and joint stiffness. Some patients may also report difficulty with swallowing, bowel and bladder abnormalities, numbness and tingling, and cognitive dysfunction.

Fibromyalgia is frequently co-morbid with psychiatric conditions such as depression and anxiety and stress-related disorders such as post-traumatic stress disorder (PTSD). However, not all people with fibromyalgia experience all associated symptoms.

Evidence from research conducted during the last three decades has revealed abnormalities within the central nervous system (CNS) affecting brain regions that may be linked both to clinical symptoms and research phenomena. These studies show a correlation but not causation of symptoms.

Fibromyalgia is considered a controversial diagnosis, due to lacking scientific consensus to its cause. Not all members of the medical community consider fibromyalgia a disease because of the absence of objective diagnostic tests.

4.3 Laboratory Results for ANA Often Drive Clinical Diagnosis

Patients are often referred to rheumatologists with vague symptoms and a positive anti-nuclear antibody (ANA) for confirmation of diagnosis and therapy. We try to emphasize to patients and referring physicians that SS is a clinical diagnosis that is confirmed by certain laboratory tests. We will often try to clarify this discrepancy about diagnosis by providing patients with information about the currently accepted clinical diagnostic criteria.

We recognize that the clinical criteria are developed for research purposes and that antibodies may precede clinical symptoms by many years. However, it is also important to emphasize that the ANA testing is much more sensitive than specific. In other words, many patients with a positive ANA may never develop any significant autoimmune disorder and that the pattern of specific autoantibodies is more closely correlated with the patient's genetic background than with specific clinical symptoms.

These diagnostic discussions (and often conflicting diagnoses among rheumatologists) must take into account that:

- *The ANA titer can differ substantially in different laboratories and even in the same laboratory when different methods are used.* This is particularly a problem when ELISA methods to detect ANA are used, in comparison to tube dilution titers using immunofluorescence assays on Hep-2 cells. Indeed, a recent *New England Journal of Medicine* "Clinical Pathologic Discussion Case" had the diagnosis revolve around differences in the method used for testing for ANA [15].
  - Thus, the same laboratory may give entirely different results on the same patient sample depending on which method is used for the assay [16, 17].
- *ANA detection in SS patients differs from SLE patients*, since the routine assays are set up for detection of SLE-associated antigens and the "positive control sera" used by the laboratory are derived from SLE patients with high titer antibodies to antigens such as double-stranded DNA [16, 17].
  - This may lead to a result in an SS patient such as a negative ANA but a positive SS-A antibody. Since the SS-A is located in the nucleus of all Hep-2 cells, how can we resolve this inconsistency [18–20]?

- For a clinical example, we used to have a diagnosis called "subacute lupus" where the ANA was negative and the antibody to SS-A was positive. It was subsequently recognized that this paradox was the result of the high "acetone" solubility of the SS-A antigen, which was removed during "overfixation" of commercially available slides [21–24]. The "control" sera for the ANA assay is generally selected from SLE patients (often chosen for their high titer to DNA or Sm/RNP) and continued to detect positive antigens, even though the SS-A antigen had been leached out. This may lead to a misleading laboratory report that the ANA is negative when the antibody to SS-A/SS-B is positive.
  - Other problems that cause discrepancy between ANA by immunofluorescence assay and ELISA include antigens in the nucleus (such as fibrillary proteins or chromatin-associated antigens) which are not well solubilized.
  - Finally, certain other antigens (such as anti-centromere or nucleolar proteins) may be present in specific areas of the cell in high enough concentrations to be easily detected by immunofluorescence method, but their level drops into the "background" noise level when the cell is solubilized for ELISA methods of detection.
- *Diagnosis of SS is defined by the patient's clinical presentation and confirmed by laboratory analysis (Tables 4.2, 4.3, and 4.4) and the clinical diagnosis should be made by the pattern of their ANA.*
  - The pattern of ANA (i.e., fine speckled or centromere or nucleolar) correlates more closely with the patient's genotype than with their clinical presentation. Thus, ANA and their patterns/specific antibodies are used to confirm a clinical diagnosis rather than being used as the basis of a "fishing expedition."
- *Not all patients fit into a nice, neat, and clean single category and often exhibit overlap features.*
  - This is important in choosing therapies. In some cases, patients may fulfill more than one set of criteria and should be considered an "overlap."

4.4 Disease Activity in Sjogren's Syndrome

After a diagnosis of SS has been confirmed, we need to use a standardized method to determine "where we have been" (organ damage index) and "where we are going" (disease activity index). This will allow comparison of treatment and prognosis among patients at different medical centers, among different ethnic groups, and establishment of registries. The European Consortium (see Chapters 5 and 30) have provided important initial steps including disease damage and activity indexes, based in parallel to our experience in SLE data collection.

- In each of these scales, particular manifestations are given a "point" value, where higher point score indicates greater severity. Computer modeling by these groups has been done to help assign the "severity [25] points" to best reflect the clinical status as judged by an expert panel (the so-called Delphi model) (Tables 4.5 and 4.6) [26].

4.5 Status of Biologic Drugs in SS Patients

Based on the dramatic success of biologic agents in rheumatoid arthritis, rheumatologists are frustrated by the relative lack of a "magic bullet" in SS and SLE with biologics. Current studies in SS using biological agents (i.e., anti-CD20 and anti-BAFF antibodies) (www.clinicaltrials.gov) are still recruiting and in progress, and several additional novel topical treatment studies are actively recruiting patients.

A number of studies using biologic agents (particularly anti-CD20) have been completed and have been reported in peer-reviewed journals (these reports will be summarized in other chapters of this book).

Table 4.5 Sjogren's syndrome disease damage index

		Score
I. Oral damage		
Decreased salivary flow	Unstimulated whole saliva collection less than 1.5 ml/15 min	1
Salivary flow impairment	Complete or almost complete, based on salivary gland scintigraphy	1
Loss of teeth	Due to characteristic changes of dry mouth	1
II. Ocular damage		
Tear flow impairment	Schirmer's-I test less than 5 mm in 5 min, without topical anesthetic	1
Structural abnormalities	Corneal ulcers, cataracts, chronic blepharitis	1
III. Extraglandular		
CNS involvement	Long-lasting stable CNS involvement	2
Peripheral neuropathy	Long-lasting stable peripheral or autonomic system impairment	1
Pleuropulmonary damage (any of the following)		2
Pleural fibrosis	Confirmed by imaging	
Interstitial fibrosis	Confirmed by imaging	
Significant irreversible functional damage	Confirmed by spirometry	
Renal impairment (any of the following)		2
Increased serum creatinine level or reduced GFR		
Tubular acidosis (urinary pH 6 and serum bicarbonate less than 15 mmol/l)		
Nephrocalcinosis		
Lymphoproliferative disease (any of the following)		5
B-cell lymphoma		
Multiple myeloma		
Waldenström's macroglobulinemia		

Ref. [25].

Table 4.6 Sjogren's syndrome disease activity index*

Constitutional symptoms		Point score
Fever	Temperature greater than 38°C, not due to infections	1
Fatigue	Sufficiently severe to affect normal activities	1
Change in fatigue	New appearance or worsening of fatigue	1
Change in salivary gland swelling	New appearance or increasing swelling of major salivary glands, not due to infection or stones	3
Articular symptoms (any of the following)		
Arthritis	Inflammatory pain in one or more joints	2
Evolving arthralgias	New appearance or worsening of joint pain without signs of articular inflammation	1

Table 4.6 (continued)

Hematologic features		
Leukopenia/lymphopenia	WBC lower than 3,500 mm^3/1,000 mm^3	1
Lymph node/spleen enlargement	Clinically palpable lymph node/spleen	2
Pleuropulmonary symptoms (any of the following)		
Pleurisy	Ground-glass appearance on computed tomography scan, not due to infection	4
Pneumonia (segmental or interstitial)		
Change in vasculitis	New appearance or worsening or recurrent flares of palpable purpura	3
Active renal involvement (any of the following)		
New or worsening proteinuria	Greater than 0.5 g/day	3
Increasing serum creatinine level		
New or worsening nephritis		
Peripheral neuropathy	Recent onset (6 months), confirmed by nerve conduction studies	1

*Ref. [26].

These double-blind studies are based on the numerous encouraging smaller studies from single-center or multi-center trials. However, it is likely that the same complexities in evaluating patient response in SS will be encountered that were seen when these agents were recently studied in double-blind studies of SLE to fulfill FDA requirements for drug approval. Both the global and patient overall evaluations are strongly influenced by symptoms of fibromyalgia that show response to both the active and placebo treatments and the final results did not fulfill their endpoints at longer endpoints of disease activity [25]. Therefore, objective damage and activity endpoints may need to be considered in a category distinct from overall global evaluation.

4.6 Ocular Treatment

Although treatment of ocular signs and symptoms is best left to the ophthalmologist, the rheumatologist will often be asked questions by the patient at the time of the office revisit (or by phone or by email) about treatment options or changes in their status. There are several key points for the rheumatologist:

- *Whether the SS patient needs to see the ophthalmologist and how soon.* In the managed care environment of medicine today, simply checking ophthalmology revisit does not specify "today" (urgent) or "next available" which may be in 6 weeks.
  - o Issues such as corneal abrasions or perforations, herpetic lesions of the eye, and vasculitic lesions including uveitis or retinal vasculitis need *immediate* attention.
  - o Issues such as blepharitis or choice of artificial tears may be more electively handled.

4.6.1 Choice of Artificial Tears

Many patients are told to go to the pharmacy and get a selection of artificial tears (Table 4.7). Most rheumatologists are not aware of the staggering array of choices that the patient sees available when they arrive at the pharmacy or grocery store. We are including Table 4.7 to help guide the choice of artificial tears that have also been discussed in more detail in the chapter by Michelson et al. [27].

Table 4.7 General rules for the dry eye patient

Artificial tears
A list showing a wide selection of artificial tear, gels, and lubricants (including their active agents and preservatives) is available on www.dryeyezone.com
An initial selection of preserved or unpreserved tears for the patient might include Refresh, GenTeal, Systane, Theratears, or their non-preserved counterpart. These recommendations for a starting selection are based on a poll of "patient preference" available on www.dryeyezone.com, as double-blind studies for comparison are not available.
Be prepared to "mix" and "match" different types of tears. The patient must be flexible in balancing the frequency of artificial tear use and viscosity to the conditions of the environment and concurrent medications.
Artificial tear use must also balance the cost of preserved versus Non-preserved tear as well as brand versus generic.
Be aware that some generic artificial tears (or tears for other conditions) may contain preservatives, especially benzalkonium chloride or thimerosal, that are poorly tolerated in the dry eye patient.
Start increasing treatment to "build" the tear film 2–3 days before the "challenge" to the eyes, as it can take several days to build the tear film and about half an hour for it to get damaged.
Avoid the use of preserved tears over four times/day.
Be aware that drops for other conditions (glaucoma, etc.) contain preservatives, and these must be included in the "four times preserved tear/day" rule.
When using generic artificial tears, be sure to carefully compare the contents.
Gels and ointments
Gels are best for nighttime use. They are thicker than artificial tears—though "liquid gels" may be somewhere in between.
Gels may not be as effective as ointments, but there is less transient blurring.
Some people do not tolerate gels, perhaps due to preservative.
Do not use excessive amounts of ointment or gel, as only a tiny amount is required.
An initial selection of ointments and gels may include Refresh PM (ointment), GenTeal Gel (may have preservative), and Lacrilube (ointment), based on user's poll (www.dryeyezone.com).
Identification of medications (including over-the-counter cold and sleep remedies) and nutritional supplements/herbs (with anti-cholinergic drying side effects) may help minimize dryness.
Recognize that other conditions cause a dry and painful eye—ranging from corneal abrasions to infections and require immediate referral to Emergency Room or Ophthalmologist (in case the patient calls or is seen by the rheumatologist with suggestive signs and symptoms).
Recognize that blepharitis (infection of the lids) may mimic a dry eye flare.
Providing patients with written information and suggestions (including by email) will help education and compliance.
Patients with dry eyes may have other causes for a sudden increase in symptoms ranging from corneal abrasions to infections (both bacterial and viral).

4.6.2 Blepharitis

A relatively common problem in the SS patient is blockage or irritation of the meibomian glands that line the lower lid (Table 4.8). This may result from overuse and irritation of preserved tears (or use of medications for concurrent problems that contain preservatives). Table 4.8 contains guidelines for the use of warm compresses and massage of the glands. This table also discusses contact allergic reactions to make-up.

4.7 Therapy of Oral Manifestations

4.7.1 Prevention of Dental Caries

Guidelines for Oral Treatment and Dental Caries Prevention in SS patients have been reviewed

Table 4.8 Blepharitis treatment*

Blepharitis is a chronic disease requiring long-term treatment to keep it under control. Treatment consists of two phases (acute phase and maintenance phase). Acute phase treatment involves intensive therapy to rapidly bring the condition under control. In the maintenance phase the goal is to indefinitely continue the minimum amount of therapy that is necessary to keep the condition quiet.
Warm compress followed by lid scrubs is the most critical element of effective blepharitis control. This therapy removes the eyelid debris (which can be colonized by bacteria), reduces the bacterial load (mechanically as well as by lysis of bacteria due to detergent action of the soap in lid scrubbing), and stabilizes the tear film by releasing oily secretions from the meibomian glands, thus reducing tear evaporation (so the dry eye symptoms are also reduced).
Warm compresses: Warm compresses heat the debris and crust on the lid margin to or above the melting point of their individual components so that they are easily removed with the lid scrubs.
Technique: Soaking a washcloth in water as warm as the eyelids can stand and then placing the cloth on the lid surface (eyelids closed) for a 5–10 min period. In the acute phase this is performed two–four times/day. We have read about variations/innovations in the way warmth may be applied to the eye. One method described is the use of a fresh boiled egg (in its shell wrapped in a washcloth). Another method described is to use a stocking filled with grains of uncooked dry rice heated in a microwave oven to a comfortable warm temperature.
Warm compresses may be combined with *eyelid massage*. This is especially important in patients who have meibomian gland dysfunction (MGD). In MGD the meibomian secretions are turbid and the gland openings are clogged. Therefore, after every 1 min of warm compresses, massaging the eyelid as follows will be useful: Gently close the eyelids. Put your index finger on the outer corner of the eyelid. Pull the eyelid toward the ear, so that the eyelids are stretched taut. Next use the index finger of the opposite hand to apply direct pressure to the taut eyelids starting at the inner aspect of the eyelid near the base of the nose. Sweep with firm but gentle pressure toward the ear. Repeat this maneuver four to five times. Remember that the goal is to apply gentle pressure to the eyelids—so just rubbing the eyelid surface will do you no good.
Lid scrubs: There are several ways of performing lid scrubbing. You can choose whichever one you are most comfortable with. The scrubbing should be directed at the base of the eyelashes on the eyelid margin. Soaps (cleansing agent used) should not have excessive perfume or lotion content. *Neutrogena bar soap*: This bar soap is used to form lather on the clean fingertips. Lather is then applied with fingertips on the eyelid margin and eyelash bases for up to 1 min (with eyelids gently closed so that soap does not enter the eye). This is followed by a facial rinse. *Johnson's baby shampoo*: The baby shampoo is first diluted one-to-one with water in a "cup" in the palm of the hand. This is then mixed by rubbing with the clean fingertips and then applied in a gentle oval scrubbing motion to the margin and eyelash bases of the closed eyelid for 1 min, followed by a fresh water facial rinse. The soap solution (bar soap or baby shampoo) can alternatively be diluted in a container (e.g., plastic cup) and scrubbing performed using a washcloth wrapped around a finger (after dipping it in the diluted soap solution). A cotton tip applicator may be used alternatively.
There are commercially available cleansing pads that are pre-soaked in a cleansing solution (*OCuSOFT Lid Scrubs* or *Novartis Eye-Scrub*). These cleansing pads are equally effective albeit more expensive method of lid scrubbing and are claimed to be less irritating to the eyelids. One study showed them to be preferred choice by patients as compared to other methods of lid scrubbing.
Antibiotic treatment: The use of an ointment on the eyelid margin immediately after lid scrubbing may help to increase patient comfort. The choice here is usually Erythromycin eye ointment or Tobradex eye ointment (steroid–antibiotic combination). In addition, the antibiotics help to further reduce the bacterial load on the eyelids. Oral *tetracyclines* (doxycycline or minocycline) can be used in recalcitrant meibomian gland dysfunction (MGD) cases. Tetracycline antibiotics affect the meibomian gland secretions, inhibit bacterial lipases as well as reduce the eyelid bacterial load.
Anti-inflammatory treatment: Castor oil has been used traditionally in folk medicine as an anti-inflammatory remedy for treatment of blepharitis. The main ingredient in castor oil is ricinoleic acid. Castor oil could either increase or decrease eyelid inflammation depending upon whether it is used only once or is used several times for many days. Eyelid inflammation may increase initially after starting treatment but with repeated use for over a week, the blepharitis inflammation will be reduced. Refresh Endura tears is a castor oil emulsion. Restasis eye drops has castor oil in addition to cyclosporine. Increasing the intake of omega-3 fatty acids (flaxseed oil supplements) may also reduce the blepharitis inflammation.
Anti-oxidant treatment: The formation of oxidants like nitric oxide in the involved eyelid margin has been speculated to play a role in blepharitis. The substance known as resveratrol is an anti-oxidant that is very effective against these nitrite type of oxidants. Grapes are particularly good sources of resveratrol. Resveratrol is found in the skin (not flesh) of grapes and is now available as a purified supplement.

Table 4.8 (continued)

Cosmetic (eye make-up) use and eyelid dermatitis (a commonly missed association)
Safe use of eye cosmetics page
Contact allergic dermatitis could be caused by many products used for eye make-up. Mascara, eye shadows, eyeliners, eyebrow pencils, etc., all have ingredients to which you could be allergic to. One could be allergic to make-up applicators and brushes. It is possible to be allergic to eye drops that you may be using or to the commercially available make-up removers and lid scrubs. Even ingredients used in nail enhancements/make-up (overlay, sculptures, etc.) can cause eyelid dermatitis when you touch the eyes. Contact allergic dermatitis of the eyelid will present as eyelid puffiness and parchment-like wrinkling of skin. Itching and redness in the involved area is possible. Allergic eyelid dermatitis may be mistaken for blepharitis. The treatment here is removing contact with the allergen, therefore blepharitis treatment will not work. As a temporary measure, a steroid ointment may help to provide relief from symptoms. Long-term steroid use on the delicate eyelid skin may result in skin atrophy, skin discoloration, or skin telangiectatic vessels.
There are important issues with mascara-containing kohl. Also called al-kahl, kajal, or surma, this color additive has been linked to lead poisoning in children and is not approved for cosmetic use in the United States. Applying surma by sharing the applicator is a major reason for the spread of Trachoma in developing countries. The FDA's Center for Food Safety and Applied Nutrition warns that kohl can be found in imported mascaras. Be sure to check the label: Sometimes "kohl" indicates the shade of a product, not the actual contents. Bacterial contamination of mascara is also common.

*http://www.agingeye.net/otheragingeye/blepharitis.php

by Wu et al. [28], based on the extensive experience with SS patients at the Dental School at University of California at San Francisco under the direction of Daniels et al. [29–31] (Table 4.9).

4.7.2 Oral Candida Prevention and Treatment

A dry mouth is not necessarily a painful mouth. Particularly in patients who have been on antibiotics, such as for upper respiratory tract infections

Table 4.9 Dental caries, prevention, and treatment

I. Background note on dental caries for SS patients and non-dental clinicians
A. *Dental caries are a destructive process caused by acid-producing bacteria called dental plaque that become attached to tooth surfaces*. The caries process is dependent upon the presence of certain sugars from the diet (particularly sucrose). The bacteria attach to the teeth and produce acids. The acids gradually dissolve those portions of the teeth that are covered by dental plaque through a process of demineralization.
B. *Decreased salivary function is thought to contribute to the dental decay process via diminished*:
• intra-oral buffering capacity;
• ability to physically wash away dental plaque and associated bacteria; and
• levels of salivary anti-bacterial enzymes and proteins.
C. *A higher risk for dental caries is seen in patients who have*
• reduced or abnormal saliva from a disease (e.g., Sjogren's syndrome),
• had radiation to their head and neck for treatment of a malignant tumor (cancer), and
• are regularly taking one or more prescription drugs that have a side effect of reducing salivary secretion.
II. Dental caries prevention and treatment
A. *Diet*
Each patient needs to understand the role of dietary sugars in dental caries development. High-caries-risk patients must eliminate dietary sugar (e.g., sucrose, glucose, and fructose) intake between meals. When recommending or purchasing commercial products, they should be labeled "*sugar-free*" (*not "sugarless," which usually contain "less" sugar*). However, under labeling regulations, "sugar-free" products may contain a small percentage of sugar (Food and Drug Administration, 2007).

Table 4.9 (continued)

Between-meal snacks that contain non-cariogenic sweetening agents should be safe, e.g., xylitol, sorbitol, saccharin, aspartame, or sucralose.
Packaged sweeteners such as Sweet n' Low®, Nutrasweet®, and Sucralose® contain a cariogenic bulking agent (dextrose), which is added to make their physical properties similar to sugar. Xylitol has a compound anti-caries effect because it is not metabolized by cariogenic bacteria (i.e., does not lead to acid production) and may shift the intra-oral bacterial population to one that is less cariogenic.
B. *Oral hygiene*
Each patient needs to learn how to effectively remove dental plaque.
This includes the use of disclosing agents (e.g., Red Cote®, 2-Tone Disclosing Tablet/Solution®, Hurriview Snap and Go®, and Agent Cool Blue Tinting Rinse®) that stain dental plaque on the teeth to make it visible and focus the correct use of a toothbrush and dental floss for removing it.
(At least) twice-daily tooth brushing with a fluoride-containing toothpaste and *daily use of dental floss between all adjoining teeth* are necessary to adequately remove dental plaque.
Sjogren's patients should carry a travel toothbrush and toothpaste and brush after meals and snacks.
For patients with limited dexterity (because of arthritis or other hand disability), electric toothbrushes, irrigators, or supplementary oral hygiene aids may be helpful.
C. *Dental topical fluoride* can be professionally applied and patient-applied. In addition to the patient using an over-the-counter fluoride-containing dentifrice (0.1% or 0.15% fluoride) twice daily, patients at high risk for developing caries should receive *supplemental forms of fluoride applied to the teeth.*
• At *dental office visits, a high-concentration fluoride should be applied*, such as 1.23% acidulated phosphate fluoride gel or foam (many brands are available) for 4 min in a tray or 2.25% fluoride varnish (Duraphat®, Duraflor®) directly onto the teeth. These applications can be repeated every 6 months or more frequently if necessary.
• Patients should be given specific instructions on the use of *self-applied fluorides* and their application demonstrated to the patient. The methods to be used depend on the severity of the patient's caries experience and/or the degree of salivary hypofunction.
• *Patients at low-to-moderate risk of caries should use a 0.05% sodium fluoride mouth rinse* (available over the counter) for 1–2 min daily, before sleep.
• *Note that some brands contain alcohol, which may be uncomfortable to those with salivary dysfunction.*
• The fluoride rinses developed for children tend to be alcohol free.
• *Patients at high risk of caries should apply 1.1% neutral (pH = 7) sodium fluoride gel* (available only by prescription) in custom-made trays for 5–10 min.
• The frequency of this application can range from weekly to daily, depending on the frequency of recurrent caries.
• Immediately after tray removal, patients should floss between all teeth to carry fluoride to the adjoining dental surfaces.
• This is best done just before going to sleep.
• Alternatively, if necessary for increased compliance, a neutral sodium fluoride dentifrice may be prescribed (Prevident 5000 Plus® or Dry Mouth®).
• The dentifrice may be less effective than tray-applied gel because the contact time with the teeth is lessened.
D. *Oral pH*
Because dental erosion and caries are acid-dependent process, the *overall oral pH is important.*
• *Normal saliva has substantial buffering capacity* (i.e., the ability to stabilize the salivary pH), but this is significantly decreased in saliva of those individuals who have the most severe salivary dysfunction.
• The critical pH has been defined for dental enamel at ~5.5 and for the root surface at ~6.3.
• Acids may come from endogenous sources (e.g., gastric reflux, bacterial metabolism) or exogenous sources (e.g., carbonated beverages, sports drinks, flavored waters, and juice).
• Strategies to increase salivary buffering capacity include the use of bicarbonate mouth rinses (CariFree Maintenance Rinse®), toothpastes, chewing gum (Orbit White®; Anderson and Orchardson, 2003), and extended-release bicarbonate lozenges (Salese®).

Table 4.9 (continued)

E. *Re-mineralizing agents*
These agents deliver calcium and phosphate to the tooth surface to begin restoration of demineralized areas (Spolsky, 2007). This approach can be effective, but only after the causes of demineralization are brought under control. There are currently four technologies available on the market:
1. *Calcium phosphopeptide and amorphous calcium phosphate* (Recaldent®; GC MI Paste with Recaldent®, Trident gum with Recaldent®)
2. *Calcium sodium phosphosilicate* (Novamin®; Dr. Collins Restore and Remineralizing Toothpaste)
3. *Amorphous calcium phosphate* (Arm and Hammer patented liquid calcium)
4. *Arginine bicarbonate and calcium carbonate* (SensiStat®)
F. *Dental restoration*
In individuals with chronic salivary dysfunction, the goal is to slow or stop the accelerated cycle of caries, restoration, and restoration failure.
• To stop this cycle, only *conservative intra-coronal restorations* should be placed initially, with the goal of simply removing carious tooth structure followed by an esthetic restorative material.
• The possibility of repairing an existing restoration, to preserve maximal tooth integrity, should be considered.
– Light-cured glass ionomer cements should be used where practical, because they release fluoride and are more resistant to marginal decay.
G. *Subgingival margins and full coronal coverage should be avoided wherever possible for initial treatment of these patients*
This is because subgingival margins are the most common location of caries in individuals with salivary hypofunction.
In addition, the location is less accessible to topical fluoride and early caries is more difficult to detect and restore in these areas.
Full veneer crowns, if ultimately necessary, should not be placed until caries are under control (i.e., the patient has been free of new carious lesions for at least 1 year).
H. *Dental recall examinations*
At each recall dental visit:
1. Visual examination of dental surfaces should be supplemented with bite wing radiographs as needed.
2. The oral mucosa should be examined for signs of candidiasis (see below).
3. The patient's dental plaque control should be reassessed by in vivo staining, and the importance of plaque control techniques should be reinforced.

Refs. [28–31].

or urine infections, a predisposition to oral candidiasis exists. This candidiasis is a low-grade erythematous candidiasis and may only be appreciated when the dentures are removed. Treatment must include not only the patient's oral symptoms but also treatment of the denture by soaking overnight and brushing with anti-fungal solutions. Another hint to the presence of oral candidiasis is the appearance of angular cheilitis and this manifestation must also be treated with topical anti-fungal creams (Tables 4.10 and 4.11).

4.7.3 Treatment of Dry and Painful Mouth

Some patients complain of painful and dry mouth that is out of proportion to their objective findings on mouth examination. This may result from a localized neuropathy called "burning mouth syndrome" that may be part of the spectrum of central sensitization or fibromyalgia symptoms. Other factors may include the role of topical mucins in providing improved viscosity as the

Table 4.10 Topical anti-fungal drugs for treating oral candidiasis

A. Nystatin vaginal tablets
• Each 10,000 units
• Use 2–4 tabs/day
• Since nystatin has a medicinal taste, may dissolve each tablet slowly in mouth using sips of water over about 5–10 min, may sip with water sweetened with nutrasweet as necessary to aid dissolution
• Treatment may take 4–6 weeks to prevent recurrence
• Partial or complete dentures must be removed during this application to permit access of the drug to all mucosal surfaces
B. Clotrimazole vaginal tablets
• Each tab 100 mg
• 1/2 tablet, b.i.d.
• Dissolve slowly in mouth, using same method as for Nystatin vaginal tablets This method is often used if there has been inadequate response to nystatin
C. Nystatin cream 10,000 U/g
• Particularly useful if patient has angular cheilitis
• Must use two–three times/day at the same time as treating oral yeast with nystatin or clotrimazole as described above
D. Nystatin topical powder
• 100,000 U/g
• Use two times/day for treatment of dentures
• Apply a fairly even coating to fitting surface of a clean, moistened denture; this supplements other intra-oral anti-fungal drugs and may be helpful in maintenance therapy
E. Dentures must be treated separately
• Dentures may be soaked in chlorhexidine (after checking that this will not discolor the product)
• Nystatin powder can be added to the liquid for overnight soaking (1/4 teaspoon)
• The denture must be brushed with nystatin and chlorhexidine to ensure removal of residual candida

Table 4.11 Oral candidiasis diagnosis and treatment

A. Diagnosis
About one third of patients with chronic hyposalivation develop oral candidiasis, usually of the chronic erythematous type (and usually not of the pseudomembranous type—white thrush).
• *Symptoms* of chronic erythematous oral candidiasis include
o a burning sensation of the mucosa,
o intolerance to acidic or spicy foods, and
o a change in taste or development of a metallic taste.
Some cases are asymptomatic.
• *Clinical signs* of candidiasis of the erythematous type include
o macular erythema on the dorsal tongue, palate, buccal mucosa, or denture-bearing mucosa,
o atrophy of the filiform papillae on the dorsal tongue, and/or
o angular cheilitis.
The diagnosis can be confirmed by fungal culture of a swab specimen, from such a mucosal lesion, revealing significant numbers of colony-forming units of a *Candida* species, usually *Candida albicans*.
B. *Treatment*
Adequate treatment usually provides significant improvement of oral symptoms, in spite of continuing oral dryness.

Table 4.11 (continued)

In patients with clinically visible salivary secretion, this is most conveniently managed with *systemic fluconazole*, one 100 mg tablet daily for 2–4 weeks, and monitoring the patient for the treatment endpoints described below.
The patient is informed that if there is no significant resolution of symptoms within 2–4 weeks, then they may be switched to a topical form of medication.
Patients with severe chronic hyposalivation and lacking visible salivary secretion usually require *topical forms of anti-fungal drugs* that *do not contain* sucrose or glucose, because they must be administered for periods of weeks or months.
These topical forms are necessary because systemically administered drugs may not reach the mouth of such patients in therapeutically adequate amounts via the saliva.
Topical drugs must not increase a patient's risk for dental caries but, currently, all commercially packaged "oral" anti-fungal drugs contain glucose or sucrose that presents a significant risk of supporting caries development when used in these patients.
• Generally, the best topical anti-fungal drug for use in patients with severe hyposalivation and remaining natural teeth is *nystatin vaginal tablets*, which contain lactose, but not sucrose or glucose.
• They must be dissolved slowly *in the mouth* for 15–20 min, two or three times/day.
• Such patients will need frequent sips of water to allow the tablet to dissolve in that time.
• *For patients wearing partial or complete dentures*, additional instructions and treatment are needed:
1. *Dentures must be removed from the mouth* before applying the anti-fungal drug.
2. *Dentures must be disinfected by soaking overnight* in a substance compatible with the denture material (e.g., 1% sodium hypochlorite for dentures without exposed metal or benzalkonium chloride diluted 1:750 in water for dentures with exposed metal) and rinsed carefully before reinserting in the mouth.
3. *Nystatin topical powder may be applied* in a thin film onto the moistened fitting surface of a denture when it is reinserted in the mouth.
• *Treatment endpoint*: Treatment should continue until the clinician has observed resolution of all the mucosal erythema, return of filiform papillae to the dorsal tongue, and resolution of associated oral symptoms (i.e., burning, intolerance to spicy foods).
• *Angular cheilitis*: The presence of angular cheilitis almost always indicates concurrent intra-oral candidiasis.
o Angular cheilitis can be treated by nystatin or clotrimazole cream, but in most cases it should not be used without concurrently treating the intra-oral infection, as described above.
• *Recurrence*: After treatment is completed, *recurrence is fairly common* and the patient must be re-treated as described above.
o After one recurrence, re-treatment should be immediately followed by maintenance therapy (e.g., continued use of half of a nystatin vaginal tablet slowly dissolved in the mouth each day, indefinitely).
o The patient with a chronic infection should be counseled on the possibility of re-infection with a previously used lipstick, lip balm, toothbrush, utensil, or other activity (e.g., oral sexual copulation).

oral membranes and tongue glide past each other. We list some guidelines for these problems below.

Table 4.12 outlines hints for dry and painful mouth.

Physicians need to be alert to medications that have anti-cholinergic side effects that exacerbate dry mouth symptoms. These drugs may include agents such as amitriptyline used for "fibromyalgia" or over-the-counter sleep remedies that contain anti-cholinergic drugs such as benadryl. Many anti-hypertensive medications and anti-seizure medications used for treatment of neuropathy may exacerbate dry mouth symptoms (Table 4.13, drugs with anti-cholinergic effects).

4.8 Summary

Symptomatic treatment of SS patients involves a wide spectrum of medical and oral medicine specialists. The issues are often "quality of life"

Table 4.12 Burning mouth and common mouth lubricants

A. Burning mouth syndrome
In some patients, the symptoms of burning mouth are disproportionate to the amount of observed dryness. In these patients, low-grade oral yeast infection must be ruled out. In particular, look under the dentures for erythematous candida infection.
In other patients, "burning" mouth syndrome may represent a local neuropathy. The use of Neurontin may be helpful in some patients. Other options include the topical use of clonazepam (0.5 mg dissolved in 2 ml water) and it is used as a mouth rinse twice daily.
B. Common products used for dry mouth
Biotene mouth rinse
Biotene mouth spray
Biotene toothpaste
Biotene gum
Oral balance gel (especially at nighttime)
Oasis oral spray
Mouth Kote oral spray
Rain Spy dry mouth spray
Thayer dry mouth spray
Farley's throat spray
Orahealth mints
Numoisyn lozenges
SalivaSure lozenges
These products are readily available at many retail stores and can be purchased online at sites such as www.amazon.com.

Table 4.13 Drugs associated with decreased salivary secretion and increased oral dryness

I. Blood pressure medications
A. α-Adrenergic blockers (clonidine, Catapres)
B. β-Adrenergic blockers (Inderal, Tenormin)
C. Combined α,β-blockers (Labetalol)
II. Anti-depressants (also used for neuropathy and other causes)
A. Amitriptyline (Elavil)
B. Nortriptyline (Pamelor)
C. Desipramine
D. Parnate, Nardil (MAO inhibitors)
E. Mellaril (dopamine blocker)
III. Muscle spasm
A. Flexeril
B. Robaxin
C. Baclofen
IV. Urologic drugs
A. Ditropan, Detrol
B. Yohimbe
V. Cardiac
A. Norpace

Table 4.13 (continued)

VI. Parkinson's
A. Sinemet (carbidopa-Levodopa)
B. Requip (robinirole)
VII. Decongestants and sleeping aids (many are over the counter)
A. Chlortrimeton
B. Pseudofed (pseudoephedirne)
C. Atarax, Benadryl

rather than "life threatening." In the limited time available for the patient at the time of their revisit, there is often not available time to deal with "quality of life" treatments such as dry eyes or dry mouth. Furthermore, it is assumed that "another specialist" will handle that problem. As a result, the patient is left without specific approaches to their symptomatic problems. This chapter provides a series of tables that might be provided to patients and their referring physicians.

References

1. Vitali C, Bombardieri S, Jonsson R, Moutsopoulos HM, Alexander EL, Carsons SE, et al. Classification criteria for Sjogren's syndrome: a revised version of the European criteria proposed by the American–European Consensus Group. Ann Rheum Dis. 2002;61(6):554–8.
2. Tan E, Cohen A, Fries J, Masi A, Mcshane D, Rothfield N, et al. The 1982 revised criteria for the classification of systemic lupus erythematosus. Arthritis Rheum. 1982;25(11):1271–1277.
3. Petri M. Review of classification criteria for systemic lupus erythematosus. Rheum Dis Clin N Am. 2005;31(2):245–54.
4. Ferri C, Valentini G, Cozzi F, Sebastiani M, Michelassi C, La Montagna G, et al. Systemic sclerosis: demographic, clinical, and serologic features and survival in 1,012 Italian patients. Medicine 2002;81(2):139.
5. Caramaschi P, Biasi D, Volpe A, Carletto A, Cecchetto M, Bambara L. Coexistence of systemic sclerosis with other autoimmune diseases. Rheumatol Int. 2007;27(4):407–410.
6. Nardi N, Brito-Zeron P, Ramos-Casals M, Aguilo S, Cervera R, Ingelmo M, et al. Circulating autoantibodies against nuclear and non-nuclear antigens in primary Sjogren's syndrome: prevalence and clinical significance in 335 patients. Clin Rheumatol. 2006;25(3):341.
7. Ramos-Casals M, Anaya J, GarcÌa-Carrasco M, Rosas J, BovÈ A, Claver G, et al. Cutaneous vasculitis in primary Sjogren syndrome: classification and clinical significance of 52 patients. Medicine 2004;83(2):96.
8. Ramos-Casals M, Jara LJ, Medina F, Rosas J, Calvo-Alen J, Mana J, et al. Systemic autoimmune diseases co-existing with chronic hepatitis C virus infection (the HISPAMEC Registry): patterns of clinical and immunological expression in 180 cases. J Intern Med. 2005;257(6):549–57.
9. Alarcon-Segovia D, Ibanez G, Hernandez-Ortiz J, Velazquez-Forero F, Gonzalez-Jimenez Y. Sjogren's syndrome in progressive systemic sclerosis (scleroderma). Am J Med. 1974;57(1):78–85.
10. Hebbar M, Janin A, Huglo D, Copin MC, Lafyatis R, Devulder B, et al. Xerostomia in systemic sclerosis: systematic evaluation by salivary scintigraphy and lip biopsy in thirty-four patients. Arthritis Rheum. 1994;37(3):439–41.
11. Janin A, Gosselin B, Gosset D, Hatron PY, Sauvezie B. Histological criteria of Sjogren's syndrome in scleroderma. Clin Exp Rheumatol. 1989;7(2):167–9.
12. Janin A, Konttinen YT, Gronblad M, Karhunen P, Gosset D, Malmstrom M. Fibroblast markers in labial salivary gland biopsies in progressive systemic sclerosis. Clin Exp Rheumatol. 1990;8(3):237–42.
13. Rasker JJ, Jayson MI, Jones DE, Matthews R, Burton JL, Rhys Davies E, et al. Sjogren's syndrome in systemic sclerosis. A clinical study of 26 patients. Scand J Rheumatol. 1990;19(1):57–65.
14. Bodolay E, Csiki Z, Szekanecz Z, Ben T, Kiss E, Zeher M, et al. Five-year follow-up of 665 Hungarian patients with undifferentiated connective tissue disease (UCTD). Clin Experimental Rheumatol. 2003;21(3):313–320.
15. Kroshinsky D, Stone JH, Bloch DB, Sepehr A. Case 5-2009—A 47-year-old woman with a rash and numbness and pain in the legs. N Engl J Med. 2009;360(7):711–720.
16. Tan EM, Feltkamp TE, Smolen JS, Butcher B, Dawkins R, Fritzler MJ, et al. Range of antinuclear antibodies in "healthy" individuals. Arthritis Rheum. 1997;40(9):1601–11.
17. Tan EM, Smolen JS, McDougal JS, Butcher BT, Conn D, Dawkins R, et al. A critical evaluation of enzyme immunoassays for detection of

antinuclear autoantibodies of defined specificities. I. Precision, sensitivity, and specificity. Arthritis Rheum. 1999;42(3):455–64.
18. Tan E, Muro Y, Pollard K. Autoantibody-defined epitopes on nuclear antigens are conserved, conformation-dependent and active site regions. Clin Exp Rheumatol. 1994;12:S27–31.
19. Tan EM. Autoantibodies to nuclear antigens (ANA): their immunobiology medicine. Adv. Immunol. 1982;33:167–240.
20. Tan EM. Antinuclear antibodies. Diagnostic markers for autoimmune diseases and probes for cell biology. Adv. Immunol. 1989;44:93–151.
21. David-Bajar KM, Bennion SD, DeSpain JD, Golitz LE, Lee LA. Clinical, histologic, and immunofluorescent distinctions between subacute cutaneous lupus erythematosus and discoid lupus erythematosus. J Invest Dermatol. 1992;99(3):251–7.
22. Fang YV, Cyran SJ, Albini B, Rostami R, Binder WL, Beutner EH. Relevance of complement fixing antinuclear antibodies. Int J Dermatol. 1999;38(2):96–100.
23. Ryhal B, DeMera RS, Shoenfeld Y, Peter JB, Gershwin ME. Are autoantibodies present in patients with subacute and chronic urticaria? J Investig Allergol Clin Immunol. 2001;11(1):16–20.
24. Sontheimer RD. Subacute cutaneous lupus erythematosus: a decade's perspective. Med Clin North Am. 1989;73(5):1073–90.
25. Merrill J, Buyon J. Rituximab: Wanted dead or alive. Arthritis Rheum. 2010;62:2188–91.
26. Vitali C, Palombi G, Baldini C, Benucci M, Bombardieri S, Covelli M, et al. Sjogren's syndrome disease damage index and disease activity index: scoring systems for the assessment of disease damage and disease activity in Sjogren's syndrome, derived from an analysis of a cohort of Italian patients. Arthritis Rheum. 2007;56(7):2223–31.
27. Michelson PE. Red eye unresponsive to treatment. West J Med. 1997;166:145–7.
28. Wu AJ. The oral component of Sjogren's syndrome: pass the scalpel and check the water. Curr Rheumatol Rep. 2003;5(4):304–10.
29. von Bultzingslowen I, Sollecito TP, Fox PC, Daniels T, Jonsson R, Lockhart PB, et al. Salivary dysfunction associated with systemic diseases: systematic review and clinical management recommendations. Oral Surg Oral Med Oral Pathol Oral Radiol Endod. 2007;103(Suppl):S57 e1–15.
30. Daniels TE, Wu AJ. Xerostomia—clinical evaluation and treatment in general practice. J Calif Dent Assoc. 2000;28(12):933–41.
31. Daniels TE. Evaluation, differential diagnosis, and treatment of xerostomia. J Rheumatol Suppl. 2000;61:6–10.

Part II

Classification Criteria and Disease Status Activity, Histology of Salivary Gland Biopsy, and Imaging

Current Concepts on Classification Criteria and Disease Status Indexes in Sjögren's Syndrome

5

Claudio Vitali, Chiara Baldini, and Stefano Bombardieri

Abstract

Different classification criteria sets have been proposed for Sjögren's syndrome (SS) by different leading experts in the field, but none of them have been widely accepted in the scientific community. Finally, the more recently proposed "American and European Consensus Group classification criteria" have achieved general consensus and this set now represents a "gold standard" to correctly classify patients with primary and secondary variants of SS. On the contrary, so far, no validated "disease status" indexes have been developed for SS. However, in the last few years, two attempts have been made on a national basis in Italy and UK to develop activity and damage criteria for SS. Nowadays, a multinational consensus is certainly needed in order to generate more largely accepted criteria to assess these disease status entities.

Keywords

Sjögren's syndrome • Classification criteria • Outcome measures • Disease activity score • Damage index • Fatigue

5.1 Introduction

Sjögren's syndrome (SS) is a common systemic autoimmune disease which primarily affects the salivary and lacrimal glands and usually leads to a persistent dryness of the mouth and eyes due to the lymphocytic infiltration and functional impairment of the exocrine glands [1, 2]. The disease is commonly included in the spectrum of connective tissue diseases (CTDs) and, together with the other members of this disease family, it shares the possibility of a multisystemic involvement with a very large range of clinical and serological manifestations. Besides the disease-specific exocrine manifestations, SS may be, in fact, characterized by constitutional symptoms, arthritis, skin, lung, renal and neurological involvement as well as by the production of a plethora of autoantibodies [3].

As SS—and CTDs in general—does not present a single distinguishing feature which can allow a correct diagnosis, the presence of a combination of clinical and laboratory manifestations is needed to identify the single disease, and all

C. Vitali (✉)
Section of Rheumatology, Department of Internal Medicine, Villamarina Hospital, Piombino, Italy
e-mail: c.vitali@yahoo.it

R.I. Fox, C.M. Fox (eds.), *Sjögren's Syndrome*, DOI 10.1007/978-1-60327-957-4_5,

these parameters have been collected in specific and sensible classification criteria sets. The purpose of the classification criteria is to distinguish patients with a disease from patients without it and from normal subjects. Ideally, classification criteria should have high sensitivity to identify the particular disease they are created for and high specificity to distinguish it from other similar diseases. Conceptually, classification criteria and diagnostic criteria could be considered equal (particularly when their sensitivity and specificity are both close to 100%). However, classification criteria are usually not completely reliable and a certain percentage of patients can be misclassified. So they do not represent the medical standing for a diagnosis and finally only the physician can make a proper diagnosis for an individual patient [4]. Therefore, classification criteria are intended to select patients for epidemiological, clinical, and therapeutic studies [4].

CTDs are chronic inflammatory diseases characterized by a relapsing remitting course. Each flare of these diseases can be spontaneously remitted or reverted by a proper therapeutic approach. If this does not happen, irreversible damage can be caused in the involved organ or system.

Activity implies reversibility of the process and it is usually characterized by inflammatory manifestations in various organs or systems. Damage represents the component of the disease process that is irreversible and can be defined as the presence of a permanent loss of function or by radiographically or histologically evident structural derangement of the compromised organ or system [4]. For this reason, the clinical course of CTDs needs to be monitored by proper instruments which can precisely and correctly measure the phase of activity and the cumulated damage. SS is generally a relatively stable, slowly progressive CTD. Nonetheless, it does not elude these rules and a certain number of patients can develop activity flares which can lead to acute involvement and to potential damage of various glandular and extraglandular organs.

Therefore, the distinction of clinical manifestations of the disease between features related to activity and those related to damage/chronicity, and the elaboration of the respective status indexes is mandatory for SS. This has historically proven to be crucial in rheumatology, in particular for clinical research on systemic autoimmune diseases and therapeutic studies [5, 6].

5.2 Comparison of the Different Classification Criteria Sets for Primary SS

Several classification criteria sets have been proposed for Sjögren's syndrome (SS) over the years by leading experts in the field, but none of them have been widely accepted in the scientific community [7–9]. The traditional criteria sets most widely used in the past for the definition of SS include the San Francisco criteria (proposed in 1975 and subsequently revised in 1984) [10, 11], the Copenhagen [12], the Japanese [13], the Greek [14], and the San Diego criteria, all proposed in 1986 [15]. The Japanese criteria have been subsequently updated over the years and the latest version was proposed in 1999 [9, 16].

Nearly all of them defined SS as an autoimmune exocrinopathy and therefore focused the efforts of the classification on the main organs involved: the lacrimal and salivary glands. Nonetheless, many important differences are appreciable when compared to each other. Table 5.1 focuses on their similarities and dissimilarities.

First, all of the criteria sets, except the Copenhagen one, used the terminology "probable" and "definite" SS, while, only the Copenhagen and the Greek criteria used the terminology "primary" SS and "secondary" SS [12, 14]. Secondly, much argumentation and concerns have dealt with the discrepancy between including in the classification criteria sets either the subjective symptoms and the objective data or exclusively the easily reproducible objective findings. Thirdly, as far as ocular tests were concerned, comparing the different criteria sets, discrepancies emerged related to the tests used, the range and the cut-off levels of normal values, and the requirement of solely one abnormal test to allow the diagnosis of keratoconjunctivitis sicca (the Greek criteria) or at least two abnormal tests (the

Table 5.1 Copenhagen criteria, Japanese criteria, Greek criteria, San Diego criteria, and San Francisco criteria: similarities and dissimilarities

	Copenhagen (1976)	Japanese (1977)	Greek (1979)	San Diego (1986)	San Francisco (1975, 1984)
Subjective dry eye	–	+	+	–	–
Subjective dry mouth	–	+	+	+	–
Exclusively objective abnormalities	+	–	–	–	+
History of parotid gland swelling	–	+	+	–	–
Ocular tests:					
-Schirmer's-I test	+(≤10 mm/5′)	+(≤10 mm/5′)	+(≤10 mm/5′)–	+(<9 mm/5′)	+(≤10 mm/5′)
-Break-up time	+(≤10 s)	–	–	–	+
-Rose Bengal (van Bijsterveld's score)	+(≥4)	+(≥2)	+(≥4)	+(≥4)	+(≥4)
-Fluorescein test	–	+	–	+	–
One abnormal test as evidence of KCS	–	–	+	–	–
At least two abnormal tests as evidence of KCS	+	+	–	+	+
Oral parameters:					
-Unstimulated whole saliva	+	–	–	+	–
-Stimulated parotid flow rate	–	–	+	+	–
-Scintigraphy	+	–	–	–	–
-Sialography	–	+	–	–	–
Minor salivary gland biopsy	>1	>1	≥2	≥2	>1
Minor salivary gland biopsy mandatory criterion	No	No	Yes	Yes	Yes
Anti-nuclear antibodies	–	–	–	+	–
Anti-SS-A/Ro	–	–	–	+	–
Anti-SS-B/La	–	–	–	+	–
IgM-RF	–	–	–	+	–
Terminology probable/definite SS	–	+	+	+	+
Terminology pSS/sSS	+	–	+	–	+

San Francisco, Copenhagen, Japanese, and San Diego criteria) (see Table 5.1) [12–15].

Similarly, various objective methods have been employed in attempts to assess the salivary components of SS. Nearly all of the five criteria sets included salivary flow rate estimation as a criterion for the diagnosis of SS salivary impairment. Sialometry was, nonetheless, performed by using different modalities. Even if both unstimulated and stimulated sialometry were not considered specific tests, they appeared to be simple and non-invasive, and thus included in the criteria as a crude assessment of the functional status of the salivary glands. Only the Japanese criteria used abnormal sialography as a criterion for salivary gland assessment in SS [13]. In contrast, the Copenhagen criteria employed salivary gland scintigraphy, which, even if rather expensive, provided a functional evaluation of all salivary glands [12]. All these criteria sets included the minor salivary gland biopsy. Both the Greek and the San Diego criteria considered the minor salivary gland biopsy to be mandatory with a focus score ≥2 as a crucial prerequisite for the diagnosis of SS [14, 15]. On the contrary, the San Diego criteria specified that an abnormal minor salivary gland biopsy was necessary only for "definite" SS, whereas the category of "probable" SS could be fulfilled in the absence of a biopsy [15]. According to the Copenhagen criteria, a patient could have been diagnosed as having SS without an abnormal salivary gland biopsy while, finally, according to the Japanese criteria, biopsy from tear glands could replace the minor salivary gland biopsy [12, 13]. As far as the modalities for performing the biopsy were concerned, all the criteria adopted the guidelines which had been previously proposed by Daniels et al. in 1975 [10], in which focal sialadenitis had been differentiated from chronic non-specific sialadenitis, defining a focus as a cluster of at least 50 mononuclear cells. To diagnose primary SS, an average focus score per 4 mm^2 was required, based on the evaluation of at least four glands. Moreover, according to Daniels the biopsy sample had to be obtained through clinically normal mucosa, and lobules characterized by non-specific infiltrates had to be excluded from the evaluation [10, 11]. The importance of focus sialadenitis was outlined by subsequent studies which confirmed that the histological criterion was highly associated with parotid flow rate, diagnosis of keratoconjunctivitis sicca, and presence of anti-nuclear or anti-Ro antibodies [11, 16–18].

Finally, for the first time, the San Diego criteria had utilized for the diagnosis of SS the presence of autoantibodies (anti-nuclear antibodies, anti-SS-A/Ro, anti-SS-B/La, and IgM-RF), pointing to the fact that the disease is autoimmune in origin [15].

Overall, in spite of their differences, these proposed classification criteria hypothetically could have been able to select and correctly classify patients affected by SS, when used by single groups of investigators. However, the major limitation of these criteria was that they had never been validated by multicenter studies or by means of standard statistical approaches, making impossible to carry out comparable epidemiological studies. Furthermore, in many cases, the sensitivity, specificity, and reliability of the procedures followed for the definition of the disease remained to be assessed.

5.3 From the Preliminary European Criteria of the Epidemiology Committee of the Commission of the European Communities to the Revised Version of the European Criteria Proposed by the American–European Consensus Group

In view of the fact that previously proposed criteria did not achieve wide acceptance, in 1988 the Epidemiology Committee of the Commission of the European Communities decided to support a multicenter study to reach a consensus on classification criteria for SS [19]. The study began in 1989 and ended in 1993 with the definition of the Preliminary European Classification Criteria for SS [20]. It is noteworthy that for the first time this study did not approach the problem using the Delphi method, which was based on the consensus of the experts, but used the same methodology and statistics which have been adopted by the American College of Rheumatology for rheumatoid arthritis (RA), deriving the criteria directly from a real patient cohort [20, 21] The European criteria were based on a six-item set and any four of these six items were considered to be required for the diagnosis. These items included (i) ocular symptoms, (ii) oral symptoms, (iii) ocular signs (defined by positive Schirmer's-I test and/or Rose Bengal score), (iv) signs of salivary gland involvement assed by parotid sialography, scintigraphy, and unstimulated salivary flow, (v) focal sialadenitis observed in lip biopsy, and (vi) presence of autoantibodies. For primary SS, the presence of four out of six items had good sensitivity (93.5%) and specificity (94%). Some exclusion criteria were also added to this classification set for SS, following the recommendations made by Fox et al. [15] and, namely, the presence of preexisting lymphoma, acquired immunodeficiency syndrome, sarcoidosis, and graft-versus-host disease. The diagnosis of secondary SS could be made when in the presence of an associated CTD, and with the exclusion of the autoantibody item, three out of the remaining five items were met [20].

The criteria set was then validated in a following survey carried out on a different population of patients and controls. The six-item criteria confirmed it had a high sensitivity (97.5%) and specificity (94.2%) [22].

After their validation, the European classification criteria achieved wide acceptance by the scientific community in view of their accuracy. In fact, when previously proposed criteria [12–15] had been used to classify patients with primary SS and controls enrolled in the European study, they all showed a very high specificity (range 97.9–100%) but a lower sensitivity (range 22.9–72.2%). This could have run the risk of selecting particular subsets of patients [20]. Other potential advantageous characteristics of the European criteria were that they distinguished between primary SS and secondary SS but avoided the concept of definite/possible SS. Nonetheless, the European criteria for the classification of SS generated extensive discussion. The key point of the debate was that these criteria could be fulfilled in the absence of either autoantibodies or positive findings on labial salivary gland biopsy and then could also be met by patients with sicca symptoms but not strictly primary SS. Furthermore, a criteria set in which two out of the six items were devoted to subjective complaints could not allow a correct classification of the patients with SS but without symptoms [9, 23, 24].

To overcome these objections and broaden the acceptance of the European classification criteria, a joint effort was undertaken by the European Study Group on Classification Criteria for SS and by a group of American experts. The analysis was performed by using a receiver operating characteristic (ROC) curve of the revised criteria. The curve was obtained by plotting the sensitivity and specificity values calculated for each different combination of positive tests. Based on this ROC curve analysis, the condition "positivity of any four out of the six items" and the condition "positivity of four out of six items with the exclusion of the cases in which both serology and histopathology were negative" showed the same accuracy (92.7%) which was the highest among those obtained by different combinations of positive items. However, the second condition had a lower sensitivity (89.5% vs 97.4%) but a higher specificity (95.2% vs 89.4%). The presence of any three of the four objective criteria items also showed a slightly lower accuracy (90.5%) but a specificity of 95.2% and a sensitivity of 84.2%. This combination was also deemed reliable to correctly classify patients with primary SS. In conclusion, the American–European Consensus Group, maintaining the previous European scheme of six items, introduced the obligatory rule that for a definite diagnosis of SS either the minor salivary gland biopsy or serology had to be positive (see Table 5.2) [25]. Other modifications were proposed and included in the European criteria set to make the item definition more precise. In particular, it was specified that Schirmer's-I test should be performed with standardized paper strips in unanesthetized closed eyes, following the European and the Japanese tradition. Moreover, as the Rose Bengal test is not available in many countries, other ocular dye scores (i.e., fluorescein stain and Lissamine Green) were proposed. These modified criteria also defined a positive minor salivary gland biopsy as the presence of at least one focus of lymphocytes, specifying that it/they had to be adjacent to normal-appearing mucous acini per 4 mm^2 glandular tissue. In particular, it was decided to add hepatitis C virus (HCV) infection as an exclusion criterion, considering that the sicca symptoms observed in this kind of patient such as extrahepatic manifestations of the virus needed to be differentiated from primary SS (see Table 5.2) [26].

The American–European Consensus Group criteria were published in 2002 and adopted as gold standard criteria in Europe and in the USA [25]. In 1999 the revised Japanese criteria for Sjögren's syndrome, advocated by the Japanese Ministry of Welfare, had been elaborated as well [27]. Compared to the American–European Consensus Group, the Japanese criteria did not include symptomatology as an item, although they stated that clinicians should be aware of the sicca symptoms. They only relied on objective test results and required at least two abnormal tests both for the diagnosis of keratoconjunctivitis sicca and xerostomia. Finally, positive

Table 5.2 American–European Consensus Group criteria. Revised international classification criteria for SS

I. *Ocular symptoms*: a positive response to at least one of the following questions:
1. Have you had daily, persistent, troublesome dry eyes for more than 3 months?
2. Do you have a recurrent sensation of sand or gravel in the eyes?
3. Do you use tear substitutes for more than three times a day?
II. *Oral symptoms*: a positive response to at least one of the following questions:
1. Have you had a daily feeling of dry mouth for more than 3 months?
2. Have you had recurrently or persistently swollen salivary glands as an adult?
3. Do you frequently drink liquids to aid in swallowing dry food?
III. *Ocular signs*: objective evidence of ocular involvement defined as a positive result for at least one of the following two tests:
1. Schirmer's-I test, performed without anesthesia ($<$5 mm in 5 min)
2. Rose Bengal score or other ocular dye score ($>$4 according to van Bijsterveld's scoring system)
IV. *Histopathology*: in minor salivary glands (obtained through normal-appearing mucosa) focal lymphocytic sialadenitis, evaluated by an expert histopathologist, with a focus score > 1, defined as a number of lymphocytic foci (which are adjacent to normal-appearing mucous acini and contain more than 50 lymphocytes) per 4 mm^2 of glandular tissue
V. *Salivary gland involvement*: objective evidence of salivary gland involvement defined by a positive result for at least one of the following diagnostic tests:
1. Unstimulated whole salivary flow ($<$1.5 mL in 15 min)
2. Parotid sialography showing the presence of diffuse sialectasis (punctate, cavitary, or destructive pattern), without evidence of obstruction in the major ducts
3. Salivary scintigraphy showing delayed uptake, reduced concentration, and/or delayed excretion of tracer
VI. *Autoantibodies*: presence in the serum of the following autoantibodies:
1. Antibodies to Ro(SS-A) or La(SS-B) antigens or both
Revised rules for classification
For primary SS
In patients without any potentially associated disease, primary SS may be defined as follows:
a. The presence of any four of the six items is indicative of primary SS, as long as either item IV (Histopathology) or VI (Serology) is positive
b. The presence of any three of the four objective criteria items (i.e., items III, IV, V, and VI)
c. The classification tree procedure represents a valid alternative method for classification, although it should be more properly used in clinical–epidemiological survey
For secondary SS
In patients with a potentially associated disease (for instance, another well-defined connective tissue disease), the presence of item I or item II plus any two from items III, IV, and V may be considered as indicative of secondary SS
Exclusion criteria
Past head and neck radiation treatment
Hepatitis C infection
Acquired immunodeficiency disease syndrome (AIDS)
Pre-existing lymphoma
Sarcoidosis
Graft versus host disease
Use of anti-cholinergic drugs (since a time shorter than fourfold the half life of the drug)

anti-SS-A/SS-B autoantibodies, which are absolute requirements for the American–European consensus Group criteria, were not mandatory for the Japanese criteria set. Overall, considering that the American–European consensus Group criteria can also be satisfied by the presence of three out of four objective criteria, the differences between the latter and the Japanese criteria are not so relevant [27]. Nowadays, looking forward to worldwide universally adopted criteria, the American Consensus Group criteria appear to be the most widely accepted tool presently available for the classification of patients with primary SS and secondary SS. A number of epidemiological studies have so far been performed that aimed at evaluating the prevalence of SS following these criteria [28–33].

5.4 Outcome Measures in SS

5.4.1 Outcome Measures in SS: A Brief History

To date, no status indexes have been proposed and adopted for SS [34]. Similarly no wide acceptance has been reached in the evaluation of generic and SS-specific measures of health status. Among the generic quality of life questionnaire, the SF-36 [35, 36] has been widely considered as the most suitable for SS. Moreover, due to the peculiarities of the clinical spectrum of SS, questionnaires specifically devoted to the assessment of sicca symptoms (i.e., Sicca Symptoms Inventory) [37] and fatigue (i.e., the Profile of Fatigue and Discomfort (PROFAD)) [38], which mostly affect the quality of life of SS patients, have been developed. The PROFAD in particular was a psychometric instrument specifically designed for SS and derived directly from specific symptoms of SS patients. The design of the PROFAD was a 16-item, 8-point scale, analyzing 6 different facets of fatigue belonging to 2 fatigue domains (somatic and mental) [38].

The history of status indexes in SS dates back to 1998 when Sutcliffe et al. [39] determined the organ damage and health status in a series of patients affected by primary SS and compared it, over the short-medium term, with patients affected by SLE and patients with both SLE and secondary SS [40]. The System Lupus International Collaborating Clinics/ACR Damage Index for Systemic Lupus Erythematosus (SLICC/ACR) damage index—an index expressly created to assess damage in SLE [41] and modified by adding sections for oral and ocular complaints—was used to assess end organ damage. The study showed that organ damage was largely restricted to the oral and ocular components within the primary SS group, whereas patients with lupus had more prominent damage within the renal, musculoskeletal, and neuropsychiatric domains. Over a longer period, in a minority of primary SS patients (11%), a second component of damage was represented by the development of lymphoma. Overall, this study demonstrated that it was possible to compare SS patients with patients affected by other autoimmune diseases and, also, that it was possible to assess, by using standardized methodology, the extent of damage in these patients.

Once demonstrated that damage could be assessed in primary SS, there arose the possibility that disease activity could also be assessed independently of damage. Two workshops were then held in Oxford (2000) and in Bethesda (2003) to start developing a preliminary core set of outcome measures to be used in randomized controlled trials and longitudinal observational studies in primary SS [42–44]. According to the workshops' consensus, the following signs and symptoms were firstly selected to be assessed in long-term studies of primary SS: (1) oral symptoms, (2) ocular symptoms, (3) oral signs, (4) ocular signs, (5) fatigue, (6) health-related quality of life measured by SF-36, and (7) IgG [45]. A number of sicca symptom questionnaires were suggested in order to assess the subjective symptoms [37, 46–47] while unstimulated salivary flow and Schirmer's-I test were proposed to assess oral and ocular signs, respectively. Analogously, for the assessment of fatigue in primary SS, the visual analog scale (VAS), the vitality score of SF-36 [36], and a number of questionnaires including the mean fluorescence intensity (MFI) [48] and the PROFAD were taken into consideration [38].

Beyond these attempts to define outcome measures for SS, more specifically defined activity and damage indexes were still lacking. Thus, there was a consensus that an effort to define these disease status entities should be made.

5.5 SS Clinical Activity Index (SCAI)—A Systemic Disease Activity Measure for Use in Clinical Trials in Primary SS and the SS Damage Index (SSDI): The UK Study

In 2007, Bowman et al. [49] initiated the development and validation of the SS Clinical Activity Index (SCAI)—a systemic disease activity measure for use in clinical trials in primary SS. This was based on the principles of the British Isles Lupus Activity Group (BILAG) [50] and a modified version was created and adopted, which included specific domains for ocular and oral lesions. In the ten domain structure of the SCAI (i.e., fatigue, constitutional symptoms, arthritis, muscle, gland swelling, skin, pulmonary, renal, neurological, and hematological domains), the items were recorded as 0 (absent), 1 (improving), 2 (the same), 3 (worse), or 4 (new) in the past 4 weeks, compared with previous disease activity. The raw scores were then converted into a "domain score" using a previously agreed scoring algorithm based on the BILAG approach (intention to treat) of "A" = requires prednisolone $\geq$ 20 mg and/or immunosuppressants, "B" = requires low-dose prednisolone/anti-malarials/NSAIDs, "C" = stable, mild disease, "D" = currently inactive but previously involved, and "E" = system never previously involved. In order to examine the validity of the proposed domain structure, a factor analysis was performed. Moreover, an external validation was made to compare the SCAI with the physician's global assessment (PhGA) as a "gold standard." In conclusion, this initial evaluation supported the potential for the SCAI as a tool for systemic activity assessment in patients with primary SS.

In order to develop a tool for longitudinal assessment of accumulated damage in patients with primary SS, to be used in both experimental trials and clinical assessment, damage data were also collected from a cohort of patients affected by primary SS [51]. As an instrument

Table 5.3 SS damage index

Ocular domain
Corneal scarring
Schirmer's-I result 0 mm/5 min in both eyes
Tear duct surgery (punctal plugs or cautery)
Oral domain
Caries
Teeth loss
Salivary gland swelling
Unstimulated salivary flow (0 mL/15 min)
Systemic domains
Neurological
Cranial neuropathy
Peripheral neuropathy
Other CNS pathology
Mononeuritis multiplex
Renal
Nephrocalcinosis
Renal tubular acidosis
Glomerular filtration rate < 50% predicted
Proteinuria >3.5 g/24 h
End-stage renal disease
Pulmonary
Pleural fibrosis
Pulmonary fibrosis
Pulmonary hypertension
Cardiovascular
Cardiomyopathy
Gastrointestinal
Chronic pancreatitis
Musculoskeletal
Erosive arthropathy
Malignancy
Paraproteinemia
Other malignancy
Macroglobulinemia
Cryoglobulinemia
Lymphoma

to collect the data, the authors revised the draft damage index derived from 2000 [42], based on the SLICC damage index. The index was completed by adding specific domains for oral and ocular involvement. Namely, damage items for ocular involvement were corneal scarring, Schirmer's-I result 0 mm/5 min in both eyes, tear duct surgery, cataract, retinal change, and chronic blepharitis, while those for oral involvement were represented by caries, teeth loss, salivary gland swelling, unstimulated salivary flow (0 mL/15 min), oral infection, parotid surgery, gum disease, oral ulceration, and dysphonia. The systemic domain was further subclassified into neurological, renal, pulmonary, cardiovascular, gastrointestinal, musculoskeletal, endocrine, and malignancy subdomains. Cross-sectional analysis of these data was subjected to a process of expert validations and a new item damage score was agreed upon, incorporating ocular, oral, and systemic domains (see Table 5.3). Total damage score correlated with disease duration at study entry, physical function as measured by SF-36, and activity as measured by the SCAI. Ocular damage score correlated with the "dry eye" domain of PROFAD–SSI.

5.6 Outcome Measures in SS: The Italian Study

Reflecting the increasing need for primary SS outcome measures within the scientific community, almost contemporary with the UK study,

Table 5.4 SS disease damage index (SSDDI)

SSDDI *Item*	*Definition*	*Score*
Oral/salivary damage		
Salivary flow impairment	Unstimulated whole saliva collection < 1.5 mL/15 min, by standard method	1
Loss of teeth	Complete or almost complete	1
Ocular damage		
Tear flow impairment	Schirmer's-I test < 5 mm in 5 min, by standard method	1
Structural abnormalities	Corneal ulcers, cataracts, chronic blepharitis	1
Neurological damage		
CNS involvement	Long-lasting stable CNS involvement	2
Peripheral neuropathy	Long-lasting stable peripheral or autonomic system impairment	1
Pleuropulmonary damage (any of the following)		2
Pleural fibrosis	Confirmed by imaging	
Interstitial fibrosis	Confirmed by imaging	
Significant irreversible functional damage	Confirmed by spirometry	
Renal impairment (any of the following)		2
Increased serum creatinine level or reduced GFR	Long-lasting stable abnormalities	
Tubular acidosis	Urinary pH > 6 and serum bicarbonate < 15 mmol/L in two consecutive tests	
Nephrocalcinosis	Confirmed by imaging	
Lymphoproliferative disease (any of the following)		5
B-cell lymphoma	Clinically and histologically confirmed	
Multiple myeloma	Clinically and histologically confirmed	
Waldenstrom's macroglobulinemia	Clinically and histologically confirmed	

Table 5.5 SS disease activity index (SSDAI)

SSDAI		
Constitutional symptoms		
Fever	≥38°C, not due to infections	1
Fatigue	Sufficiently severe to affect normal activities	1
Change in fatigue	New appearance or worsening of fatigue	1
Change in salivary gland swelling	New appearance or increasing swelling of major salivary glands, not due to infection or stones	3
Articular symptoms (any of the following)		2
Arthritis	Inflammatory pain in ≥1 joint	
Evolving arthralgias	New appearance or worsening of joint pain without signs of articular inflammation	
Hematologic features		
Leukopenia/lymphopenia	<3,500 mm^3/<1,000 mm^3	1
Lymph node/spleen enlargement	Clinically palpable lymph node/spleen	2
Pleuropulmonary symptoms (any of the following)		4
Pleurisy	Confirmed by imaging, not due to infection	1
Pneumonia (segmental or interstitial)	Ground-glass appearance on computed tomography scan, not due to infection	2
Change in vasculitis	New appearance or worsening or recurrent flares of palpable purpura	3
Active renal involvement (any of the following)		2
New or worsening proteinuria	>0.5 g/day	
Increasing serum creatinine level	Above the normal limits	
New or worsening nephritis	Glomerular or interstitial, histologically defined	
Peripheral neuropathy	Recent onset (<6 months), confirmed by nerve conduction studies	1

an Italian study was undertaken similarly aimed at constructing indexes to define and measure disease damage and disease activity in SS [52]. Twelve Italian centers participated in the study from February 2004 to May 2006. Data from 206 Italian patients with primary SS were collected and analyzed in order to select the individual clinical variables and the combination of variables that represent the most valid predictors of damage and disease activity. The disease had to be active to some degree in at least 50% of the patients enrolled in the study. Investigators judged the level of disease activity in each patient on the basis of their clinical experience, and according to the instructions provided in the study protocol guidelines, and clarified during the preliminary educational meetings. Patients who were classified as having active disease at the time of enrollment were evaluated a second time by the same investigator after 3 months. A total of 108 items were evaluated, which had been classified into 15 domains, according to the affected organ or system. Univariate and multivariate analyses were performed to select the clinical and serologic variables that were the best predictors of damage and of disease activity, and these variables were used to construct the SS disease damage index (SSDDI) and the SS disease activity index (SSDAI) (see Tables 5.4 and 5.5). The weight of each variable in the indexes was determined by using multivariate regression models. The construct validity of each instrument was confirmed by the close correlation of the derived index scores with the physician's global assessment (external gold standard) of the respective disease states. Finally, the accuracy of the SSDAI in distinguishing patients initially classified by the investigators as having active or very active disease from those classified as having inactive or mildly/moderately active disease was assessed by ROC curve analysis. For this purpose, an SSDAI score of ≥5 had high sensitivity (86.5%) and specificity (87.6%). In its final version, the SSDDI scale included 6 domains and 15 items, while the SSDAI included 8 domains and 15 items. Both SSDDI and SSDAI demonstrated construct validity and SSDAI appeared also to be sensitive to change [52].

Overall, both the SCAI/SSDI and the SSDAI/SSDDI represented exploratory attempts to define activity and damage criteria for SS. Despite their potential limitations, which were mainly related to the fact that some rare disease manifestations might have not been observed in "national" patient cohorts, they both specifically reflected the need of the scientific community to have at disposal validated status indexes in primary Sjögren's syndrome (pSS). Ultimately they served as the basis of a multinational collaborative project, which the European League Against Rheumatism (EULAR) has recently fostered for the development and validation of outcome measures in pSS [53].

5.7 Late-Breaking Update: The EULAR Project

During the last few years, the EULAR has promoted an international multicenter collaborative project aimed at developing consensus disease activity indexes for SS to be used in both clinical trials and daily practice. To date, two different tools have been proposed: a systemic activity score (ESSDAI: EULAR SS disease activity index) for the assessment of the global activity of primary SS [54] and a SS patient's activity score (ESSPRI: EULAR SS patient reported index) for collecting the main symptomatic features of the disease (dryness, fatigue, and arthralgias) [55]. The two indexes have been created with the aim of reflecting the dichotomous nature of SS, which may be characterized by both subjective glandular symptoms and severe multiorgan involvement. The ESSDAI was intended for clinicians to assess systemic activity of pSS patients and was not designed to evaluate patients' symptoms and complaints. On the other hand, the ESSPRI was mainly focused on measuring patients' dryness, pain, and fatigue. The two indexes resulted from the collaboration of, respectively, 39 and 21 European and North American SS experts, headed by a steering committee which included two experts in clinical epidemiology. The development of the ESSDAI and of the ESSPRI had required several steps. For the ESSDAI the steering committee members prepared a preliminary selection of domains significantly associated with SS disease activity on the basis of their clinical experience, literature review, and previous work. This proposal was submitted to the experts and 12 organ-specific "domains," contributing to disease activity, were identified. For each domain, features of disease activity were classified in three or four levels according to their severity. A total of 720 realistic clinical vignettes generated from 96 real patients were then analyzed in a multiple regression model to estimate the weight of each domain; the physician global assessment was used as the dependent variable of the model. In 2010, the ESSDAI was published and later, during the same year, its sensitivity to change and accuracy were assessed [56]. In the study, the ESSDAI seemed to detect changes in SS activity more accurately than the SSDAI and the SCAI and, noteworthy, for patients with stable disease activity, the ESSDAI did not show erroneous improvement.

In 2011, the ESSPRI was also published after that 230 patients participated in the construction of this patient-self-administered questionnaire. Domains relevant to patients were selected based on literature review and previous PROfile of FAtigue and Discomfort (PROFAD) and Sicca Symptoms Inventory (SSI) questionnaires. Identified key patient symptoms included fatigue, mental fatigue, pain, and dryness. These symptoms were easily and efficiently measured by visual analog scales (0–10 patient's global assessment—PtGA). In multivariate analysis dryness, pain, and fatigue, but not mental fatigue, were significantly associated with PtGA. Thus, ESSPRI was redefined as the mean of the three scales: dryness, pain, and fatigue.

In summary, to date, the first part of the EULAR project has been completed and the ESSDAI and the ESSPRI have been developed as recently reported in three different papers [54–56]. At the present, in order to adopt the ESSPRI and ESSDAI for assessing the therapy effectiveness in clinical trials, the validation of these scoring systems is ongoing. ESSDAI and ESSPRI still require to be validated in terms of feasibility, face and construct validity, reliability, and sensitivity to change and this phase of the EULAR project has recently begun.

In conclusion, after the achievement of a general consensus on the more recently proposed "American and European Consensus Group classification criteria," nowadays, it is to be hoped that efforts continue. The ultimate goal will be the elaboration of validated "disease status" indexes to better understand the natural history, prognosis, functional consequences, and response to treatment of SS. The project is ongoing at the moment; nonetheless, it is likely that in a near future internationally accepted outcome measures will be available for SS as they are for many of the other systemic autoimmune diseases.

References

1. Fox RJ. Sjögren's syndrome. Lancet 2005;366: 321–31.
2. Binard A, Devauchelle-Pensec V, Fautrel B, Jousse S, Youinou P, Saraux A. Epidemiology of Sjögren's syndrome: where are we now? Clin Exp Rheumatol. 2007;25:1–4.
3. Kassan SS, Mutsopoulos HM. Clinical manifestations and early diagnosis of Sjögren syndrome. Arch Intern Med. 2004;164:1275–84.
4. Fries JF, Hochberg MC, Medsger TA Jr, Hunder GG, Bombardier C. Criteria for rheumatic disease. Different types and different functions. The American College of Rheumatology Diagnostic and Therapeutic Criteria Committee. Arthritis Rheum. 1994;37:454–62.
5. Wolfe F., Lassere M, van der Heijde D et al. Preliminary core set of domains and reporting requirements for longitudinal observational studies in rheumatology. J Rheumatol. 1999;26:484–9.
6. Felson DT, Anderson JJ, Boers M, et al. The American College of Rheumatology preliminary core set of disease activity measures for rheumatoid arthritis clinical trials. The Committee on Outcome Measures in Rheumatoid Arthritis Clinical Trials. Arthritis Rheum. 1993;36:729–40.
7. Ramos Casals M, Tzioufas AG, Font J. Primary Sjögren's syndrome: new clinical and therapeutic concepts. Ann Rheum Dis. 2005;64:347–54.
8. Moutsopoulos HM, Chused T, Mann D, et al. Sjögren's syndrome (sicca syndrome): current issues. Ann Intern Med. 1980;92:212–26
9. Fox RI, Saito I. Criteria for diagnosis of Sjögren's syndrome. Rheum Dis North Am. 1994;20: 391–407.
10. Daniels TE, Silverman S, Michalski JP, Greenspan JS, Sylvester RA, Talal N. The oral component of Sjögren's syndrome. Oral Surg Oral Med Oral Pathol. 1975;39:875–85.
11. Daniels TE. Labial salivary gland biopsy in Sjögren's syndrome: assessment as a diagnostic criterion in 362 suspected cases. Arthritis Rheum. 1984; 27:147–56.
12. Manthorpe R, Oxholm P, Prause JU, Schiodt M. The Copenhagen criteria for Sjögren's syndrome. Scand J Rheumatol. 1986;(Suppl 61):19–21.
13. Homma M, Tojo T, Akizuki M, Yamagata H. Criteria for Sjögren's syndrome in Japan. Scand J Rheumatol. 1986;(Suppl 61):26–27.
14. Skopouli FN, Drosos AA, Papaioannou T, Moutsopoulos HM. Preliminary diagnostic criteria for Sjögren's syndrome. Scand J Rheumatol. 1986;(Suppl 61):22–25.
15. Fox RI, Robinson CA, Curd JG, Kozin F, Howell FV. Sjögren's syndrome. Proposed criteria for classification. Arthritis Rheum. 1986;29:577–85.
16. Fujibayashi T, SugaiS, Myasaka N, Tojo T, Miyawaki S, Ichikawa Y, et al. Criteria for the diagnosis of Sjögren's syndrome [Japanese criteria III]. Annual reports of research group of autoimmune disease 1999;135–8.
17. Atkinson JC, Travis WD, Slocum L, Ebbs WL, Fox PC. Serum anti-SS-B/La and IgA rheumatoid factor are markers of salivary gland disease activity in primary Sjögren's syndrome. Arthritis Rheum. 1992;35:1368–72.
18. Daniels TE, Witcher JP. Association of patterns of labial salivary gland inflammation with keratoconjunctivitis sicca. Analysis of 618 patients with suspected Sjögren's syndrome. Arthritis Rheum. 1994;6:869–77.
19. Workshop on diagnostic criteria for Sjögren's syndrome: I. Questionnaires for dry eye and dry mouth. II. Manual of methods and procedures. Clin Exp Rheumatol. 1989;7:212–9.
20. Vitali C, Bombardieri S, Moutsopoulos HM, Balestrieri G, Bencivelli W, Bernstein RM, Bjerrum

KB, Braga S, Coll J, de Vita S, et al. Preliminary criteria for the classification of Sjögren's syndrome. Results of a prospective concerted action supported by the European community. Arthritis Rheum. 1993;36:340–7.
21. Arnett FC, Edworthy SM, Bloch DA, McShane DJ, Fries JF, Cooper NS, Healey LA, Kaplan SR, Liang MH, Luthra HS, Medsger TA, Mitchell DM, et al. The 1987 revised American association criteria for classification of rheumatoid arthritis. Arthritis Rheum. 1988;31:315–24.
22. Vitali C, Bombardieri S, Moutsopoulos HM, Coll J, Gerli R, Hatron PY, Kater L, Konttinen YT, Manthorpe R, Meyer O, Mosca M, Ostuni P, Pellerito RA, Pennec Y, Porter SR, Richards A, Sauvezie B, Schiødt M, Sciuto M, Shoenfeld Y, Skopouli FN, Smolen JS, Soromenho F, Tishler M, Wattiaux MJ, et al. Assessment of the European classification criteria for Sjögren's syndrome in a series of clinically defined cases: results of a prospective multicentre study. The European Study Group on Diagnostic Criteria for Sjögren's Syndrome. Ann Rheum Dis. 1996;55:116–121.
23. Fox RI, Saito I. Summary of the IVth International Sjögren's syndrome meeting. Arthritis Rheum. 1994;37:771–2.
24. Fox RI. Fifth international symposium on Sjögren's syndrome. Arthritis Rheum. 1996;39:195–6
25. Vitali C, Bombardieri S, Jonsson R, Moutsopoulos HM, Alexander EL, Carson SE, Daniels TE, Fox PC, Fox RI, Kassan SS, Pillemer SR, Talal N, Weismanet MH. Classification criteria for Sjögren's syndrome: a revised version of the European criteria proposed by the American–European Consensus Group. Ann Rheum Dis. 2002;61:554–8.
26. Ramos-Casals M, Garcia Carrasco M, Cervera R, Rosas J, Trejo O, dela Red G, et al. Hepatitis C virus infection mimicking primary Sjögren's syndrome. A clinical and immunologic description of 35 cases. Medicine (Baltimore). 2001;80:1–8.
27. Manthorpe R. Sjögren's syndrome criteria. American–European and Japanese Groups' criteria compared and contrasted. Ann Rheum Dis. 2002;61:482–4
28. Brun JG, Madland TM, Gjesdal CB, Bertelsen LT. Sjögren's syndrome in an out-patient clinic: classification of patients according to the preliminary European criteria and the proposed modified European criteria. Rheumatology (Oxford). 2002;41: 301–4.
29. Sánchez-Guerrero J, Pérez-Dosal MR, Cárdenas-Velázquez F, Pérez-Reguera A, Celis-Aguilar E, Soto-Rojas AE, Avila-Casado C. Prevalence of Sjögren's syndrome in ambulatory patients according to the American–European Consensus Group criteria. Rheumatology (Oxford). 2005;44:235–40.
30. Zhao Y, Kang J, Zheng WJ, Zhou W, Guo XP, Gao Y, Dong Y. Evaluation of international classification criteria (2002) for primary Sjögren's syndrome in Chinese patients. Chin Med Sci J. 2005;20:190–3.
31. Alamanos Y, Tsifetaki N, Voulgari PV, Venetsanopoulou AI, Siozos C, Drosos AA. Epidemiology of primary Sjögren's syndrome in north-west Greece, 1982–2003. Rheumatology. 2006;45:187–91.
32. Kabasakal Y, Kitapcioglu G, Turk T, Oder G, Durusoy R, Mete N, Egrilmez S, Akalin T. The prevalence of Sjögren's syndrome in adult women. Scand J Rheumatol. 2006;35:379–83.
33. Haugen AJ, Peen E, Hultén B, Johannessen AC, Brun JG, Halse AK, Haga HJ. Estimation of the prevalence of primary Sjögren's syndrome in two age-different community-based populations using two sets of classification criteria: the Hordaland Health Study. Scand J Rheumatol. 2008;37:30–4.
34. Vitali C. Measurement of disease activity and damage in Sjögren's syndrome. Rheum Dis Clin North Am. 2008;34:963–71.
35. Pollard L, Choy EH, Scott DL. The consequences of rheumatoid arthritis: quality of life measures in the individual patient. Clin Exp Rheumatol. 2005;23(Suppl. 39): S43–S52.
36. Strombeck B, Ekdahl C, Manthorpe R, Wikstrom I, Jacobson L. Health related quality of life in primary Sjögren's syndrome, rheumatoid arthritis, fibromyalgia compared to normal population data using SF-36. Scand J Rheumatol. 2000;29:20–8.
37. Bowman AJ, Booth DA, Blatts RG, Field A, Rostron J, The UK Sjögren's Interest Group. Validation of the Sicca Symptoms Inventory for clinical studies of Sjögren's syndrome. J Rheumatol. 2003;30:1259–66.
38. Bowman AJ, Booth DA, Platts RG, The UK Sjögren's Interest Group. Measurement of fatigue and discomfort in primary Sjögren's syndrome using a new questionnaire tool. Rheumatology. 2004;43:758–64.
39. Sutcliffe N, Stoll T, Pyke S, Isenberg DA. Functional disability and end organ damage in patients with systemic lupus erythematosus (SLE), SLE and Sjögren's syndrome (SS) and primary Sjögren's syndrome. J Rheumatol. 1998;25:63–8.
40. Stewart AL, Hays RD, Ware JE. The MOS short-form general health survey. Med Care. 1988;26:724–35.
41. Gladman D, Ginzler E, Goldsmith C, et al. The development and initial validation of the systemic lupus international collaborating clinics/American College of Rheumatology damage index for systemic lupus erythematosus. Arthritis Rheum. 1996;39:363–9.
42. Bowman S, Pillemer S, Jonsson R, et al. Revisiting Sjögren's syndrome in the new millennium: perspectives on assessment and outcome measures. Report of a workshop held on 23 March 2000 at Oxford, UK. Rheumatology (Oxford). 2001;40:1180–8.
43. Asmussen KH, Bowman S. Outcome measures in Sjögren's syndrome. Rheumatology (Oxford). 2001;40:1085–8.
44. Bowman S. Collaborative research into outcome measures in Sjögren's syndrome. Update on disease assessment. Scand J Rheumatol. 2002;31(Suppl 116):23–7.

45. Pillemer SR, Smith J, Fox PC, Bowman SJ. Outcome measures for Sjögren's syndrome, April 10–11, 2003, Bethesda, Maryland, USA. J Rheumatol. 2004;31:143–9.
46. Schiffman RM, Christianson MD, Jacobson G, Hirsch JD, Reins BL. Reliability and validity of the ocular surface disease index. Arch Ophthalmol. 2000;118:615–21.
47. Thomson WM, Chalmers JM, Spencer AJ, Williams SM. The xerostomia inventory: a multi-item approach to measuring dry mouth. Comm Dent Health. 1999;159:174–81.
48. Smets EM, Garssen B, Bonke B, De Haes JC. The multidimensional fatigue inventory (MFI), psychometric qualities of an instrument to assess fatigue. J Psychosom Res. 1995;39:315–25.
49. Bowman SJ, Sutcliffe N, Isenberg DA, Goldblatt F, Adler M, Price E, Canavan A, Hamburger J, Richards A, Rauz S, Regan M, Gadsby K, Rigby S, Jones A, Mathew R, Mulherin D, Stevenson A, Nightingale P. Sjogren's systemic clinical activity index (SCAI)—a systemic disease activity measure for use in clinical trials in primary Sjogren's syndrome. Rheumatology (Oxford). 2007;46:1845–51.
50. Hay EM, Bacon PA, Gordon C, et al. The BILAG index: a reliable and valid instrument for measuring clinical disease activity in systemic lupus erythematosus. Q J Med. 1993;86:447–58.
51. Barry RJ, Sutcliffe N, Isenberg DA, Price E, Goldblatt F, Adler M, Canavan A, Hamburger J, Richards A, Regan M, Gadsby K, Rigby S, Jones A, Mathew R, Mulherin D, Stevenson A, Nightingale P, Rauz S, Bowman SJ. The Sjogren's syndrome damage index—a damage index for use in clinical trials and observational studies in primary Sjogren's syndrome. Rheumatology. 2008;47:1193–8.
52. Vitali C, Palombi G, Baldini C, Benucci M, Bombardieri S, Covelli M, Del Papa N, De Vita S, Epis O, Franceschini F, Gerli R, Govoni M, Maddali Bongi S, Maglione W, Migliaresi S, Montecucco C, Orefice M, Priori R, Tavoni A, Valesini G. Sjögren's syndrome disease damage index and disease activity index: scoring systems for the assessment of disease damage and disease activity in Sjögren's syndrome, derived from an analysis of a cohort of Italian patients. Arthritis Rheum. 2007;56: 2223–31.
53. Vitali C. Measurement of disease activity and damage in Sjögren's syndrome. Rheum Dis Clin North Am. 2008;34:963–71.
54. Seror R, Ravaud P, Bowman SJ, Baron G, Tzioufas A, Theander E, Gottenberg JE, Bootsma H, Mariette X, Vitali C. EULAR Sjögren's Task Force. EULAR Sjogren's syndrome disease activity index: development of a consensus systemic disease activity index for primary Sjogren's syndrome. Ann Rheum Dis. 2010;69:1103–9.
55. Seror R, Ravaud P, Mariette X, Bootsma H, Theander E, Hansen A, Ramos-Casals M, Dörner T, Bombardieri S, Hachulla E, Brun JG, Kruize AA, Praprotnik S, Tomsic M, Gottenberg JE, Devauchelle V, Devita S, Vollenweider C, Mandl T, Tzioufas A, Carsons S, Saraux A, Sutcliffe N, Vitali C, Bowman SJ, On behalf of the EULAR Sjögren's Task Force. EULAR Sjogren's syndrome patient reported index (ESSPRI): development of a consensus patient index for primary Sjogren's syndrome. Ann Rheum Dis. 2011;70:968–72.
56. Seror R, Mariette X, Bowman S, Baron G, Gottenberg JE, Boostma H, Theander E, Tzioufas A, Vitali C, Ravaud P, European League Against Rheumatism Sjögren's Task Force. Accurate detection of changes in disease activity in primary Sjögren's syndrome by the European League Against Rheumatism Sjögren's Syndrome Disease Activity Index. Arthritis Care Res (Hoboken). 2010;62:551–8.

Histopathology and Glandular Biopsies in Sjögren's Syndrome

6

Roland Jonsson, Kathrine Skarstein, and Malin V. Jonsson

Abstract

The glandular inflammatory lesion in Sjögren's syndrome (SS) is a distinctive but not pathognomonic chronic lymphocytic adenitis best characterized in salivary glands. The glands are readily accessible; decreased function gives rise to prominent clinical symptoms and signs; and the glands are affected in almost all patients. A labial salivary gland biopsy specimen can be very disease specific for SS if it is obtained through normal-appearing mucosa, includes ≥5 separate glands separated from their surrounding connective tissue, is interpreted after lobes or glands showing non-specific changes are excluded, demonstrates focal sialadenitis in all or most of the glands in the specimen, and has a focus score that provides a diagnostic threshold. Such glandular biopsies can also provide tissue diagnosis for conditions that can resemble SS clinically, particularly sarcoidosis and amyloidosis. The characteristic pathologic lesion is part of classification criteria for SS and probably provides the best single criterion in terms of its disease sensitivity and specificity, convenience, availability, and low risk. More recently, studies have found germinal center reactions in the glandular biopsies indicating a more severe disease phenotype.

Keywords

Acinar • Chronic inflammation • Degeneration • Ductal • Fibrosis • Focus score • Focal sialadenitis • Lymphocytes • Mononuclear cells • Salivary gland

R. Jonsson (✉)
Broegelmann Research Laboratory, The Gade Institute, University of Bergen, Bergen, Norway; Department of Rheumatology, Haukeland University Hospital, Bergen, Norway
e-mail: roland.jonsson@gades.uib.no

6.1 Introduction

All organs affected by Sjögren's syndrome (SS) display a potentially progressive mononuclear lymphoid cell infiltration. These circumscribed and most often well-defined infiltrates presumably give rise to functional derangements of

R.I. Fox, C.M. Fox (eds.), *Sjögren's Syndrome*, DOI 10.1007/978-1-60327-957-4_6,

the affected organ and to the diverse clinical presentations/features of the syndrome. The inflammatory-related pathologic findings include (1) focal mononuclear cell adenitis of salivary, lacrimal, eccrine, and mucosal glands; (2) primary biliary cirrhosis, sclerosing cholangitis, pancreatitis, and atrophic gastritis; (3) interstitial nephritis; (4) lymphocytic interstitial pneumonitis; (5) peripheral vasculitis; and (6) progression to pseudolymphoma or a B-cell lymphoma (MALT lymphoma).

6.2 Benign Lymphoepithelial Lesion in Salivary Glands

The salivary glands are the most and best-studied organs in SS. This is due to the fact that the glands are readily accessible; decreased function gives rise to prominent clinical symptoms and signs; and the glands are affected in almost all patients. In a great number of patients, the major salivary glands become enlarged and histopathology usually reveals a benign lymphoepithelial lesion [1]. Historically this lesion, first described by Mikulicz (1892) and named by Godwin (1952), is characterized by lymphocytic replacement of the salivary epithelium and by the presence of so-called epimyoepithelial islands.

Histomorphology helps to distinguish this benign lesion from lymphoma [2]. The origin of these islands has been shown to be epithelial but without clear evidence of myoepithelial cells. With regard to the terms "Mikulicz disease" or "Mikulicz syndrome" applied to salivary or lacrimal gland swelling caused by SS, these are so ambiguous and ill-defined that they are recommended not to be used [3]. The solitary diagnosis of salivary benign lymphoepithelial lesion should suggest the presence of SS and additional diagnostic steps should be taken.

The typical histological finding in glandular biopsies is a progressive focal infiltration of mononuclear lymphoid cells (Fig. 6.1). This correlates largely to the reduced salivary secretion [4]. However, the mechanisms leading to attraction and accumulation and the biological role of the infiltrating cells remain undefined [5]. The infiltrating cells may interfere with glandular function at several levels: destruction of glandular structures by cell-mediated mechanisms; secretion of cytokines that activate pathways related to interferons (IFNs); local production of autoantibodies, etc.

The progression of SS to extraglandular B-cell lymphoma is well documented [6–8] and is further presented in Chapter 17. The incidence of non-Hodgkin's lymphoma (NHL), which may be of the MALT type, is in the range of 4–5% [9]. Previous estimates of a more than 40-fold increased risk of NHL were probably too high, as a recent large linked registry study showed

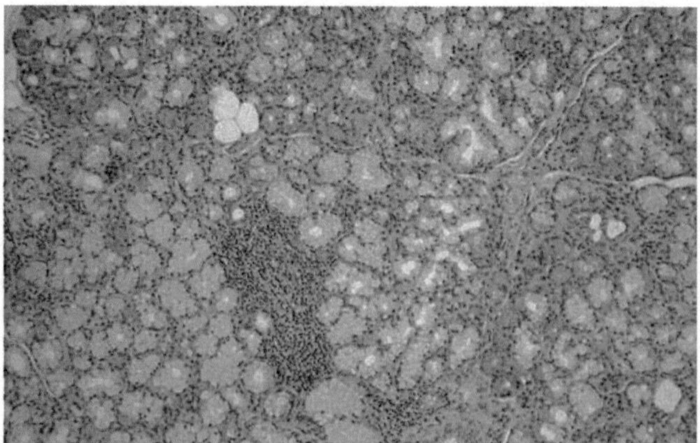

Fig. 6.1 Minor salivary gland tissue sections obtained from a patient with Sjögren's syndrome. Periductal focal mononuclear cell infiltrates are surrounded by normal salivary gland tissue. Note the varying size of the infiltrates; smaller infiltrate indicated by *arrowheads*, larger indicated by *arrows*

a 16-fold increased risk [10]. Predictive factors for lymphoproliferative disease are skin vasculitis/palpable purpura, low C3 and C4, $CD4^+$ T lymphocytopenia and a low $CD4^+/CD8^+$ T-cell ratio, and parotid enlargement at first study visit [10, 11].

6.2.1 Major Salivary Gland Biopsy in Sjögren's Syndrome

Major salivary gland biopsies, more specifically, parotid gland biopsies have not been common for the diagnosis of SS mainly because these procedures carry the potential surgical risks of damage to the facial nerve, cutaneous fistula, and scarring. In addition, parotid gland biopsies are not included in the established classification criteria for diagnosing SS [12]. Consequently, validated histopathological diagnostic criterions based on the biopsy of the parotid gland are lacking.

Earlier studies have reported that diagnosing the salivary component of SS from major salivary gland specimens is problematic as major salivary glands from individuals who do not have SS also commonly contain lymphocytic foci [13]. Examinations of a high number of post-mortem specimen evaluated by focus scoring lymphocytic foci occurred commonly and equally in submandibular, parotid, and lacrimal glands [14]. Inflammatory foci in subjects who had no history of rheumatic disease in both parotid and submandibular glands have been reported in other studies [15, 16].

Lymphomas associated with SS often arise in the parotid gland [9], and in cases where a malignant tumor is suspected a parotid biopsy is performed. Most often lymphoma has been diagnosed in patients with atypical or persistent parotid salivary gland swelling, and biopsy of the affected gland histopathologically confirmed the diagnosis of MALT lymphoma [17, 18]. Incidentally, localization of lymphoma in the labial glands has also been reported [19, 20], underlining the need for degree of awareness of the possibility of lymphoma in salivary gland biopsies from patients with features of SS. In cases where a malignant tumor is suspected a parotid biopsy is compulsory.

Recently, Pijpe et al. [21] proposed that histopathology of the parotid gland should be included in the classification criteria for SS as an alternative for labial glands. Biopsies from both labial and parotid glands of a series of 35 patients suspected for SS were performed in order to assess the value of the parotid biopsy as diagnostic tool for primary SS. Based on these data histopathological conditions of the minor and major glands were reported to be comparable. As discussed, the approach presents some limitations, in particular related to the fact that parotid biopsy requires specific surgical skills/expertise and labial biopsy is more easily performed. However, the diagnostic potential of a parotid biopsy should be reconsidered. Accordingly, there is need for larger comparative studies of labial and parotid glands to find out the best diagnostic tools for histopathologic evaluation of SS [22].

6.3 Minor Salivary Gland Biopsy in Sjögren's Syndrome—A Comparison of Biopsy Techniques

In principal, three methods of performing minor salivary gland biopsies have been described. A skin trephine ("punch") to remove a core of tissue either from the lip or the palate is rapid and easily done, but most often does not provide enough glandular tissue for examination. Removing an ellipse of labial mucosa that includes all tissue above the orbicularis oris muscle may damage sensory nerves and is very unpredictable with regard to representative glandular material for analysis [23].

The third method, labial salivary gland biopsy by obtaining separate glands, has become the most important in establishing the diagnosis of Sjögren's syndrome. It is performed preferentially according to the procedure described by Daniels (Fig. 6.2) [24, 25]. After local anesthesia, a 1.5–2-cm linear incision in normal-appearing labial mucosa is made parallel to the vermilion

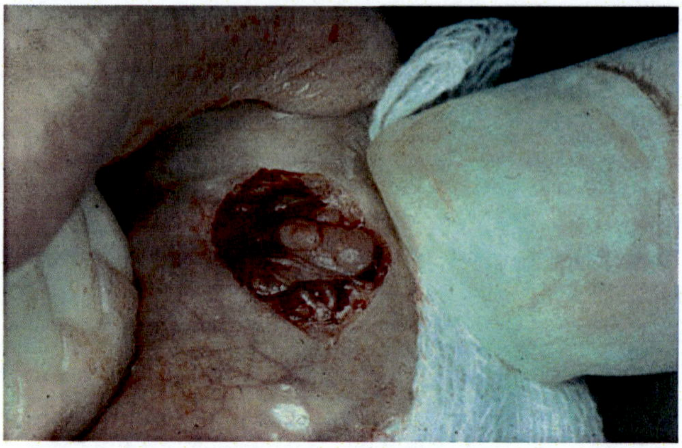

Fig. 6.2 Biopsy procedure for minor labial salivary glands. The area is numbed with adrenaline-containing local anesthesia. A 1.5–2-cm linear incision in normal-appearing labial mucosa is then made parallel to the vermilion border in the middle of the lower lip, between the midline and the corner of the mouth. At least five lobes of labial glands are then obtained by blunt dissection, providing enough minor glands for routine diagnosis and with a low risk of sensory nerve damage

border in the middle of the lower lip, between the midline and the corner of the mouth. At least five lobes of labial glands are then obtained by blunt dissection, which can be separately processed for routine and, if desired, be additionally processed for immunomorphological and/or transcriptomic/proteomic analysis. The advantage with this method is that it provides enough minor glands for routine diagnosis, carries a low risk of sensory nerve damage, and allows a midplane histologic section to be prepared simultaneously for all glands in the specimen.

With any of the techniques described, labial midline biopsies should be avoided because there are few minor glands in the midline of the lip.

The incidence of permanent sensory loss or long-term numbness with labial biopsy varies between different studies [20, 24, 26, 27]. When comparing the morbidity (pain, sensory loss, and motor function) of different biopsy techniques one should be aware of the importance of using independent clinicians in the assessment of the adverse effects. It has been demonstrated that the incision biopsy of the parotid gland in experienced hands is a safe procedure showing only temporarily hypoesthesia [21, 28]. Nevertheless, in skilled hands both labial and parotid gland biopsies will result in minimal adverse effects.

After routine histologic fixation and preparation (embedding in paraffin at a level such that a section can be cut through the approximate midplane of each gland), the biopsy is examined/evaluated according to a method in which a focus is defined as an accumulation of at least 50 inflammatory mononuclear cells per 4 mm^2 (Fig. 6.3) [25]. According to the original and revised European criteria [12, 29], a biopsy is positive if the focus score is more than or equal to 1 per 4 mm^2, whereas the California criteria define a positive biopsy as more than 1 focus per 4 mm^2 [30]. Occasionally, islands of degenerating epithelium (lymphoepithelial lesions) together with chronic inflammatory cells are seen in labial gland biopsies (Fig. 6.4), but such structures are more common in the major glands. One differential diagnostic feature is the presence of granulomatous inflammation, which is seen with sarcoidosis but not with Sjögren's syndrome (Fig. 6.4).

When evaluating the biopsies for focus scoring certain exclusions have to be made: (1) lobes with duct dilation and extravasated polymorphonuclear leukocytes, (2) extensive degeneration, and (3) extensive fatty replacement or fibrosis of glandular tissue.

Focal mononuclear cell inflammation may be observed in cases of obstructed salivary glands

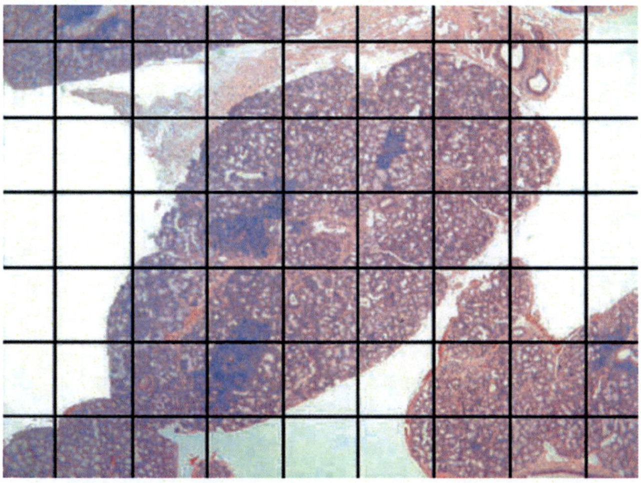

Fig. 6.3 Determining the degree of inflammation by focus score. When assessing focus score, a grid is commonly used to determine the total area of the glandular tissue. The number of foci containing 50 or more cells is then quantified. Focus score is then calculated as the number of focal mononuclear cell infiltrates per 4 mm^2 of intact minor salivary gland tissue

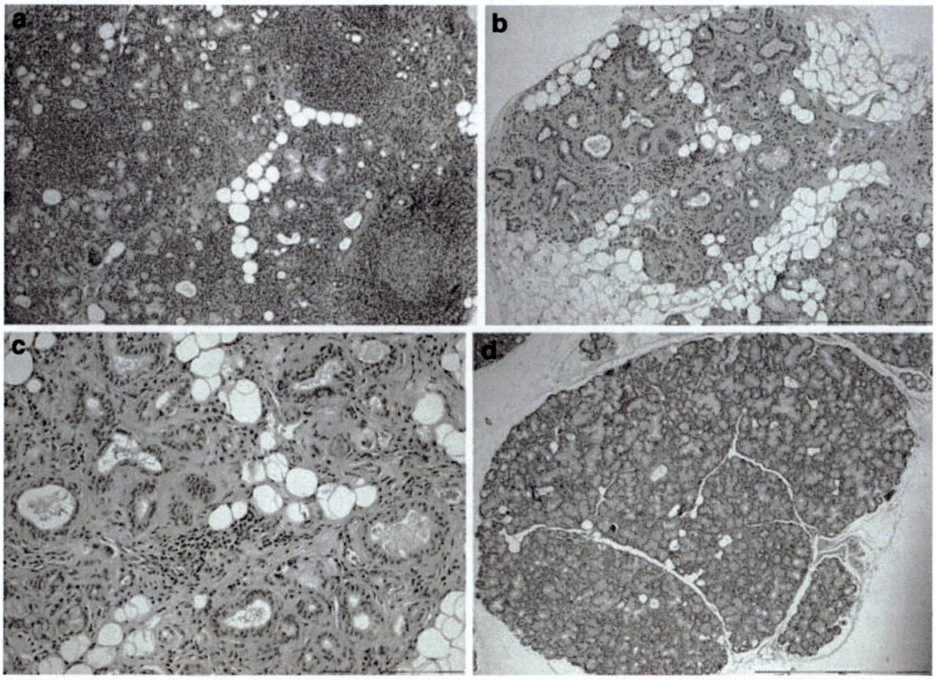

Fig. 6.4 Variants of minor salivary gland histomorphology. **a** Focal infiltrates and germinal center formation. **b** Fat cell degeneration, atrophy of acinar cells, and periductal fibrosis. **c** Atrophic areas of salivary gland tissue infiltrated by plasma cells. **d** Normal salivary gland tissue

(mucocele/mucous retention cyst) or under traumatized mucosa (biting). The biopsy should therefore be obtained from clinically healthy and normal-appearing mucosa.

Chisholm and Mason [31] introduced a grading system for semiquantitative assessment of chronic inflammation in labial gland biopsies. They found that more than 1 focus of lymphoid mononuclear cells per 4 mm^2 area of gland was found only in SS patients and was not present in post-mortem specimens. In general, focal infiltration is an uncommon finding in labial glands except in SS. However, studies of submandibular glands have shown a high prevalence of lymphocytic foci [32].

The focus scoring utilized most often today builds on the grading studies by Chisholm and Mason [31]. This scoring enumerates scores from 1 to 12 foci per 4 mm^2 [33] and found that there was a significant positive correlation between higher focus scores and larger foci. Within the foci the proportion of plasma cell or activated lymphocytes decreased sharply as focus size increased. A number of studies by Daniels followed on this theme [24, 25, 34]. Most subsequent studies have verified a high sensitivity of the labial gland biopsies in SS and present figures as 68 and 81%, respectively [35, 36]. The specificity of a positive labial salivary gland biopsy is 86.2%, and the sensitivity is 82.4% in patients with primary Sjögren's syndrome diagnosed according to the European criteria [37].

6.3.1 Characteristics of Focal Mononuclear Cell Infiltration in Labial Minor Salivary Glands

6.3.1.1 Focal Infiltration

The focal infiltration of lymphoid cells in the salivary glands is mostly a slow, progressive process in Sjögren's syndrome, as demonstrated by an increase in the focus score over time [4]. The focus score is associated with the presence of keratoconjunctivitis sicca and autoantibodies [34, 38], whereas the correlation with xerostomia is less evident [4].

Although the methodology in assessing the focus score of labial salivary glands is standardized and regarded as an important diagnostic tool in the histopathological evaluation, its reproducibility between the different pathologists and at different section levels within the same samples seems to be low [39, 40]. To overcome the problem with non-homogenous distribution of the inflammatory infiltrates in the glands and the sample size, a multilevel analysis of labial glands was proposed [41]. The authors concluded that the evaluation of a cumulative focus score on three different section levels on labial salivary gland biopsy could improve the diagnostic accuracy of the criteria set used for SS classification, especially in biopsies with a baseline focus score between 1 and 2.

Another recent study [20] did a retrospective analysis of 452 patients who underwent minimally invasive minor salivary gland biopsy as a part of an evaluation of SS in order to evaluate the efficacy of labial biopsy in diagnostic routine application. Taking in mind the limitations of retrospective studies, their data showed that multilevel examination improved the contribution of labial salivary gland biopsy to SS diagnosis. In contrast, others reported persistence of focus score at different section levels in a smaller cohort of primary SS patients ($n = 24$) [42].

The histopathological characteristics of labial salivary glands in SS are those of a primary lymphocytic infiltrate in otherwise generally normal-appearing glands and include (1) focal aggregates of at least 50 lymphocytes, plasma cells, and macrophages, adjacent to and replacing normal-appearing acini and (2) consistent presence of these foci in all or most of the glands in the specimen, but with variability in the number of foci per gland [23]. Larger foci often exhibit formation of germinal centers in approximately one-fourth of patients in larger cohorts of SS patients [43–45].

Another pattern of inflammation in labial salivary gland biopsy is chronic sialadenitis, characterized by scattered mononuclear cell infiltration without focal aggregates and accompanied by degenerative changes such as acinar atrophy, ductal hyperplasia, fibrosis, and/or fatty infiltration

(Fig. 6.4). This pattern is not considered to be associated with primary SS and often progresses to glandular atrophy and xerostomia.

6.3.1.2 Ectopic Germinal Center Formation

Germinal centers (GCs) were defined as well-circumscribed inflammatory foci containing at least 50 mononuclear cells, presenting with a dark and light zone, within otherwise normal salivary gland epithelium [44]. Densely packed proliferating cells (centroblasts) are localized in the dark zone. The dark zone is surrounded by the proposed GC light zone which is more richly supplied with follicular dendritic cells and less densely packed with cells (centrocytes) [46].

Such lymphoid neogenesis has previously described with the presence of ectopic follicles/GC in 20–25% of patients with SS [43–45, 47–49]. Similar features have been described in other autoimmune diseases such as rheumatoid arthritis (RA) [50], myasthenia gravis [51], multiple sclerosis [52], during chronic *Helicobacter pylori* infections in gastric mucosa [53], in chronic inflammatory disorders of the liver [54], Hashimotos disease [55], and in oral buccal mucosa related to amalgam fillings and lichenoid reactions [56, 57].

Germinal center formation was investigated in more detail [48], and the contemporary existence of GC and focal interaction (FI) was disclosed. GCs were characterized by B-cell and T-cell organization, increased levels of proliferating cells, follicular dendritic cell networks, and the localization of plasma cells in a mantel zone-like area.

6.3.1.3 Clinical Implications of Ectopic Germinal Center Formation

By morphology, GC-like structures were detected in 47/169 of patients [44]. Focus score, IgG levels, and RF titres were elevated compared to the GC− patients. Mean unstimulated salivary flow was reduced in the GC+ patients [44].

An association of GC development with increased risk of B-cell lymphomas has been proposed [9], wherein formation of proliferating GCs were thought to contribute to malignant transformation and development of MALT lymphoma. The estimated life-time risk of lymphoma in SS has been estimated to be 5–10% [9, 11], but in general mortality is not significantly increased compared to the general population [58]. Patients with SS and chronic *H. pylori* infection are at increased risk for developing lymphomas, possibly related to prolonged lymphocytic activation in the target organ(s) of these patients [59, 60]. In a recent study, significant predictors of lymphoproliferative disease were purpura/skin vasculitis, low levels of complement factors C3/C4, $CD4^+$ T lymphocytopenia and a low $CD4^+/CD8^+$ T-cell ratio [11, 61].

Results from Refs. [43, 44] indicate a certain clinical immunological phenotype for SS patients with ectopic lymphoid organization, which warrant further studies. Whether ectopic GC identifies patients at risk to develop lymphoma remains to be seen in prospective studies.

6.4 Late Breaking Update

Several studies regarding histopathological features in the minor salivary glands have been published since the submission of this manuscript in late 2008 and its publishing in 2011. In this section we present some of these contributions.

Histopathological studies of the minor salivary glands have unraveled an interest in both the infiltrating inflammatory cells and the salivary gland epithelium. Stromal changes such as fat/adipose tissue, both in the form of degenerative changes as a consequence of chronic "burned out" inflammation [62] and as a possible source of chemokines [63] as resident adipocytes, expressed CXCL12 in the minor salivary glands of patients with pSS, possibly providing survival niches for long-lived plasma cells.

A recently published study [64] investigated lymphoid organization (Fig. 6.4) in labial salivary gland tissue biopsies available from two Swedish pSS patient cohorts ($n = 175$), by light microscopy in a blinded study in order to identify

GC-like structures as a sign of ectopic lymphoid tissue formation and organization. At diagnosis, 25% of pSS patients were found to have GC-like structures in their salivary glands, corresponding to previous [43–45, 48] and more recent findings in other cohorts [62, 65, 66]. Through a linkage study with the Swedish cancer registry 7 of 175 patients studied (14% of GC+ and 0.8% of GC-) went on to develop NHL in a total of 1855 patient years at risk, with a median onset of 7 years following the initial diagnostic salivary gland biopsy. Six of these seven patients had GC-like structures at diagnosis; the remaining patient was GC negative at the time of diagnosis ($p = 0.001$). In a Greek study investigating major infiltrating cells in salivary gland infiltrates of various severity three of seven cases with lymphoma also presented with GC-like structures in the minor salivary glands ($p = 0.005$) [65].

In a Norwegian cohort of pSS ($n = 141$), interleukin (IL)-17, IL-1RA, IL-15, macrophage inflammatory protein 1 (MIP-1), eotaxin, interferon (IFN), and IL-4 levels were significantly increased in the 27 (23%) patients with ectopic germinal center formation (GC+) in the salivary glands compared with the GC- patients ($n = 70$). In addition, minor differences in cytokine levels were found when comparing age groups [62]. Increased titers of Th17-associated cytokines, IL-17, IL-1, and the IL-23 subunit IL-12p40, were speculated to indicate a higher activity of these cells in GC+ patients.

Taken together, these findings indicate an important role for the minor salivary gland biopsy in the diagnostic evaluation for primary Sjögren's syndrome – a highly predictive and easy to obtain marker for NHL development. Furthermore, such a marker may allow for risk stratification of patients and the possibility to initiate preventive B-cell directed therapy.

References

1. Seifert G, Sobin LH. Histological typing of salivary gland tumors. 2nd ed. Berlin: Springer; 1991, pp. 107–8.
2. Morgan WS, Castleman B. A clinicopathologic study of Mikulicz's disease. Am J Pathol. 1953 May-Jun;29(3):471–503.
3. Batsakis JG. The pathology of head and neck tumors: the lymphoepithelial lesion and Sjögren's syndrome, Part 16. Head Neck Surg. 1982 Nov-Dec;5(2):150–63.
4. Jonsson R, Kroneld U, Backman K, Magnusson B, Tarkowski A. Progression of sialadenitis in Sjögren's syndrome. Br J Rheumatol. 1993 Jul;32(7):578–81.
5. Delaleu N, Jonsson MV, Jonsson R. Disease mechanisms of Sjögren's syndrome. Drug Disco Today Disease Mech [Review]. 2004;1(3):329–36.
6. Anderson LG, Talal N. The spectrum of benign to malignant lymphoproliferation in Sjögren's syndrome. Clin Exp Immunol. 1972 Feb;10(2):199–221.
7. Kassan SS, Thomas TL, Moutsopoulos HM, Hoover R, Kimberly RP, Budman DR, et al. Increased risk of lymphoma in sicca syndrome. Ann Intern Med. 1978 Dec;89(6):888–92.
8. Zulman J, Jaffe R, Talal N. Evidence that the malignant lymphoma of Sjögren's syndrome is a monoclonal B-cell neoplasm. N Engl J Med. 1978 Nov 30;299(22):1215–20.
9. Voulgarelis M, Dafni UG, Isenberg DA, Moutsopoulos HM. Malignant lymphoma in primary Sjögren's syndrome: a multicenter, retrospective, clinical study by the European Concerted Action on Sjögren's Syndrome. Arthritis Rheum. 1999 Aug;42(8):1765–72.
10. Theander E, Henriksson G, Ljungberg O, Mandl T, Manthorpe R, Jacobsson LT. Lymphoma and other malignancies in primary Sjögren's syndrome: a cohort study on cancer incidence and lymphoma predictors. Ann Rheum Dis. 2006 Jun;65(6):796–803.
11. Ioannidis JP, Vassiliou VA, Moutsopoulos HM. Long-term risk of mortality and lymphoproliferative disease and predictive classification of primary Sjögren's syndrome. Arthritis Rheum. 2002 Mar;46(3):741–7.
12. Vitali C, Bombardieri S, Jonsson R, Moutsopoulos HM, Alexander EL, Carsons SE, et al. Classification criteria for Sjögren's syndrome: a revised version of the European criteria proposed by the American-European Consensus Group. Ann Rheum Dis. 2002 Jun;61(6):554–8.
13. Batsakis JG. Tumors of the head and neck: clinical and pathological considerations. 2nd ed. Baltimore, MD: Williams & Wilkins; 1979, pp. 105–12.
14. Waterhouse JP. Focal adenitis in salivary and lacrimal glands. Proc R Soc Med. 1963 Oct;56:911–8.
15. Waterhouse JP, Doniach I. Post-mortem prevalence of focal lymphocytic adenitis of the submandibular salivary gland. J Pathol Bacteriol. 1966 Jan;91(1):53–64.
16. Scott J. The incidence of focal chronic inflammatory changes in human submandibular salivary glands. J Oral Pathol. 1976 Nov;5(6):334–46.

17. Klussmann JP, Wagner M, Guntinas-Lichius O, Müller A. Detection of HHV-8 sequences and antigens in a MALT lymphoma associated with Sjögren's syndrome. J Oral Pathol Med. 2003;32:243–5.
18. De Vita S, De Marchi G, Sacco S, Gremese E, Fabris M, Ferraccioli G. Preliminary classification of nonmalignant B cell proliferation in Sjögren's syndrome: perspectives on pathobiology and treatment based on an integrated clinico-pathologic and molecular study approach. Blood Cells Mols Dis. 2001;27: 757–66.
19. Van Mello NM, Pillemer SR, Tak PP, Sankar V. B cell MALT lymphoma diagnosed by labial minor salivary gland biopsy in patients screened for Sjögren's syndrome. Ann Rheum Dis. 2005 Mar;64(3):471–3.
20. Caporali R, Bonacci E, Epis O, Bobbio-Pallavicini F, Morbini P, Montecucco C. Safety and usefulness of minor salivary gland biopsy: retrospective analysis of 502 procedures performed at a single center. Arthritis Rheum. 2008 May 15;59(5):714–20.
21. Pijpe J, Kalk WW, van der Wal JE, Vissink A, Kluin PM, Roodenburg JL, et al. Parotid gland biopsy compared with labial biopsy in the diagnosis of patients with primary Sjögren's syndrome. Rheumatology (Oxford). 2007 Feb;46(2):335–41.
22. Caporali R, Bonacci E, Epis O, Morbini P, Montecucco C. Comment on: parotid gland biopsy compared with labial biopsy in the diagnosis of patients with primary Sjögren's syndrome. Rheumatology (Oxford). 2007 Oct;46(10):1625–6.
23. Daniels TE, Aufdemorte TB, Greenspan JS. Histopathology of Sjögren's syndrome. In: Talal N, Moutsopoulos HM, Kassan SS, editors. Sjögren's syndrome – clinical and immunological aspects. Berlin: Springer; 1987, pp. 41–52.
24. Daniels TE. Labial salivary gland biopsy in Sjögren's syndrome. Assessment as a diagnostic criterion in 362 suspected cases. Arthritis Rheum. 1984;27(2):147–56.
25. Daniels TE. Salivary histopathology in diagnosis of Sjögren's syndrome. Scand J Rheumatol Suppl. 1986;61:36–43.
26. Richards A, Mutlu S, Scully C, Maddison P. Complications associated with labial salivary gland biopsy in the investigation of connective tissue disorders. Ann Rheum Dis. 1992 Aug;51(8):996–7.
27. Friedman JA, Miller EB, Huszar M. A simple technique for minor salivary gland biopsy appropriate for use by rheumatologists in an outpatient setting. Clin Rheumatol. 2002 Aug;21(4):349–50.
28. Biasi D, Mocella S, Caramaschi P, Carletto A, Baracchino F, Colletti V, et al. Utility and safety of parotid gland biopsy in Sjögren's syndrome. Acta Otolaryngol. 1996 Nov;116(6):896–9.
29. Vitali C, Bombardieri S, Moutsopoulos HM, Balestrieri G, Bencivelli W, Bernstein RM, et al. Preliminary criteria for the classification of Sjogren's syndrome. Results of a prospective concerted action supported by the European Community. Arthritis Rheum. 1993 Mar;36(3):340–7.
30. Fox RI, Robinson CA, Curd JG, Kozin F, Howell FV. Sjögren's syndrome. Proposed criteria for classification. Arthritis Rheum. 1986 May;29(5): 577–85.
31. Chisholm DM, Mason DK. Labial salivary gland biopsy in Sjögren's disease. J Clin Pathol. 1968 Sep;21(5):656–60.
32. Chisholm DM, Waterhouse JP, Mason DK. Lymphocytic sialadenitis in the major and minor glands: a correlation in postmortem subjects. J Clin Pathol. 1970 Nov;23(8):690–4.
33. Greenspan JS, Daniels TE, Talal N, Sylvester RA. The histopathology of Sjögren's syndrome in labial salivary gland biopsies. Oral Surg Oral Med Oral Pathol. 1974 Feb;37(2):217–29.
34. Daniels TE, Whitcher JP. Association of patterns of labial salivary gland inflammation with keratoconjunctivitis sicca. Analysis of 618 patients with suspected Sjögren's syndrome. Arthritis Rheum. 1994 Jun;37(6):869–77.
35. Whaley K, Williamson J, Chisholm DM, Webb J, Mason DK, Buchanan WW. Sjögren's syndrome. I. Sicca components. Q J Med. 1973 Apr;42(166): 279–304.
36. Takeda Y. Histopathological studies of the labial salivary glands in patients with Sjogren's syndrome. Part I: light microscopic study. Bull Tokyo Med Dent Univ. 1980/03/01 ed 1980:9–25.
37. Vitali C, Moutsopoulos HM, Bombardieri S. The European Community Study Group on diagnostic criteria for Sjögren's syndrome. Sensitivity and specificity of tests for ocular and oral involvement in Sjögren's syndrome. Ann Rheum Dis. 1994 Oct;53(10):637–47.
38. Atkinson JC, Travis WD, Slocum L, Ebbs WL, Fox PC. Serum anti-SS-B/La and IgA rheumatoid factor are markers of salivary gland disease activity in primary Sjögren's syndrome. Arthritis Rheum. 1992 Nov;35(11):1368–72.
39. Vivino FB, Gala I, Hermann GA. Change in final diagnosis on second evaluation of labial minor salivary gland biopsies. J Rheumatol. 2002 May;29(5): 938–44.
40. Al-Hashimi I, Wright JM, Cooley CA, Nunn ME. Reproducibility of biopsy grade in Sjögren's syndrome. J Oral Pathol Med. 2001 Aug;30(7): 408–12.
41. Morbini P, Manzo A, Caporali R, Epis O, Villa C, Tinelli C, et al. Multilevel examination of minor salivary gland biopsy for Sjögren's syndrome significantly improves diagnostic performance of AECG classification criteria. Arthritis Res Ther. 2005;7(2):R343–8.
42. Scardina GA, Spano G, Carini F, Spicola M, Valenza V, Messina P, et al. Diagnostic evaluation of serial sections of labial salivary gland biopsies in Sjögren's syndrome. Med Oral Pathol Oral Cir Bucal. 2007 Dec;12(8):E565–8.
43. Jonsson MV, Skarstein K. Follicular dendritic cells confirm lymphoid organization in the minor salivary

glands of primary Sjögren's syndrome. J Oral Pathol Med. 2008 Oct;37(9):515–21.
44. Jonsson MV, Skarstein K, Jonsson R, Brun JG. Serological implications of germinal center-like structures in primary Sjögren's syndrome. J Rheumatol. 2007 Oct;34(10):2044–9.
45. Salomonsson S, Jonsson MV, Skarstein K, Brokstad KA, Hjelmström P, Wahren-Herlenius M, et al. Cellular basis of ectopic germinal center formation and autoantibody production in the target organ of patients with Sjögren's syndrome. Arthritis Rheum. 2003 Nov;48(11):3187–201.
46. Janeway CA, Travers P, Walport M, Schlomchik M. Immunobiology: the immune system in health and disease. 6th ed. New York: Garland Science Publishing; 2005, p. 378.
47. Amft N, Curnow SJ, Scheel-Toellner D, Devadas A, Oates J, Crocker J, et al. Ectopic expression of the B cell-attracting chemokine BCA-1 (CXCL13) on endothelial cells and within lymphoid follicles contributes to the establishment of germinal center-like structures in Sjögren's syndrome. Arthritis Rheum. 2001 Nov;44(11):2633–41.
48. Jonsson MV, Szodoray P, Jellestad S, Jonsson R, Skarstein K. Association between circulating levels of the novel TNF family members APRIL and BAFF and lymphoid organization in primary Sjögren's syndrome. J Clin Immunol. 2005 May;25(3): 189–201.
49. Stott DI, Hiepe F, Hummel M, Steinhauser G, Berek C. Antigen-driven clonal proliferation of B cells within the target tissue of an autoimmune disease. The salivary glands of patients with Sjögren's syndrome. J Clin Invest. 1998 Sep 1;102(5):938–46.
50. Takemura S, Braun A, Crowson C, Kurtin PJ, Cofield RH, O'Fallon WM, et al. Lymphoid neogenesis in rheumatoid synovitis. J Immunol. 2001 Jul 15;167(2):1072–80.
51. Sims GP, Shiono H, Willcox N, Stott DI. Somatic hypermutation and selection of B cells in thymic germinal centers responding to acetylcholine receptor in myasthenia gravis. J Immunol. 2001 Aug 15;167(4):1935–44.
52. Serafini B, Rosicarelli B, Magliozzi R, Stigliano E, Aloisi F. Detection of ectopic B-cell follicles with germinal centers in the meninges of patients with secondary progressive multiple sclerosis. Brain Pathol. 2004 Apr;14(2):164–74.
53. Mazzucchelli L, Blaser A, Kappeler A, Schärli P, Laissue JA, Baggiolini M, et al. BCA-1 is highly expressed in *Helicobacter pylori*-induced mucosa-associated lymphoid tissue and gastric lymphoma. J Clin Invest. 1999 Nov;104(10):R49–54.
54. Grant AJ, Goddard S, Ahmed-Choudhury J, Reynolds G, Jackson DG, Briskin M, et al. Hepatic expression of secondary lymphoid chemokine (CCL21) promotes the development of portal-associated lymphoid tissue in chronic inflammatory liver disease. Am J Pathol. 2002 Apr;160(4):1445–55.
55. Armengol MP, Juan M, Lucas-Martin A, Fernandez-Figueras MT, Jaraquemada D, Gallart T, et al. Thyroid autoimmune disease: demonstration of thyroid antigen-specific B cells and recombination-activating gene expression in chemokine-containing active intrathyroidal germinal centers. Am J Pathol. 2001 Sept;159(3):861–73.
56. Larsson Å, Warfvinge G. The histopathology of oral mucosal lesions associated with amalgam or porcelain-fused-to-metal restorations. Oral Dis. 1995 Sep;1(3):152–8.
57. Larsson Å, Warfvinge G. Immunohistochemistry of 'tertiary lymphoid follicles' in oral amalgam-associated lichenoid lesions. Oral Dis. 1998 Sep;4(3):187–93.
58. Theander E, Manthorpe R, Jacobsson LT. Mortality and causes of death in primary Sjögren's syndrome: a prospective cohort study. Arthritis Rheum. 2004 Apr;50(4):1262–9.
59. Raderer M, Osterreicher C, Machold K, Formanek M, Fiebiger W, Penz M, et al. Impaired response of gastric MALT-lymphoma to *Helicobacter pylori* eradication in patients with autoimmune disease. Ann Oncol. 2001 Jul;12(7):937–9.
60. Streubel B, Huber D, Wohrer S, Chott A, Raderer M. Frequency of chromosomal aberrations involving MALT1 in mucosa-associated lymphoid tissue lymphoma in patients with Sjögren's syndrome. Clin Cancer Res. 2004 Jan 15;10(2):476–80.
61. Theander E, Henriksson G, Ljungberg O, Mandl T, Manthorpe R, Jacobsson LT. Lymphoma and other malignancies in primary Sjögren's syndrome. A cohort study on cancer incidence and lymphoma predictors. Ann Rheum Dis. 2005 Nov 10;65: 796–803.
62. Reksten TR, Jonsson MV, Szyszko EA, Brun JG, Jonsson R, Brokstad KA. Cytokine and autoantibody profiling related to histopathological features in primary Sjögren's syndrome. Rheumatology (Oxford). 2009;48(9):1102–6.
63. Szyszko EA, Brokstad KA, Øijordsbakken G, Jonsson MV, Jonsson R, Skarstein K. Salivary glands of primary Sjögren's syndrome patients express factors vital for plasma cell survival. Arthritis Res Ther. 2011;13(1):R2.64.
64. Theander E, Vasaitis L, Baecklund E, Nordmark G, Warfvinge G, Liedholm R, et al. Lymphoid organisation in labial salivary gland biopsies is a possible predictor for the development of malignant lymphoma in primary Sjögren's syndrome. Ann Rheum Dis. 2011;(70): In press.
65. Christodoulou MI, Kapsogeorgou EK, Moutsopoulos HM. Characteristics of the minor salivary gland infiltrates in Sjögren's syndrome. J Autoimmun. 2010;34(4):400–7.
66. Le Pottier L, Devauchelle V, Fautrel A, Daridon C, Saraux A, Youinou P, et al. Ectopic germinal centers are rare in Sjögren's syndrome salivary glands and do not exclude autoreactive B cells. J Immunol. 2009;182(6):3540–7.

Imaging Technology in Sjögren's Syndrome: Non-invasive Evaluation of the Salivary Glands

7

Jonn Terje Geitung and Malin V. Jonsson

Abstract

The assessment of salivary gland involvement in Sjögren's syndrome is traditionally based on the presence of focal mononuclear cell infiltrates in the salivary glands and by measures of salivary secretion (sialometry) as well as subjective symptoms of oral dryness (xerostomia). Although a salivary gland biopsy is considered to be the gold standard, other methods are needed in cases where a biopsy cannot be performed or need to be supplemented. Through the recent years, existing techniques have been improved and new imaging techniques developed. There is both a need and a possibility to use other traditional methods such as scintigraphy as well as computer tomography, ultrasound, and magnetic resonance imaging.

Keywords

Computer tomography • Imaging • Magnetic resonance imaging • Non-invasive • Scintigraphy • Sialography • Ultrasound

Salivary gland tissue in Sjögren's syndrome is characterized by focal mononuclear cell infiltration, loss of salivary gland acinar epithelial tissue, and degenerative changes such as fibrosis. This makes functional imaging like scintigraphy and MRI obvious choices [1, 2]. In contrast to the histopathological evaluation where the minor or parotid salivary glands are examined, the gland of choice for functional evaluation is the major salivary glands, i.e., the parotid glands and/or the submandibular glands. In cases where the labial salivary gland biopsy is insufficient or not possible to perform, there is a potential diagnostic role for sialographic and scintigraphic examinations [3].

Important to imaging techniques is also the typical pattern of parotid gland ducts, where the conventional X-ray sialography is still considered the gold standard for showing changes [4, 5]. It has, however, in part been replaced by MR sialography.

Imaging procedures have had rapid progress throughout recent years, both with improvements in existing techniques and development of new imaging techniques. In addition to sialometry [see Chapter 14, Oral and Dental Manifestations

J.T. Geitung (✉)
Haraldsplass Deaconess University Hospital, Bergen, Norway
e-mail: jtgeit@online.no; jonn.terje.geitung@haraldsplass.no

R.I. Fox, C.M. Fox (eds.), *Sjögren's Syndrome*, DOI 10.1007/978-1-60327-957-4_7,

of Sjögren's syndrome] sialography has traditionally been used to evaluate the salivary component. Nuclear medicine (scintigraphy) has had a role in the diagnosis of Sjögren's syndrome and is considered an important diagnostic tool. The presence of objective salivary gland involvement is defined by either unstimulated whole salivary flow of less than or equal to 1.5 mL/15 min, diffuse sialectasis by parotid sialography, or salivary scintigraphy showing delayed uptake, reduced concentration, and/or delayed excretion of tracer [6]. Other imaging methods are available but not established as routine in diagnosing Sjögren's syndrome. The available imaging methods are conventional radiographs (including sialography), computer tomography (CT), ultrasound (US), magnetic resonance imaging (MRI), and nuclear medicine (scintigraphy). These will be further described below.

7.1 Conventional Radiographs

7.1.1 Sialography

Conventional X-rays are commonly used for examinations of joints, bones, and lungs. This does not give direct information concerning Sjögren's syndrome but information concerning other effects of the disease. It is also a part of the diagnosis and follow-up of patients with rheumatic diseases. However, as a primary diagnostic examination for Sjögren's syndrome, plain X-ray is not indicated. CT and MRI are also used for other organs in connection with Sjögren's syndrome and rheumatic diseases but will not be dealt with here.

For Sjögren's syndrome in particular, only sialography has a diagnostic yield, showing the ducts of the salivary glands [5]. The examination is performed by installing a contrast medium into the salivary ducts and then exposing radiographs of the area at different angles. It is a very good procedure for determining the architecture and configuration of the glandular ducts. In patients with Sjögren's syndrome, the characteristic finding is a snowstorm-like or Christmas tree pattern. In cases where the glandular tissue is severely damaged, complete absence of structures may be observed. Sialography is a well-established method, but has its limitations as it is time-consuming and may be painful and risky. In patients with severe salivary gland dysfunction, sialography is even contraindicated; due to reduced salivary flow, the contrast medium injected may remain in the gland [7]. It is a cumbersome method to perform, may be uncomfortable to the patient, and similar diagnostic results may now be achieved with MR sialography [8].

Sialography is not suited for repetition and, therefore, not applicable for patient follow-up. Various stages of sialectasis can be detected in patients with Sjögren's syndrome, and an abnormal result was determined in 72–86% of patients. Second only to lip biopsy and histopathological evaluation of the salivary glands, parotid sialography yielded the highest accuracy for the diagnosis of patients with Sjögren's syndrome [9]. However, in a healthy population, 15–29% of otherwise healthy and asymptomatic individuals may also demonstrate sialectasis, and chronic sialadenitis of other causes may also show the same pattern, diminishing the value of the test, reviewed in [10].

7.2 Computer Tomography

As conventional radiographs, CT is also based on ionizing radiation with an X-ray tube rotating around the patient. CT will thus expose patients to a significant radiation dose, and this may exclude younger patients.

At first, this technique gave cross-sectional slices. Today CT provides a volume that can be analyzed in different planes as well as three-dimensionally, all with a high spatial resolution. It is in many ways an excellent method but not for Sjögren's syndrome. CT is the best method for detecting stones in the salivary ducts and is often used for preoperative staging of tumors in the salivary glands [11]. CT may also be used for sialography, providing a three-dimensional view of the ductal system. However, the tissue resolution is not sufficient for detecting tissue changes in the salivary glands, such as fibrosis [12].

7.3 Ultrasound

The salivary glands are situated superficially and thus well situated for the use of high frequency transducers (Fig. 7.1a, b). Ultrasound is based on sound waves, like SONAR. Piezoelectric crystals emit and receive sound, and the higher the frequency, the better the spatial resolution. The development of transducers has provided both high spatial and tissue resolution, giving excellent examinations of the salivary glands, and changes in tissue due to inflammation may be seen [13]. The salivary ducts can also be visualized, but the anatomical overview is difficult. One investigation compared US and scintigraphy and found US to be better [14] while another found US to be equivalent to MRI [15]. Ultrasound is easily available and "comfortable" to the patient as well as providing good access to the parotid and submandibular glands. Accordingly, it is natural that during the development of ultrasound, several investigations on ultrasound and Sjögren's syndrome have been made [16].

7.4 Magnetic Resonance Imaging

The patient lies in a large *magnet*, the patient's nuclear spin will then align parallel or antiparallel to the magnetic field. A radio frequency is sent to the patient. The frequency will be chosen as to obtain *resonance* with given atoms. When the radio frequency is off, one measures given time constants in order to find the amount of given atoms, mainly hydrogen atoms. The making of an *image* is based on this information. MRI gives better tissue resolution, but poorer spatial resolution, than CT and provides a similar anatomic overview. It too is used for preoperative staging of tumors, but due to better tissue resolution, it is better than CT in detecting and delineating pathologic changes in soft tissues (Fig. 7.2a, b) [11, 17].

A large number of articles concerning MR–sialography and Sjögren's syndrome have been published [18, 19]. Dynamic MR sialography, by stimulating with citric acid, has been introduced as an improved method for Sjögren's syndrome [20]. When performing MRI of the parotid glands, a small coil with a small field of view is used. This gives a high tissue and spatial resolution, not only for the parotid glands, but for labial salivary glands as well [21]. It has been called MR microscopy of the salivary glands [22]. This method provides a resolution at least as good as ultrasound, a better overview over the entire glands and salivary ducts (MR sialography, Fig. 7.3), and may with contrast media provide information regarding function.

The recent development of MRI in the diagnosis of Sjögren's syndrome is toward functional examinations, using perfusion techniques and diffusion-weighted techniques [2, 23, 24]. MR spectroscopy has been used for improving

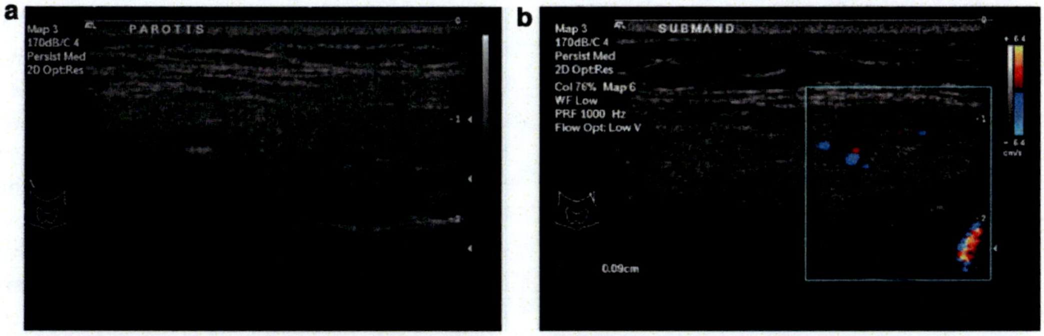

Fig. 7.1 Ultrasound. **a** Longitudinal high-resolution image showing a normal parotid gland, illustrating how well the structure of the gland is seen. **b** We see a slightly dilated duct in a submandibular gland of patient (marked with *crosses*)

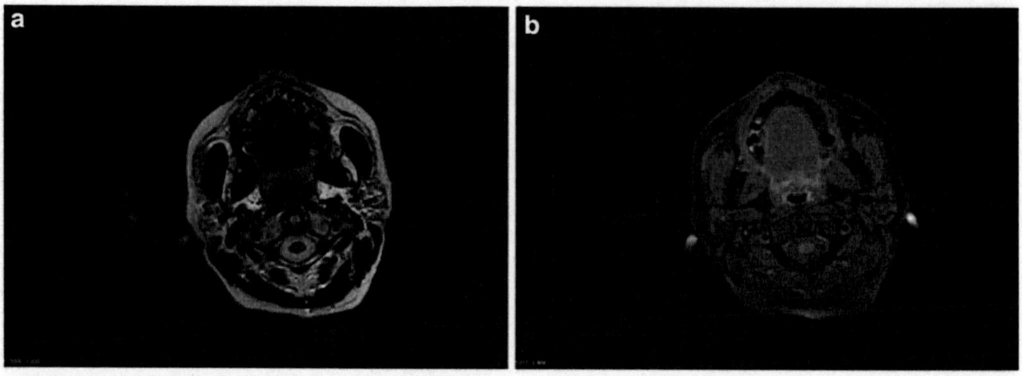

Fig. 7.2 MRI. The figure shows very irregular parotid ducts bilaterally, a typical finding in a patient with severe symptoms of Sjögren' syndrome. **a** Axial T1 weighted MR image clearly showing the irregular parotid glands. Some of the submandibular glands may be seen as well and appear to be just as irregular. **b** Axial image with fat saturation technique, showing the same patient as in (**a**)

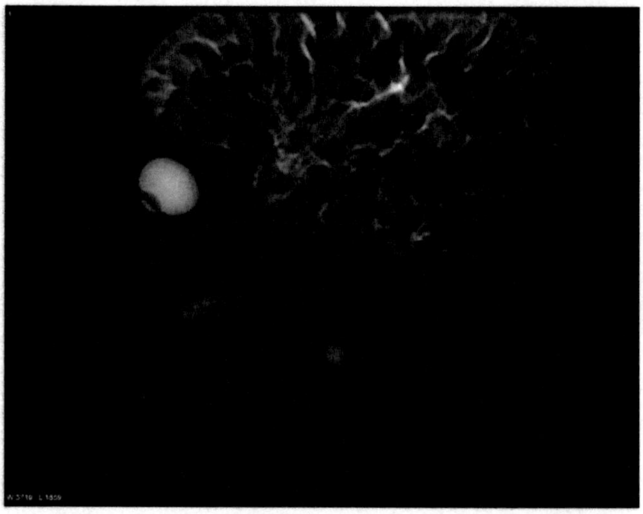

Fig. 7.3 MR sialogram. Sagittal MR image with contrast, showing a slightly irregular parotid duct. We also see a cyst in contact with the duct, a typical finding in Sjögren's syndrome. We do, however, not see a "Christmas" tree, but still it shows the same pattern as can be observed in conventional sialograms

diagnosis of tumors but so far not in Sjögren's syndrome. Although a time-consuming and expensive method to perform, requiring experienced interpretation of the images, at present MRI represents state-of-the-art in imaging of the salivary glands and possibly the primary imaging modality for Sjögren's syndrome.

7.5 Nuclear Medicine

7.5.1 Scintigraphy

Scintigraphy is a method used to evaluate the function of the salivary glands. Technetium 99m Tc-sodium pertechnetate (^{99m}Tc-PT) is used, and the velocity and density of this marker is observed and evaluated in the salivary glands. The radioactively marked fluid is injected intravenously, and the examination is performed when/as the marker is expected to be in or pass the glands. Several registrations are necessary to achieve a dynamic examination. The examination is a registration of the amount of radioactively marked substance. In regard to Sjögren's syndrome, scintigraphy is commonly used to determine whether the patient responds to stimulation or not. A dynamic scintigraphy will give information about the function of the salivary glands [25].

To the authors' knowledge, studies regarding the function of salivary glands in Sjögren's syndrome, with positron emission tomography (PET), have not yet been performed. PET has a potential for functional imaging that in the future may give information not obtainable by other methods.

The resolution of scintigraphy is not comparable to the other imaging methods previously mentioned. However, functional studies providing a quantitative evaluation of parotid function still make scintigraphy a frequently used imaging method for Sjögren's syndrome [1, 25, 26]. Reported sensitivity of scintigraphy ranges from 75 to 87%, but has low specificity [27–29]. In addition, scintigraphy may only be performed in a hospital setting, thus limiting the accessibility and applicability. Furthermore, there may be difficulties in the ability of the procedures to differentiate between uptake and secretory failure. Scintigraphy is, as sialography, unsuited for repetition [30]. Nonetheless, one study indicates that scintigraphy still is better than ultrasound as a diagnostic tool for Sjögren's syndrome [29]. Scintigraphy is an accepted imaging method in overall approaches for diagnosing Sjögren's syndrome [30, 31].

7.6 Comparison of Nuclear Medicine, Ultrasound, and MRI

MRI and US may detect small amounts of fibrotic tissue or edema in glands. With contrast media they may also provide information regarding function of the salivary glands, more so MRI than US. MRI may also give an excellent anatomic overview. Both MRI and US have excellent spatial and tissue resolution.

Nuclear medicine provides a dynamic examination, making it possible to quantify function. The impression, however, is that MRI is the better method, but both availability and the need of expertise may have limited the application and use of this method. In addition, so may also costs and time consumption.

Scintigraphy, on the other hand, is a well-established method and incorporated in diagnostic approaches. One may expect ultrasound to challenge that position as it is becoming more easily available and has proven to be of equal diagnostic value. However, ultrasound is more user-dependent than the other methods and is not as easily documented as compared to scintigraphy.

An overview of current methods is provided in Table 7.1.

Table 7.1 A review of current methods

Topic	Scintigraphy	MRI	US	Clinical comparisons
Functional information	+++ Detection of isotopes	+(+) Examination of perfusion and diffusion	+ Perfusion	Scintigraphy superior
Morphological information	+ Low resolution	+++ Excellent both tissue and spatial resolution	++ Excellent tissue resolution but problems with anatomic overview	MRI superior in resolution and in making anatomical "maps"
Existing experience	+++	+	++	Scintigraphy is a well-established method. Ultrasound is also widely used, whereas the use of MRI most likely will increase
Seeing the ducts	–	+++ MRI sialography	(+)	MRI is the only one of these methods showing the ductal structures

References

1. Umehara I, Yamada I, Murata Y, Takahashi Y, Okada N, Shibuya H. Quantitative evaluation of salivary gland scintigraphy in Sjögren's syndrome. J Nucl Med. 1999;40:64–9.
2. Roberts C, Parker CJ, Rose CJ, et al. Glandular function in Sjögren syndrome: assessment with dynamic contrast-enhanced MR imaging and tracer kinetic modeling—initial experience. Radiology. 2008;246:845–53.
3. Lindvall AM, Jonsson R. The salivary gland component of Sjögren's syndrome: an evaluation of diagnostic methods. Oral Surg Oral Med Oral Pathol. 1986;62(1):32–42.
4. Rubin P, Holt JF. Secretory sialography in diseases of the major salivary glands. Am J Roentgenol. 1957;77:575–98.
5. Whaley K, Blair S, Low PS, Chisholm DM, Wick WC, Buchanan WW. Sialographic abnormalities in Sjögren's syndrome, rheumatoid arthritis and connective tissue diseases. Clin Radiol. 1972;23: 474–82.
6. Vitali C, Bombardieri S, Jonsson R, et al. Classification criteria for Sjögren's syndrome: a revised version of the European criteria proposed by the American-European Consensus Group. Ann Rheum Dis. 2002;61(6):554–8.
7. Valdez IH, Fox PC. Diagnosis and management of salivary dysfunction. Crit Rev Oral Biol Med. 1993;4(3–4):271–7.
8. Tonami H, Ogawa Y, Matobe M, et al. MR sialography in patients with Sjögren syndrome. Am J Neuroradiol. 1998;19:1199–203.
9. Vitali C, Bombardieri S, Moutsopoulos HM, et al. Assessment of the European classification criteria for Sjögren's syndrome in a series of clinically defined cases: results of a prospective multicentre study. The European Study Group on Diagnostic Criteria for Sjögren's Syndrome. Ann Rheum Dis. 1996;55(2):116–21.
10. Soto-Rojas AE, Kraus A. The oral side of Sjögren syndrome. Diagnosis and treatment. A review. Arch Med Res. 2002;33(2):95–106.
11. Lee YY, Wong KT, King AD, Ahuja AT. Imaging of salivary gland tumours. Eur J Radiol. 2008;66:419–36.
12. de Clerck LS, Corthouts R, Francx L, et al. Ultrasonography and computer tomography of the salivary glands in the evaluation of Sjögren's syndrome. Comparison with parotid sialography. J Rheumatol. 1988;15:1777–81.
13. Riente L, Delle Sedie A, Filippucci E, et al. Ultrasound imaging for rheumatologist XIV. Ultrasound imaging in connective tissue diseases. Clin Exp Rheumatol. 2008;26:230–3.
14. Salaffi F, Carotti M, Iagnocco A, et al. Ultrasonography of salivary glands in primary Sjögren's syndrome: a comparison with contrast sialography and scintigraphy. Rheumatology. 2008; 47:1244–9.
15. El Miedany YM, Ahmed I, Mourad HG, et al. Quantitative ultrasonography and magnetic resonance imaging of the parotid gland: can they replace the histopathologic studies in patients with Sjögren's syndrome? Joint Bone Spine 2004;71: 29–38.
16. Wernicke D, Hess H, Gromnica-Ihle E, Krause A, Schmidt WA. Ultrasonography of salivary glands—a highly specific imaging procedure for diagnosis of Sjögren's syndrome. J Rheumatol. 2008;35: 285–93.
17. Thoeny HC. Imaging of salivary gland tumours. Cancer Imaging 2007;30:52–62.
18. Tonami H, Higashi K, Matoba M, Yokota H, Yamamoto I, Sugai S. A comparative study between MR sialography and salivary gland scintigraphy in the diagnosis of Sjögren syndrome. J Comput Assist Tomogr. 2001;25:262–8.
19. Takagi Y, Sumi M, Van Cauteren M, Nakamura T. Fast and high-resolution MR sialography using a small surface coil. J Magn Reson Imaging. 2005;22:29–37.
20. Morimoto Y, Habu M, Tomoyose T, et al. Dynamic magnetic resonance sialography as a new diagnostic technique for patients with Sjögren's syndrome. Oral Dis. 2006;12:408–14.
21. Sumi M, Yamada T, Takagi Y, Nakamura T. MR imaging of labial glands. Am J Neuroradiol. 2007;28:1552–6.
22. Takagi Y, Sumi M, Sumi T, Ichikawa Y, Nakamura T. MR Microscopy of the parotid glands in patients with Sjögren's syndrome: quantitative MR diagnostic criteria. Am J Neuroradiol. 2005;26: 1207–14.
23. Simon-Zoula SC, Boesch C, De Keyzer F, Thoeny HC. Functional imaging of the parotid glands using blood oxygenation level dependent (BOLD)-MRI at 1.5 T and 3 T. J Magn Reson Imaging. 2008;27: 43–8.
24. Kawai Y, Sumi M, Kitamori H, Takagi Y, Nakamura T. Diffusion-weighted MR microimaging of the lacrimal glands in patients with Sjögren's syndrome. Am J Roentgenol. 2005;184:1320–5.
25. Nishiyama S, Miyawaki S, Yoshinaga Y. A study to standardize quantitative evaluation of parotid gland scintigraphy in patients with Sjögren's syndrome. J Rheumatol. 2006;33:2470–74.
26. Henrikssen AM, Nossent HC. Quantitative salivary gland scintigraphy can distinguish patients with primary Sjögren's syndrome during the evaluation of sicca symptoms. Clin Rheumatol. 2007;26: 1837–41.
27. Markusse HM, Pillay M, Breedveld FC. The diagnostic value of salivary gland scintigraphy in patients suspected of primary Sjögren's syndrome. Br J Rheumatol. 1993;32(3):231–35.

28. Hermann GA, Vivino FB, Goin JE. Scintigraphic features of chronic sialadenitis and Sjögren's syndrome: a comparison. Nucl Med Commun. 1999;20(12):1123–32.
29. Decuzzi M, Tatulli F, Giampaolo M, et al. Sialoscintigraphy versus ultrasonography of the salivary glands in patients first diagnoses with Sjögren's syndrome. Hell J Nucl Med. 2006;9:103–5.
30. Coll J, Rubiés-Prat, Gutiérrez-Cebollada, Tomás S. Sjögren's syndrome: a stepwise approach to the use of diagnostic tests. Ann Rheum Dis. 1992;51: 607–10.
31. Brito-Zerón P, Ramos-Casals M, Bove A, Sentis J, Font J. Predicting adverse outcomes in primary Sjögren's syndrome: identification of prognostic factors. Rheumatology 2007;46:1359–62.

Part III

Mechanisms of Pathogenesis

Genomics and Viruses in Sjögren's Syndrome

8

Kathy L. Moser and John B. Harley

Abstract

Contributions from both genetic and environmental factors to the etiology of Sjögren's syndrome (SS) are being discovered, though their roles in disease pathogenesis remain obscure. An important key to fully understand how genetic variation leads to disease is to comprehensively test all potential variation for association. Extraordinary developments in our understanding of the inherent variation present in the human genome and rapid advances in the technical capacity to evaluate this variation are moving us closer to understanding the genetic etiology for numerous complex diseases. In particular, major shifts in the past few years from small candidate gene studies to large genome-wide screens for association of human variation with disease have been remarkably successful. Dozens of new disease associations previously thought intractable to discovery have now been identified in complex diseases. Although the genetics of SS remains vastly unexplored, rapid advances in our understanding of related autoimmune diseases illustrate the potential complexity of the expected genetic landscape for SS with several emerging themes. First, multiple genes contribute to increasing disease risk. Second, many genes have now been associated with multiple autoimmune disorders. Third, the frequencies of some disease-associated variants are relatively common while others are rare within populations. In addition, the frequency of any given disease risk allele often varies between different racial groups. Fourth, certain disease variants are more strongly associated with clinically recognizable disease subgroups or manifestations as opposed to more general susceptibility risk to disease. Overall, studies in autoimmune diseases related to SS provide an encouraging glimpse into the potential for success in establishing the genetic basis for SS. We discuss how genetics is transforming our understanding of autoimmunity with relevance to SS and review evidence

K.L. Moser (✉)
Arthritis and Immunology Program, Oklahoma Medical Research Foundation, Oklahoma City, OK, USA
e-mail: moserk@omrf.org

R.I. Fox, C.M. Fox (eds.), *Sjögren's Syndrome*, DOI 10.1007/978-1-60327-957-4_8,

suggesting how environmental influences on susceptible genetic backgrounds may conspire to generate disease. We also discuss recent advances in transcriptional profiling and proteomic studies, which are beginning to provide global views of gene or protein expression profiles. Collectively, the broad views offered by these powerful and complementary approaches are revealing important disease-associated pathways and enhancing our understanding of the etiological mechanisms in SS.

Keywords
Sjögren's syndrome • Genetics • Genomics • Proteomics • Viruses

8.1 Introduction

Essentially all human traits, including susceptibility to disease, are governed by genetics and influenced to varying degrees by environmental exposures. Indeed, a new era has emerged during the past decade in our basic understanding of human genomes and our technical capacity to detect and characterize genetic variation. The application of modern genetic and genomic tools is revealing revolutionary insights into disease mechanisms for a multitude of complex diseases. Importantly, the comprehensive and unbiased nature of genome-wide screens removes the severe limitations imposed by employing more traditional hypothesis-driven candidate gene studies as the only approach to genetic discovery. Using genome-wide association (GWA) study approaches, tremendous progress has recently been made in identifying dozens of genetic loci that confer risk to autoimmune phenotypes, including systemic lupus erythematosus (SLE), rheumatoid arthritis (RA), multiple sclerosis (MS), and Crohn's disease. These successes provide unequivocal evidence that modern genetic studies using state-of-the-art tools can lead to novel and important insights into disease pathogenesis.

In contrast, the genetic factors associated with SS are virtually unexplored. Large-scale studies in SS are in the very earliest stages of planning and implementation. Despite the current lack of comprehensive genetic studies in SS, collective evidence from mouse models, family studies, candidate gene studies, and genetic findings in related diseases (e.g., SLE and RA) support an underlying etiology with complex genetic architecture. In this chapter, we review the existing evidence to support genetic contributions to SS, summarize the evidence for the few candidate genes studied to date, and briefly describe potential environmental influences that may interact with genetic risk loci to promote development of disease. We also discuss emerging genomic and proteomic data that provide useful insight into the underlying signaling pathways that are dysregulated in SS.

8.2 Evidence Supporting a Genetic Component in SS

Twin studies and family-based studies are often used as a first step toward estimating the relative influence of genetic versus environmental influences on disease. Studies demonstrating increased concordance rates of disease among monozygotic twins and familial aggregation showing that a phenotype clusters in families at rates above the population prevalence are often taken as evidence to support a genetic etiology. Such reports in SS are extremely limited. A few case reports of twins with SS have been published, but reliable twin concordance rates have not been estimated [1–4]. Scofield et al. reported a case of monozygotic twins with Sjögren's syndrome who both had increased serum levels of anti-60-kDa Ro/SS-A autoantibodies [4]. A set of adolescent dizygotic twins, both with shared diagnosis of primary SS (pSS), were described in

2005 by Houghton et al. [3]. Interestingly, one of the two sisters presented with pulmonary symptoms, uncommon in pediatric pSS. Using SLE and RA as closely related traits to estimate the potential genetic contribution to SS, if we may use SLE and RA to make a crude guess, then twin concordance could be expected to be between those of RA (15%) and SLE (25%), with a female sibling or fraternal twin rate of 2–4% and estimated odds of female sibling concordance (λ(lambda)$_s$) between 8 and 20.

Several families consisting of multiple individuals with SS have been described [5–10]. SS patient family histories commonly include relatives with other autoimmune diseases (30–35%) and most often include SS (12%), autoimmune thyroid disease (AITD, 14%), RA (14%), and SLE (5–10%) [8, 11]. Multiple sclerosis has also been shown to cluster with SS in families [12]. In a large family study of SLE, 8 out of 60 members were found to share a diagnosis of SLE. Among individuals with SLE, all shared positive antinuclear autoantibodies (ANAs), six shared pleuritis and malar rash, five reported photosensitivity, and four shared nephritis. Of the 51 relatives who contributed samples and for which results were obtained, 29% had autoantibodies and 18% had autoimmune disease including 1 with SS [10]. These studies provide supportive evidence that underlying disease mechanisms among related autoimmune diseases are likely to be shared. This is also intuitively expected considering that so many immunologic, immunogenetic, and clinical features of SS are found in nearly every other autoimmune rheumatic disease.

Additional support for a genetic component to SS has been obtained from mouse models. Approximately 20 models have been reported and are reviewed in detail elsewhere [13]. At present, no individual mouse model fully represents the majority of key disease manifestations of human disease. However, most models available develop sialadenitis and/or dacryoadenitis, so these models do constitute valuable tools for evaluating initiation of disease, various components of the overall SS phenotype such as autoantibody production, and the effects of immune manipulation. While genetic mapping in mouse models of SS is far from complete, several genes have been identified. For example, the NFS/sld mouse develops sialadenitis that is characterized by inflammatory lesions containing $CD3^+$ and $CD4^+$ cells with few $CD8^+$ and B cells. The mice carry an autosomal recessive gene, *sld*, and autoimmunity appears to be driven by reactivity against the cytoskeletal protein α(alpha)-fodrin [14, 15]. However, no anti-Ro/SS-A or anti-La/SS-B is detected in the NFS/sld model [16]. Another model, the aly/aly mouse, carries an autosomal recessive alymphoplasia (aly) mutation mapped to a gene that codes for an NF-κ(kappa)B-inducing kinase [17]. $CD4^+$ T cells infiltrate the lacrimal and salivary glands at 3 months, but no autoantibodies against nuclear elements or salivary gland have been identified [18]. Another model includes the Id3 knockout in which T-cell receptor-mediated thymic selection at the time of T-cell development is disrupted. Mice deficient in Id3 develop anti-Ro/SS-A and anti-La/SS-B antibodies, dry eyes and mouth, and experience lymphocyte infiltration in lacrimal and salivary glands [19]. Recovery of salivary function and improvements of histopathology were observed following treatment of a CD20 monoclonal antibody that depleted B lymphocytes [20]. Perhaps the Id3 knockout model will prove to be a useful animal model to guide immunotherapy development in pSS patients.

As with the majority of SS mouse models, dissection of the genetic loci that drives lymphocytic infiltration, aberrant cytokine production, development of autoantibodies, and glandular dysfunction will provide important tools for understanding complex pathogenic mechanisms in human disease. Likewise, identification of causal genes in humans will be of extraordinary benefit for fully informing the development of mouse models that more accurately represents human disease.

8.3 Technological Influences on Gene Discovery

Traditional scientific inquiry is hypothesis-driven. From a genetics perspective, the kinds of studies considered standard just a few years ago included genotyping of one or a few variants within a given candidate gene for a few hundred subjects. To provide perspective on how increased technical capacity for genotyping has led to the remarkable success of discovery-based approaches in disease gene mapping, we summarize key features of the human genome and describe important advances in our understanding of variation.

The human genome contains approximately 3 billion base pairs of genetic sequence. Approximately 21,000 genes are encoded, the majority of which give rise to multiple messenger RNA (mRNA) transcripts and protein isoforms through processes such as alternative splicing or post-translational modifications. Naturally occurring genetic variation in the human genome is abundant, dispersed throughout the genome, and includes single-nucleotide polymorphisms (SNPs), variable number short tandem repeats (VNTRs), insertion/deletions (indels), and gene copy number variation (CNV). Across all classes of variation type, approximately 90% of sites that are polymorphic between any two copies of the human genome are SNPs [21].

Within the human genome, approximately 90% of heterozygosity is attributable to some 10–15 million variants (primarily SNPs) considered to be common as defined by population allele frequencies >1%. The remaining 10% are considered rare or even absent (i.e., monomorphic) in certain populations [22, 23]. The large contribution of common variation to human heterogeneity is the result of the shared ancestry and population history of human populations with important implications for disease gene mapping. The majority of genetic variation arose before the dramatic expansion and dispersal of the African population 10,000–40,000 years ago and is shared by all humans.

This shared ancestry of humans explains the extensive correlation among nearby chromosomal variants, termed linkage disequilibrium (LD) or haplotypes. Studies have shown that throughout much of the genome, a high degree of ancestral LD is observed (termed "haplotype blocks"), with only 3–5 common haplotypes accounting for ~90% of the genetic variation observed at any given region [21, 24]. Disease variants that were deleterious during evolution (such as mutations that cause early-onset severe diseases) are typically rare, due to selection. Conversely, disease variants that act after reproduction may have been neutral or subject to balancing selection (e.g., sickle cell and malaria). In such cases, the genetic variation underlying disease may be common.

An important implication of the patterns of variation in the genome for association studies is that a relatively small number of variants can often be informative surrogates for nearby variants and essentially "tag" the common variation within a large interval. Thus, not all variation needs to be genotyped in order to detect a genetic association effect. Indeed, genotyping of about 1% (~1 million) of all SNPs can "capture" the great majority of the association effects originating from the ~10 million variants present in the human genome. Genotyping technologies have been built around selecting the most informative subset of SNPs based on these patterns of LD for screening the genome. On the other hand, not every genetic association detected with the screening SNPs in a genome scan means the true disease causal variant has been genotyped. A screening SNP may simply be in LD with the nearby true causal variant and serving as an informative marker. Additional genotyping ("fine mapping") and sequencing are nearly always required to more precisely determine the true causal variant detected in association studies.

A rapid and unprecedented swell of new genetic discoveries has been fostered by the development of affordable, high-throughput genotyping technology. Microarray-based platforms that provide technical capacity for genome-wide association (GWA) studies interrogating between 300,000 and 500,000 SNPs have been exceptionally fruitful for prostate cancer, breast cancer, and autoimmune diseases such as T1D, RA, and SLE [25–30]. For example, we now recognize over 30 genes/loci in which robust genetic association with SLE is established [31]. In Crohn's disease, association with more than 30 genes/loci has also been identified [32]. Ongoing studies are expected to continue to reveal numerous additional genes that contribute

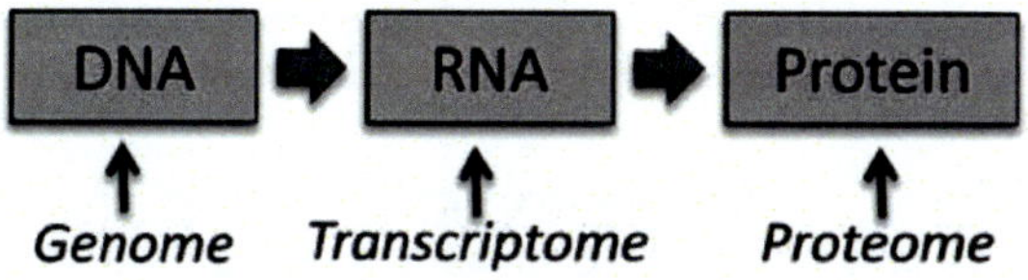

Fig. 8.1 Components of genomic studies amenable to high-throughput technologies. Genetic studies using genome-wide association approaches to characterize variation in DNA can test >1 million variants using microarrays. Gene expression studies also employ microarray technology to measure levels of mRNA transcripts for essentially every gene, defined as the transcriptome. Proteomic studies use large-scale methods such as mass spectrometry to characterize structure and function of the entire set of proteins

to SLE and other autoimmune diseases related to SS.

More recently, further increases in throughput for genotyping technology allow simultaneous interrogation of over 1 million genetic variants in a single experiment and often within an economic realm of feasibility to include several hundreds, if not thousands, of subjects. Advances in genotyping technologies that allow high throughput, unbiased interrogation of essentially all genes are complemented by parallel technologies that interrogate RNA transcripts or proteins at the genome-wide level using cost-effective approaches (Fig. 8.1). These tremendously more comprehensive, discovery-based approaches allow detection of novel genes, transcripts, and proteins that are associated with disease but have never before been hypothesized to have a role in disease.

8.4 Lessons from SLE and Other Autoimmune Diseases

Numerous genetic loci that are associated with more than one autoimmune disease have been identified in recent years, confirming a basis for shared etiology. Associations of certain human leukocyte antigen (*HLA*) loci, such as *HLA-DR* variants (alleles), have been extensively reported in SS, SLE, RA, and others [33]. The list of non-HLA genes implicated in multiple autoimmune diseases also continues to grow. Examples include association of *CTLA-4* with AITD; type 1 diabetes (T1D); celiac disease; Wegener's granulomatosis; SLE; vitiligo; Addison's disease, and RA [34–41]; *PD-1* with RA, T1D, and SLE [42]; and *PTPN22* with SLE, RA, and T1D; Graves's disease and Hashimoto's thyroiditis [43–48]; *CTLA-4* (cytotoxic T-lymphocyte antigen 4), *PTPN22* (protein tyrosine phosphatase, non-receptor type 22), and *PD-1* (programmed death 1) are all expressed in lymphocytes and play important regulatory roles during immune responses. Interestingly, *IRF5* (interferon regulatory factor 5) and *STAT4* (signal transducer and activator of transcription 4) are genes strongly associated with SLE and implicated in multiple autoimmune diseases including recent data suggesting association with pSS [49]. Both *IRF5* and *STAT4* regulate innate immune responses involving interferon pathway signaling. Murine studies are also consistent with models of multigenic inheritance, and numerous susceptibility loci have been identified that are shared across different autoimmune mouse models for SS as well as for other autoimmune diseases [50].

Of the diseases most commonly thought to overlap with SS, SLE has received the most attention in comparison studies and provides a model of the expectations for genetic studies in SS. Genetic studies in SLE are perhaps the most advanced and successful in terms of overall progress toward understanding etiology, largely due to recent GWA studies [31, 51]. Before 2007, there were nine established SLE susceptibility genes identified through candidate gene studies or family-based linkage approaches. Among the more than 30 genetic associations now recognized in SLE, 3 major biological themes are confirmed by the specific genes involved: immune complex processing, Toll-like receptor (TLR) function and type-I interferon (IFN) signaling, and signal transduction in lymphocytes (reviewed in Harley et al. [51] and Moser et al. [31]). Multiple genes from each of these three pathways are associated with SLE. Genes involved in immune complex processing include Fc receptors (e.g., *FcGR2A, FcGR3B, FcGR3A*), complement components (e.g., *C4A, C4B, C2, C1q*), and others (e.g., *CRP, ITGAM*). Genes involved in TLR/IFN pathways include *IRF5*,

STAT4, *SPP1*, *IRAK1*, *TREX1*, and *TNFAIP3*. In addition to *HLA-DR*, other genes involved in lymphocyte signal transduction include *BLK*, *LYN*, *BANK1*, *TNFSF4*, and *FcGR2B*. Additional genes of unknown function have been identified that will undoubtedly expand on these themes as our understanding progresses (e.g., *ICA1*, *SCUBE1*, and *PXK*). Importantly, ongoing studies are in progress that indicate many additional novel associations with SLE will be established.

Familial clustering and sharing of clinical and serological features of SS with SLE, RA, and other autoimmune diseases has long been the foundation for suspecting shared etiology. For example, subsets of patients with SLE or SS may manifest similar symptoms (commonly including arthralgias, myalgias, fatigue, rashes, and visceral involvement from vasculitis) or serological abnormalities such as ANAs, anti-Ro/SS-A, or anti-La/SS-B autoantibodies [52]. Certain features of SS are more commonly shared with RA patients, such as production of rheumatoid factor (RF) antibodies. Identification of genetic loci that influence expression of specific "subphenotypes," such as particular autoantibody specificities, kidney disease, and others, is beginning to emerge and will likely lead to deeper understanding of why such clustering of disease features occurs.

An important consideration when reviewing the current state of our genetic understanding in SLE is that the bulk of discoveries have been made in European-derived populations. Additional layers of the complex genetic architecture for SLE provided by other populations are only beginning to be delineated. The relative contribution from rare variants and structural variants such as CNVs is largely unknown as well. Interestingly, genetic effects influenced by gender or age are also possible and supported by studies of SPP1 (osteopontin), showing strongest association in men as well as in women with early-onset disease [53]. Thus, we are most likely still viewing the "tip of the iceberg" for total number of genes that influence risk of developing SLE and the heterogeneous subphenotypes characteristic of this complex disease.

8.5 Genes Implicated in SS

There is no reason to suspect that the genetics of SS will be significantly less complex than the picture emerging for related diseases such as SLE, and it will be fascinating to eventually understand where the genetic similarities and differences lie. Large-scale genetic studies in SS, either with respect to number of variants tested or sample sizes evaluated, have not been done. In the meantime, the relatively few genetic studies performed to date are consistent with association of multiple genes with SS, several of which are well established in other autoimmune diseases.

Current literature includes approximately 30 genetic studies in SS, nearly all of which describe testing a total of about 20 candidate genes. This reflects less than 0.1% of the estimated 21,000 genes in the human genome. In addition, sample sizes included in the SS genetic studies reported to date are typically less than 200 cases and controls. These studies are profoundly underpowered, from a statistical perspective, to detect the small effect sizes (OR = <1.3) generally anticipated. Consequently, such small studies are usually unreliable. Replication of genetic effects has also been problematic and is not surprising given the limitations of studies reported to date. By contrast, the largest ongoing genetic studies in SLE are evaluating nearly 20,000 subjects assembled by the constructive cooperation of multiple groups around the world.

While the size and scope of the SS studies reported to date are far removed from the large-scale studies being conducted for numerous other autoimmune diseases, they do suggest several genes that warrant more rigorous studies evaluating larger cohort sizes that are statistically robust and fine mapping to more comprehensively characterize the genetic effects.

Historically, genetic studies in SS were dominated by evaluations of the HLA region prior to 1995 (reviewed by Cobb et al. [54]). Evidence for association between SS and several non-HLA genes has been reported (Table 8.1), some of which have been associated with primary SS

Table 8.1 Putative non-HLA candidate genes associated with SS

Locus	Population (SS case sample size)	References
ApoE	Finnish (63)	[55]
BAFF	Australian (112)	[56]
CCR5	Czech (39)	[57]
Fas	Norwegian (70)	[58]
FasL	Norwegian (70)	[58]
GSTM1	Japanese (106)	[59]
HA-1	Mixed Caucasian (88)	[60]
IgKM	Australian (26)	[61]
IkBα(alpha)	Taiwan (98)	[62]
IkBβ(beta)	Columbian (67)	[63]
IL-1RN	French (36)	[64]
IL-1RA	Northern European (36)	[64]
IL-10	Finnish (66)	[65]
	Spanish (63)	[66]
	Japanese (47)	[67]
IL-4Rα(alpha)	Korean (45)	[68]
IRF5	French (100–212)	[69, 70]
	Swedish (228)	[71]
	Norwegian (140)	[71]
MBL	Japanese (104)	[72]
	Japanese (101)	[73]
	Spanish (81)	[74]
PTPN22	Columbian (70)	[75]
STAT4	US Caucasian (124)	[49]
	Swedish (228)	[71]
	Norwegian (140)	[71]
TcRBV	United Kingdom (61)	[76]
TGF-β(beta)1	French (129)	[77]
TNF-α(alpha)	French (35)	[78]
52 kDa Ro/SS-A	Norwegian (70)	[79]
	Japanese (111)	[80]

and/or various forms of secondary SS or specific autoantibodies. As summarized below, pathways involve both innate and adaptive arms of the immune system and broadly include interferon signaling, cytokines, antigen presentation, lymphocyte signaling, and apoptosis.

The role of innate immune disease mechanisms in SS and other autoimmune diseases has received increased attention over the last several years. Dysregulation of interferon pathways in particular has emerged as a major focus. In SS, overexpression of type-I IFN-inducible genes (the "interferon signature") has been detected in salivary gland tissue, lacrimal gland tissue, and peripheral blood [81–84]. Interferon regulatory factor 5 (*IRF5*), a member of a family of transcription factors, acts downstream of Toll-like receptors and type-I IFN stimulation to promote the expression of proinflammatory cytokines, including IFN-α(alpha) [85, 86]. Association of *IRF5* with SS has now been demonstrated in independent cohorts [69–71]. There is a 5-bp insertion/deletion polymorphism located in the promoter that may increase expression levels of *IRF5* in SS. In SLE, this gene has been associated in genetic studies of Asian, Caucasian, Hispanic, and African–American populations with several independent genetic effects conferring risk [87–93], supporting complex patterns of how various polymorphisms relate to specific SLE-related phenotypes [94]. Additional studies will be required to more fully understand the role of this important risk factor for SS and related autoimmune diseases.

Mannose-binding lectin (MBL), a serum protein, is also important in innate immune mechanisms. MBL is critical for host recognition of microorganisms and contains a domain that can bind to the receptor collectin on the surface of phagocytes aiding in phagocytosis [95]. MBL also mediates the activation of the complement pathway by lectin [95]. A mutation in codon 54 of the *MBL* gene, in addition to other MBL polymorphisms, affects serum levels [72]. Wang et al. reported a higher allele frequency of wild-type *MBL* codon 54 in Japanese SS patients than controls [72]. Tsutsumi et al. found homozygosity for the codon 54 mutation to be associated with SS in a separate cohort of Japanese SS cases and controls [95]. Neither Mullighan [96] nor Aittoniemi [97] could confirm association between *MBL* polymorphisms and SS. A recent study reported by Ramos-Casals et al. included evaluation of clinical and immunological manifestations of disease and suggested that patients with *MBL*-low genotypes have milder disease [74].

Alterations of cytokine expression patterns in SS have been described and are potentially influenced by genetic variants [98]. Association of SS with polymorphisms in interleukin *(IL)-10, IL-6, IL-1RA, IL-4Rα(alpha), TNF-α(alpha)*, interferon gamma *(IFN-γ(gamma))*, *BAFF*, and transforming growth factor-beta 1 *(TGF-β(beta)1)* have been reported but in many cases not confirmed in independent studies [54]. Small sample sizes, population differences, and incomplete evaluation of the genetic variation across these loci are likely to contribute to the difficulties with confirmation of reported associations. As larger studies are eventually performed, establishing association with these genes and understanding functional consequences of relevant variants may help explain specific features of SS such as increases in T-cell/B-cell proliferation and antibody production (e.g., *BAFF, IL-10, IL-6, IL-4Rα(alpha)*). Additional studies may also shed light on the role of cytokines in specific disease manifestations. For example, the interleukin 4 receptor alpha *(IL-4Rα(alpha))* gene has been evaluated in several studies of SS, suggesting association with disease susceptibility as well as parotid gland enlargements, increased levels of rheumatoid factor, and other immunological markers [68, 99].

Transforming growth factor-beta1 (TGF-β(beta)1) has also been implicated in the pathogenesis of SS [78]. TGF-β(beta)1 is a profibrotic, immunosuppressive cytokine expressed by many cell types and is known to be under-expressed in salivary glands of SS patients as compared to controls [77]. Gottenberg et al. analyzed a number of cytokine gene polymorphisms, including *TGF-β(beta)1*, and identified a variant with increased allele frequency in SS patients with anti-La/SS-B autoantibodies and patients who carry the *HLA-DRB1*3* haplotype [77]. They hypothesized that both the *TGF-β(beta)1* polymorphism and the *HLA-DRB1*3* haplotype act in combination to promote the production of anti-La/SS-B autoantibodies.

Adaptive immune responses in SS are influenced by antigen presentation. In humans, the major histocompatability complex (MHC) region on chromosome 6 contains 140 genes between flanking genetic markers *MOG* and *COL11A2* [100]. The subset of *HLA* genes located within the MHC region is the most well-characterized, encode cell surface antigen-presenting proteins, and are well-documented risk factors for the development of autoimmune disorders [101, 102]. Associations of *HLA* alleles (mostly Class II genes, *HLA-DR, or HLA-DQ*) have been described, and specific alleles vary in different ethnic groups with SS [103]. In most studies, when an HLA association with SS was demonstrable, a stronger association could be found to the anti-Ro/SS-A and anti-La/SS-B autoantibody responses. The HLA class I genetic associations with SS are less powerful than the HLA associations at *HLA-DR* and *HLA-DQ*. Other genes within the MHC region, such as *TNF-α(alpha)* and *TAP2*, may be more strongly associated in patients who are seropositive for anti-Ro/SS-A. All of these studies are complicated by extensive LD structure in this region of the genome, increasing the difficulty in pinpointing true causal variants. Studies in SLE have also indicated associations with these loci, and ongoing efforts suggest that more than one independent effect originates from this region. Detailed studies across the MHC locus in SS are needed to further clarify the physical genetics so that their etiologic role can be addressed.

Polymorphisms that shape the autoantibody repertoire may be important in SS. The anti-Ro52 autoantibody was discovered and demonstrated to be present in SS by Ben-Chetrit et al. [104]. Curiously, a polymorphism in intron 1 of the *Ro52* autoantigen has also associated with SS by Nakken et al. in SS patients positive for anti-Ro/SS-A [79]. Similarly, Imanishi et al. reported a polymorphism in intron 3 that may influence the presence of anti-SS-A/Ro52 antibody in SS patients [80]. Recent studies by Espionosa et al. have shown that Ro52 is an important negative regulator of proinflammatory cytokine production regulated by IRF transcription factors through the IL23–Th17 pathway [105]. Furthermore, allotypes, originally defined by allospecific sera, are heritable differences in antibody structure and may contribute to genetic risk. Whittingham et al. reported evidence for association of anti-La/SS-B autoantibodies with *KM(1)* allotype in SS [61]. This discovery was replicated 20 years later by Pertovaara et al. [55], but not in another study of comparable sample size [106]. Finally, Lawson et al. observed a decreased frequency of the deleted/deleted genotype of the T-cell receptor beta variable *(TCRβV)* gene in SS patients compared to controls [76].

Lymphocyte signaling molecules that regulate proliferation, activation, and effector functions have been identified as candidates in SS. *STAT4* (signal transducer and activator of transcription 4) is a lymphocyte signal transduction molecule involved in IL-12 and IL-13 signaling [49]. *STAT4*, a member of the STAT family of transcription factors, encodes a protein that transmits signals induced by interleukin-12, type-I IFNs (thus linking innate and adaptive immunity), interleukin-23, and other cytokines. Upon activation by cytokines, STAT4 stimulates transcription of IFN-γ(sigma), a key inducer of T-cell differentiation into type-I T-helper cells. The protein encoded by *STAT4* is required to regulate T-helper cell responses [107, 108]. SNPs in the *STAT4* gene have also been found to be strongly associated with SLE and RA [94].

Another signaling molecule, protein tyrosine phosphatase non-receptor type-22 (*PTPN22*), has been suggested as a candidate gene in SS. *PTPN22* is expressed primarily in lymphoid tissues. This gene encodes for the protein Lyp that dephosphorylates kinases Lck, Fyn, and Zap-70, all known to have prominent roles in T-cell signaling. This protein also interacts with Src tyrosine kinases (Csk) and the adaptor molecule Grb2 leading to downregulation of T-cell signaling [109]. In a collection of SS Colombian cases and matched controls, Gomez et al. found the 1858 T allele to be a risk factor for SS [75]. However, an independent study by Ittah et al. found no significant difference in the 1858 T allele frequency [109]. This allele has been shown to interrupt the interaction of Lyp and Csk leading to aberrant activation of T cells [109]. Criswell et al. also reported no association with SS in their collection of 265 multiplex autoimmune families [110]. The 1858 T allele of *PTPN22* is associated with multiple autoimmune diseases including type 1 diabetes [44], RA [43, 47, 110–112], juvenile idiopathic arthritis [112, 113], SLE [26, 47, 110, 114], Graves' disease [48, 115], myasthenia gravis [116], generalized vitiligo [117], and Wegener's granulomatosis [118]. Additional studies in larger cohorts of SS patients should be evaluated to more definitively determine the potential role of this important "autoimmunity" locus in SS.

Cytotoxic T-lymphocyte-associated antigen 4 (CTLA-4) is another important negative regulator of immune responses in T cells. CTLA-4 acts to suppress T-cell activation and proinflammatory cytokine production [119]. CTLA-4 can also trigger apoptosis of activated

T cells [119]. In 2006, Downie-Doyle et al. reported association of *CTLA*-4+49G/A and CT60 haplotypes with susceptibility to SS [119]. Soon afterward, Gottenberg et al. reported results from two separate cohorts of SS patients and controls [120]. In the first cohort, allele frequency differences between patients and controls were observed for the *CTLA*-4+49G/A allele but not *CTLA*-4 CT60. In a second cohort, however, allelic distributions for both *CTLA*-4+49G/A and CT60 variants were not significantly different between SS patients and controls [120]. Inconsistencies between studies may be due in part to analytical differences between haplotype versus single SNP analyses. The +49A:CT60G haplotype has also been associated with SLE; however, association with additional haplotypes has also been observed but remains to be fully defined [121, 122].

An important role for apoptosis has long been hypothesized in SS. FAS and FAS ligand (TNF receptor superfamily, member 6) have been implicated in the pathogenesis of various diseases of the immune system, including SS. These cell surface molecules are responsible for transducing a death signal into the cytoplasm, leading to apoptosis [58]. Bolstad et al. observed significant differences in frequencies of three *FAS* alleles in patients compared to controls [58]. However, Mullighan et al. did not find FAS alleles associated with SS in their collection [123].

Other associations have been reported with SS, but have yet to be replicated. One such example is the glutathione-*S*-transferase MI (*GSTM1*) and *GSTT1* genes. In Japanese patients, 57.5% of SS patients shared a *GSTM1* homozygous null genotype compared to 44.1% of controls and were found to have higher levels of anti-Ro/SS-A autoantibodies [59]. Another example was reported in a study of Finnish Caucasian patients with SS, where the apolipoprotein E (*ApoE*) epsilon4 allele was found to be associated with early onset of SS [124].

Thus, much work remains to firmly establish and characterize genes that confer risk to developing SS and related disease manifestations. We have an abundance of evidence that the necessary genetic tools are in hand waiting to be applied to SS. Assembling large cohorts of carefully evaluated patients will be necessary and will require collaborative international efforts. The value in using discovery-based approaches can then be realized and followed by studies that are hypothesis-driven in both humans and highly relevant mouse models.

8.6 Viral Influences in SS

In addition to a potentially complex genetic architecture in SS, the etiology of SS is certain to be further complicated by "environmental" factors such as viruses. Monozygotic twin concordance rates, although not formally measured in SS, are less than 35% in related diseases such as SLE [31]. Understanding how pathogens interact with an autoimmune-prone genetic background to result in expression of disease manifestations is critical for a more complete understanding of etiology. In a recent review, Munz et al. discuss in detail multiple mechanisms by which viral infections may trigger autoimmune disease or vice versa [125]. Prevailing hypotheses for potential autoimmune disease mechanisms triggered by infection include (1) adjuvant effect of pathogens in priming autoreactive immune responses; (2) molecular mimicry; and (3) bystander activation of autoreactive cells and epitope spreading. On the other hand, evidence also supports mechanisms in which autoimmune disease could affect anti-viral responses through (1) bystander activation; (2) increased pathogen replication; and (3) redistribution of anti-viral immune responses to sites of autoimmune inflammation. Support for each of these mechanisms has been observed in various autoimmune diseases and with respect to various viruses. Of course, the role of viruses in inducting, promoting, sustaining, or exacerbating infections in any autoimmune disease could be complicated by the influence of more than one virus acting simultaneously or sequentially to generate a specific phenotype.

In SS, numerous infectious agents have been considered and include Epstein–Barr virus (EBV), human T-cell leukemia virus 1 (HTLV1), hepatitis C (HepC), endogenous retroviral particles, and coxsackieviruses [126]. Specific evidences supporting these candidate viruses vary, but generally include small studies aimed at detecting viral nucleic acids or proteins or serological evidence of past infection. Controversial results have been reported for virtually all viruses studied to date in SS and association with any single virus has not been firmly established. Other lines of evidence to support role of viral infections in SS include such properties as the ability of certain viruses to directly infect cells in the salivary gland and/or immune system, sequence similarities between viral proteins and autoantigens (particularly Ro/SS-A and La/SS-B) that may promote autoantibody production through a molecular mimicry mechanism, elevation of viral antibodies or viral sequences in SS patients, association between viral infection and lymphocyte transformation into lymphoma, and association of symptoms mimicking SS following viral infection [126, 127]. Regardless of the specific virus, mechanisms of host–virus relationships that control or perpetuate latency and re-activation cycles of viral replication and inflammatory responses (such as production of IFNs) are complex but likely to be important in SS.

The complex set of possible host–environment interactions spreading over a lifetime undoubtedly contributes to difficulties in study design and the ability to establish robust associations with a particular virus. Perhaps the most significant insight into understanding this relationship comes from a variety of studies in SLE consistent with a role for EBVs that are potentially informative for SS [127, 128]. A model developed from studies during the past decade is depicted in Fig. 8.2. First, genetic predisposition could include numerous potential variants that influence subsequent steps in this model. Specific variants in genes that are involved in activation and regulation of IFN responses (e.g., *IRF5* or *STAT4*), antigen presentation and specificity (e.g., T-cell receptors and *HLA*), and lymphocyte function (e.g., *PTPN22* and *BAFF*) would be required to increase risk of developing autoimmunity after the necessary environmental exposures are encountered. As previously discussed, more than 30 genes in SLE have now been identified, illustrating that the predisposing genetic backgrounds are likely to be quite complex. Next, serologic exposure and evidence of viral EBV DNA have been shown to be highly associated with SLE in children and adults, consistent with a necessary but not sufficient role of viral infection. Furthermore, studies in patients where samples were available prior to development of autoimmune responses provide compelling evidence for cross-reactive responses between EBV and SLE/SS autoantigen responses as a critical step. A single first epitope targeted by anti-Ro autoimmune responses in SLE is TKYKQRNGWSHKD, which then spreads over time to possibly more than 20 different secondary epitopes. Antibodies that bind the initial Ro epitope have been shown to cross-react to an EBV epitope, GGSGSGPRHRDGVRR of the viral EBNA-1 protein. Another important and interesting finding was originally reported by Arbuckle et al., showing that the development of anti-Ro and anti-La precedes the appearance of clinical manifestations and diagnosis of SLE by more than 3 years [129]. In SS, low levels of anti-Ro and anti-La have been associated with subclinical dry eyes and dry mouth in otherwise apparently healthy individuals. Progressive production toward high levels of these autoantibodies would be expected to result in fully blown autoimmune disease.

Similar models for EBV and other viruses have also been suggested in SS. For example, cross-reactivity between another Ro epitope and a peptide derived from the Coxsackievirus 2B protein has been reported in SS patients [130]. Of course, not all SS patients produce anti-Ro autoantibodies. Indeed, associations of HCV with SS appear to be enriched in patients who are negative for anti-Ro, reviewed by Ramos-Casals et al. [131]. In both SS and HCV-associated lymphomas and lymphoproliferative diseases, cross-reactivities or molecular mimicry have been suggested based on similarity of antigen receptor gene segments expressed [132].

Thus, multiple viruses are potentially associated with SS, and our understanding of their role in contributing to SS is far from complete. Interactions with genetic factors that contribute

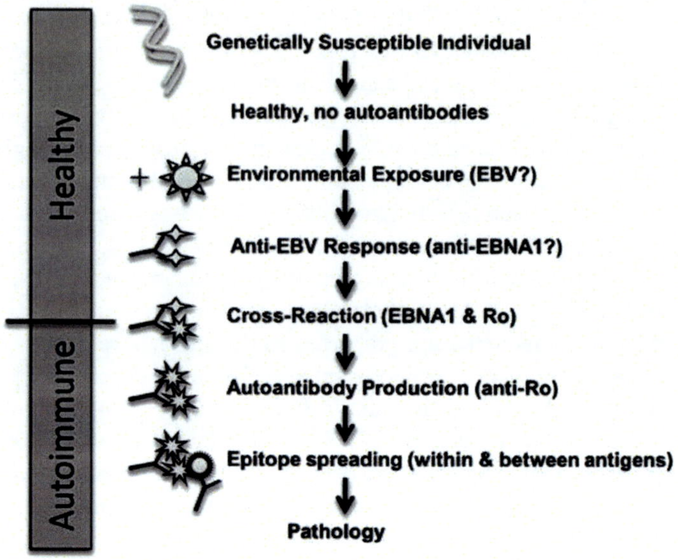

Fig. 8.2 Potential model for development of autoimmunity through molecular mimicry of EBV EBNA-1 and Ro epitopes

to overall risk of disease as well as progression at each step shown in Fig. 8.2 are likely to exist but yet to be fully elucidated.

8.7 Insights from Genomic and Proteomic Studies

Biological networks and pathways that define human physiology are immensely complex. As opposed to the traditional "reductionist" view of dissecting individual components of a disease state, understanding mechanisms of disease that take into consideration these complexities is fast becoming the focus of a relatively new area that has emerged in the last decade of "systems biology." Either subtle or significant alterations in normal levels of gene expression and/or their protein products may correlate with disease states. Two major approaches developed in recent years provide opportunities to gain further insight into etiology of disease. The first is transcriptional or gene expression profiling, which measures levels of mRNA at a global level. The second is proteomics, which has similar goals for the detection of comprehensive sets of proteins. Both have been applied in SS and are facilitating the identification of important disease-related pathways.

High-throughput transcriptional profiling using microarray technology has been applied to SS, SLE, RA, and numerous other complex diseases. These studies aim to comprehensively characterize patterns of gene expression in isolated cells from normal and diseased tissues. Studies in SS, SLE, and RA have demonstrated characteristic peripheral blood cell (PBC) gene expression fingerprints or "signatures." A prominent signature that has been repeatedly observed in autoimmune phenotypes including SS is marked by overexpression of interferon (IFN)-inducible genes [133]. In SS, our group has evaluated PBC gene expression patterns using microarrays that interrogate over 22,000 mRNA transcripts and identified IFN signaling as the most significantly dysregulated pathway in PBCs [81]. This IFN signature appears to be most prominent in the subset of patients who produce anti-Ro/anti-La autoantibodies. We also identified additional pathways that are dysregulated in peripheral blood cells of SS patients including B-cell and T-cell receptor signaling, insulin-like growth factor 1, granulocyte macrophage colony-stimulating factor, peroxisome proliferator-activated receptor-a/retinoid X receptor-α, and PI3/AKT signaling.

Several gene expression profiling studies of salivary gland tissue and saliva in human SS have also been reported. One of the most consistent findings across all these studies is the dysregulation of IFN pathways. In a study by Hjelmervik et al., patients with primary SS and controls with symptoms of SS but no objective criteria were evaluated [83]. RNA was extracted from minor salivary gland tissue and hybridized to cDNA microarrays with features representing ~16,000 transcripts. The highest ranked transcripts were from the T-cell receptor β(beta) locus and numerous other genes consistent with a chronic inflammatory state. Genes involved in IFN responses were also noted. In addition, downregulation of the expression of carbonic anhydrase II was also found. This gene is essential in saliva production, and secretion may thus contribute to direct functional abnormalities in SS. Using a similar study design, Gottenberg et al. also evaluated minor salivary gland tissue and identified genes implicating IFN-mediated innate immune mechanisms in the pathogenesis of pSS [82]. This study also demonstrated the presence of plasmacytoid dendritic cells, a major producer of IFN, in salivary gland tissue of all SS patients but none in the controls. More recently, IFN-related gene expression patterns were also reported in a third study of three pSS and three controls [134]. Furthermore, activation of IFN-related pathways in saliva has also been reported using both transcriptional profiling and proteomic approaches [84]. Finally, a recent study evaluating gene expression profiles in salivary gland epithelial cells revealed significant dysregulation of apoptotic and IFN pathways. These data were then coupled with genome-wide association study to identify chromosomal regions that appear to harbor genetic loci that influence quantitative transcript levels associated with SS [135]. Future studies will be necessary to further test the candidates identified.

Conclusion

Genomic studies in SS strongly support the role of innate and adaptive immune mechanisms in the pathogenesis of SS. A proposed model suggests that genetic susceptibility involves specific variants in a potentially long list of genes. Genes involved in innate immune mechanisms, such as apoptosis, IFN signaling, cytokine levels, expression of autoantigens, and T-cell and B-cell function, are all likely to be important. Initial triggers of autoimmunity may involve several mechanisms such as molecular mimicry between certain viruses and common autoantigens in SS. Once cross-reactive autoantibodies are produced and immune responses mature, continued stimulation by immune complexes (and perhaps viruses) of TLRs in salivary glands and downstream signaling pathways may be dysregulated and contribute to the persistence of what is observed as the IFN signature [82]. Other pathways, such as apoptosis and lymphocyte signaling, contribute to the overall complex etiology of SS.

Identifying the genetic factors that cause SS lags far behind the remarkable progress that has recently been observed in other closely related autoimmune diseases. Full leveraging of the powerful tools available for genetic discovery has been hampered by lack of large, well-characterized cohorts of patients. SS genetics investigators are working toward assembling the samples and data needed to launch large-scale genetics studies with the expectation that fundamental new knowledge about this complex disease will be discovered, allowing for more precise definition of pathogenic mechanisms leading to the overall SS phenotype as well as clinically heterogeneous subsets of patients. Important opportunities for rapid translation into improved diagnostic and therapeutic approaches for SS and its spectrum diseases are certain to follow.

References

1. Besana C, Salmaggi C, Pellegrino C, et al. Chronic bilateral dacryo-adenitis in identical twins: a possible incomplete form of Sjogren syndrome. Eur J Pediatr. 1991;150:652–5.
2. Bolstad AI, Haga HJ, Wassmuth R, Jonsson R. Monozygotic twins with primary Sjogren's syndrome. J Rheumatol. 2000;27:2264–6.
3. Houghton KM, Cabral DA, Petty RE, Tucker LB. Primary Sjogren's syndrome in dizygotic adolescent twins: one case with lymphocytic interstitial pneumonia. J Rheumatol. 2005;32:1603–6.
4. Scofield RH, Kurien BT, Reichlin M. Immunologically restricted and inhibitory anti-Ro/SSA in monozygotic twins. Lupus 1997;6:395–8.
5. Boling EP, Wen J, Reveille JD, Bias WB, Chused TM, Arnett FC. Primary Sjogren's syndrome and autoimmune hemolytic anemia in sisters. A family study. Am J Med. 1983;74:1066–71.
6. Lichtenfeld JL, Kirschner RH, Wiernik PH. Familial Sjogren's syndrome with associated primary salivary gland lymphoma. Am J Med. 1976;60:286–92.
7. Mason AM, Golding PL. Multiple immunological abnormalities in a family. J Clin Path. 1971;24:732–5.
8. Reveille JD. The molecular genetics of systemic lupus erythematosus and Sjogren's syndrome. Curr Opin Rheumatol. 1992;4:644–56.
9. Sabio JM, Milla E, Jimenez-Alonso J. A multicase family with primary Sjogren's syndrome. J Rheumatol. 2001;28:1932–4.
10. Sestak AL, Shaver TS, Moser KL, Neas BR, Harley JB. Familial aggregation of lupus and autoimmunity in an unusual multiplex pedigree. J Rheumatol.1999;26:1495–9.
11. Reveille JD, Wilson RW, Provost TT, Bias WB, Arnett FC. Primary Sjogren's syndrome and other autoimmune diseases in families. Prevalence and immunogenetic studies in six kindreds. Annl Intern Med. 1984;101:748–56.
12. de Seze J, Devos D, Castelnovo G, et al. The prevalence of Sjogren syndrome in patients with primary progressive multiple sclerosis. Neurology 2001;57:1359–63.
13. Soyfoo MS, Steinfeld S, Delporte C. Usefulness of mouse models to study the pathogenesis of Sjogren's syndrome. Oral Dis. 2007;13:366–75.
14. Hayashi Y, Kojima A, Hata M, Hirokawa K. A new mutation involving the sublingual gland in NFS/N mice. Partially arrested mucous cell differentiation. Am J Path. 1988;132:187–91.
15. Ishimaru N, Yoneda T, Saegusa K, et al. Severe destructive autoimmune lesions with aging in murine Sjogren's syndrome through Fas-mediated apoptosis. Am J Path. 2000;156:1557–64.
16. Haneji N, Hamano H, Yanagi K, Hayashi Y. A new animal model for primary Sjogren's syndrome in NFS/sld mutant mice. J Immunol. 1994;153:2769–77.
17. Shinkura R, Kitada K, Matsuda F, et al. Alymphoplasia is caused by a point mutation in the mouse gene encoding Nf-kappa b-inducing kinase. Nat Genet. 1999;22:74–7.
18. Tsubata R, Tsubata T, Hiai H, et al. Autoimmune disease of exocrine organs in immunodeficient alymphoplasia mice: a spontaneous model for Sjogren's syndrome. Eur J Immunol. 1996;26:2742–8.
19. Li H, Dai M, Zhuang Y. A T cell intrinsic role of Id3 in a mouse model for primary Sjogren's syndrome. Immunity 2004;21:551–60.
20. Hayakawa I, Tedder TF, Zhuang Y. B-lymphocyte depletion ameliorates Sjogren's syndrome in Id3 knockout mice. Immunology 2007;122:73–9.
21. Gabriel SB, Schaffner SF, Nguyen H, et al. The structure of haplotype blocks in the human genome. Science 2002;296:2225–9.
22. Kruglyak L, Nickerson DA. Variation is the spice of life. Nat Genet. 2001;27:234–6.
23. Reich DE, Gabriel SB, Altshuler D. Quality and completeness of SNP databases. Nat Genet. 2003;33:457–8.
24. Reich DE, Cargill M, Bolk S, et al. Linkage disequilibrium in the human genome. Nature 2001;411:199–204.
25. Easton DF, Pooley KA, Dunning AM, et al. Genome-wide association study identifies novel breast cancer susceptibility loci. Nature 2007;447:1087–93.
26. Harley JB, Alarcon-Riquelme ME, Criswell LA, et al. Genome-wide association scan in women with systemic lupus erythematosus identifies susceptibility variants in *ITGAM, PXK, KIAA1542* and other loci. Nat Genet. 2008;40:204–10.
27. Hom G, Graham RR, Modrek B, et al. Association of systemic lupus erythematosus with C8orf13-BLK and ITGAM-ITGAX. N Engl J Med. 2008;358:900–9.
28. McCarthy MI, Abecasis GR, Cardon LR, et al. Genome-wide association studies for complex traits: consensus, uncertainty and challenges. Nat Rev. 2008;9:356–69.
29. Todd JA, Walker NM, Cooper JD, et al. Robust associations of four new chromosome regions from genome-wide analyses of type 1 diabetes. Nat Genet. 2007;39:857–64.
30. Wellcome-Trust-Case–Control-Consortium. Genome-wide association study of 14,000 cases of seven common diseases and 3,000 shared controls. Nature 2007;447:661–78.
31. Moser KL, Kelly JA, Lessard CJ, Harley JB. Recent insights into the genetic basis of systemic lupus erythematosus. Genes Immun. 2009;10:373–9.

32. Barrett JC, Hansoul S, Nicolae DL, et al. Genome-wide association defines more than 30 distinct susceptibility loci for Crohn's disease. Nat Genet. 2008;40:955–62.
33. Graham RR, Ortmann WA, Langefeld CD, et al. Visualizing human leukocyte antigen class II risk haplotypes in human systemic lupus erythematosus. Am J Hum Genet. 2002;71:543–53.
34. Barreto M, Santos E, Ferreira R, et al. Evidence for CTLA4 as a susceptibility gene for systemic lupus erythematosus. Eur J Hum Genet. 2004;12: 620–6.
35. Blomhoff A, Kemp EH, Gawkrodger DJ, et al. CTLA4 polymorphisms are associated with vitiligo, in patients with concomitant autoimmune diseases. Pigment Cell Res. 2005;18:55–8.
36. Blomhoff A, Lie BA, Myhre AG, et al. Polymorphisms in the cytotoxic T lymphocyte antigen-4 gene region confer susceptibility to Addison's disease. J Clin Endocrinol Metab. 2004;89:3474–6.
37. Furugaki K, Shirasawa S, Ishikawa N, et al. Association of the T-cell regulatory gene CTLA4 with Graves' disease and autoimmune thyroid disease in the Japanese. J Hum Genet. 2004;49: 166–8.
38. Hunt KA, McGovern DP, Kumar PJ, et al. A common CTLA4 haplotype associated with coeliac disease. Eur J Hum Genet. 2005;13: 440–4.
39. Lee CS, Lee YJ, Liu HF, et al. Association of CTLA4 gene A–G polymorphism with rheumatoid arthritis in Chinese. Clin Rheumatol. 2003;22: 221–4.
40. Torres B, Aguilar F, Franco E, et al. Association of the CT60 marker of the CTLA4 gene with systemic lupus erythematosus. Arthritis Rheum. 2004;50:2211–5.
41. Zhou Y, Huang D, Paris PL, Sauter CS, Prock KA, Hoffman GS. An analysis of CTLA-4 and proinflammatory cytokine genes in Wegener's granulomatosis. Arthritis Rheum. 2004;50: 2645–50.
42. Prokunina L, Alarcon-Riquelme M. The genetic basis of systemic lupus erythematosus—knowledge of today and thoughts for tomorrow. Hum Mol Genet. 2004;13 (Spec No 1):R143–48.
43. Begovich AB, Carlton VE, Honigberg LA, et al. A missense single-nucleotide polymorphism in a gene encoding a protein tyrosine phosphatase (PTPN22) is associated with rheumatoid arthritis. Am J Hum Genet. 2004;75:330–7.
44. Bottini N, Musumeci L, Alonso A, et al. A functional variant of lymphoid tyrosine phosphatase is associated with type I diabetes. Nat Genet. 2004;36:337–8.
45. Ladner MB, Bottini N, Valdes AM, Noble JA. Association of the single nucleotide polymorphism C1858T of the PTPN22 gene with type 1 diabetes. Hum Immunol. 2005;66:60–4.
46. Onengut-Gumuscu S, Ewens KG, Spielman RS, Concannon P. A functional polymorphism (1858C/T) in the PTPN22 gene is linked and associated with type I diabetes in multiplex families. Genes Immun. 2004;5:678–80.
47. Orozco G, Sanchez E, Gonzalez-Gay MA, et al. Association of a functional single-nucleotide polymorphism of PTPN22, encoding lymphoid protein phosphatase, with rheumatoid arthritis and systemic lupus erythematosus. Arthritis Rheum. 2005;52:219–24.
48. Velaga MR, Wilson V, Jennings CE, et al. The codon 620 tryptophan allele of the lymphoid tyrosine phosphatase (LYP) gene is a major determinant of Graves' disease. J Clin Endocrinol Metabol. 2004;89:5862–5.
49. Korman BD, Alba MI, Le JM, et al. Variant form of *STAT4* is associated with primary Sjogren's syndrome. Genes Immun. 2008;9:267–70.
50. Marrack P, Kappler J, Kotzin BL. Autoimmune disease: why and where it occurs. Nat Med. 2001;7:899–905.
51. Harley IT, Kaufman KM, Langefeld CD, Harley JB, Kelly JA. Genetic susceptibility to SLE: new insights from fine mapping and genome-wide association studies. Nat Rev Genet. 2009;10:285–90.
52. Fox RP, Michelson P, Wallace DJ. Dubois' lupus erythematosus: Sjogren's syndrome. Philadelphia, PA: Lippincott, Williams, & Wilkins; 2007, pp. 775–8.
53. Han S, Guthridge JM, Harley IT, et al. Osteopontin and systemic lupus erythematosus association: a probable gene–gender interaction. PLoS One 2008;3:e0001757.
54. Cobb BL, Lessard CJ, Harley JB, Moser KL. Genes and Sjogren's syndrome. Rheum Dis Clin N Am. 2008;34:847–68, vii.
55. Pertovaara M, Hurme M, Antonen J, Pasternack A, Pandey JP. Immunoglobulin KM and GM gene polymorphisms modify the clinical presentation of primary Sjogren's syndrome. J Rheumatol. 2004;31:2175–80.
56. Nossent JC, Lester Z, Zahra D, Mackey CR, Rischmueller M. Polymorphism in the 5′ regulatory region of the B-lymphocyte activating factor gene is associated with the Ro/La autoantibody response and serum BAFF levels in primary Sjogren's syndrome. Rheumatology 2008;47:1311–6.
57. Petrek M, Cermakova Z, Hutyrova B, et al. CC chemokine receptor 5 and interleukin-1 receptor antagonist gene polymorphisms in patients with primary Sjogren's syndrome. Clin Exp Rheumatol. 2002;20:701–3.
58. Bolstad AI, Wargelius A, Nakken B, Haga HJ, Jonsson R. Fas and Fas ligand gene polymorphisms in primary Sjogren's syndrome. J Rheum. 2000;27:2397–405.
59. Morinobu A, Kanagawa S, Koshiba M, Sugai S, Kumagai S. Association of the glutathione

S-transferase M1 homozygous null genotype with susceptibility to Sjogren's syndrome in Japanese individuals. Arthritis Rheum. 1999;42: 2612–5.
60. Harangi M, Kaminski WE, Fleck M, et al. Homozygosity for the 168His variant of the minor histocompatibility antigen HA-1 is associated with reduced risk of primary Sjogren's syndrome. Eur J Immunol. 2005;35:305–17.
61. Whittingham S, Propert DN, Mackay IR. A strong association between the antinuclear antibody anti-La (SS-B) and the kappa chain allotype Km(1). Immunogenetics 1984;19:295–9.
62. Ou TT, Lin CH, Lin YC, et al. IkappaBalpha promoter polymorphisms in patients with primary Sjogren's syndrome. J Clin Immunol. 2008;28: 440–4.
63. Castiblanco J, Anaya JM. The IkappaBL gene polymorphism influences risk of acquiring systemic lupus erythematosus and Sjogren's syndrome. Hum Immunol. 2008;69:45–51.
64. Perrier S, Coussediere C, Dubost JJ, Albuisson E, Sauvezie B. IL-1 receptor antagonist (IL-1RA) gene polymorphism in Sjogren's syndrome and rheumatoid arthritis. Clin Immunopathol. 1998;87:309–13.
65. Hulkkonen J, Pertovaara M, Antonen J, Lahdenpohja N, Pasternack A, Hurme M. Genetic association between interleukin-10 promoter region polymorphisms and primary Sjogren's syndrome. Arthritis Rheum. 2001;44:176–9.
66. Font J, Garcia-Carrasco M, Ramos-Casals M, et al. The role of interleukin-10 promoter polymorphisms in the clinical expression of primary Sjogren's syndrome. Rheumatology 2002;41:1025–30.
67. Origuchi T, Kawasaki E, Ide A, et al. Ann Rheum Dis. 2003;62:1117–8.
68. Youn J, Hwang SH, Cho CS, et al. Association of the interleukin-4 receptor alpha variant Q576R with Th1/Th2 imbalance in connective tissue disease. Immunogenetics 2000;51:743–6.
69. Miceli-Richard C, Comets E, Loiseau P, Puechal X, Hachulla E, Mariette X. Association of an *IRF5* gene functional polymorphism with Sjogren's syndrome. Arthritis Rheum. 2007;56:3989–94.
70. Miceli-Richard C, Gestermann N, Ittah M, et al. The CGGGG insertion/deletion polymorphism of the *IRF5* promoter is a strong risk factor for primary Sjogren's syndrome. Arthritis Rheum. 2009;60:1991–7.
71. Nordmark G, Kristjansdottir G, Theander E, et al. Additive effects of the major risk alleles of *IRF5* and *STAT4* in primary Sjogren's syndrome. Genes Immun. 2009;10:68–76.
72. Wang ZY, Morinobu A, Kanagawa S, Kumagai S. Polymorphisms of the mannose binding lectin gene in patients with Sjogren's syndrome. Annl Rheum Dis. 2001;60:483–6.
73. Tsutsumi A, Sasaki K, Wakamiya N, et al. Genes Immun. 2001;2:99–104.
74. Ramos-Casals M, Brito-Zeron P, Soria N, et al. Mannose-binding lectin-low genotypes are associated with milder systemic and immunological disease expression in primary Sjogren's syndrome. Rheumatology 2009;48:65–9.
75. Gomez LM, Anaya JM, Gonzalez CI, et al. PTPN22 C1858T polymorphism in Colombian patients with autoimmune diseases. Genes Immun. 2005;6: 628–31.
76. Lawson CA, Donaldson IJ, Bowman SJ, et al. Analysis of the insertion/deletion related polymorphism within T cell antigen receptor beta variable genes in primary Sjogren's syndrome. Annl Rheum Dis. 2005;64:468–70.
77. Gottenberg JE, Busson M, Loiseau P, et al. Association of transforming growth factor beta1 and tumor necrosis factor alpha polymorphisms with anti-SSB/La antibody secretion in patients with primary Sjogren's syndrome. Arthritis Rheum. 2004;50:570–80.
78. Guggenbuhl P, Veillard E, Quelvenec E, et al. Analysis of TNFalpha microsatellites in 35 patients with primary Sjogren's syndrome. Joint Bone Spine 2000;67:290–5.
79. Nakken B, Jonsson R, Bolstad AI. Polymorphisms of the Ro52 gene associated with anti-Ro 52-kd autoantibodies in patients with primary Sjogren's syndrome. Arthritis Rheum. 2001;44: 638–46.
80. Imanishi T, Morinobu A, Hayashi N, et al. A novel polymorphism of the SSA1 gene is associated with anti-SS-A/Ro52 autoantibody in Japanese patients with primary Sjogren's syndrome. Clin Exp Rheumatol. 2005;23:521–4.
81. Emamian ES, Leon JM, Lessard CJ, et al. Peripheral blood gene expression profiling in Sjogren's syndrome. Genes Immun. 2009;10:285–96.
82. Gottenberg JE, Cagnard N, Lucchesi C, et al. Activation of IFN pathways and plasmacytoid dendritic cell recruitment in target organs of primary Sjogren's syndrome. Proc Nat Acad Sci USA. 2006;103:2770–5.
83. Hjelmervik TO, Petersen K, Jonassen I, Jonsson R, Bolstad AI. Gene expression profiling of minor salivary glands clearly distinguishes primary Sjogren's syndrome patients from healthy control subjects. Arthritis Rheum. 2005;52:1534–44.
84. Hu S, Wang J, Meijer J, et al. Salivary proteomic and genomic biomarkers for primary Sjogren's syndrome. Arthritis Rheum. 2007;56: 3588–600.
85. Takaoka A, Yanai H, Kondo S, et al. Integral role of IRF-5 in the gene induction programme activated by Toll-like receptors. Nature 2005;434: 243–9.
86. Taniguchi T, Ogasawara K, Takaoka A, Tanaka N. IRF family of transcription factors as regulators of host defense. Ann Rev Immunol. 2001;19: 623–55.

87. Demirci FY, Manzi S, Ramsey-Goldman R, et al. Association of a common interferon regulatory factor 5 (*IRF5*) variant with increased risk of systemic lupus erythematosus (SLE). Annl Hum Genet. 2007;71:308–11.
88. Graham RR, Kozyrev SV, Baechler EC, et al. A common haplotype of interferon regulatory factor 5 (*IRF5*) regulates splicing and expression and is associated with increased risk of systemic lupus erythematosus. Nat Genet. 2006;38:550–5.
89. Kelly JA, Kelley JM, Kaufman KM, et al. Interferon regulatory factor-5 is genetically associated with systemic lupus erythematosus in African Americans. Genes Immun. 2008;9:187–94.
90. Kozyrev SV, Lewen S, Reddy PM, et al. Structural insertion/deletion variation in *IRF5* is associated with a risk haplotype and defines the precise *IRF5* isoforms expressed in systemic lupus erythematosus. Arthritis Rheum. 2007;56:1234–41.
91. Reddy MV, Velazquez-Cruz R, Baca V, et al. Genetic association of *IRF5* with SLE in Mexicans: higher frequency of the risk haplotype and its homozygozity than Europeans. Hum Genet. 2007;121:721–7.
92. Shin HD, Sung YK, Choi CB, Lee SO, Lee HW, Bae SC. Replication of the genetic effects of IFN regulatory factor 5 (*IRF5*) on systemic lupus erythematosus in a Korean population. Arthritis Res Ther. 2007;9:R32.
93. Sigurdsson S, Nordmark G, Goring HH, et al. Polymorphisms in the tyrosine kinase 2 and interferon regulatory factor 5 genes are associated with systemic lupus erythematosus. Am J Hum Genet. 2005;76:528–37.
94. Remmers EF, Plenge RM, Lee AT, et al. *STAT4* and the risk of rheumatoid arthritis and systemic lupus erythematosus. N Engl J Med. 2007;357:977–86.
95. Tsutsumi A, Sasaki K, Wakamiya N, et al. Mannose-binding lectin gene: polymorphisms in Japanese patients with systemic lupus erythematosus, rheumatoid arthritis and Sjogren's syndrome. Genes Immun. 2001;2:99–104.
96. Mullighan CG, Heatley S, Bardy PG, Lester S, Rischmueller M, Gordon TP. Lack of association between mannose-binding lectin gene polymorphisms and primary Sjogren's syndrome. Arthritis Rheum. 2000;43:2851–2.
97. Aittoniemi J, Pertovaara M, Hulkkonen J, et al. The significance of mannan-binding lectin gene alleles in patients with primary Sjogren's syndrome. Scand J Rheumatol. 2002;31:362–5.
98. Roescher N, Tak PP, Illei GG. Cytokines in Sjogren's syndrome. Oral Dis. 2009;15:519–26.
99. Ramos-Casals M, Font J, Brito-Zeron P, Trejo O, Garcia-Carrasco M, Lozano F. Interleukin-4 receptor alpha polymorphisms in primary Sjogren's syndrome. Clin Exp Rheumatol. 2004;22:374.
100. Complete sequence and gene map of a human major histocompatibility complex. The MHC Sequencing Consortium. Nature 1999;401:921–3.
101. Merriman TR, Todd JA. Genetics of autoimmune disease. Curr Opin Immunol. 1995;7:786–92.
102. Nepom GT. MHC and autoimmune diseases. Immunology 1993;59:143–64.
103. Bolstad AI, Jonsson R. Genetic aspects of Sjogren's syndrome. Arthritis Res. 2002;4:353–9.
104. Ben-Chetrit E, Chan EK, Sullivan KF, Tan EM. A 52-kD protein is a novel component of the SS-A/Ro antigenic particle. J Exp Med. 1988;167:1560–71.
105. Espinosa A, Dardalhon V, Brauner S, et al. Loss of the lupus autoantigen Ro52/Trim21 induces tissue inflammation and systemic autoimmunity by disregulating the IL-23–Th17 pathway. J Exp Med. 2009; 206:1661–71.
106. Downie-Doyle S, Lester S, Bardy P, Gordon T, Rischmueller M, Pile K. Immunoglobulin kappa light chain gene alleles are not associated with primary Sjogren's syndrome. Genes Immun. 2002;3(Suppl 1):S63–5.
107. Morinobu A, Gadina M, Strober W, et al. *STAT4* serine phosphorylation is critical for IL-12-induced IFN-gamma production but not for cell proliferation. Proc Nat Acad Sci USA. 2002;99: 12281–6.
108. Nishikomori R, Usui T, Wu CY, Morinobu A, O'Shea JJ, Strober W. Activated *STAT4* has an essential role in Th1 differentiation and proliferation that is independent of its role in the maintenance of IL-12R beta 2 chain expression and signaling. J Immunol. 2002;169:4388–98.
109. Ittah M, Gottenberg JE, Proust A, et al. No evidence for association between 1858 C/T single-nucleotide polymorphism of PTPN22 gene and primary Sjogren's syndrome. Genes Immun. 2005;6:457–8.
110. Criswell LA, Pfeiffer KA, Lum RF, et al. Analysis of families in the Multiple Autoimmune Disease Genetics Consortium (MADGC) collection: the PTPN22 620 W allele associates with multiple autoimmune phenotypes. Am J Hum Genet. 2005;76:561–71.
111. Lee AT, Li W, Liew A, et al. The PTPN22 R620W polymorphism associates with RF positive rheumatoid arthritis in a dose-dependent manner but not with HLA-SE status. Genes Immun. 2005;6: 129–33.
112. Viken MK, Amundsen SS, Kvien TK, et al. Association analysis of the 1858C>T polymorphism in the PTPN22 gene in juvenile idiopathic arthritis and other autoimmune diseases. Genes Immun. 2005;6:271–3.
113. Hinks A, Barton A, John S, et al. Association between the PTPN22 gene and rheumatoid arthritis and juvenile idiopathic arthritis in a UK population: further support that PTPN22 is an autoimmunity gene. Arthritis Rheum. 2005;52:1694–9.
114. Kyogoku C, Langefeld CD, Ortmann WA, et al. Genetic association of the R620W polymorphism of protein tyrosine phosphatase PTPN22 with human SLE. Am J Hum Genet. 2004;75:504–7.

115. Smyth D, Cooper JD, Collins JE, et al. Replication of an association between the lymphoid tyrosine phosphatase locus (LYP/PTPN22) with type 1 diabetes, and evidence for its role as a general autoimmunity locus. Diabetes 2004;53:3020–3.
116. Vandiedonck C, Capdevielle C, Giraud M, et al. Association of the PTPN22*R620W polymorphism with autoimmune myasthenia gravis. Annl Neurol. 2006;59:404–7.
117. Canton I, Akhtar S, Gavalas NG, et al. A single-nucleotide polymorphism in the gene encoding lymphoid protein tyrosine phosphatase (PTPN22) confers susceptibility to generalised vitiligo. Genes Immun. 2005;6:584–7.
118. Jagiello P, Aries P, Arning L, et al. The PTPN22 620 W allele is a risk factor for Wegener's granulomatosis. Arthritis Rheum. 2005;52:4039–43.
119. Downie-Doyle S, Bayat N, Rischmueller M, Lester S. Influence of CTLA4 haplotypes on susceptibility and some extraglandular manifestations in primary Sjogren's syndrome. Arthritis Rheum. 2006;54:2434–40.
120. Gottenberg JE, Loiseau P, Azarian M, et al. CTLA-4+49A/G and CT60 gene polymorphisms in primary Sjogren syndrome. Arthritis Res Ther. 2007;9:R24.
121. Graham DS, Wong AK, McHugh NJ, Whittaker JC, Vyse TJ. Evidence for unique association signals in SLE at the CD28-CTLA4-ICOS locus in a family-based study. Hum Mol Genet. 2006;15: 3195–205.
122. Lester S, Downie-Doyle S, Rischmueller M. CTLA4 polymorphism and primary Sjogren's syndrome. Arthritis Rheum. 2006;54:2434–40.
123. Mullighan CG, Heatley S, Lester S, Rischmueller M, Gordon TP, Bardy PG. Fas gene promoter polymorphisms in primary Sjogren's syndrome. Annl Rheum Dis. 2004;63:98–101.
124. Pertovaara M, Lehtimaki T, Rontu R, Antonen J, Pasternack A, Hurme M. Presence of apolipoprotein E epsilon4 allele predisposes to early onset of primary Sjogren's syndrome. Rheumatology 2004;43:1484–7.
125. Munz C, Lunemann JD, Getts MT, Miller SD. Antiviral immune responses: triggers of or triggered by autoimmunity? Nat Rev Immunol. 2009;9: 246–58.
126. Triantafyllopoulou A, Moutsopoulos H. Persistent viral infection in primary Sjogren's syndrome: review and perspectives. Clin Rev Allergy Immunol. 2007;32:210–4.
127. Toussirot E, Roudier J. Epstein–Barr virus in autoimmune diseases. Best Pract Res Clin Rheumatol. 2008;22:883–96.
128. Harley JB, Harley IT, Guthridge JM, James JA. The curiously suspicious: a role for Epstein–Barr virus in lupus. Lupus 2006;15:768–77.
129. Arbuckle MR, McClain MT, Rubertone MV, et al. Development of autoantibodies before the clinical onset of systemic lupus erythematosus. N Engl J Med. 2003;349:1526–33.
130. Stathopoulou EA, Routsias JG, Stea EA, Moutsopoulos HM, Tzioufas AG. Cross-reaction between antibodies to the major epitope of Ro60 kD autoantigen and a homologous peptide of Coxsackie virus 2B protein. Clin Exp Immunol. 2005;141:148–54.
131. Ramos-Casals M, Munoz S, Zeron PB. Hepatitis C virus and Sjogren's syndrome: trigger or mimic? Rheum Dis Clin North Am. 2008;34:869–84, vii.
132. De Re V, De Vita S, Gasparotto D, et al. Salivary gland B cell lymphoproliferative disorders in Sjogren's syndrome present a restricted use of antigen receptor gene segments similar to those used by hepatitis C virus-associated non-Hodgkins's lymphomas. Eur J Immunol. 2002;32: 903–10.
133. Baechler EC, Batliwalla FM, Reed AM, et al. Gene expression profiling in human autoimmunity. Immunol Rev. 2006;210:120–37.
134. Wakamatsu E, Matsumoto I, Yasukochi T, et al. Overexpression of phosphorylated STAT-1alpha in the labial salivary glands of patients with Sjogren's syndrome. Arthritis Rheum. 2006;54:3476–84.
135. Perez P, Anaya JM, Auilera S, Urzua U, Munroe D, Molina C, Hermosos MA, Cherry JM, Alliende C, Olea N, Ruiz-Narvaez E, Gonzalez MJ. Gene expression and chromosomal location for susceptibility to Sjogren's syndrome. J Autoimmun. 2009;33:99–108.

Autoantibodies and Autoantigens in Sjögren's Syndrome

9

Kazuhisa Nozawa, Minoru Satoh, Seunghee Cha, Yoshinari Takasaki, and Edward K.L. Chan

Abstract

Over the past 30 plus years since the identification of the now classic anti-SS-A/Ro and anti-SS-B/La autoantibodies in Sjögren's syndrome, there have been a few new and interesting autoantibodies including anti-fodrin, anti-M3 muscarinic receptor, anti-NA14, and other autoantibodies that are reported to be closely linked to this disease. This chapter describes the current data available for the specificities of these antibodies, their usefulness in diagnosis and prognosis of the disease, and hypotheses on the nature of autoantibody production.

Keywords

Autoantigen • Autoantibody • Systemic autoimmune disease • Sjögren's syndrome SS-A/Ro • SS-B/La • NA14 • M3 muscarinic receptor • Fodrin • Apoptosis

Abbreviations

AGAs	anti-Golgi complex antibodies
APCs	antigen-presenting cells
ANA	santi-nuclear antibodies
CHB	congenital heart block
GC	germinal center
M3R	muscarinic type 3 receptor
NA14	nuclear autoantigen 14 kDa
PM/DM	polymyositis/dermatomyositis
RA	rheumatoid arthritis
SLE	systemic lupus erythematosus
SS	Sjögren's syndrome
SSc	scleroderma

E.K.L. Chan (✉)
Department of Oral Biology, University of Florida College of Dentistry, Gainesville, FL, USA
e-mail: echan@ufl.edu

9.1 Introduction

Sjögren's syndrome (SS) is a systemic autoimmune disease in which the immune response is activated to attack and destroy the exocrine glands that produce tears and saliva [1, 2]. The disease may be isolated (primary SS) or it may occur in association with other rheumatic diseases (secondary SS) such as rheumatoid arthritis (RA), scleroderma (SSc), and systemic lupus erythematosus (SLE). The etiology of SS remains unknown, but the pathogenesis of exocrine cell damage is apparently multifactorial involving

R.I. Fox, C.M. Fox (eds.), *Sjögren's Syndrome*, DOI 10.1007/978-1-60327-957-4_9,

Table 9.1 Prevalence of autoantibodies in Sjögren's syndrome

Autoantibodies	Prevalence in primary Sjögren's syndrome (%)	References
Non-organ specific		
Anti-SS-A/Ro	60–75	[7]
Anti-SS-B/La	25–50	[7, 198]
Anti-M3 muscarinic receptor	63	[197]
Anti-α-fodrin	40–70	[120, 129]
Rheumatoid factor	60–80	[199]
Anti-neutrophil cytoplasmic	10–25	[200, 201]
Anti-phospholipid	20	[202]
Anti-centromere	2–20	[124]
Anti-mitochondrial	13	[203]
Organ specific		
Anti-smooth muscle	62	[198]
Anti-thyroid	28	[204]
Anti-salivary duct	Rare	[205]

both environmental and genetic factors. One of the central clues comes from the observation that the immune system in SS targets a restricted and highly specific group of intracellular autoantigens [3–5]. The disease is characterized by hypergammaglobulinemia and the presence of the non-organ-specific autoantibodies such as anti-SS-A/Ro, anti-SS-B/La, and various kinds of organ-specific autoantibodies. Table 9.1 summarizes the autoantibodies often recognized in patients with SS along with their prevalence. Unique feature of autoantibody production in SS is that prevalence of organ-specific autoantibodies is relatively high compared to other systemic autoimmune diseases, suggesting that organ-specific autoantibodies may play a role in the disease pathogenesis of SS.

The intracellular autoantigens targeted by the high-titer autoantibody response are a diverse group of macromolecules that are ubiquitously expressed [4]. In systemic autoimmune diseases, many of these cellular antigens are components of protein–nucleic acid complexes but otherwise share no obviously common features in terms of subcellular distribution, protein structure, or function [6]. In spite of the diversity, the specificity of the autoimmune response is remarkably predictive of disease phenotype, such that specific autoantibodies have become useful diagnostic and prognostic biomarkers [7–10]. The predominant target autoantigens in SS are the ribonucleoprotein autoantigens SS-A/Ro and SS-B/La [3], which are included in the disease diagnostic criteria [11]. Although autoantibodies to SS-A/Ro and SS-B/La are indicative of SS, their presence, especially in the case of anti-SS-A/Ro antibodies, is not specific since they are found with some frequency in patients with other systemic autoimmune diseases such as SLE [3, 7]. Two additional autoantigens, α-fodrin [12] and muscarinic type 3 receptor (M3R) [13, 14], were identified more recently as targets for SS-specific autoantibodies. Although the interests of many researchers have focused on these autoantibodies, they have not been yet established as SS-specific autoantibodies for clinical diagnostic use. Furthermore, there have been many reports of other less prevalent autoantibodies such as nuclear mitotic apparatus protein

(NuMA) [15, 16], members of golgin autoantigen protein family [17], poly-(ADP)-ribose polymerase (PARP) [18], 90-kDa nucleolar organizer region protein (NOR90/hUBF) [19], p80-coilin [20], nuclear autoantigen of 14 kDa (NA14) [21, 22], and many others that have been described in SS. However, they are mostly not restricted to SS. Here, we review the representative autoantibodies frequently recognized in patients with SS and discuss the major factors for autoantibody production in relationship to the pathogenesis of SS.

9.2 Autoantigens and Autoantibodies in Sjögren's Syndrome

9.2.1 Anti-SS-A/Ro and Anti-SS-B/La Antibodies

Anti-SS-A/Ro and anti-SS-B/La are the most clinically important and best-characterized autoantibodies in SS [3]. The SS-A/Ro autoantigen was first identified as a specific precipitin in the Ouchterlony double-immunodiffusion assay and later shown to be the 60-kDa protein (Ro60) existing as ribonucleoprotein complexes with four small hY (human cytoplasmic) RNA molecules [23–26]. In anti-nuclear antibody assay performed in clinical laboratories, anti-SS-B/La and anti-SS-A/Ro are often reported as nuclear speckles and/or nucleolar staining (Fig. 9.1). The cellular function for Y RNAs remains unknown but Ro60 protein is currently postulated to play roles in small RNA quality control and the enhancement of cell survival following exposure to ultraviolet irradiation [27]. Anti-SS-B/La antibodies were first defined by immunodiffusion in association with SS-A/Ro precipitins [24, 28]. SS-B/La is a distinct 47-kDa protein (Fig. 9.2a) and associates with a variety of small RNAs derived from RNA polymerase III including Ro hY RNAs, pre-5S RNA, pre-tRNAs as well as many viral RNAs [29, 30]. The SS-B/La protein has been described to have multiple functions including as a transcription termination factor for RNA polymerase [31, 32] and a factor in mediating the correct ribosome translational start sites [33]. Anti-SS-B/La antibodies are almost invariably accompanied by anti-SS-A/Ro antibodies, reflecting the physical

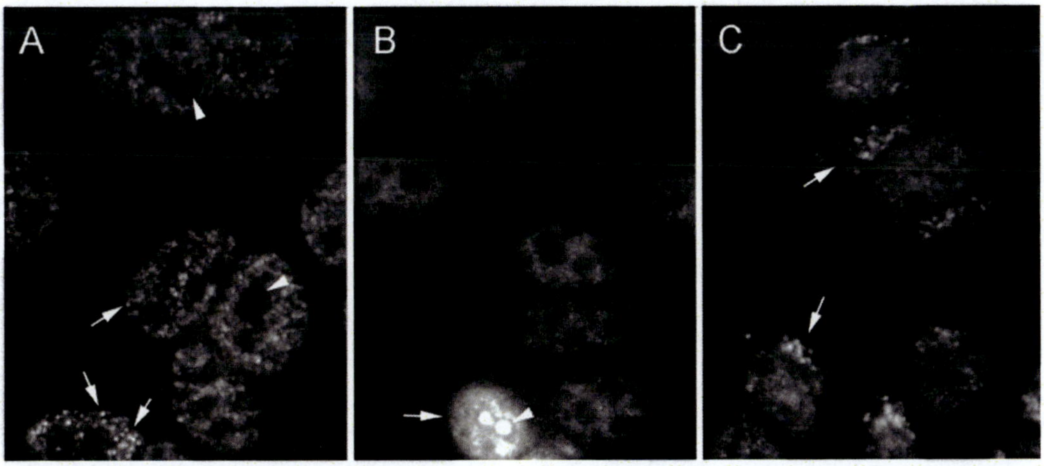

Fig. 9.1 Nuclear and nucleolar staining of SS-A/Ro sera in different HEp-2 cell substrates. **a** HEp-2 cells from BION, Inc. showed discrete nuclear speckles (*arrows*) while the nucleoli (*arrowheads*) were negative when stained by human prototype anti-SS-A/Ro serum Ge at 1:200 dilution. **b** The HEP2000 cells (Ro60-transfected HEp-2 cells, Immunoconcept) stained similarly with serum Ge gave nuclear speckles in untransfected cells and much brighter staining in transfected cells (*arrow*) showing intense homogeneous nucleolar staining (*arrowhead*). **c** HEp-2 showed an interesting serum Pa containing both anti-SS-A/Ro (nuclear speckles) and anti-golgin-245 autoantibody (Golgi staining, *arrows*)

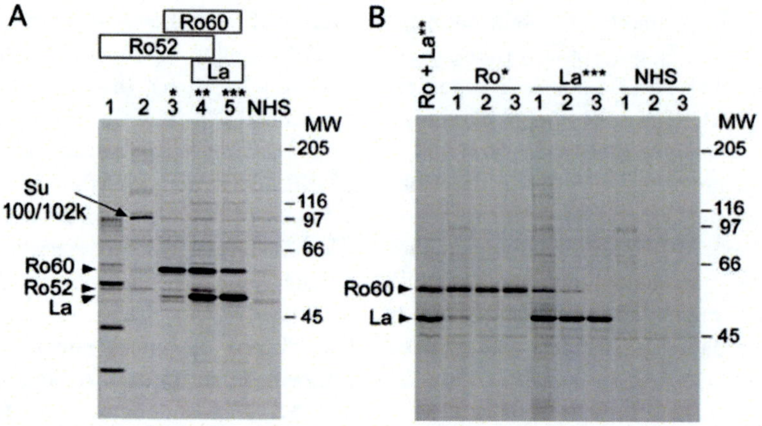

Fig. 9.2 Immunoprecipitation analysis of human anti-SS-A/Ro and anti-SS-B/La sera. **a** Five sera (lanes 1–5) containing various levels of anti-SS-A/Ro and anti-SS-B/La and a control normal human serum (NHS) were analyzed by immunoprecipitation using cell lysates from human K562 cells metabolically labeled with $[^{35}S]$-methionine. Ro60, Ro52, and SS-B/La (La) can be differentiated using gels with acrylamide:bisacrylamide ratio 166:1 [195, 196]. **b** Effects of different concentration of NaCl on the interaction of Ro60 (Ro) and La. $[^{35}S]$-Methionine-labeled K562 cell extract was prepared using NET/NP40 buffer (0.15 M or 0.75 M NaCl, 2 mM EDTA, 50 mM Tris–HCl pH 7.5, 0.3% NP40), immunoprecipitated with anti-Ro60 or anti-La prototype serum, or normal human serum (NHS), and washed using the same buffer with different concentrations of NaCl. NaCl concentrations of the buffer used were as follows: lane 1: cell extract 0.15 M, washing 0.15 M; lane 2: cell extract 0.15 M, washing 0.75 M; lane 3: cell extract 0.75 M, washing 0.75 M. Ro + La: anti-Ro60 + La prototype serum under the condition 3. *, **, and *** in panels **a** and **b** indicate the use of the same serum

association of these molecules in SS-A/Ro and SS-B/La ribonucleoprotein particle complex, but anti-SS-A/Ro antibodies frequently occur in the absence of anti-SS-B/La antibodies.

It has been shown that most anti-Ro60-positive sera also react with a structurally unrelated 52-kDa protein (Ro52, also known as TRIM21) [26, 34, 35]. There has been report of association of Ro60 and Ro52 via direct protein–protein interaction [36]; however, the interaction may be weak or transient and was not observed by other investigators (Fig. 9.2b) [37]. In 2006, the laboratories of Kamitani and Wahren-Herlenius independently reported that Ro52 is an E3 ubiquitin ligase [38, 39]. Thus it is possible that Ro60 and/or SS-B/La are substrates for Ro52-mediated ubiquitinylation and somehow they are stabilized during certain disease states and the complexes contribute to the formation of autoantibodies to these components.

The reported prevalence of anti-SS-A/Ro and SS-B/La antibodies depends on the method and sensitivity of detection. Overall, anti-SS-A/Ro antibodies occur in approximately 60–75% of patients with primary SS and also observed in secondary SS (Table 9.1). Anti-SS-B/La antibodies have been reported to occur in up to 50% of primary SS patients. Kelly et al. reported that the presence of anti-SS-A/Ro antibodies identified patients with more severe systemic diseases [31]. Davidson et al. described that parotid swelling and lymphadenopathy were more common in anti-SS-A/Ro and anti-SS-B/La antibodies-positive patients and the risk of developing non-Hodgkin's lymphoma was higher in this group compared to anti-SS-A/Ro and anti-SS-B/La antibodies seronegative patients [32]. It is interesting that a recent study including 321 SS patients showed that among anti-SS-A/Ro, anti-SS-B/La, and anti-fodrin antibodies, anti-SS-B/La antibodies were strongly correlated to organ involvement and cytopenias, and thus could serve as a prognostic marker in primary SS [40].

Considerations regarding the role of anti-SS-A/Ro and anti-SS-B/La antibodies in the pathogenesis of SS include (1) their association with high frequency of severe salivary gland destruction and hematologic disorder such as thrombocytopenia, leukopenia, and hypergammaglobulinemia [41, 42]; (2) aberrant expression pattern of Ro60 and SS-B/La in labial salivary glands and conjunctival epithelial cells from SS patients [43–45]; (3) salivary enrichment of anti-SS-A/Ro and SS-B/La antibodies in patients with SS, suggesting local production in salivary glands [46, 47]; and (4) presence of anti-Ro52, anti-Ro60, anti-SS-B/La autoantibodies-producing cells in salivary glands of patients with SS [48, 49].

Gordon et al. have proposed to divide the pathogenesis of SS-A/Ro and SS-B/La in SS to consist of three steps starting with the initiation of autoimmunity, diversification of autoantibodies, and antibody-mediated tissue injury [50]. In the initiation step, the key finding is that intracellular autoantigens including SS-A/Ro and SS-B/La are clustered in membrane blebs (apoptotic bleb) at the surface of apoptotic cells. It has been proposed that apoptotic cells serve as a source of immunogen of intracellular proteins for the production of autoantibodies [51]. Redistribution of SS-A/Ro and SS-B/La polypeptide into the blebs may produce neo-epitopes during apoptosis via exposure of cryptic epitopes or molecular modifications (posttranslational modification—discussed in a subsequent section) such as oxidation, proteolytic cleavage, or conformational changes [51–53] and they termed the neo-epitopes induced by apoptosis as "apotopes" [50]. In genetically susceptible individuals, the generation of non-tolerized epitopes of SS-A/Ro and SS-B/La may initiate an autoimmune response, particularly in situations of increased apoptosis or where the clearance of apoptotic cells is impaired [54–56]. To date, there are several interesting reports on apotopes and posttranslational modification of Ro60 and SS-B/La [53, 57–59]. Traditional mapping techniques of ELISA or immunoblotting have identified three immunodominant epitopes of SS-B/La: LaA (aa 1–107), LaC (aa 111–242), and LaL2/3 (aa 346–408) [60–62]. Passively transferred of IgG specific for LaA and LaC could bind cell membrane of apoptotic cells in a murine xenograft model, whereas IgG specific for LaL2/3 did not bind and identical findings were observed in cultured human fetal cardiocytes rendered apoptotic in vitro [63]. Therefore, LaA and LaC are exposed as apotopes while the LaL2/3 epitope remains masked, presumably by maintaining an intracellular location in apoptotic cells. Furthermore, sera from mothers of infants with congenital heart block (CHB) react with LaA and LaC, indicating that these apotopes may be targets of maternal autoantibodies [63].

The presence of anti-Ro52 without anti-Ro60 antibodies has been correlated with SS, whereas the presence of both anti-Ro52 and anti-Ro60 antibodies, or anti-Ro60 antibodies alone, has been correlated with other rheumatic diseases such as SLE [64]; however, these have not remained consistent findings. In the study of Ro60 apotopes, a surprising report showed that Ro60 apotope was highly specific for a subset of SLE patients with anti-Ro60 alone without anti-SS-B/La, but not detected in anti-Ro60-positive patients with primary SS, irrespective of the presence of anti-SS-B/La [65]. Interestingly, SLE patients with anti-Ro60 antibodies alone have been shown to have a high risk of nephritis and seizures than those with both anti-Ro60 and anti-SS-B/La antibodies [66], raising the possibility that specificity for Ro60 apotopes may predict clinical outcomes toward SLE. In contrast to Ro60, Ro52 has been reported to be not detected on cell surface of early and late apoptotic cells using human Jurkat and HeLa cell lines [57]. This contrasts with earlier studies, in which surface binding of anti-Ro52 antibodies to apoptotic fetal cardiocytes and impairment of their clearance were reported [55, 67]. These observations suggest that translocation of Ro52 to the cell membrane may be cell-type specific or caused by a mechanism unique to methods in the experimental induction of apoptosis [68–70]. Alternatively, Ro52 may be translocated to the surface of apoptotic HeLa and Jurkat cells but have no attachment site to anchor it to the cell surface. Therefore, maternal anti-Ro52 antibody may also contribute to CHB by binding to live cardiomyocytes and inducing calcium overload and apoptosis [71, 72].

Once the initiation step of autoantibodies production is established, it has been thought that intrastructural–intermolecular epitope spreading occurs for the diversification of anti-SS-A/Ro and anti-SS-B/La autoimmune responses [73]. Spreading of the immune response appears to be a common theme in autoimmune diseases. The clustering of autoantibody specificity in patients with SS is thought to arise by a process of B-cell epitope spreading between components of SS-A/Ro-SS-B/La ribonucleoprotein complexes after the initiation of immunity to a single component of this structure. Such spreading has been reported in mice immunized with SS-A/Ro or SS-B/La proteins or corresponding shorter synthetic peptides [74–78] and rabbits following immunization with Ro60 peptide [79]. The B-cell epitope spreading in patients and experimental animals is hypothesized to result from collaboration between T and B cells specific for epitopes on the SS-A/Ro and SS-B/La polypeptides non-covalently linked together in a ribonucleoprotein particle, a mechanism that has been termed intramolecular–intrastructural help [80]. McClain et al. reported that early Ro60 response in lupus crossreacts with a peptide of the latent viral protein Epstein–Barr virus nuclear antigen (EBNA-1), suggesting that molecular mimicry plays a role in the initiation step [81].

After the establishment of autoimmune response, some pathological autoantibodies may subsequently have a capability of causing tissue destruction. Although a mechanism of the tissue destruction of anti-SS-A/Ro and SS-B/La autoantibodies has not been elucidated, some new observation concerned with the tissues destruction of anti-SS-A/Ro and SS-B/La autoantibodies has been reported in the CHB model [67]. In a fetus diagnosed with isolated CHB, evaluation of the maternal serum almost invariably reveals the presence of autoantibodies against SS-A/Ro and SS-B/La and in vitro and in vivo studies suggest that one pathogenic cascade linking the antibodies to eventual scarring may be induced via apoptosis. Clancy et al. reported that nuclear injury and the translocation of SS-A/Ro and SS-B/La antigens to the fetal cardiomyocyte plasma membrane were common downstream events of Fas and TNF receptor ligation, requiring caspase activation [67]. These investigators also showed that cultured fetal cardiomyocytes expressed phosphatidylserine receptors (PSRs), which are known to mediate phagocytosis of apoptotic cells, and the phagocytic uptake was blocked by anti-PSR antibodies and was significantly inhibited following pre-incubation of apoptotic cardiomyocytes with IgG from anti-SS-A/Ro and anti-SS-B/La autoantibodies-positive mother of a CHB child. These investigators proposed that resident cardiomyocytes participate in the physiologic clearance of apoptotic cardiomyocytes and that the clearance is inhibited by opsonization via maternal autoantibodies, resulting in accumulation of apoptotic cells, promoting inflammation, and subsequent scaring [67]. The report by Kuhn et al. also provides evidence in support of a role for SS-A/Ro and SS-B/La antigens in apoptotic clearance in the epidermis of patients with cutaneous lupus erythematosus after ultraviolet irradiation [82]. Interestingly, in Ro60 knockout mice, it has been reported that UVB irradiation resulted in significantly increased numbers of apoptotic cells compared with wild-type mice [83]. One interpretation of these data is that Ro60 is involved in cell survival, and thus increased apoptosis is a reflection of the loss of survival signals, with the net effect being exaggerated apoptosis. Furthermore, SS-A/Ro and SS-B/La may have dual functions depending on whether they are intracellular protein in live cells or translocated to the cell surface of apoptotic cells. In any case, tissue destruction mediated by the binding of SS-A/Ro and SS-B/La antibodies to apoptotic cells and leading to perturbation of their clearance is currently an attractive hypothesis for the autoimmune pathogenesis. Further studies will be needed to define the molecular pathways whereby SS-A/Ro and SS-B/La are redistributed to the cell surface during apoptosis, identification of the functional domains on the apotopes involved in physiological clearance, and characterization of their interactions with molecular chaperones and counter receptors.

9.2.2 Anti-muscarinic Type 3 Receptor (M3R) Autoantibodies

One of the potentially very important breakthroughs in the understanding of defective secretion in SS originated from studies in 1996 and

1997. In the first study, the binding of a radiolabeled muscarinic type 3 receptor (M3R) agonist [^{3}H]-quinuclidinyl benzilate (QNB) to M3R of purified rat parotid gland membranes was inhibited in a non-competitive manner when the membrane was pre-incubated with primary SS sera [84], suggesting that circulating antibodies against rat parotid gland M3R were present in the sera of primary SS. Studies using a mouse model further defined that sialadenitis is to be due, in part, to a general loss of neurotransmitter responsiveness in the salivary gland cells rather than lymphocytic infiltration [85, 86]. Other studies later have also demonstrated the presence and functional/pathological roles of anti-M3R autoantibodies in human sera as well as in animal models of SS [13, 14, 87–95]. The classical model (apoptosis model), which claims defective secretory function in SS is a consequence of cytotoxic immune response that causes apoptosis of fluid secreting acinar cells, is challenged by an alternative model that mainly emphasizes functional suppression by anti-M3R autoantibodies [96]. The latter model can explain why patients who are free of lymphocytic infiltration in the salivary glands still develop severe dryness.

Acetylcholine (Ach) mediates important physiological responses such as muscle contraction, salivary and tear secretion, and cardiac rate through a family of muscarinic receptors. Muscarinic receptors, G-protein-coupled seven transmembrane receptors, are widely distributed throughout the human body and mediate distinct physiological functions according to location and receptor subtype. Five distinct muscarinic receptor subtypes (M1–M5) are known to exist, although the exact location and functional roles of all subtypes have not been fully elucidated to date [97]. Human and rodent studies identified that both M1 and M3 receptors are present in the salivary glands, whereas the parotid glands express predominantly M3 receptors [98–100], playing a pivotal role in the production of saliva by serous and mucous cells of the acinar structures [101]. Therefore, it was anticipated that the impairment of this pathway by anti-M3R autoantibodies may lead to defective secretion in patients positive for the autoantibodies. The regulation of saliva secretion via M3R in the acinar cells and the consequence of anti-M3R antibody on secretion is illustrated in Fig. 9.3.

Some of the controversies regarding anti-M3R autoantibodies lie in their prevalence and specificity. The prevalence of these receptors ranged from anywhere between 9 and 90%, depending on the sensitivity of assay systems developed and targeted epitopes on M3R [93, 102, 103]. ELISA (or its variants) has been the most common screening method for this antibody and linear peptides were not suitable for detection or inhibition studies, indicating that M3R epitope(s) is discontinuous or conformational [104]. In fact, the highest prevalence originated from a study utilizing GST-fusion recombinant peptides which allow dimerization of linear peptides and thus may maintain a native tertiary structure found in vivo [102]. Although the critical epitope(s) of M3R have not been clearly defined to date, the dominant epitope was presumed to be present in the second extracellular cellular loop (aa 213–228) where a receptor and ligand-binding site is located [87]. However, later studies pointed out other potential M3R epitopes such as the third extracellular loop (aa 514–527) [105] or second extracellular loop encompassing the transmembrane domain (aa 213–237) [92]. More importantly, it is still questionable if anti-M3R binding is specific to M3R, as indicated by a study where anti-peptide M3R (aa 208–228) antibodies strongly bind to M1R [103]. Nonetheless, full mapping of M3R epitopes, improvement of sensitivity/specificity of assays, proper and well-defined selection of disease and healthy controls, and large patient-oriented studies will allow more consistent findings and thorough information on prevalence and specificity.

Does the presence of the anti-M3R autoantibody guarantee secretory hypofunction? Antagonistic roles of anti-M3R antibodies in M3R-mediated pathway have been tested in various ways. Infusion of purified serum IgG or F(ab′)2 fragments from parental NOD mice or human primary SS patients, but not serum IgG from healthy controls, alters stimulated saliva production [14]. Anti-M3R antibody reversibly

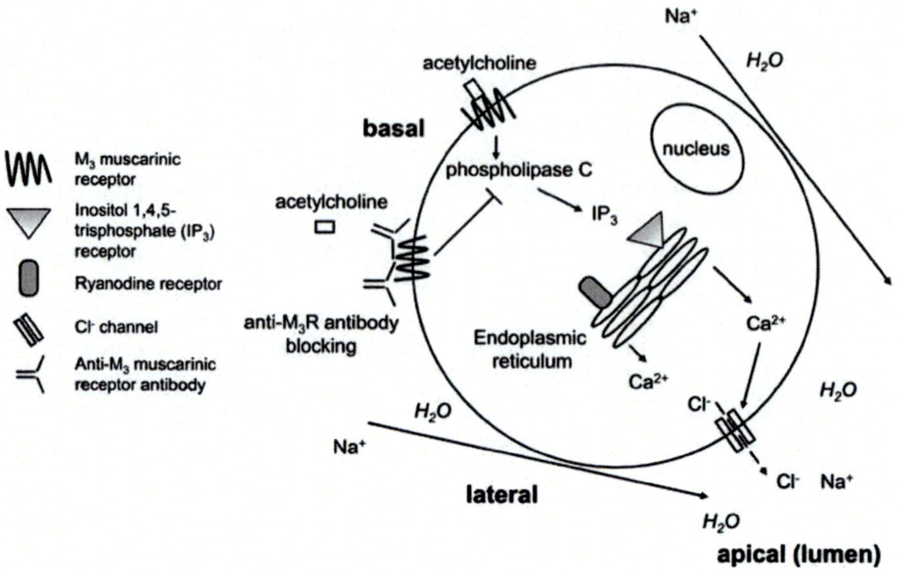

Fig. 9.3 Autoantibody influencing saliva secretion mediated by acetylcholine muscarinic type 3 receptor (M3R) signaling in acinar cells. Binding of acetylcholine to the M3R stimulates phospholipase C to generate inositol 1,4,5-triphosphate (IP3). IP3 binds to and opens the IP3 receptor on the endoplasmic reticulum at the apical pole of the cell, causing the release of Ca^{2+}. Release of Ca^{2+} stimulates Ca^{2+}-induced Ca release via IP3 receptor and ryanodine receptor which both amplify and propagate the Ca^{2+} signal. Increased Ca^{2+} activates the apical membrane Cl^- channel. Efflux of Cl^- into acinus lumen draws Na^+ across the cell to maintain electroneutrality, and the resulting osmotic gradient generates fluid secretion. Autoantibodies to M3R may influence its activity and potentially signal apoptosis. Modified from Dawson et al. [197]

inhibited carbachol-evoked increase in intracellular calcium in both mouse and human acinar cells by approximately 50% [106]. Functional assays utilizing mouse bladder smooth muscle supported the hypothesis that chronic stimulation of membrane-bound M3R can result in desensitization of the receptor [91]. Furthermore, inhibitory function of anti-M3R antibody on postganglionic cholinergic neurotransmission appears to be reversed when intravenous IgGs from healthy adults were present. Anti-idiotypic antibodies present in pooled IgG neutralized patient IgG-mediated inhibition of M3R cholinergic neurotransmission, providing a rationale for IVIg as a treatment of autonomic dysfunction in patients with SS [107].

Presence of putative autoantibodies against cell surface M3R expressed in the exocrine glands strongly indicates that SS also has a characteristic of not only systemic non-organ-specific autoimmune diseases but also organ-specific autoimmune disease characterized by anti-receptor antibodies such as those described in myasthenia gravis and Grave's disease [108]. Receptor dysregulation by anti-M3R autoantibodies rather than direct damage to the cells via apoptosis may have a key role in the development of salivary gland hypofunction through the functional suppression of the M3R pathway (Fig. 9.3). Other potential factors contributing to the pathogenesis have been proposed including cytokines, cholinesterase [109, 110], and aquaporins [111, 112]. Interestingly, there has been accumulating evidence for additional roles of anti-M3R autoantibodies in interstitial cystitis, mild cognitive impairment, overactive bladder syndrome, and autonomic nervous system dysfunction involving gastrointestinal and the urinary systems observed in patients with SS [88, 113–115]. Wide distribution of M3R in various organs and high homology among these receptors make autoantibody involvement in those clinical symptoms sound convincing although further investigation and/or verification is required.

9.2.3 Anti-α-fodrin Antibody

α-Fodrin belongs to the family of α-spectrin family and has been known, alternatively, as non-erythroid α-spectrin (also called calspectin or α-spectrin ΠΣ1) [116]. In humans, four spectrin genes have been identified, which include α-spectrin and β-spectrin genes [116]. Genes for fodrin encode proteins that are approximately 60% identical to their erythroid counterparts [117]. α-Fodrin is expressed ubiquitously in non-erythroid tissues and is similar to erythroid spectrin in some respects, including immunochemical reactivity, rod-like appearance on electron microscopy, tetramer formation, and ability to bind actin and ankyrin [118]. Unlike erythroid spectrin, α-fodrin is not uniformly distributed along the cell membrane. Although the current understanding of the function of α-fodrin is incomplete, it has been suggested that α-fodrin maintains the spatial organization of specialized membrane proteins and mediates their attachment to the actin cytoskeleton [116]. Interestingly, α-fodrin is known to associate with membrane ion channels and pumps such as Na^+/K^+-ATPase in salivary gland via various ankyrin species [119]. In mice, α-fodrin is a 240-kDa protein forming a heterodimer with β-fodrin and it has been shown that α-fodrin is cleaved by caspase-3 into small fragments of 150 and 120 kDa [120–122]. Haneji et al. identified the 120-kDa α-fodrin as an organ-specific autoantigen from salivary gland of NFS/sld mouse, a mouse model of human SS [12]. Subsequently, Yanagi et al. reported that, in NOD mice, specific autoantibody production was found against 120-kDa α-fodrin, and that it was closely related to autoimmune sialadenitis, which resembles human SS [123]. Current data suggest that fragmented α-fodrin appears as a result of apoptosis and raises the possibility that apoptotic signal might take part in the mechanism to produce anti-α-fodrin autoantibody in the pathogenesis in SS [124, 125]. In human, it has also been reported that anti-α-fodrin antibody is predominantly detected in the sera from SS patients compared to SLE, suggesting that anti-α-fodrin autoantibody is valuable for the diagnosis of SS [126]. Although antibody against β-fodrin also has been described, clinical associations have not been reported [127]. Witte et al. also reported that IgA antibodies against α-fodrin are useful markers for SS [128]. The frequency of anti-α-fodrin antibodies in SS varies between 40 and 70% [129]. Although anti-α-fodrin autoantibodies originally were described as SS-specific autoantibodies, recent data have shown that anti-α-fodrin autoantibodies are present in 10–30% of patients with active inflammatory diseases, such as RA or SLE and 2% in healthy blood donor [129, 130]. In a 2005 review article, it was concluded that anti-α-fodrin clearly involved in the pathogenesis of murine models of SS but there were conflicting data regarding the prevalence and significance of anti-α-fodrin in human SS [120]. In the same year, Sordet et al. reported that anti-α-fodrin antibodies are not useful diagnostic markers for SS [131]. Also in 2005, Ruiz-Tiscar et al. reported that the frequency of anti-α-fodrin in SS is lower than previously reported but there are some anti-α-fodrin-positive SS patients who are negative for anti-SS-A/Ro [132]. However, in a 2008 study using 321 primary SS patients, investigators reported that antibodies to α-fodrin were not diagnostically superior to conventional anti-SS-A/Ro and anti-SS-B/La testing [40]. One possible explanation regarding the current discrepancy in the literature is that the production of anti-fodrin autoantibody in SS may be more specific in Asians or specifically Japanese population than others.

9.2.4 Antibodies to Nuclear Protein NA14

We have reported a novel class of coiled-coil-rich proteins that are recognized as cytoplasmic organelle-associated autoantigens in systemic autoimmune diseases [17, 133]. These include a family of Golgi complex autoantigens known as "golgins" such as giantin [134], golgin-245 (see Fig. 9.1c) [135], Golgi-associated microtubule-binding protein (GMAP-210) [136], golgin-95/GM130 [137], golgin-160 [137], and golgin-97 [138], endosomal proteins EEA1 [139] and CLIP-170 [140], and centrosomal proteins pericentrin [141], ninein [142], and Cep250 and Cep110 [143]. The mitotic organelles are also known to be associated with coiled-coil-rich autoantigens, including NuMA [15, 16, 144], and centromere-associated proteins CENP-E [143, 145, 146] and CENP-F [147, 148]. These cytoplasmic organelle-associated autoantigens are proteins with high molecular masses and high content of coiled-coil domain and autoantibodies against these proteins have been often recognized in patients with SS although their prevalence is generally low at 1–2%. It is not clear why coiled-coil-rich proteins can selectively elicit autoimmune response; however, one possibility is that physical features of coiled-coils are more stable or resistance to proteases and their enhanced stability promotes the induction and production of antibodies in certain disease states. The immune response appears to be not merely directed at crossreactive coiled-coil structures, because the human autoimmune response to coiled-coil-rich proteins appears to be highly specific [134, 149].

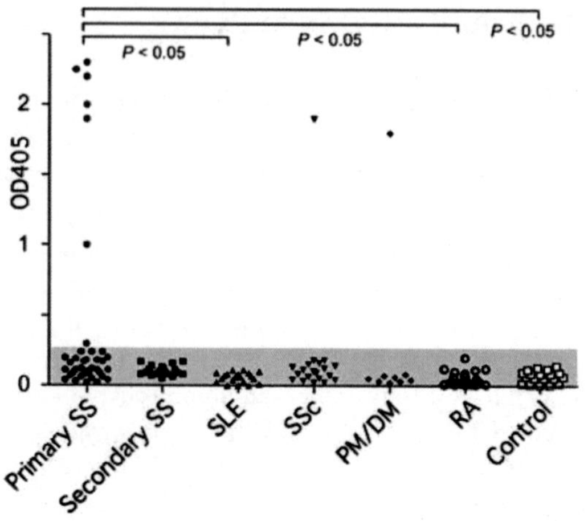

Fig. 9.4 Autoantibodies to nuclear antigen NA14 are detected primarily in primary Sjögren's syndrome. ELISA analysis of anti-NA14 in rheumatic disease cohorts using recombinant NA14 as antigen. Sera were tested at 1:1000 dilution and the cut-off value designating a positive reaction was the mean $OD_{405\ nm}$ of normal healthy controls plus five standard deviations. Statistical analysis was performed by Kruskal–Wallis with Dunn's multiple comparison test

Nuclear autoantigen 14 kDa (NA14) was originally identified as a novel coiled-coil autoantigen recognized by an autoimmune serum from a patient with SS [21]; in fact, the same SS patient serum was used to screen a cDNA library and another coiled-coil-rich Golgi-associated microtubule-binding protein (GMAP-210) was cloned and characterized [136]. Transfected NA14 localized to the nucleus and thus NA14 was reported as a nuclear autoantigen [21]. However, more recent reports showed that NA14 proteins also localized to centrosomes and play an important role in cell division and proliferation [150, 151].

There was no report regarding the prevalence of autoantibodies to NA14 in systemic autoimmune diseases until our published study [22]. In this study, anti-NA14 autoantibodies were determined in patients with various rheumatic diseases from cohorts in both United States and Japan. Figure 9.4 shows representative data from our US cohort only. The combined prevalence of anti-NA14 were 18/132 (13.6%) primary SS, 0/50 (0%) secondary SS, 2/100 (2%) SLE, 1/43 (2.3%) SSc, 0/54 RA (0%), and 1/29 (3.4%) PM/DM. Anti-NA14 antibody-positive sera were observed most frequently in primary SS. Interestingly, none of the secondary SS patients had autoantibodies to NA14. There were no obvious differences observed between patient cohorts in Japan and United States. Although a few anti-NA14-positive sera were observed in other rheumatic diseases like SLE, SSc, and PM/DM, anti-NA14 autoantibodies were almost exclusively observed in only primary SS compared to other rheumatic diseases. Our data showed that anti-NA14 antibodies appeared independent of anti-SS-A/Ro and anti-SS-B/La antibodies and 36.4% (4/11) of anti-NA14-positive sera was negative for anti-SS-A/Ro and anti-SS-B/La antibodies. It has been proposed that primary SS negative for SS-A/Ro and SS-B/La antibodies represents immunologically distinct populations compared to SS-A/Ro and SS-B/La antibody-positive population. Primary SS may be divided into clinically distinct groups based on the presence of specific autoantibodies such as anti-SS-A/Ro antibodies. Although we have not analyzed the clinical characteristics of anti-NA14 antibody-positive patients, the detection of anti-NA14 antibodies may provide useful information with primary SS and future studies will be needed to examine correlations with clinical activities.

9.3 Major Factors of Autoantibody Production in Sjögren's Syndrome

The autoimmune etiopathogenic model of SS is based on the existence of altered immune system incapable of discriminating between "foreign" and "self" macromolecules. The abnormal autoimmune response may be initiated by the altered/abnormal self-antigens expressed at the epithelium of exocrine glands or other organs through a specific combination of intrinsic and exogenous factors. The abnormal responses of both T and B cells against autoantigens may contribute to the histopathological lesions characteristically observed in SS and to alteration in the production of cytokines and chemokines, thereby helping to perpetuate the autoimmune lesion. Later activation of tissue damage leads to chronic inflammation of exocrine glands, with fibrosis and loss of physiological function. Various recent studies have contributed to a better understanding of these autoimmune etiopathogenic processes. Figure 9.5 summarizes a four-step working hypothesis on the major factors for autoantibody production and how they may contribute to the pathogenesis of SS.

9.3.1 Initiation Phase

The first step is the initiation phase required for the supply of autoantigens. The major source of autoantigen may derive from increased apoptosis

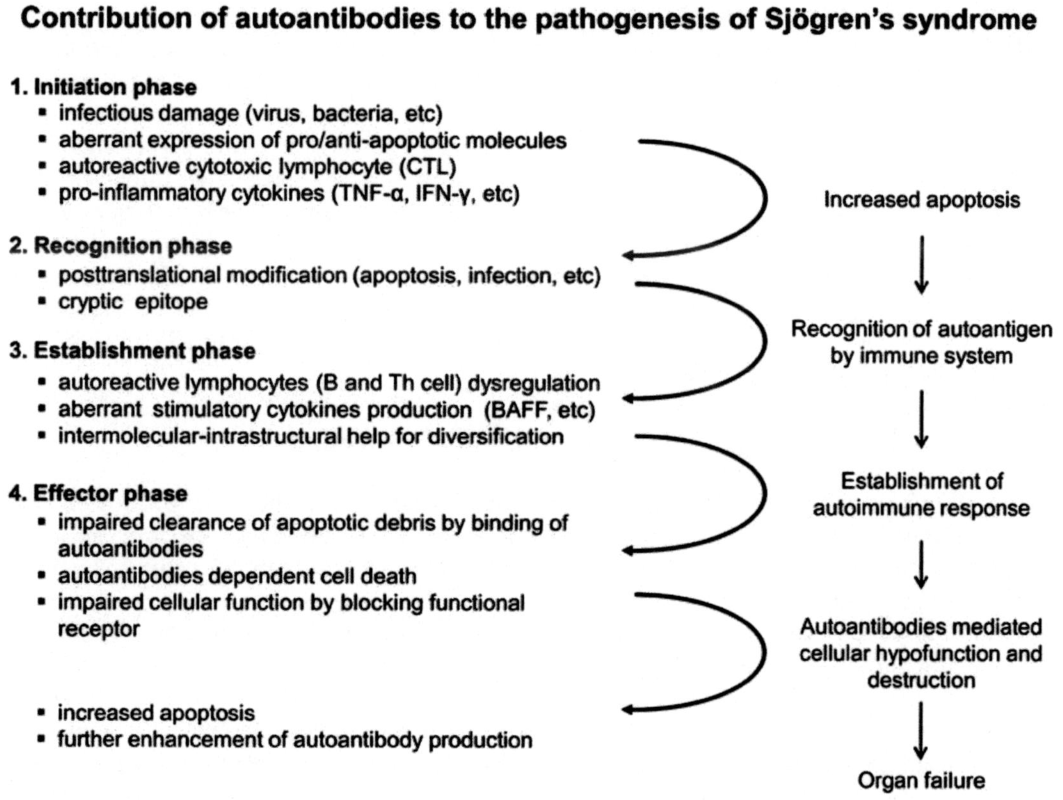

Fig. 9.5 Outline of the putative contributions of autoantibodies to the pathogenesis of Sjögren's syndrome. See text for discussion

in acinar and other unknown target cells induced by various factors such as viral or bacterial infection, dysregulation of apoptotic pathway, autoreactive cytotoxic T cells, and pro-inflammatory cytokines. The released autoantigens from apoptotic cells are physiologically not recognized by immune system and immune response is not evoked. In keeping with the trend of research into the role of apoptosis in disease pathogenesis, a variety of studies have been published in relation to SS [152]. Using in situ techniques, it has been shown that apoptosis is enhanced in glandular tissue from SS patients as compared with both normal controls and patients with nonspecific sialadenitis [153, 154]. A greater amount of apoptosis has been observed in acinar and ductal epithelial cells compared to the infiltrating lymphocytes. There is greater cellular expression of pro-apoptotic molecules in acinar and ductal cells (CD95/Fas) than the anti-apoptotic proteins Bcl-2 and Bcl-XL [153, 154]. Although aberrant pro-inflammatory cytokines like IFN-γ and TNF-α have also been shown to modulate Fas-mediated apoptosis in SS [155, 156], cell-mediated death is considered to play a central role for the Fas-mediated cytotoxic cell damage of acinar/ductal cells by Fas ligand. Fas ligands on activated T cells or soluble Fas ligands released by activated T cells are both known to mediate apoptosis [157]. However, the incidence of apoptosis in SS is still somewhat controversial since it has been reported that Fas-induced apoptosis is uncommon in SS [158]. It is unclear whether increased apoptosis in other cell types may contribute to the development of autoantibodies in SS. Indeed, the serum levels of soluble Fas ligand are reported to be elevated in patients with SS [159], suggesting that other organ involvement cannot be ruled out.

Certain viruses such as HTLV-1, EBV, HIV-1, HHV-6, and HCV have been reported in SS [124]. Some viruses, such as EBV, are known to cause B-cell or T-cell hyperactivation rather than apoptosis. Furthermore, molecular mimicry of viral-related molecules has been suggested in the pathway of autoantibody production. The SS-A/Ro and SS-B/La autoantigens have been found to share sequence similarities with some viral proteins. It has been shown that there is homology between six regions of Ro60 and the nucleocapsid protein of vesicular stomatitis virus [160]. Some of the immunoreactive regions within the SS-B/La protein have been found to have homology with proteins of EBV, HHV-6, and HIV-1 [161]. Although there is no direct evidence that specific viral infection led to increased apoptosis in tissues of SS patients, not all SS patients are positive for anti-viral antibodies, and presumably as many virally infected individuals do not develop SS, it remains possible that these viruses promote autoantibody production through molecular mimicry.

Aberrant activation of autoreactive lymphocytes might be one of the causing factors for the progression to increased apoptosis. Immunohistological analysis of salivary gland-infiltrating cells normally shows a predominance of T cells. Most T cells in the lymphocytic infiltrates are CD45 RO+ memory phenotype $CD4^+$ T cells and express the α/β T-cell receptor and LFA-1. These $CD4^+$ T cells may contribute to B-cell hyperreactivity. In addition, salivary acinar cells are not just innocent bystanders since they can also serve as active participants in the immune process by upregulating cytokines, MHC class II, and/or co-stimulatory molecules. Active and constant antigen presentation by salivary epithelial cells as antigen-presenting cells may be associated with germinal center (GC) formation in about 17% of patients with SS [162–165].

9.3.2 Recognition Phase

As discussed above, aberrant regulation of apoptosis occurs in tissues of exocrine glands or other affected organs of SS patients. Increased apoptosis serves not only as source of autoantigens but also changes non-immunogenic antigens to potentially immunogenic autoantigens by posttranslational modifications that can expose cryptic epitopes. Posttranslational modifications occur in a variety of proteins of eukaryotic cells and are significant for a number of cellular functions and the maintenance of homeostasis. It has long been hypothesized that posttranslationally modified self-proteins could act as means to induce autoimmunity [166]. After the modified self-proteins are taken up, digested, and processed in antigen-presenting cells (APCs), potentially self-reactive T and B cells can recognize them, resulting in the breaking of tolerance. One explanation for the mechanisms of loss of tolerance to unmodified proteins following immune response to cryptic epitope is through a process called epitope spreading in part contributed by intermolecular–intrastructural help [80]. The immune response may spread to unmodified self-proteins and thus generating an autoimmune reaction [166]. The most frequently observed posttranslational modifications include glycosylation, phosphorylation, acetylation, citrullination, and cleavage by apoptosis [5, 149, 167–169]. Several studies have shown that posttranslational modifications can affect autoantibodies binding onto different autoantigens in various systemic autoimmune diseases [5, 149, 167–169]. Interests in Ro60 epitope (aa 169–190) have been renewed recently, as McClain et al. demonstrated that this sequence could be involved, through molecular mimicry mechanisms with viral proteins, in the initiation of the autoimmune response [81]. They also showed that purified antibodies against the epitope cross-reacted with the peptide aa 58–72 sequence of the latent viral protein Epstein–Barr virus nuclear antigen-1 (EBNA-1). Phosphorylation of the linear B-cell epitope of SS-B/La (aa 349–368) enhances autoantibody binding and its relative avidity [59]. Although susceptibility to efficient cleavage by a caspase is a frequent feature of several SS autoantigens, it is not a universal feature of all the autoantigens. For example, caspase-mediated proteolytic cleavage SS-A/Ro has not been observed [170]. Thus Rosen and co-workers have speculated alternative mechanisms such as cleavage by granzyme B, which is another effector protease especially in cell killing mediated by $CD8^+$ cytotoxic T lymphocytes and natural killer cells [5]. Furthermore, it is known that apoptosis also can mediate not only proteolytic cleavage but also citrullination or oxidation [171]. For example, oxidized low-density lipoproteins have been found on apoptotic cells, and mice immunized with apoptotic cells develop high titers of autoantibodies to various oxidized epitopes, whereas mice immunized with viable or necrotic cell do not [172]. These data indicate that the posttranslationally modified self-antigens found on apoptotic cell are "neoantigens" capable of eliciting an immune response.

9.3.3 Establishment Phase: Autoreactive T and B Lymphocytes Dysregulation and Aberrant Cytokines Production

The production and persistence of autoantibodies in autoimmune conditions may be caused by immune dysregulation with autoreactive T-lymphocyte and B-lymphocyte hyperactivation and aberrant cytokines production. Infiltrating lymphocytes and dendritic cells in affected tissues interact with salivary gland epithelial cells and contribute to the perpetuation and progression of the disease. In this context, dysregulation of cytokines production (e.g., Th1/Th2 imbalance, elevated BAFF production) and chronic B-cell hyperactivity are consistent and prominent immunoregulatory abnormalities in SS [2, 173–176]. Recent studies have demonstrated the B-cell hyperactivity in the inflamed tissues, especially in SS patients with detectable ectopic GC-like structures [177]. Similar ectopic lymphoid structures have also been described in the target tissues of several other autoimmune conditions that are accompanied by B-cell disturbance such as RA [178, 179], SLE [178, 180], and chronic autoimmune thyroiditis [181, 182]. Delineation of common and diverse mechanisms of SS may underlie the B-cell disturbances, and the development of ectopic GC-like structures in SS entities should be important for our understanding of their immunopathogenesis.

Chronic focal periductal lymphocytic sialadenitis is a hallmark of SS and it is generally thought to be a stepwise process [2, 173, 174]. This process may include (1) a sequence of scattered tiny perivascular lymphoid infiltrates, (2) subsequent development of the typical focal periductal lymphoid sialadenitis/formation of ectopic GC-like structures, and (3) eventually the destruction and replacement of the affected glandular tissue [177]. In this process, cytokine and/or autoantibody-mediated endocrine glandular tissue dysfunction may occur [106, 183]. These ectopic GC-like structures of the inflamed tissues bear a histological resemblance to the native GCs that are physiologically generated from primary B-cell follicles of secondary lymphoid organs during T-cell-dependent immune response. The ectopic GC-like structures contain T and B cells aggregate with proliferating lymphocytes, a network of follicular dendritic cells, and activated endothelial cells with the morphology of high endothelial venules [163, 179, 180, 184, 185]. Hanson et al. have explained abnormal B-cell differentiation pathways resulting in autoantibody production from the ectopic lymphoid tissues by "niche" theory [177]. The ectopic GCs represent a niche where B cells, which are recruited by chemokines into the microenvironment of chronically inflamed tissues, may escape from peripheral check points against autoreactivity and are abnormally stimulated. B cells may proliferate and incompletely differentiate via T-cell-dependent or independent pathway into memory B cells and plasma cells, resulting in autoantibody production. Furthermore, the autoreactive B cells may be additionally stimulated by cytokines such as BAFF.

9.3.4 Establishment Phase: Intermolecular–Intrastructural Help

Autoantigens are usually macromolecular complexes such as SS-A/Ro and SS-B/La, and linkages of autoimmune response among the components of the complex are often observed in patients with SS and other systemic autoimmune diseases [186, 187]. For instance, anti-Sm antibodies always occur with anti-U1RNP, and anti-SS-B/La is also associated with antibodies against SS-A/Ro and the Y5 small RNA molecule [188–190]. This phenomenon was also observed in autoantibodies to PCNA [191]. Such linked sets of autoantibodies, reacting with multiple components of the same macromolecular complex, may be the products of intermolecular–intrastructural help, which plays a key role in the immune system [192]. The importance of intermolecular–intrastructural help in the progression of autoimmunity is also supported by peptide immunization studies in SS-A/Ro and SS-B/La antigen–antibody systems in which mice immunized with recombinant murine SS-B/La develop not only anti-SS-B/La antibodies but also anti-SS-A/Ro antibodies [74, 76]; conversely, immunization with SS-A/Ro causes the production of both anti-SS-B/La and anti-SS-A/Ro antibodies [74, 76]. Gordon et al. have also reported similar results in which sera from mice immunized by Ro52 and Ro60 showed reactivity against the fragment of SS-B/La protein [73]. The explanation for these observations is that T cells specific for the immunized antigen can provide help to B cells carrying receptor for other components such as in the case of SS-A/Ro-SS-B/La complex. Alternatively, or in addition, the spread of autoimmunity to other proteins within a macromolecular complex may come from distinct products of the antigen processing by APC [193, 194]. This suggests that activated autoreactive B cells (or professional APC) can prime autoreactive T cells.

9.3.5 Effector Phase

Although tissue destruction mediated by autoreactive cytotoxic T cells and aberrant cytokines such as TNF-α is considered as major factor of the tissue damage of SS, antibody-mediated tissue destruction is also believed to play an important role in the process. Clancy et al. recently reported novel effector mechanisms of tissue destruction mediated by autoantibodies [67]. They demonstrated that anti-SS-A/Ro and anti-SS-B/La antibodies bound to apoptotic cardiomyocytes caused an impaired clearance of the apoptotic cells. Blocking physiologic apoptotic cell clearance by autoantibody binding of apoptotic cells would be expected to skew the pool of IgG autoantibody–apoptotic cell complexes toward pro-inflammatory reaction by infiltrating macrophages [67]. If inhibitory (or stimulatory) antibodies are produced against functional receptors on cell surface such as M3R, the cellular functions will be impaired by the autoantibodies resulting in tissue hypofunction (or hyperfunction) and organ failure. The autoantibody-mediated cellular destruction and hypofunction eventually result in organ failure such as dry eye and/or dry mouth. It is important that autoantibody-induced tissue damage may further increase apoptosis and amplify the autoantibody production, contributing to the diseases progression of SS.

Acknowledgments This work was supported in part by NIH Grant AI47859.

References

1. Papiris SA, Tsonis IA, Moutsopoulos HM. Sjogren's syndrome. Semin Respir Crit Care Med. 2007;28:459–71.
2. Fox RI. Sjogren's syndrome. Lancet. 2005; 366:321–31.
3. Chan EKL, Andrade LEC. Antinuclear antibodies in Sjögren's syndrome. Rheum Dis Clin North Am. 1992;18:551–70.
4. Tan EM, Chan EKL, Sullivan KF, et al. Antinuclear antibodies (ANAs): diagnostically specific immune markers and clues toward the understanding of systemic autoimmunity. Clin Immunol Immunopathol. 1988;47:121–41.
5. Rosen A, Casciola-Rosen L. Altered autoantigen structure in Sjogren's syndrome: implications for the pathogenesis of autoimmune tissue damage. Crit Rev Oral Biol Med. 2004;15:156–64.
6. Tan EM. Autoantibodies in pathology and cell biology. Cell. 1991;67:841–2.
7. von Mühlen CA, Tan EM. Autoantibodies in the diagnosis of systemic rheumatic diseases. Semin Arthritis Rheum. 1995;24:323–58.
8. Scofield RH. Autoantibodies as predictors of disease. Lancet 2004;363:1544–6.
9. Bizzaro N, Tozzoli R, Shoenfeld Y. Are we at a stage to predict autoimmune rheumatic diseases? Arthritis Rheum. 2007;56:1736–44.
10. Shoenfeld Y, Tincani A. Autoantibodies—the smoke and the fire. Autoimmunity 2005;38:1–2.
11. Vitali C, Bombardieri S, Jonsson R, et al. Classification criteria for Sjogren's syndrome: a revised version of the European criteria proposed by the American–European Consensus Group. Ann Rheum Dis. 2002;61:554–8.
12. Haneji N, Nakamura T, Takio K, et al. Identification of alpha-fodrin as a candidate autoantigen in primary Sjögren's syndrome. Science 1997;276: 604–7.
13. Waterman SA, Gordon TP, Rischmueller M. Inhibitory effects of muscarinic receptor autoantibodies on parasympathetic neurotransmission in Sjogren's syndrome. Arthritis Rheum. 2000;43:1647–54.
14. Robinson CP, Brayer J, Yamachika S, et al. Transfer of human serum IgG to nonobese diabetic $Ig\mu^{null}$ mice reveals a role for autoantibodies in the loss of secretory function of exocrine tissues in Sjögren's syndrome. Proc Natl Acad Sci USA. 1998;95: 7538–43.
15. Andrade LEC, Chan EKL, Peebles CL, et al. Two major autoantigen–antibody systems of the mitotic spindle apparatus. Arthritis Rheum. 1996;39: 1643–53.
16. Price CM, McCarty GA, Pettijohn DE. NuMA protein is a human autoantigen. Arthritis Rheum. 1984;27:774–9.
17. Chan EKL, Fritzler MJ. Golgins: coiled-coil proteins associated with the Golgi complex. Electronic J Biotechnol. 1998;1:1–10.
18. Yamanaka H, Willis EH, Penning CA, et al. Human autoantibodies to poly(adenosine diphosphate-ribose) polymerase. J Clin Invest. 1987;80:900–4.
19. Chan EKL, Imai H, Hamel JC, et al. Human autoantibody to RNA polymerase I transcription factor hUBF. Molecular identity of nucleolus organizer region autoantigen NOR-90 and ribosomal RNA transcription upstream binding factor. J Exp Med. 1991;173:1239–44.
20. Andrade LEC, Chan EKL, Raska I, et al. Human autoantibody to a novel protein of the nuclear coiled body. Immunological characterization and cDNA cloning of p80-coilin. J Exp Med. 1991;173: 1407–19.
21. Ramos-Morales F, Infante C, Fedriani C, et al. NA14 is a novel nuclear autoantigen with a coiled-coil domain. J Biol Chem. 1998;273:1634–9.
22. Nozawa K, Ikeda K, Satoh M et al. Autoantibody to NA14 is an independent marker primarily for Sjögren's syndrome. Front Biosci. 2009;14: 3733–9.
23. Clark G, Reichlin M, Tomasi TB. Characterization of a soluble cytoplasmic antigen reactive with sera from patients with systemic lupus erythematosus. J Immunol. 1969;102:117–22.
24. Alspaugh MA, Tan EM. Antibodies to cellular antigens in Sjögren's syndrome. J Clin Invest. 1975;55:1067–73.
25. Wolin SL, Steitz JA. The Ro small cytoplasmic ribonucleoproteins: identification of the antigenic protein and its binding site on the Ro RNAs. Proc Natl Acad Sci USA. 1984;81:1996–2000.
26. Chan EKL, Buyon JP. The SS-A/Ro antigen. In: van Venrooij WJ, Maini RN, editors. Manual

of biological markers of disease. Dordrecht, Netherlands: Kluwer; 1994. pp. 1–18.
27. Chen X, Wolin SL. The Ro 60 kDa autoantigen: insights into cellular function and role in autoimmunity. J Mol Med. 2004;82:232–9.
28. Mattioli M, Reichlin M. Characterization of a soluble nuclear ribonucleoprotein antigen reactive with SLE sera. J Immunol. 1971;107:1281–90.
29. Pruijn GJM. The La (SS-B) antigen. In: van Venrooij WJ, Maini RN, editors. Manual of biological markers of disease. Netherlands: Kluwer; 1994, pp. 1–14.
30. Maraia RJ, Bayfield MA. The La protein–RNA complex surfaces. Mol Cell. 2006;21:149–52.
31. Gottlieb E, Steitz JA. The RNA binding protein La influences both the accuracy and the efficiency of RNA polymerase III transcription in vitro. EMBO J. 1989;8:841–50.
32. Rinke J, Steitz JA. Precursor molecules of both human 5S ribosomal RNA and transfer RNAs are bound by a cellular protein reactive with anti-La lupus antibodies. Cell 1982;29:149–59.
33. Meerovitch K, Svitkin YV, Lee HS, et al. La autoantigen enhances and corrects aberrant translation of poliovirus RNA in reticulocyte lysate. J Virol. 1993;67:3798–807.
34. Ben-Chetrit E, Chan EKL, Sullivan KF, et al. A 52-kD protein is a novel component of the SS-A/Ro antigenic particle. J Exp Med. 1988;167:1560–71.
35. Chan EKL, Hamel JC, Buyon JP, et al. Molecular definition and sequence motifs of the 52-kD component of human SS-A/Ro autoantigen. J Clin Invest. 1991;87:68–76.
36. Slobbe RL, Pluk W, van Venrooij WJ, et al. Ro ribonucleoprotein assembly in vitro. Identification of RNA–protein and protein–protein interactions. J Mol Biol. 1992;227:361–6.
37. Boire G, Gendron M, Monast N, et al. Purification of antigenically intact Ro ribonucleoproteins; biochemical and immunological evidence that the 52-kD protein is not a Ro protein. Clin Exp Immunol. 1995;100:489–98.
38. Espinosa A, Zhou W, Ek M, et al. The Sjogren's syndrome-associated autoantigen Ro52 is an E3 ligase that regulates proliferation and cell death. J Immunol. 2006;176:6277–85.
39. Wada K, Kamitani T. Autoantigen Ro52 is an E3 ubiquitin ligase. Biochem Biophys Res Commun. 2006;339:415–21.
40. Locht H, Pelck R, Manthorpe R. Diagnostic and prognostic significance of measuring antibodies to alpha-fodrin compared to anti-Ro-52, anti-Ro-60, and anti-La in primary Sjogren's syndrome. J Rheumatol. 2008;35:845–9.
41. Atkinson JC, Travis WD, Slocum L, et al. Serum anti-SS-B/La and IgA rheumatoid factor are markers of salivary gland disease activity in primary Sjogren's syndrome. Arthritis Rheum. 1992;35:1368–72.
42. Gerli R, Muscat C, Giansanti M, et al. Quantitative assessment of salivary gland inflammatory infiltration in primary Sjogren's syndrome: its relationship to different demographic, clinical and serological features of the disorder. Br J Rheumatol. 1997;36:969–75.
43. Barcellos KS, Nonogaki S, Enokihara MM, et al. Differential expression of Ro/SSA 60 kDa and La/SSB, but not Ro/SSA 52 kDa, mRNA and protein in minor salivary glands from patients with primary Sjogren's syndrome. J Rheumatol. 2007;34:1283–92.
44. de Wilde PC, Kater L, Bodeutsch C, et al. Aberrant expression pattern of the SS-B/La antigen in the labial salivary glands of patients with Sjogren's syndrome. Arthritis Rheum. 1996;39:783–91.
45. Yannopoulos DI, Roncin S, Lamour A, et al. Conjunctival epithelial cells from patients with Sjogren's syndrome inappropriately express major histocompatibility complex molecules, La(SSB) antigen, and heat-shock proteins. J Clin Immunol. 1992;12:259–65.
46. Horsfall AC, Rose LM, Maini RN. Autoantibody synthesis in salivary glands of Sjogren's syndrome patients. J Autoimmun. 1989;2:559–68.
47. Halse AK, Marthinussen MC, Wahren-Herlenius M, et al. Isotype distribution of anti-Ro/SS-A and anti-La/SS-B antibodies in plasma and saliva of patients with Sjogren's syndrome. Scand J Rheumatol. 2000;29:13–9.
48. Tengner P, Halse AK, Haga HJ, et al. Detection of anti-Ro/SSA and anti-La/SSB autoantibody-producing cells in salivary glands from patients with Sjogren's syndrome. Arthritis Rheum. 1998;41:2238–48.
49. Halse A, Tengner P, Wahren-Herlenius M, et al. Increased frequency of cells secreting interleukin-6 and interleukin-10 in peripheral blood of patients with primary Sjogren's syndrome. Scand J Immunol. 1999;49:533–8.
50. Reed JH, Jackson MW, Gordon TP. B cell apotopes of the 60-kDa Ro/SSA and La/SSB autoantigens. J Autoimmun. 2008;31:263–7.
51. Casciola-Rosen LA, Anhalt G, Rosen A. Autoantigens targeted in systemic lupus erythematosus are clustered in two populations of surface structures on apoptotic keratinocytes. J Exp Med. 1994;179:1317–30.
52. Utz PJ, Anderson P. Posttranslational protein modifications, apoptosis, and the bypass of tolerance to autoantigens. Arthritis Rheum. 1998;41:1152–60.
53. Pan ZJ, Davis K, Maier S, et al. Neo-epitopes are required for immunogenicity of the La/SS-B nuclear antigen in the context of late apoptotic cells. Clin Exp Immunol. 2006;143:237–48.

54. Rosen A, Casciola-Rosen L, Ahearn J. Novel packages of viral and self-antigens are generated during apoptosis. J Exp Med. 1995;181:1557–61.
55. Miranda-Carus ME, Askanase AD, Clancy RM, et al. Anti-SSA/Ro and anti-SSB/La autoantibodies bind the surface of apoptotic fetal cardiocytes and promote secretion of TNF-alpha by macrophages. J Immunol. 2000;165:5345–51.
56. Lipham WJ, Redmond TM, Takahashi H, et al. Recognition of peptides that are immunopathogenic but cryptic. Mechanisms that allow lymphocytes sensitized against cryptic peptides to initiate pathogenic autoimmune processes. J Immunol. 1991;146:3757–62.
57. Reed JH, Neufing PJ, Jackson MW, et al. Different temporal expression of immunodominant Ro60/60 kDa-SSA and La/SSB apotopes. Clin Exp Immunol. 2007;148:153–60.
58. Huang M, Ida H, Kamachi M, et al. Detection of apoptosis-specific autoantibodies directed against granzyme B-induced cleavage fragments of the SS-B (La) autoantigen in sera from patients with primary Sjogren's syndrome. Clin Exp Immunol. 2005;142:148–54.
59. Terzoglou AG, Routsias JG, Moutsopoulos HM, et al. Post-translational modifications of the major linear epitope 169–190aa of Ro60 kDa autoantigen alter the autoantibody binding. Clin Exp Immunol. 2006;146:60–5.
60. Gordon TP, Greer M, Reynolds P, et al. Estimation of amounts of anti-La(SS-B) antibody directed against immunodominant epitopes of the La(SS-B) autoantigen. Clin Exp Immunol. 1991;85:402–6.
61. Chan EKL, Francoeur AM, Tan EM. Epitopes, structural domains, and asymmetry of amino acid residues in SS-B/La nuclear protein. J Immunol. 1986;136:3744–9.
62. Chan EKL, Tan EM. The small nuclear ribonucleoprotein SS-B/La binds RNA with a conserved protease-resistant domain of 28 kilodaltons. Mol Cell Biol. 1987;7:2588–91.
63. Neufing PJ, Clancy RM, Jackson MW, et al. Exposure and binding of selected immunodominant La/SSB epitopes on human apoptotic cells. Arthritis Rheum. 2005;52:3934–42.
64. Ben-Chetrit E, Fox RI, Tan EM. Dissociation of immune responses to the SS-A (Ro) 52-kd and 60-kd polypeptides in systemic lupus erythematosus and Sjögren's syndrome. Arthritis Rheum. 1990;33:349–55.
65. Reed JH, Jackson MW, Gordon TP. A B cell apotope of Ro 60 in systemic lupus erythematosus. Arthritis Rheum. 2008;58:1125–9.
66. Malik S, Bruner GR, Williams-Weese C, et al. Presence of anti-La autoantibody is associated with a lower risk of nephritis and seizures in lupus patients. Lupus. 2007;16:863–6.
67. Clancy RM, Neufing PJ, Zheng P, et al. Impaired clearance of apoptotic cardiocytes is linked to anti-SSA/Ro and -SSB/La antibodies in the pathogenesis of congenital heart block. J Clin Invest. 2006;116:2413–22.
68. Saegusa J, Kawano S, Koshiba M, et al. Oxidative stress mediates cell surface expression of SS-A/Ro antigen on keratinocytes. Free Radic Biol Med. 2002;32:1006–16.
69. Gerl V, Hostmann B, Johnen C, et al. The intracellular 52-kd Ro/SSA autoantigen in keratinocytes is up-regulated by tumor necrosis factor alpha via tumor necrosis factor receptor I. Arthritis Rheum. 2005;52:531–8.
70. Dorner T, Hucko M, Mayet WJ, et al. Enhanced membrane expression of the 52 kD Ro(SSA) and La(SSB) antigens by human keratinocytes induced by TNF alpha. Ann Rheum Dis. 1996;54: 904–9.
71. Salomonsson S, Sonesson SE, Ottosson L, et al. Ro/SSA autoantibodies directly bind cardiomyocytes, disturb calcium homeostasis, and mediate congenital heart block. J Exp Med. 2005;201: 11–7.
72. Wahren-Herlenius M, Sonesson SE. Specificity and effector mechanisms of autoantibodies in congenital heart block. Curr Opin Immunol. 2006;18:690–6.
73. Gordon TP, Kinoshita G, Cavill D, et al. Restricted specificity of intermolecular spreading to endogenous La (SS-B) and 60 kDa Ro (SS-A) in experimental autoimmunity. Scand J Immunol. 2002;56:168–73.
74. Topfer F, Gordon T, McCluskey J. Intra- and intermolecular spreading of autoimmunity involving the nuclear self-antigens La (SS-B) and Ro (SS-A). Proc Natl Acad Sci USA. 1995;92: 875–9.
75. Keech CL, Gordon TP, McCluskey J. The immune response to 52-kDa Ro and 60-kDa Ro is linked in experimental autoimmunity. J Immunol. 1996;157:3694–9.
76. Tseng CE, Chan EKL, Miranda E, et al. The 52-kd protein as a target of intermolecular spreading of the immune response to components of the SS-A/Ro-SS-B/La complex. Arthritis Rheum. 1997;40: 936–44.
77. Reynolds P, Gordon TP, Purcell AW, et al. Hierarchical self-tolerance to T cell determinants within the ubiquitous nuclear self-antigen La (SS-B) permits induction of systemic autoimmunity in normal mice. J Exp Med. 1996;184:1857–70.
78. Scofield RH, Kaufman KM, Baber U, et al. Immunization of mice with human 60-kd Ro peptides results in epitope spreading if the peptides are highly homologous between human and mouse. Arthritis Rheum. 1999;42: 1017–24.
79. Scofield RH, Henry WE, Kurien BT, et al. Immunization with short peptides from the sequence of the systemic lupus erythematosus-associated 60-kDa Ro autoantigen results in anti-Ro

ribonucleoprotein autoimmunity. J Immunol. 1996;156:4059–66.
80. Fatenejad S, Craft J. Intrastructural help in diversification of humoral autoimmune responses. Clin Exp Immunol. 1996;106:1–4.
81. McClain MT, Heinlen LD, Dennis GJ, et al. Early events in lupus humoral autoimmunity suggest initiation through molecular mimicry. Nat Med. 2005;11:85–9.
82. Kuhn A, Herrmann M, Kleber S, et al. Accumulation of apoptotic cells in the epidermis of patients with cutaneous lupus erythematosus after ultraviolet irradiation. Arthritis Rheum. 2006;54:939–50.
83. Xue D, Shi H, Smith JD, et al. A lupus-like syndrome develops in mice lacking the Ro 60-kDa protein, a major lupus autoantigen. Proc Natl Acad Sci USA. 2003;100:7503–8.
84. Bacman S, Sterin-Borda L, Camusso JJ, et al. Circulating antibodies against rat parotid gland M3 muscarinic receptors in primary Sjogren's syndrome. Clin Exp Immunol. 1996;104:454–9.
85. Yamamoto H, Sims NE, Macauley SP, et al. Alterations in the secretory response of non-obese diabetic (NOD) mice to muscarinic receptor stimulation. Clin Immunol Immunopathol. 1996;78: 245–55.
86. Yamamoto H, Ishibashi K, Nakagawa Y, et al. Detection of alterations in the levels of neuropeptides and salivary gland responses in the non-obese diabetic mouse model for autoimmune sialoadenitis. Scand J Immunol. 1997;45:55–61.
87. Cavill D, Waterman SA, Gordon TP. Antibodies raised against the second extracellular loop of the human muscarinic M3 receptor mimic functional autoantibodies in Sjogren's syndrome. Scand J Immunol. 2004;59:261–6.
88. Wang F, Jackson MW, Maughan V, et al. Passive transfer of Sjogren's syndrome IgG produces the pathophysiology of overactive bladder. Arthritis Rheum. 2004;50:3637–45.
89. Gordon TP, Bolstad AI, Rischmueller M, et al. Autoantibodies in primary Sjogren's syndrome: new insights into mechanisms of autoantibody diversification and disease pathogenesis. Autoimmunity 2001;34:123–32.
90. Kovacs L, Feher E, Bodnar I, et al. Demonstration of autoantibody binding to muscarinic acetylcholine receptors in the salivary gland in primary Sjogren's syndrome. Clin Immunol. 2008;128: 269–76.
91. Cha S, Singson E, Cornelius J, et al. Muscarinic acetylcholine type-3 receptor desensitization due to chronic exposure to Sjogren's syndrome-associated autoantibodies. J Rheumatol. 2006;33:296–306.
92. Naito Y, Matsumoto I, Wakamatsu E, et al. Muscarinic acetylcholine receptor autoantibodies in patients with Sjogren's syndrome. Ann Rheum Dis. 2005;64:510–1.
93. Gao J, Cha S, Jonsson R, et al. Detection of anti-type 3 muscarinic acetylcholine receptor autoantibodies in the sera of Sjogren's syndrome patients by use of a transfected cell line assay. Arthritis Rheum. 2004;50:2615–21.
94. Nguyen KH, Brayer J, Cha S, et al. Evidence for antimuscarinic acetylcholine receptor antibody-mediated secretory dysfunction in nod mice. Arthritis Rheum. 2000;43:2297–306.
95. Ishikawa Y, Eguchi T, Skowronski MT, et al. Acetylcholine acts on M3 muscarinic receptors and induces the translocation of aquaporin5 water channel via cytosolic Ca^{2+} elevation in rat parotid glands. Biochem Biophys Res Commun. 1998;245:835–40.
96. Dawson LJ, Fox PC, Smith PM. Sjogrens syndrome—the non-apoptotic model of glandular hypofunction. Rheumatology (Oxford) 2006;45:792–8.
97. Abrams P, Andersson KE, Buccafusco JJ, et al. Muscarinic receptors: their distribution and function in body systems, and the implications for treating overactive bladder. Br J Pharmacol. 2006;148:565–78.
98. Culp DJ, Luo W, Richardson LA, et al. Both M1 and M3 receptors regulate exocrine secretion by mucous acini. Am J Physiol. 1996;271:C1963–72.
99. Watson EL, Abel PW, DiJulio D, et al. Identification of muscarinic receptor subtypes in mouse parotid gland. Am J Physiol. 1996;271:C905–13.
100. Beroukas D, Goodfellow R, Hiscock J, et al. Up-regulation of M3-muscarinic receptors in labial salivary gland acini in primary Sjogren's syndrome. Lab Invest. 2002;82:203–10.
101. Baum BJ. Principles of saliva secretion. Ann NY Acad Sci. 1993;694:17–23.
102. Kovacs L, Marczinovits I, Gyorgy A, et al. Clinical associations of autoantibodies to human muscarinic acetylcholine receptor 3(213–228) in primary Sjogren's syndrome. Rheumatology (Oxford) 2005;44:1021–5.
103. Schegg V, Vogel M, Didichenko S, et al. Evidence that anti-muscarinic antibodies in Sjogren's syndrome recognise both M3R and M1R. Biologicals 2008;36:213–22.
104. Cavill D, Waterman SA, Gordon TP. Failure to detect antibodies to extracellular loop peptides of the muscarinic M3 receptor in primary Sjogren's syndrome. J Rheumatol. 2002;29:1342–4.
105. Koo NY, Li J, Hwang SM, et al. Functional epitope of muscarinic type 3 receptor which interacts with autoantibodies from Sjogren's syndrome patients. Rheumatology (Oxford). 2008;47: 828–33.
106. Dawson LJ, Stanbury J, Venn N, et al. Antimuscarinic antibodies in primary Sjogren's syndrome reversibly inhibit the mechanism of fluid secretion by human submandibular salivary acinar cells. Arthritis Rheum. 2006;54:1165–73.

107. Cavill D, Waterman SA, Gordon TP. Antiidiotypic antibodies neutralize autoantibodies that inhibit cholinergic neurotransmission. Arthritis Rheum. 2003;48:3597–602.
108. Fox RI, Konttinen Y, Fisher A. Use of muscarinic agonists in the treatment of Sjogren's syndrome. Clin Immunol. 2001;101:249–63.
109. Dawson LJ, Christmas SE, Smith PM. An investigation of interactions between the immune system and stimulus-secretion coupling in mouse submandibular acinar cells. A possible mechanism to account for reduced salivary flow rates associated with the onset of Sjogren's syndrome. Rheumatology (Oxford) 2000;39:1226–33.
110. Dawson LJ, Caulfield VL, Stanbury JB, et al. Hydroxychloroquine therapy in patients with primary Sjogren's syndrome may improve salivary gland hypofunction by inhibition of glandular cholinesterase. Rheumatology (Oxford) 2005;44:449–55.
111. Tsubota K, Hirai S, King LS, et al. Defective cellular trafficking of lacrimal gland aquaporin-5 in Sjogren's syndrome. Lancet 2001;357:688–9.
112. Beroukas D, Hiscock J, Jonsson R, et al. Subcellular distribution of aquaporin 5 in salivary glands in primary Sjogren's syndrome. Lancet 2001;358: 1875–6.
113. Kovacs L, Papos M, Takacs R, et al. Autonomic nervous system dysfunction involving the gastrointestinal and the urinary tracts in primary Sjogren's syndrome. Clin Exp Rheumatol. 2003;21:697–703.
114. Orman B, Sterin-Borda L, De Couto PA, et al. Anti-brain cholinergic autoantibodies from primary Sjogren syndrome sera modify simultaneously cerebral nitric oxide and prostaglandin biosynthesis. Int Immunopharmacol. 2007;7: 1535–43.
115. van de Merwe JP. Interstitial cystitis and systemic autoimmune diseases. Nat Clin Pract Urol. 2007;4:484–91.
116. Winkelmann JC, Forget BG. Erythroid and nonerythroid spectrins. Blood 1993;81:3173–85.
117. Moon RT, McMahon AP. Generation of diversity in nonerythroid spectrins. Multiple polypeptides are predicted by sequence analysis of cDNAs encompassing the coding region of human nonerythroid alpha-spectrin. J Biol Chem. 1990;265:4427–33.
118. Bennett V. Spectrin-based membrane skeleton: a multipotential adaptor between plasma membrane and cytoplasm. Physiol Rev. 1990;70:1029–65.
119. Koob R, Zimmermann M, Schoner W, et al. Colocalization and coprecipitation of ankyrin and Na^+,K^+-ATPase in kidney epithelial cells. Eur J Cell Biol. 1988;45:230–37.
120. Witte T. Antifodrin antibodies in Sjogren's syndrome: a review. Ann NY Acad Sci. 2005;1051:235–9.
121. Bizzaro N, Villalta D, Tonutti E. Low sensitivity of anti-alpha-fodrin antibodies in patients with primary Sjogren's syndrome. J Rheumatol. 2004;31:2310–11.
122. Maruyama T, Saito I, Hayashi Y, et al. Molecular analysis of the human autoantibody response to alpha-fodrin in Sjogren's syndrome reveals novel apoptosis-induced specificity. Am J Pathol. 2004;165:53–61.
123. Yanagi K, Ishimaru N, Haneji N, et al. Anti-120-kDa alpha-fodrin immune response with Th1-cytokine profile in the NOD mouse model of Sjögren's syndrome. Eur J Immunol. 1998;28:3336–45.
124. Nakamura H, Kawakami A, Eguchi K. Mechanisms of autoantibody production and the relationship between autoantibodies and the clinical manifestations in Sjogren's syndrome. Transl Res. 2006;148:281–8.
125. Miyazaki K, Takeda N, Ishimaru N, et al. Analysis of in vivo role of alpha-fodrin autoantigen in primary Sjogren's syndrome. Am J Pathol. 2005;167:1051–59.
126. Watanabe T, Tsuchida T, Kanda N, et al. Anti-alpha-fodrin antibodies in Sjögren's syndrome and lupus erythematosus. Arch Dermatol. 1999;135: 535–9.
127. Kuwana M, Okano T, Ogawa Y, et al. Autoantibodies to the amino-terminal fragment of beta-fodrin expressed in glandular epithelial cells in patients with Sjogren's syndrome. J Immunol. 2001;167:5449–56.
128. Witte T, Matthias T, Arnett FC, et al. IgA and IgG autoantibodies against alpha-fodrin as markers for Sjogren's syndrome. Systemic lupus erythematosus. J Rheumatol. 2000;27:2617–20.
129. Witte T, Matthias T, Bierwirth J, et al. Antibodies against alpha-fodrin are associated with sicca syndrome in the general population. Ann NY Acad Sci. 2007;1108:414–7.
130. Chen Q, Li X, He W, et al. The epitope study of alpha-fodrin autoantibody in primary Sjogren's syndrome. Clin Exp Immunol. 2007;149: 497–503.
131. Sordet C, Gottenberg JE, Goetz J, et al. Anti-{alpha}-fodrin autoantibodies are not useful diagnostic markers of primary Sjogren's syndrome. Ann Rheum Dis. 2005;64:1244–5.
132. Ruiz-Tiscar JL, Lopez-Longo FJ, Sanchez-Ramon S, et al. Prevalence of IgG anti-{alpha}-fodrin antibodies in Sjogren's syndrome. Ann NY Acad Sci. 2005;1050:210–16.
133. Nozawa K, Fritzler MJ, Chan EKL. Unique and shared features of Golgi complex autoantigens. Autoimmun Rev. 2005;4:35–41.
134. Nozawa K, Fritzler MJ, von Mühlen CA, et al. Giantin is the major Golgi autoantigen in human anti-Golgi complex sera. Arthritis Res Ther. 2004;6:R95-R102.
135. Fritzler MJ, Lung CC, Hamel JC, et al. Molecular characterization of golgin-245: a novel Golgi

complex protein containing a granin signature. J Biol Chem. 1995;270:31262–8.
136. Infante C, Ramos-Morales F, Fedriani C, et al. GMAP-210, A *cis*-Golgi network-associated protein, is a minus end microtubule-binding protein. J Cell Biol. 1999;145:83–98.
137. Fritzler MJ, Hamel JC, Ochs RL, et al. Molecular characterization of two human autoantigens: unique cDNAs encoding 95- and 160-kD proteins of a putative family in the Golgi complex. J Exp Med. 1993;178:49–62.
138. Griffith KJ, Chan EKL, Lung CC, et al. Molecular cloning of a novel 97-kd Golgi complex autoantigen associated with Sjögren's syndrome. Arthritis Rheum. 1997;40:1693–702.
139. Selak S, Chan EKL, Schoenroth L, et al. Early endosome antigen. 1: an autoantigen associated with neurological diseases. J Investig Med. 1999;47:311–8.
140. Griffith KJ, Ryan JP, Senécal JL, et al. The cytoplasmic linker protein CLIP-170 is a human autoantigen. Clin Exp Immunol. 2002;127:533–8.
141. Doxsey SJ, Stein P, Evans L, et al. Pericentrin, a highly conserved centrosome protein involved in microtubule organization. Cell 1994;76:639–50.
142. Bouckson-Castaing V, Moudjou M, Ferguson DJ, et al. Molecular characterisation of ninein, a new coiled-coil protein of the centrosome. J Cell Sci. 1996;109:179–90.
143. Mack GJ, Rees J, Sandblom O, et al. Autoantibodies to a group of centrosomal proteins in human autoimmune sera reactive with the centrosome. Arthritis Rheum. 1998;41:551–8.
144. Price CM, Pettijohn DE. Redistribution of the nuclear mitotic apparatus protein (NuMA) during mitosis and nuclear assembly. Properties of purified NuMA protein. Exp Cell Res. 1986;166: 295–311.
145. Rattner JB, Rees J, Arnett FC, et al. The centromere kinesin-like protein, CENP-E. An autoantigen in systemic sclerosis. Arthritis Rheum. 1996;39: 1355–61.
146. Yen TJ, Li G, Schaar BT, et al. CENP-E is a putative kinetochore motor that accumulates just before mitosis. Nature 1992;359:536–9.
147. Rattner JB, Rao A, Fritzler MJ, et al. CENP-F is a ca 400 kDa kinetochore protein that exhibits a cell-cycle dependent localization. Cell Motil Cytoskel. 1993;26:214–26.
148. Liao H, Winkfein RJ, Mack G, et al. CENP-F is a protein of the nuclear matrix that assembles onto kinetochores at late G2 and is rapidly degraded after mitosis. J Cell Biol. 1995;130:507–18.
149. Nozawa K, Casiano CA, Hamel JC, et al. Fragmentation of Golgi complex and Golgi autoantigens during apoptosis and necrosis. Arthritis Res. 2002;4:R3.
150. Errico A, Claudiani P, D'Addio M, et al. Spastin interacts with the centrosomal protein NA14, and is enriched in the spindle pole, the midbody and the distal axon. Hum Mol Genet. 2004;13: 2121–32.
151. Pfannenschmid F, Wimmer VC, Rios RM, et al. *Chlamydomonas* DIP13 and human NA14: a new class of proteins associated with microtubule structures is involved in cell division. J Cell Sci. 2003;116:1449–62.
152. Humphreys-Beher MG, Peck AB, Dang H, et al. The role of apoptosis in the initiation of the autoimmune response in Sjogren's syndrome. Clin Exp Immunol. 1999;116:383–7.
153. Manganelli P, Quaini F, Andreoli AM, et al. Quantitative analysis of apoptosis and bcl-2 in Sjogren's syndrome. J Rheumatol. 1997;24:1552–7.
154. Kong L, Ogawa N, Nakabayashi T, et al. Fas and Fas ligand expression in the salivary glands of patients with primary Sjogren's syndrome. Arthritis Rheum. 1997;40:87–97.
155. Gannot G, Bermudez D, Lillibridge D, et al. Fas and Fas-mediated effects on a human salivary cell line in vitro: a model for immune-mediated exocrine damage in Sjogren's syndrome. Cell Death Differ. 1998;5:743–50.
156. Kulkarni K, Selesniemi K, Brown TL. Interferon-gamma sensitizes the human salivary gland cell line, HSG, to tumor necrosis factor-alpha induced activation of dual apoptotic pathways. Apoptosis 2006;11:2205–15.
157. Ju ST, Panka DJ, Cui H, et al. Fas(CD95)/FasL interactions required for programmed cell death after T-cell activation. Nature 1995;373:444–8.
158. Ohlsson M, Skarstein K, Bolstad AI, et al. Fas-induced apoptosis is a rare event in Sjogren's syndrome. Lab Invest. 2001;81:95–105.
159. Nozawa K, Kayagaki N, Tokano Y, et al. Soluble Fas (APO-1, CD95) and soluble Fas ligand in rheumatic diseases. Arthritis Rheum. 1997;40:1126–9.
160. Scofield RH, Harley JB. Autoantigenicity of Ro/SSA antigen is related to a nucleocapsid protein of vesicular stomatitis virus. Proc Natl Acad Sci USA. 1991;88:3343–7.
161. Haaheim LR, Halse AK, Kvakestad R, et al. Serum antibodies from patients with primary Sjogren's syndrome and systemic lupus erythematosus recognize multiple epitopes on the La(SS-B) autoantigen resembling viral protein sequences. Scand J Immunol. 1996;43:115–21.
162. Salomonsson S, Jonsson MV, Skarstein K, et al. Cellular basis of ectopic germinal center formation and autoantibody production in the target organ of patients with Sjogren's syndrome. Arthritis Rheum. 2003;48:3187–201.
163. Szodoray P, Alex P, Jonsson MV, et al. Distinct profiles of Sjogren's syndrome patients with ectopic salivary gland germinal centers revealed by serum cytokines and BAFF. Clin Immunol. 2005;117: 168–76.

164. Jonsson MV, Skarstein K. Follicular dendritic cells confirm lymphoid organization in the minor salivary glands of primary Sjogren's syndrome. J Oral Pathol Med. 2008;37:515–21.
165. Jonsson MV, Skarstein K, Jonsson R, et al. Serological implications of germinal center-like structures in primary Sjogren's syndrome. J Rheumatol. 2007;34:2044–9.
166. Wu CT, Gershwin ME, Davis PA. What makes an autoantigen an autoantigen? Ann NY Acad Sci. 2005;1050:134–45.
167. Casciola-Rosen L, Andrade F, Ulanet D, et al. Cleavage by granzyme B is strongly predictive of autoantigen status: implications for initiation of autoimmunity. J Exp Med. 1999;190:815–26.
168. Doyle HA, Mamula MJ. Post-translational protein modifications in antigen recognition and autoimmunity. Trends Immunol. 2001;22:443–9.
169. Utz PJ, Hottelet M, Schur PH, et al. Proteins phosphorylated during stress-induced apoptosis are common targets for autoantibody production in patients with systemic lupus erythematosus. J Exp Med. 1997;185:843–54.
170. Casiano CA, Martin SJ, Green DR, et al. Selective cleavage of nuclear autoantigens during CD95 (Fas/APO-1)-mediated T cell apoptosis. J Exp Med. 1996;184:765–70.
171. Doyle HA, Mamula MJ. Posttranslational modifications of self-antigens. Ann NY Acad Sci. 2005;1050:1–9.
172. Chang MK, Binder CJ, Miller YI, et al. Apoptotic cells with oxidation-specific epitopes are immunogenic and proinflammatory. J Exp Med. 2004;200:1359–70.
173. Kassan SS, Moutsopoulos HM. Clinical manifestations and early diagnosis of Sjogren syndrome. Arch Intern Med. 2004;164:1275–84.
174. Hansen A, Lipsky PE, Dorner T. Immunopathogenesis of primary Sjogren's syndrome: implications for disease management and therapy. Curr Opin Rheumatol. 2005;17:558–65.
175. Mitsias DI, Tzioufas AG, Veiopoulou C, et al. The Th1/Th2 cytokine balance changes with the progress of the immunopathological lesion of Sjogren's syndrome. Clin Exp Immunol. 2002;128:562–8.
176. Hagiwara E, Pando J, Ishigatsubo Y, et al. Altered frequency of type 1 cytokine secreting cells in the peripheral blood of patients with primary Sjogren's syndrome. J Rheumatol. 1998;25:89–93.
177. Hansen A, Lipsky PE, Dorner T. B cells in Sjogren's syndrome: indications for disturbed selection and differentiation in ectopic lymphoid tissue. Arthritis Res Ther. 2007;9:218.
178. Zintzaras E, Voulgarelis M, Moutsopoulos HM. The risk of lymphoma development in autoimmune diseases: a meta-analysis. Arch Intern Med. 2005;165:2337–44.
179. Schroder AE, Greiner A, Seyfert C, et al. Differentiation of B cells in the nonlymphoid tissue of the synovial membrane of patients with rheumatoid arthritis. Proc Natl Acad Sci USA. 1996;93:221–5.
180. Hutloff A, Buchner K, Reiter K, et al. Involvement of inducible costimulator in the exaggerated memory B cell and plasma cell generation in systemic lupus erythematosus. Arthritis Rheum. 2004;50:3211–20.
181. Hsi ED, Singleton TP, Svoboda SM, et al. Characterization of the lymphoid infiltrate in Hashimoto thyroiditis by immunohistochemistry and polymerase chain reaction for immunoglobulin heavy chain gene rearrangement. Am J Clin Pathol. 1998;110:327–33.
182. Ansell SM, Grant CS, Habermann TM. Primary thyroid lymphoma. Semin Oncol. 1999;26:316–23.
183. Jonsson MV, Delaleu N, Brokstad KA, et al. Impaired salivary gland function in NOD mice: association with changes in cytokine profile but not with histopathologic changes in the salivary gland. Arthritis Rheum. 2006;54:2300–5.
184. Jonsson MV, Szodoray P, Jellestad S, et al. Association between circulating levels of the novel TNF family members APRIL and BAFF and lymphoid organization in primary Sjogren's syndrome. J Clin Immunol. 2005;25:189–201.
185. Daridon C, Pers JO, Devauchelle V, et al. Identification of transitional type II B cells in the salivary glands of patients with Sjogren's syndrome. Arthritis Rheum. 2006;54:2280–8.
186. Tan EM. Antinuclear antibodies: diagnostic markers for autoimmune diseases and probes for cell biology. Adv Immunol. 1989;44:93–151.
187. Hardin JA. The lupus autoantigens and the pathogenesis of systemic lupus erythematosus. Arthritis Rheum. 1986;29:457–60.
188. Mattioli M, Reichlin M. Heterogeneity of RNA protein antigens reactive with sera of patients with systemic lupus erythematosus. Arthritis Rheum. 1974;17:421–9.
189. Boulanger C, Chabot B, Menard HA, et al. Autoantibodies in human anti-Ro sera specifically recognize deproteinized hY5 Ro RNA. Clin Exp Immunol. 1995;99:29–36.
190. Boire G, Craft J. Human Ro ribonucleoprotein particles: characterization of native structure and stable association with the La polypeptide. J Clin Invest. 1990;85:1182–90.
191. Kogure T, Takasaki Y, Takeuchi K, et al. Autoimmune responses to proliferating cell nuclear antigen multiprotein complexes involved in cell proliferation are strongly associated with their structure and biologic function in patients with systemic lupus erythematosus. Arthritis Rheum. 2002;46:2946–56.
192. Lake P, Mitchison NA. Associative control of the immune response to cell surface antigens. Immunol Commun. 1976;5:795–805.

193. Lin RH, Mamula MJ, Hardin JA, et al. Induction of autoreactive B cells allows priming of autoreactive T cells. J Exp Med. 1991;173:1433–9.
194. Mamula MJ, Janeway CA, Jr. Do B cells drive the diversification of immune responses? Immunol Today. 1993;14:151–2.
195. McCauliffe DP, Wang L, Satoh M, et al. Recombinant 52 kDa Ro(SSA) ELISA detects autoantibodies in Sjogren's syndrome sera that go undetected by conventional serologic assays. J Rheumatol. 1997;24:860–6.
196. Buyon JP, Slade SG, Chan EKL, et al. Effective separation of the 52 kDa SSA/Ro polypeptide from the 48 kDa SSB/La polypeptide by altering conditions of polyacrylamide gel electrophoresis. J Immunol Methods. 1990;129:207–210.
197. Dawson L, Tobin A, Smith P, et al. Antimuscarinic antibodies in Sjogren's syndrome: where are we, and where are we going? Arthritis Rheum. 2005;52:2984–95.
198. Nardi N, Brito-Zeron P, Ramos-Casals M, et al. Circulating auto-antibodies against nuclear and non-nuclear antigens in primary Sjogren's syndrome: prevalence and clinical significance in 335 patients. Clin Rheumatol. 2006;25:341–6.
199. Jonsson R. Sjögren's syndrome. In: Koopman WJ, Moreland LW, editors. Arthritis and allied conditions: A textbook of rheumatology. 15th ed. Philadelphia, PA: Lippincott Williams & Wilkins; 2005, pp. 1681–706.
200. Font J, Ramos-Casals M, Cervera R, et al. Antineutrophil cytoplasmic antibodies in primary Sjogren's syndrome: prevalence and clinical significance. Br J Rheumatol. 1998;37:1287–91.
201. Hauschild S, Schmitt WH, Csernok E, et al. ANCA in systemic vasculitides, collagen vascular diseases, rheumatic disorders and inflammatory bowel diseases. Adv Exp Med Biol. 1993;336:245–51.
202. Asherson RA, Fei HM, Staub HL, et al. Antiphospholipid antibodies and HLA associations in primary Sjogren's syndrome. Ann Rheum Dis. 1992;51:495–8.
203. Manthorpe R, Permin H, Tage-Jensen U. Autoantibodies in Sjogren's syndrome. With special reference to liver-cell membrane antibody (LMA). Scand J Rheumatol. 1979;8:168–72.
204. D'Arbonneau F, Ansart S, Le BR, et al. Thyroid dysfunction in primary Sjogren's syndrome: a long-term followup study. Arthritis Rheum. 2003;49:804–9.
205. Goldblatt F, Beroukas D, Gillis D, et al. Antibodies to AB blood group antigens mimic anti-salivary duct autoantibodies in patients with limited sicca symptoms. J Rheumatol. 2000;27:2382–8.

B-cell Epitopes of Sjögren's Syndrome-Related Autoantigens Ro/SSA and La/SSB

10

Athanasios G. Tzioufas, John G. Routsias, and Haralampos M. Moutsopoulos

Abstract

A common laboratory finding in Sjögren's syndrome (SS) is the presence of autoantibodies against intracellular autoantigens. These autoantibodies usually target the Ro/La RNP complex, consisting of at least three proteins, the Ro52, La, and Ro60 autoantigens non-covalently associated with one of the four small, uridine-rich hY RNAs (human cYtoplasmic RNAs). In this review, we first provide a brief overview of the antigenic determinant types that have been identified on the corresponding autoantigens. The antibody targets of autoantigens include primary, secondary, tertiary, and quarternary structure epitopes as well as cryptotopes and neoepitopes. We next focus on the functional, structural, and antigenic features of the components of the Ro/La ribonucleoprotein particle and address the clinical value of the autoantibodies against them. We also discuss in detail the regulation of autoantibody production via idiotypic/anti-idiotypic network and the diversification of their specificity via epitope spreading. Finally, we describe the ability of post-translational modifications to induce autoreactive immune attack via the generation of neoepitopes and we summarize the potential of synthetic epitopes for future development of new diagnostic tests and novel therapeutic strategies.

Keywords

Sjögren's syndrome • Ro/SSA • La/SSB • B-cell epitopes • Anti-idiotypic antibodies • Autoantigens

10.1 Introduction

Over the past several years, different laboratories have tried to define the fine specificity of autoantibodies to intracellular antigens by identifying within the antigen moiety the antigenic determinants (or B-cell epitopes), preferentially recognized by autoantibodies. Characterization of B-cell epitopes might give useful information on putative mechanisms of autoantibody production, such as molecular mimicry (sequence or structural molecular similarity that leads to cross-reactivity between antigens from a foreign agent

A.G. Tzioufas (✉)
Department of Pathophysiology, School of Medicine, University of Athens, Athens, Greece
e-mail: agtzi@med.uoa.gr

R.I. Fox, C.M. Fox (eds.), *Sjögren's Syndrome*, DOI 10.1007/978-1-60327-957-4_10,

and self-proteins) and epitope spreading (expansion of a B-cell autoreactive clone from a single determinant to other sites on the autoantigen) [1]. Furthermore, definition of B-cell epitopes with high sensitivity and specificity may allow development of immunoassays based on single epitopes (usually produced as synthetic peptides) that can be utilized for detection of autoantibodies. When used as antigenic substrates in diagnostic assays, synthetic peptides have several advantages over recombinant antigens. In contrast to in vivo production of recombinant proteins, peptide synthesis is a controlled chemical process that leads to high purity and homogenous, stable antigen preparations, allowing generation of highly sensitive and specific assays [2]. Such laboratory test systems can be useful for defining subgroups of a disease and may offer important information on the prognosis and natural course of the disease [3]. Furthermore, clinically relevant peptides, corresponding to B-cell epitopes, have been proposed as potentially useful in the treatment of autoimmune diseases via the use of immobilized peptides to remove pathogenic autoantibodies or as vaccine components [4, 5].

The identification of B-cell epitopes of autoantigens has raised an array of questions. Do autoimmune epitopes constitute a few dominant sequences or do they represent multiple disparate regions on a single autoantigen? Are frequency and significance of epitope spreading important for maintenance and perpetuation of the autoimmune response? Are the molecular structures of epitopes suitable to provide support for the hypothesis of epitope mimicry as a trigger for autoimmunity? Does knowledge of epitopes provide information on the regulation of the autoimmune response? In this review, we will discuss the clinical and biological relevance of epitopes to Ro/SSA and La/SSB, major autoantigens in Sjögren's syndrome (SS).

10.2 Classification of B-cell Epitopes of Intracellular Autoantigens

The B-cell epitopes are classified according to their structure as follows (Fig. 10.1):

1. *Primary structure epitopes (identified also as linear epitopes)* are composed of sequential amino acids. Such epitopes have been identified by synthetic peptide mapping in the majority of autoantigens discussed here, including Ro60, Ro52, La, Sm B, Sm D, RNP70, and Scl-70.
2. *Secondary structure epitopes* are formed by amino acids distributed in simple three-dimensional structures, such as α(alpha)-helices or β(beta)-sheets. They reside in a local α(alpha)-helical secondary structure

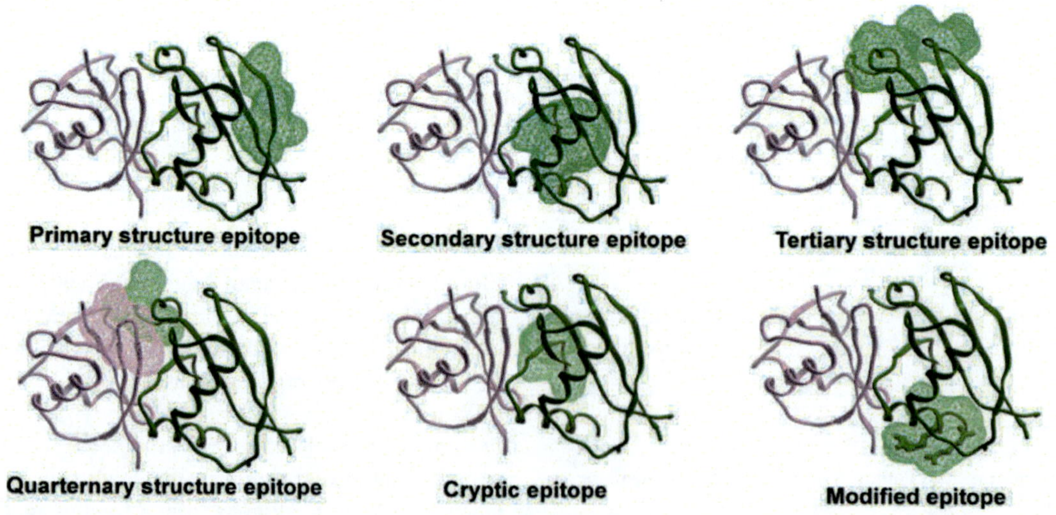

Fig. 10.1 Types of the epitopes according to their structure

stretch with all amino acids relevant for antibody binding located on one side of the helix. Other secondary structure epitopes have been described in Ro52 and Ro60 leucine zipper and zinc finger motifs, in patients with neonatal lupus and primary SS, respectively.

3. *Tertiary structure epitopes* are formed by distant regions of the protein sequence coming together in the tertiary structure. Such conformational epitopes may be the main targets of some autoantibodies (e.g., anti-Ro60).
4. *Quaternary structure epitopes* consist of amino acids distributed over different subunits within a macromolecular complex, interacting transiently or permanently to form a structure recognized by the autoantibody. Such epitopes have been identified in the Ro/La RNP complexes as well as in nucleosome subunits composed of histones and DNA elements.
5. *Cryptic epitopes (cryptotopes)* are usually linear epitopes hidden in the native structure of the autoantigen. They become accessible to antibody binding after disruption of the three-dimensional structure by denaturation, proteolytic degradation, or chemical modification of the autoantigen. These epitopes are observed in a number of nuclear autoantigens.
6. *Modified epitopes (neoepitopes)* contain post-translationally modified amino acid residues [6]. Examples of these modifications include (1) serine, threonine, and tyrosine phosphorylation; (2) lysine acetylation or ubiquitination; (3) cysteine lipidation or oxidation (disulfide-bond formation); (4) glutamic acid methylation or gamma-carboxylation; (5) glutamine deamidation; (6) asparagine (N-linked) and serine/threonine (O-linked) glycosylation; (7) arginine citrullination or symmetric/asymmetric dimethylation; and (8) proteolytic cleavage or degradation. In some instances, side chain modifications of specific amino acids, such as citrullination of arginine residues, are responsible for epitope high-affinity binding [7]. Such modified amino acids have been reported in a variety of human nuclear proteins, including the Sm antigens D1 and D3 [8], fibrillarin [9], and nucleolin [10].

10.2.1 Ro/La RNP Particles

In patients with systemic lupus erythematosus (SLE) and SS, the Ro/La RNP is one of the main targets of autoantibodies (Fig. 10.1). Human Ro/La RNP is composed of one of the four small, uridine-rich hY RNAs (*h*uman c*Y*toplasmic *RNA*s) non-covalently associated with at least three proteins, the Ro52, La, and Ro60 autoantigens [11, 12]. Additional components of the complex have been identified recently as the proteins calreticulin [13] and nucleolin [14]. The localization of these complexes is exclusively cytoplasmic but their protein components can be found in the nucleus as well.

10.2.2 La/SSB

The La/SSB antigen is a 47-kDa phosphoprotein that associates with a variety of small RNAs, including 5S cellular RNA and tRNA, 7S RNA, and hY RNAs, all transcribed by RNA polymerase III. In molecular level, it binds a short poly-uridylate sequence (poly-U) that exists at the 3 end of almost all nascent pol III transcripts (and in mature hY RNAs) [15–17]. In this regard La mediates transcript release from RNA polymerase III and facilitates multiple rounds of transcription/reinitiation by RNA polymerase III. In addition to immature RNA polymerase III products and hY RNAs, La can bind to viral RNAs (e.g., adenovirus VA, Epstein–Barr encoded RNAs (EBER)) and the RNA component of telomerase complex [18, 19]. La/SSB autoantigen has additional cellular functions: (1) La is an essential factor for cap-independent translation (La binds to internal ribosomal entry site (IRES) elements of the 5′-untranslated region of viral or human mRNAs promoting their cap-independent translation at the correct AUG) [20]; (2) La acts as an adenosine triphosphate (ATP)-dependent helicase able to melt RNA–DNA hybrids [21]; (3) La unwinds double-stranded RNA inhibiting the double-stranded RNA-dependent activation of protein kinase PKP [22]; (4) La can associate with telomerase and influence telomere homeostasis in vivo [18]; and (5) La is an RNA chaperone capable of transient bipartite (5′-end and 3′-end) binding of nascent RNA transcripts (e.g., tRNA precursors) [23].

Structurally, human La is a multidomain protein that contains the La motif in its N-terminal region, a typical RNA recognition motif (RRM) in its central part, and an unusual RRM, encompassing residues 229–326 (RRM_3). The latter is followed by a long, flexible polypeptide that contains a short basic motif (SBM), a regulatory phosphorylation site on Ser^{366}, and a nuclear localization signal (NLS). Recently, the three-dimensional structure of the La motif, the central RRM, and the carboxyl-terminal RNA recognition domain of the autoantigen was solved [24, 25] (Fig. 10.2). The La motif folds into a winged-helix motif elaborated by the insertion of three helices. The central RRM consists of a four-strand β(beta)-sheet attached to two α(alpha)-helices, while the C-terminal RRM folds to generate a five-stranded, anti-parallel β(beta)-sheet surface that is terminated by a long α(alpha)-helix. It seems that both the La motif and the adjacent central RRM are required for high-affinity poly-U RNA binding and that the C-terminal RRM, in conjunction with the SBM downstream, contributes to La interactions with non-poly-U RNA targets such as viral RNAs and TOP (terminal oligopyrimidine) mRNAs [24, 26].

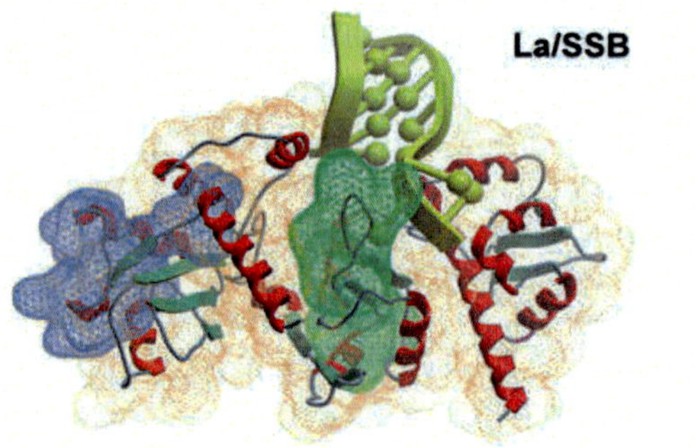

Fig. 10.2 Modeled structure of the human La region 5–326aa in complex with part of the hY1-RNA (shown in *yellow ribbons*), containing the La motif, the central RRM, and carboxyl-terminal RRM (RRM_3). The epitopes 145–164 and 289–308 are represented with *green and blue wire surface*

During the last decade, the target epitopes of anti-La/SSB autoantibodies have been mapped (Fig. 10.3). Early efforts to identify epitopes on the La antigen began by using enzymatic digestion of the native protein and large recombinant fragments. In this regard, antigenic sites covering the larger part of La autoantigen were identified. These sites were called LaA (amino acids 1–107, 1–107aa), LaC (111–242aa), and LaL2/3 (346–408aa) [27]. Later, more detailed and analytical epitope mapping revealed the exact localization of its antigenic determinants. Some of the La epitopes were found to reside in functional regions of the autoantigen, like the RNA recognition motif (RRM) and the ATP-binding site [28–30]. The interaction of hY RNA with the RRM motif, however, did not affect autoantibody binding in the same region [28]. In contrast, the interaction of the ATP-binding site with ATP abolishes autoantibody binding at the same part of the protein [29]. B-cell epitope mapping of La/SSB was also performed in our laboratory using 20-*mer* synthetic peptides overlapping

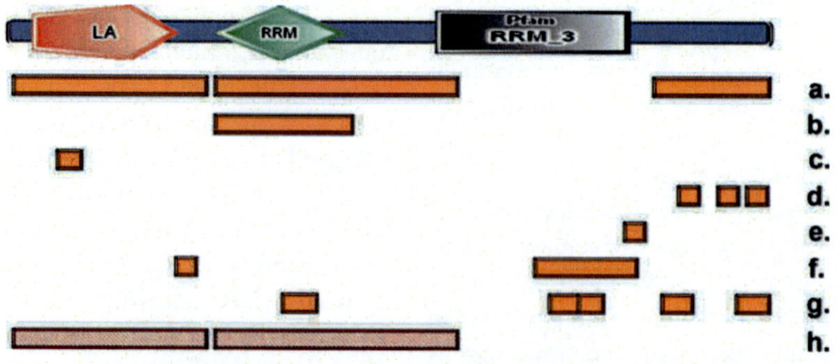

Fig. 10.3. Schematic representation of autoepitopes of the La48 kDa protein. **a.** [27, 30]. **b.** [28]. **c.** [93]. **d.** [29]. **e.** [94]. **f.** [31]. **g.** [34, 35] (apotopes). Domain organization: LA = La motif (N-terminal RRM), RRM: RNA = recognition motif (central RRM), RRM_3: RNA recognition motif (N-terminal RRM)

eight amino acids and covering the whole sequence of the protein. Peptides highly antigenic were those spanning the sequences; HKAFKGSI (147–154aa), NGNLQLRNKEVT (291–302aa), VTWEVLEGEVEKEALKKI (301–318aa), and GSGKGKVQFQGKKTKF (349–364aa) [31].

The first epitope (147–154aa) is located in the center of the RRM motif (112–183aa) while the second and third epitopes (291–302aa and 301–318aa) are located within the RRM_3 motif (231–334aa). The fourth epitope (349–364aa) is the most sensitive and specific epitope for the detection of autoantibodies, demonstrating a sensitivity and specificity of greater than 90% [32]. The existence of autoantibodies to the La/SSB epitope, 349–364aa, is also positively associated with longer disease duration, recurrent or permanent parotid gland enlargement, and a higher proportion of non-exocrine manifestations compared to SS patients without autoantibodies [33]. Additional epitopes have also been identified in other parts of the molecule by various investigators using recombinant fragments of La/SSB or synthetic peptides (Fig. 10.3). Their existence is believed to be correlated with the extended intramolecular spreading of epitopes to the whole La/SSB molecule that occurs during the course of the disease.

Recent studies reported the recognition of "apotopes" (epitopes expressed on apoptotic cells) by anti-La/SSB autoantibodies [34, 35]. It is well known that Ro and La antigens translocate to surface blebs during apoptosis. It seems that the La antigen is translocated during late apoptosis, since anti-La autoantibodies can bind exclusively to late apoptotic cells. The apotopes of La are located in the amino terminal 60% of the protein (comprising LaA and LaC fragments) [34], which possesses La, RRM, and RRM_3 motifs (see Fig. 10.3g), but detailed information about the fine location of the apotopes is not currently available.

10.2.3 The Ro60 Autoantigen

Ro60 antigen is found in virtually all vertebrate cells and the nematode *Caenorhabditis elegans*

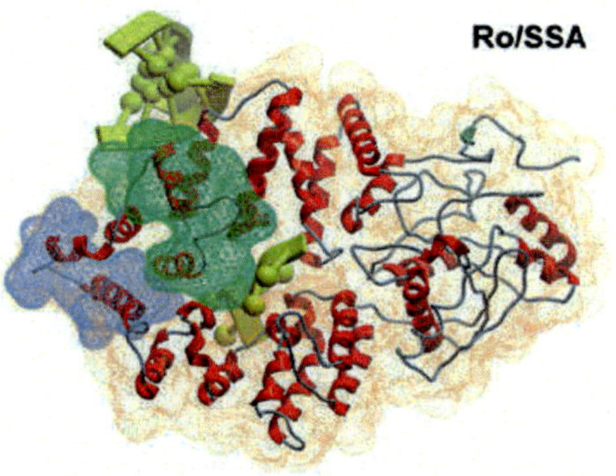

Fig. 10.4 Modeled structure of the human Ro60 complexed with RNAs (shown in *yellow ribbons*). The epitopes 169–190 and 211–232 are represented with *green and blue wire surface*

[36] and functions in the quality control and the discard pathway for nascent transcripts synthesized by RNA polymerase III (e.g., 5S rRNA precursors). In this regard, Ro60 binds misfolded small RNAs (e.g., 5S RNA), leading them to degradation. Recently, the structure of *Xenopus laevis* Ro60, 78% identical to human Ro60, was solved and found to consist of two distinct domains (Fig. 10.4) [37]. One domain is similar to the von Willebrand Factor A (vWFA) domain, which is found in proteins that function in cell adhesion. The other domain consists of a series of alpha(α)-helical repeats (HEAT repeats) that are arranged orbicularly around an inner hole of 10–15 Å ("doughnut"-like structure). This hole most probably holds the 3′-ends of misfolded RNAs, while the YRNAs bind to conserved residues to the outside of the "doughnut." Another conserved role for the Ro60 in facilitating cell survival after ultraviolet irradiation has recently emerged from studies in radiation-resistant eubacterium *Deinococcus radiodurans* [38] and mammalian cells lacking Ro60 [39]. Studies of mice lacking the Ro60 kDa protein suggest also that the normal function of Ro may be important for the prevention of autoimmune disease [39]. In these studies, mice lacking Ro were found to develop autoantibodies and membranoproliferative glomerulonephritis.

Epitopes of Ro60 have been defined previously using a variety of epitope mapping procedures [1, 40] (Fig. 10.5). Three major studies

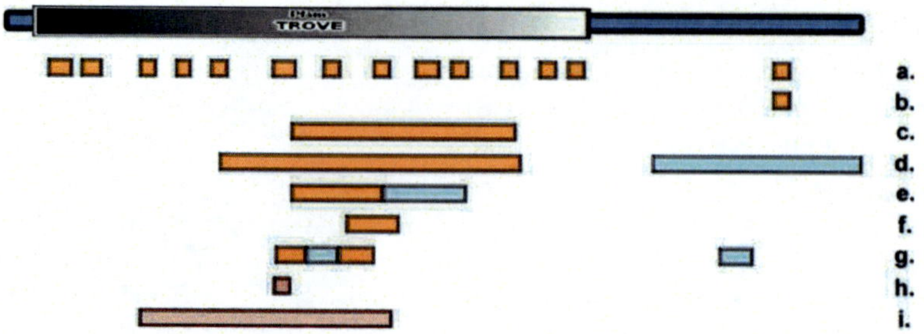

Fig. 10.5 Schematic representation of autoepitopes of the Ro60 kDa protein. **a** [44, 45, 95–97]. **b** [44]. **c** [43]. **d** [41]. **e** Veldhoven [98]. **f** [40]. **g** [47]. **h** [48] (initial pre-disease epitope in SLE). **i** [51] (apotope). Major epitopes are shown in *orange*, minor epitopes are shown in *cyan*. Domain organization: TROVE = domain found in RNA-binding components of Telomerase, Ro, and Vault RNPs

[41–43] using recombinant fragments of Ro60 identified a major epitope within the central part of the molecule (within 181–320aa, 139–326aa, and 155–295aa regions of the sequence, respectively). The exact locations of the antigenic determinants were revealed only after the application of synthetic peptides. Wahren-Herlenius et al. [40] identified a major epitope using synthetic peptide 216–245aa. Scofield and associates, using synthetic octapeptides, identified numerous epitopes covering the entire length of Ro60 [44, 45]; most probably due to epitope spreading to the entire length of Ro60 antigen that had occurred in the sera used in this study. The same investigators reported that one of the peptides (485–492aa) shared sequence similarity with the N-protein of vesicular stomatitis virus (VSV) and speculated that VSV might be involved in the pathogenesis of SLE [41]. However, in a subsequent study, the population of anti-Ro60 antibodies directed against the above-mentioned region was found to be limited [46]. In our laboratory, epitope mapping with synthetic peptides revealed the precise antigenic regions of Ro60, in the 169–190aa and 211–232aa parts of the antigen [47]. One of them, the 169–190aa epitope (originally described as SLE-associated epitope), was recently found to be the initial pre-disease target of autoantibodies in individuals who developed SLE several years later [48]. Our recent results indicate that although the 169–190aa and 211–232aa epitopes were identified as small peptide moieties (22aa in length), their recognition by autoantibodies is conformation-dependent, and their antigenicity is dramatically enhanced upon interaction with the molecular chaperone, calreticulin [49]. Other studies in our laboratory have identified an epitope within the zinc finger motif of the Ro60 protein. Synthetic peptide analogues corresponding to this region, 301–327aa, were reacted with the majority of anti-Ro/SSA and La/SSB-positive sera from patients with primary SS in the absence of zinc ions. In contrast, the native form of the zinc finger domain, in the presence of zinc ions, could bind to Ro52 but not to autoantibodies [50]. Recently the "apotopes" of Ro60, which are recognized by anti-Ro60 autoantibodies in the surface of apoptotic cells, were defined [51].

Ro60 autoantigen is translocated in the membrane early in apoptosis (before the translocation of La antigen) [35]. The apotopes of Ro60 are located within a large region spanning the residues 82–244 of the protein (about one-third of the molecule comprising Huntingtin, elongation factor 3 (EF3), protein phosphatase 2A(pp_2A) and the yeast PI3-kinase TOR1 (HEAT) repeats, including the hY RNA recognition sites) [34, 51]. Similar with La there are no detailed apotope mapping currently available. Interestingly, Ro60 apotopes are recognized in a greater extent by anti-Ro60 antibodies of SLE sera (62%) as compared with anti-Ro60 antibodies with SS sera (20%). More distinguishable are the sera with anti-Ro60 antibodies alone (commonly found in SLE sera) which recognize the apotope at 92%, while the sera where anti-Ro60 antibodies are accompanied by anti-La antibodies (usually SS sera) recognize the apotope at only 13% [51]. Similar disease specificity of the epitopes was reported in the initial epitope mapping of the antigen by our group (epitopes 169–90 and 211–232 were characterized as SLE and SS-related epitopes, respectively) [47] and this discrimination of the anti-Ro60 specificities was attributed by the presence of accompanying anti-La antibodies by another group [52].

10.2.4 The Ro52 Autoantigen

Ro52 functions as a transcription modulator due to its domain organization [53]. The two zinc finger motifs in Ro52 are not of the types that promote binding of nucleic acid but instead usually promote protein–protein interactions [54]. DNA-binding activity has, however, been suggested for Ro52, and a consensus-binding motif has been described. In line with many other really interesting new gene (RING)-containing proteins, a role for Ro52 in ubiquitination has been suggested [55]. Ro52 can also homodimerize through its leucine zipper domain [56]. The epitopes of Ro52 have been mapped in various studies with different methods (Fig. 10.6). The major immunoreactivity of Ro52 autoantigen was identified, using recombinant Ro52 fusion proteins, in the middle coiled-coil region of Ro52 [57–59]. The 190–245aa region of the sequence was reactive with almost all anti-Ro52-positive sera and was independent of associated diseases [58]. An epitope spanning the 200–239aa region of Ro52, which contains the complete leucine zipper, has also been identified [60]. High levels of autoantibodies against this epitope were associated with NLE and congenital heart block [61]. These autoantibodies can bind directly to the cell surfaces of cardiomyocytes in primary culture and cause dysregulation of the Ca^{2+} homeostasis, which is followed by apoptosis [62].

10.2.5 The Multifunctional Chaperone Calreticulin

The protein calreticulin is an exemplary multifunctional molecule of the endoplasmic reticulum capable of interacting with proteins, peptides, sugars, and nucleic acids [63]. The exact mode of interaction with other Ro/La RNP complex components is controversial since it has been found to interact with Ro52, hY RNA, and the epitopes of Ro60 autoantigen [13, 49]. Some of the numerous functions of calreticulin include (1) regulation of Ca^{2+} homeostasis; (2) chaperoning of glycoproteins in the endoplasmic reticulum to ensure proper folding; (3) action as a stress protein; (4) regulation of integrin-mediated adhesion (surface calreticulin); (5) modification of gene expression by binding to the glucocorticoid receptor; (6) a role as a component of cytotoxic T-lymphocyte/natural killer cell (CTL/NK)

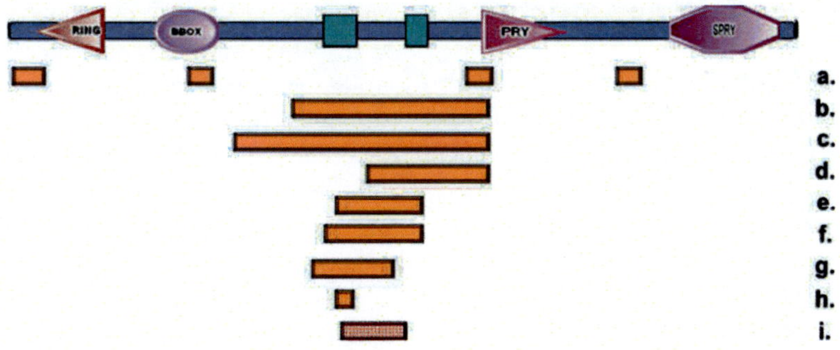

Fig. 10.6 Schematic representation of autoepitopes of the Ro52 kDa protein. **a** [99]. **b** [100]. **c** [57]. **d** [101]. **e** [58]. **f** [102]. **g** [59]. **h** [103]. **g** [61] (CHB-related epitope). Domain organization: RING = type of zinc finger domain involved in protein–protein interactions, BBOX = B-Box zinc finger associated with RING finger and a coiled-coil motif to form the so-called tripartite motif that is commonly found in transcription factors, SPRY = domain named from SPla and RYanodine Receptor, PRY = domain associated with SPRY domain. Segments of low compositional complexity are shown in *green*

granules; and (7) action as C1q receptor (surface calreticulin) [63]. Its immunoreactivity, which is rather limited, involves antigenic regions in the N terminus (1–24aa) and the central part of the molecule (193–207aa, 253–282aa) [64, 65]. Previous studies showed that animal immunization with Ro60 (but not with La) autoantigen led to spreading of immunity to calreticulin indicating that calreticulin is associated with a subpopulation of Ro particles from which La has already dissociated [66].

In addition, it was found that when Ro epitopes are complexed together with calreticulin, the antigenicity of the complex is increased compared to that of calreticulin or the Ro epitopes alone [49]. Using complexes of highly purified human calreticulin with the linear epitopes of Ro60, almost all positive anti-Ro60 sera were found to bind strongly onto the newly formed conformation of the epitopes [49]. When calreticulin or the linear epitopes of Ro60 were tested individually with the same sera, the prevalence of positive reactions was much lower. These observations suggest conformation-dependent enhancement of antigenicity of the Ro60 epitopes upon interaction with the chaperone protein calreticulin. Such complexes can potentially be used as substrates for the efficient detection of autoantibodies.

10.3 Clinical Significance of Epitopes in Sjögren's Syndrome and Specific HLA Associations

The clinical significance of autoantibodies to linear epitopes of Ro/SSA and La/SSB was investigated in a European multicenter study, which examined sera from 88 patients with primary Sjögren's syndrome (pSS). It was found that autoantibodies to the La/SSB epitope, p349–364aa, were associated with longer disease duration ($p < 0.05$), recurrent or permanent parotid gland enlargement ($p < 0.005$), and a higher proportion of non-exocrine manifestations ($p < 0.005$) compared to patients without autoantibodies. In addition, the presence of anti-Ro/SSA and anti-La/SSB autoantibodies was associated with the presence of HLA-DRB1*03 and DQB1*02 ($p = 0.038$ and $p = 0.034$, respectively). This association was even more prominent and extended to HLA-DQA1*0501 when patients were stratified according to the presence of autoantibodies to discrete La/SSB B-cell epitopes in comparison with autoantibody-negative patients ($p < 0.01$). In particular, they were found also to be highly associated with the alleles HLA-DQB1*02 and HLA-DQA1*0501 as well as with the presence of a shared amino acid motif in the region 59–69aa of DQB1 first domain ($p < 0.01$). Therefore, it appears that HLA-restricted presentation of La/SSB peptide determinants is crucial for development of autoimmune response against La/SSB [33].

10.4 B-cell Epitopes for the Investigation of the Autoimmune Response

10.4.1 Complementary Epitopes and Anti-idiotypic Antibodies

The idiotypic network theory was proposed by Nobel laureate Niels Jerne [67], who hypothesized that antibodies could act as antigens and elicit anti-antibodies (called anti-idiotypic antibodies). When anti-idiotypic antibodies target the antigen-binding sites of the idiotypic antibodies, then they can either (a) compete with the antigen for the same binding site (Ab2_anti-idiotypic antibodies according to Jerne's classification) or (b) elicit anti-anti-idiotypic antibodies with similar antigenic specificity with the idiotypic antibodies [68]. Thus, anti-idiotypic antibodies can either "neutralize" idiotypic antibodies or elicit antibodies with the same antigenic specificity of idiotypic antibodies. In fact, under these conditions, an anti-idiotypic network is established that regulates the production of idiotypic antibodies. Based on the detailed knowledge of the antigenic structures that are recognized by autoantibodies, one can design complementary epitopes that are expected to be recognized by anti-idiotypic antibodies, using the "molecular

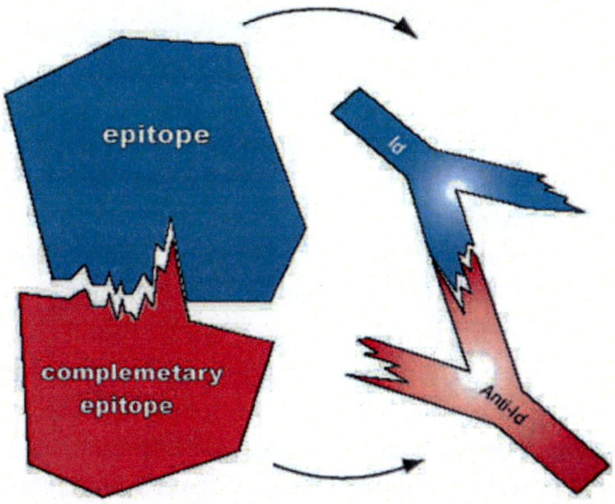

Fig. 10.7 Schematic representation of the similarity of epitopes and complementary epitopes with regions located in $F(ab)_2$ of anti-idiotypic and idiotypic antibodies, respectively

recognition" theory [69]. According to this theory, a sense peptide, transcribed and translated from a nucleotide sequence read in the $5' \rightarrow 3'$ direction, binds to its complementary peptide counterpart and is transcribed and translated in frame with that of its sense peptide from a nucleotide sequence read in the $5' \rightarrow 3'$ direction on the opposite DNA strand. Interestingly, many experimental data suggest that these interacting peptides have the ability to generate and detect interacting pairs of idiotypic and anti-idiotypic antibodies [70] (Fig. 10.7).

Recent findings indicate that autoimmunity can be initiated through an immune response against a peptide that is complementary to the autoantigen [71]. Pedergraft and co-workers demonstrated that a subset of proteinase 3 (PR3)-ANCA patients harbors antibodies directed against the protein product of the middle fragment (105–201aa) of the antisense RNA of PR3, termed complementary PR3 or cPR3 [72]. These antibodies were not present in patients with anti-MPO autoantibodies (myeloperoxidase (MPO)-ANCA), SLE patients, or healthy controls. It was also demonstrated that human anti-cPR3 and anti-PR3 antibodies are an idiotypic–anti-idiotypic pair, that mice immunized with cPR3 develop anti-cPR3 and anti-human PR3 antibodies, and that complementary PR3 transcripts are present in peripheral leukocyte RNA from a subset of ANCA patients [71, 72]. Recent studies in our laboratory have demonstrated that in SLE and SS there is also an active idiotypic–anti-idiotypic network targeting the two major B-cell epitopes of La/SSB and their complementary peptides [73]. The anti-idiotypic antibodies were isolated using the complementary epitopes and were found to bind anti-La/SSB antibodies, competing with La/SSB epitopes for their antigen-binding site. In some cases, these anti-idiotypic antibodies were capable of completely masking anti-La/SSB antibodies, abolishing their anti-La/SSB reactivity. A specific procedure, developed with the use of complementary peptides for the release of anti-La/SSB antibodies from their anti-idiotypic counterpart, was applied in 44 anti-La (−), anti-Ro/ANA (+) sera from patients with SLE and SS. Ninety-four percent of SS sera and 80% of SLE sera were found to be negative for anti-epitope 349–364aa antibodies prior to the treatment with complementary epitope. After treatment, all SS and SLE sera became positive for anti-epitope 349–364aa antibodies, while none of the normal sera exhibited a positive reaction. Heating without addition of complementary epitope 349–364aa had no effect on patient sera reactivity. Thus, virtually all anti-Ro/ANA (+) sera possess hidden anti-La/SSB antibodies that can be unmasked by treatment with the complementary epitope. Animal studies also demonstrated that mice immunized with complementary epitopes of La/SSB develop anti-human La/SSB antibodies [74]. Thus, the complementary epitopes of La/SSB appear to have the potential to induce an autoimmune response against La/SSB autoantigen.

In recent work from our laboratory, the role of anti-idiotypic antibodies to anti-La/SSB in the pathogenesis of neonatal lupus syndrome (NLS) was investigated [75]. We found that mothers giving birth to a healthy child and with no history of a child with NLS exhibited statistically significant higher prevalence of anti-idiotypic activity to autoantibodies against the major B-cell epitope of La/SSB compared to mothers carrying a child with NLS or mothers giving birth to a healthy child but who previously gave birth to a child with NLS. Thus, the

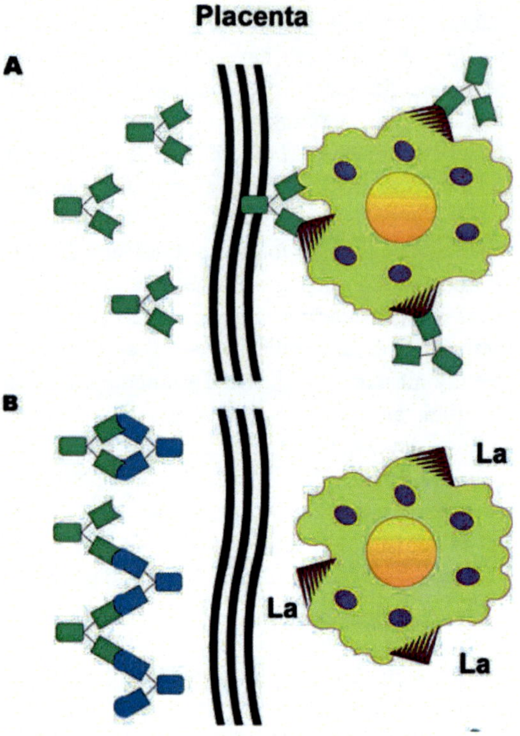

Fig. 10.8 Proposed mechanism for the role of anti-idiotypic antibodies in CHB. **a** In CHB pathogenic maternal anti-La autoantibodies enter the fetal circulation via the placenta and bind to the La autoantigen exposed on the surface of apoptotic cardiomyocytes. **b** The presence of anti-idiotypic antibodies to autoantibodies against La/SSB can protect the fetus by blocking the entrance of pathogenic antibodies to its circulation

presence of anti-idiotypic antibodies to autoantibodies against La/SSB seems to protect the fetus, most probably by blocking the entrance of pathogenic maternal autoantibodies via the placenta (Fig. 10.8) [75].

10.4.2 Early Epitope Recognition in Autoimmune Diseases and Epitope Spreading

Autoimmunity typically commences when tolerance to self-antigens is lost, a phenomenon that has fascinated immunologists for more than a century. During the past few decades, innovative methodologies for screening and analyzing cellular and biochemical processes have led to an extensive body of literature that characterizes human autoimmune diseases on multiple levels. Nevertheless, the precise etiology of most human autoimmune diseases remains largely unexplained, and the initiating immunogens are unclear.

In SLE, the onset and progression of autoantibody development before clinical diagnosis have been studied. Using the US Department of Defense Serum Repository with over 30 million specimens prospectively collected from 5 million US Armed Forces personnel, Arbuckle et al. evaluated serum samples obtained from 130 persons before they received a diagnosis of SLE [76]. They found that in 115 of the 130 patients with SLE (88%), at least 1 SLE autoantibody tested was present before the diagnosis (up to 9.4 years earlier; mean, 3.3 years). ANA, APL, anti-Ro, and anti-La antibodies were present earlier than anti-Sm and anti-snRNP antibodies. Anti-dsDNA antibodies were found later than ANA and earlier than anti-snRNP antibodies. The earliest autoantibodies detected in the pre-clinical period, as individuals progressed toward clinical SLE, were antibodies to Ro60 (mean, 3.7 years before the disease onset).

McClain et al. mapped the initial, pre-disease target of the anti-Ro60 autoantibody response to the region, 169–180aa (TKYKQRNGWSHK), of the autoantigen [48]. This region belongs to the SLE-related 169–190aa epitope, previously identified by Routsias et al. [47]. This 169–180aa epitope was found by McClain and co-workers to cross-react with a peptide (GGSGSGPRHRDGVRR, 58–72aa) from the latent viral protein Epstein–Barr virus nuclear antigen-1 (EBNA-1) [48]. Notably, no areas of primary sequence homology exist between EBNA-1 58–72aa and Ro169–180aa although these peptides have similar high isoelectric points (12.0 and 10.5, respectively). However, animals immunized with either the 169–180, epitope of Ro60 or the cross-reactive EBNA-1 epitope progressively developed autoantibodies binding multiple epitopes of Ro and spliceosomal autoantigens. These animals eventually developed some of the clinical symptoms of lupus, such as leukopenia, thrombocytopenia, or renal dysfunction. Although these experiments indicate a possible cross-reaction between the initial epitope of Ro60 and the 58–72aa region of EBNA-1, any involvement of Epstein–Barr virus in the pathogenesis of SLE has to be proved. In addition, other possible cross-reactions of Ro60 169–180aa epitope with various xenoantigens have to be studied (e.g., the Ro60 169–176aa, TKYKQRNG, with that of L-polymerase 53–60aa, TKYKIRNG of human parainfluenza virus 1).

After the initial response against Ro60 autoantigen, autoantibody targets can be expanded to the whole Ro60 by a procedure known as epitope spreading. The term epitope spreading was introduced in the early 1990s to describe the ability of the B-cell and T-cell immune response to diversify, at the level of specificity, from a single determinant to many sites on an autoantigen [77]. This process is not a feature restricted to systemic autoimmune diseases but is a common characteristic of the natural immune response mounted against some pathogens. Our studies with rabbit immunizations revealed that immunization with a single synthetic epitope of La/SSB produced epitope spreading to other B-cell epitopes of the molecule. Yiannaki et al. showed that immunization of rabbits with an antigenic peptide of La autoantigen led to antibodies to multiple epitopes of La [78]. These results demonstrate that loss of tolerance to a single antigenic determinant of the autoantigen can begin an autoimmune response that virtually recreates the humoral autoimmune specificity seen in human SLE. Clues to the mechanisms involved in the aforementioned production of cross-reactive antibodies to the common spliceosomal proteins have been reported by Monneaux et al. [79, 80]. According to their model, a consensus sequence (the RNP motif) conserved in many nuclear, nucleolar, and cytoplasmic antigens plays the role of a "driver" epitope. Cross-reactive autoantibodies targeting this epitope have the potential to spread the autoimmune response to other RNA-binding proteins through molecular mimicry. Subsequently, intramolecular spreading to these specific proteins can occur. This hypothesis is based on the observation that this "driver" epitope sequence in the RNP motif is recognized by $CD4^+$ T cells from lupus mice and is often targeted by autoantibodies very early during the course of the disease [79, 81]. Remarkably, this sequence is present in components of Ro/La RNP, such as Ro60 (119–131aa), La (146–158aa), and nucleolin (346–358aa, 517–529aa) as well as in spliceosomal proteins, such as RNP70 (139–151aa) and RNP A (47–59aa, 239–251aa). Several other sequences might also be considered as important "initiator" sequences, e.g., the recurring proline-rich sequence, PPPGMRPP, present in several snRNPs or the dimethylarginine-modified CRG repeats present on the B, D1, and D3 autoantigens [82].

10.4.3 Post-translational Modifications (PTMs) of B-cell Epitopes

The majority of mammalian proteins have PTMs, which potentially can be recognized by the immune system as self-neoepitopes. PTMs are either driven by enzymes or occur spontaneously, but the extent of protein modification varies in inflammatory and autoimmune disorders. These associations have been known for sometime, but their effects on disease etiology are still unclear. Two amino acid modifications have been described as targets of systemic autoimmunity.

1. *Arginine modifications.* Arginine residues are susceptible to three forms of modification: methylation, deimination, and citrullination. Two of them have been correlated with systemic autoimmunity.
   a. *Dimethylation*: The Sm proteins D1, D3, and B/B′ contain a C-terminal rich in arginine and glycine residues that is conserved in most eukaryotic organisms. Studies using mass spectrometry and sequencing of the C terminus of these Sm proteins have shown that repeated RG dipeptide regions in Sm D1 and Sm D3 and repeated GRG triplets in Sm B/B′ contain symmetric dimethylarginine residues [83, 84]. Dimethylation of arginine residues of the major Sm D1 and Sm D3 autoepitopes

remarkably increases binding by SLE autoantibodies. Moreover, a particular Sm D3 peptide represents a highly specific substrate for detecting a subclass of anti-Sm antibodies by ELISA [85]. Thus, symmetrical dimethylarginine residues act as targets for autoantibodies in SLE. It was recently shown that the same autoantigens contain asymmetric dimethylarginine in addition to the already-reported symmetric dimethylarginine residues [86]. The effect of this modification in autoantibody binding has not been studied yet.

b. *Citrullination*: Removal of the imine group from an arginine residue produces citrulline, which lacks the positive charge of arginine. This reaction is catalyzed by the peptidylarginine deiminase (PAD) family of enzymes. Citrulline has recently attracted interest as an autoantibody target in RA [87]. One of the major autoantigens in RA, filaggrin, is citrullinated by PAD and provides several targets for autoantibody binding. However, citrullination of B-cell epitopes of Ro 60, spanning the sequence 212–232aa, in the arginine residues, did not reveal alterations in antibody-binding capacity [88].

2. *Serine/Threonine Phosphorylation*: Phosphorylation is the most common and ubiquitous form of enzyme-mediated PTM. It has been implicated in the recognition of nuclear autoantigens by the immune system in SLE. In fact, phosphorylated components of U1 snRNP particles are specifically recognized by autoantibodies of SLE patients and $CD4^+$ T cells from lupus-prone mice (MRL/lpr mice). La protein can be phosphorylated at position 366. La phosphorylated at serine 366 is nucleoplasmic and is associated with nascent RNA polymerase III transcripts while non-phosphorylated La is cytoplasmic and is associated with a subset of mRNAs that contain 5′-terminal oligopyrimidine (5′-TOP) [89]. Thus, La exists in distinct states that differ in subcellular localization and is associated with RNAs, which can be discriminated by serine 366 phosphorylation. Proteomic analyses of parotid glands of patients with Sjögren's syndrome and controls revealed that patients with Sjögren's syndrome express only the phosphorylated forms of the molecule [90]. This specific phosphorylation resides within an antigenic determinant of La/SSB. This major B-cell epitope was previously identified in our laboratory and was found to reside in the 349–368aa region of La/SSB [31]. Our studies indicate that the antigenicity of the epitope is significantly enhanced upon phosphorylation of serine 366 [91].

10.5 Summary and Future Directions

The extensive study of B-cell epitopes of intracellular autoantigens provides useful insights into the diagnosis, classification, and prognosis of autoimmune diseases. The successful development of diagnostic assays is hindered by a number of factors concerning epitope recognition in autoimmune disorders, such as cross-reactivity, epitope spreading, epitope masking, and epitope modification. Issues regarding the simultaneous analysis of a large number of autoantibody specificities in a single test also have to be considered. The analysis of B-cell epitopes of autoantigens provides clues to overcome these problems.

1. Autoantibody screening test methodologies can be improved using large-scale arrays with specific autoantigen epitopes. These arrays are able to perform large-scale multiplex characterizations of autoantibody responses against structurally diverse autoantigens [92]. Chemical modifications of autoepitopes can provide better antigenic substrates mimicking naturally occurring PTMs. The lesson of citrullinated peptides taught us that recombinant proteins are not always the preferred substrate for autoantibody detection and that synthetic peptides can be successfully used in diagnostic assays if the exact structure of the autoantibody target is known [3].
2. Complementary peptides can efficiently neutralize anti-idiotypic antibodies, enhancing

the interaction of the idiotypic autoantibodies with their target epitope. The analysis of B-cell epitopes of autoantigens provides a better understanding of the origin and evolution of autoimmune response. In this regard, foreign epitopes, mimicking complementary epitopes or post-translationally modified peptides, could be the initiating agents of autoimmune disease. In addition, the spreading of autoimmune response from the initial epitope to others can be utilized for monitoring the evolution of autoimmune disease. Finally, the analysis of B-cell epitopes of autoantigens can provide potential therapeutic regimens, using epitopes with high specificity as vaccines, as tolerogens, or as modifiers of the autoimmune response via the idiotypic–anti-idiotypic network.

References

1. Moutsopoulos MN, Routsias JG, Vlachoyiannopoulos PG, Tzioufas AG, Moutsopoulos HM. B-cell epitopes of intracellular autoantigens: myth and reality. Mol Med. 2000;6(3):141–51.
2. Van Regenmortel MH. Synthetic peptides versus natural antigens in immunoassays. Ann Biol Clin. 1993;51(1):39–41.
3. Routsias JG, Tzioufas AG, Moutsopoulos HM. The clinical value of intracellular autoantigens B-cell epitopes in systemic rheumatic diseases. Clin Chim Acta. 2004;340(1–2):1–25.
4. Arnon R, Ben-Yedidia T. Old and new vaccine approaches. Int Immunopharmacol. 2003;3(8):1195–204.
5. Sela M, Mozes E. Therapeutic vaccines in autoimmunity. Proc Natl Acad Sci USA. 2004;101 (Suppl 2):14586–92.
6. Doyle HA, Mamula MJ. Post-translational protein modifications in antigen recognition and autoimmunity. Trends Immunol. 2001;22(8): 443–9.
7. Elkon KB. Epitope mapping of autoantigens using recombinant proteins and synthetic peptides. Clin Exp Rheumatol. 1989;7(Suppl 3):S63–8.
8. Brahms H, Raymackers J, Union A, de Keyser F, Meheus L, Luhrmann R. The C-terminal RG dipeptide repeats of the spliceosomal Sm proteins D1 and D3 contain symmetrical dimethylarginines, which form a major B-cell epitope for anti-Sm autoantibodies. J Biol Chem. 2000;275(22):17122–9.
9. Aris JP, Blobel G. cDNA cloning and sequencing of human fibrillarin, a conserved nucleolar protein recognized by autoimmune antisera. Proc Natl Acad Sci USA. 1991;88(3):931–5.
10. Lapeyre B, Amalric F, Ghaffari SH, Rao SV, Dumbar TS, Olson MO. Protein and cDNA sequence of a glycine-rich, dimethylarginine-containing region located near the carboxyl-terminal end of nucleolin (C23 and 100 kDa). J Biol Chem. 1986;261(20):9167–73.
11. Ben-Chetrit E, Chan EK, Sullivan KF, Tan EM. A 52-kD protein is a novel component of the SS-A/Ro antigenic particle. J Exp Med. 1988;167(5): 1560–71.
12. Slobbe RL, Pluk W, van Venrooij WJ, Pruijn GJ. Ro ribonucleoprotein assembly in vitro. Identification of RNA–protein and protein–protein interactions. J Mol Biol. 1992;227(2):361–6.
13. Cheng ST, Nguyen TQ, Yang YS, Capra JD, Sontheimer RD. Calreticulin binds hYRNA and the 52-kDa polypeptide component of the Ro/SS-A ribonucleoprotein autoantigen. J Immunol. 1996;156(11):4484–91.
14. Fouraux MA, Bouvet P, Verkaart S, van Venrooij WJ, Pruijn GJ. Nucleolin associates with a subset of the human Ro ribonucleoprotein complexes. J Mol Biol. 2002;320(3):475–88.
15. Maraia RJ, Kenan DJ, Keene JD. Eukaryotic transcription termination factor La mediates transcript release and facilitates reinitiation by RNA polymerase III. Mol Cell Biol. 1994;14(3):2147–58.
16. Peek R, Pruijn GJ, van der Kemp AG, van Venrooij WJ. Subcellular distribution of Ro ribonucleoprotein complexes and their constituents. J Cell Sci. 1993;106(Pt 3):929–35.
17. Simons FH, Pruijn GJ, van Venrooij WJ. Analysis of the intracellular localization and assembly of Ro ribonucleoprotein particles by microinjection into *Xenopus laevis* oocytes. J Cell Biol. 1994;125(5):981–8.
18. Ford LP, Shay JW, Wright WE. The La antigen associates with the human telomerase ribonucleoprotein and influences telomere length in vivo. RNA 2001;7(8):1068–75.
19. van Venrooij WJ, Pruijn GJ. Ribonucleoprotein complexes as autoantigens. Curr Opin Immunol. 1995;7(6):819–24.
20. Ray PS, Das S. La autoantigen is required for the internal ribosome entry site-mediated translation of Coxsackievirus B3 RNA. Nucleic Acids Res. 2002;30(20):4500–8.
21. Bachmann M, Pfeifer K, Schroder HC, Muller WE. Characterization of the autoantigen La as a nucleic acid-dependent ATPase/dATPase with melting properties. Cell 1990;60(1):85–93.
22. Xiao Q, Sharp TV, Jeffrey IW, et al. The La antigen inhibits the activation of the interferon-inducible protein kinase PKR by sequestering and unwinding double-stranded RNA. Nucleic Acids Res. 1994;22(13):2512–8.

23. Fan H, Goodier JL, Chamberlain JR, Engelke DR, Maraia RJ. 5′ processing of tRNA precursors can be modulated by the human La antigen phosphoprotein. Mol Cell Biol. 1998;18(6):3201–11.
24. Alfano C, Sanfeliced D, Babon J, et al. Structural analysis of cooperative RNA binding by the La motif and central RRM domain of human La protein. Nat Struc Mol Biol. 2004;11(4):323–9.
25. Jacks A, Babon J, Kelly G, et al. Structure of the C-terminal domain of human La protein reveals a novel RNA recognition motif coupled to a helical nuclear retention element. Structure 2003;11(7):833–43.
26. Maraia RJ, Intine RV. Recognition of nascent RNA by the human La antigen: conserved and divergent features of structure and function. Mol Cell Biol. 2001;21(2):367–79.
27. McNeilage LJ, Macmillan EM, Whittingham SF. Mapping of epitopes on the La(SS-B) autoantigen of primary Sjogren's syndrome: identification of a cross-reactive epitope. J Immunol. 1990;145(11):3829–35.
28. Rischmueller M, McNeilage LJ, McCluskey J, Gordon T. Human autoantibodies directed against the RNA recognition motif of La (SS-B) bind to a conformational epitope present on the intact La (SS-B)/Ro (SS-A) ribonucleoprotein particle. Clin Exp Immunol. 1995;101(1):39–44.
29. Troster H, H Bartsch H, Klein R, et al. Activation of a murine autoreactive B cell by immunization with human recombinant autoantigen La/SS-B: characterization of the autoepitope. J Autoimmun. 1995;8(6):825–42.
30. Weng YM, McNeilage J, Topfer F, McCluskey J, Gordon T. Identification of a human-specific epitope in a conserved region of the La/SS-B autoantigen. J Clin Invest. 1993;92(2):1104–8.
31. Tzioufas AG, Yiannaki E, Sakarellos-Daitsiotis M, Routsias JG, Sakarellos C, Moutsopoulos HM. Fine specificity of autoantibodies to La/SSB: epitope mapping, and characterization. Clin Exp Immunol. 1997;108(2):191–8.
32. Yiannaki EE, Tzioufas AG, Bachmann M, et al. The value of synthetic linear epitope analogues of La/SSB for the detection of autoantibodies to La/SSB; specificity, sensitivity and comparison of methods. Clin Exp Immunol. 1998;112(1):152–8.
33. Tzioufas AG, Wassmuth R, Dafni UG, et al. Clinical, immunological, and immunogenetic aspects of autoantibody production against Ro/SSA, La/SSB and their linear epitopes in primary Sjogren's syndrome (pSS): a European multicentre study. Ann Rheum Dis. 2002;61(5):398–404.
34. Reed JH, Jackson MW, Gordon TP. B cell apotopes of the 60-kDa Ro/SSA and La/SSB autoantigens. J Autoimmun. 2008;31(3):263–7.
35. Reed JH, Neufing PJ, Jackson MW, et al. Different temporal expression of immunodominant Ro60/60 kDa-SSA and La/SSB apotopes. Clin Exp Immunol. 2007;148(1):153–60.
36. Chen X, Wolin SL. The Ro 60 kDa autoantigen: insights into cellular function and role in autoimmunity. J Mol Med. 2004;82(4):232–9.
37. Stein AJ, Fuchs G, Fu C, Wolin SL, Reinisch KM. Structural insights into RNA quality control: the Ro autoantigen binds misfolded RNAs via its central cavity. Cell 2005;121(4):529–39.
38. Chen X, Quinn AM, Wolin SL. Ro ribonucleoproteins contribute to the resistance of *Deinococcus radiodurans* to ultraviolet irradiation. Genes Dev. 2000;14(7):777–82.
39. Xue D, Shi H, Smith JD, et al. A lupus-like syndrome develops in mice lacking the Ro 60-kDa protein, a major lupus autoantigen. Proc Natl Acad Sci USA. 2003;100(13):7503–8.
40. Wahren-Herlenius M, Muller S, Isenberg D. Analysis of B-cell epitopes of the Ro/SS-A autoantigen. Immunol Today. 1999;20(5):234–40.
41. McCauliffe DP, Yin H, Wang LX, Lucas L. Autoimmune sera react with multiple epitopes on recombinant 52 and 60 kDa Ro(SSA) proteins. J Rheumatol. 1994;21(6):1073–80.
42. Saitta MR, Arnett FC, Keene JD. 60-kDa Ro protein autoepitopes identified using recombinant polypeptides. J Immunol. 1994;152(8):4192–202.
43. Wahren M, Ruden U, Andersson B, Ringertz NR, Pettersson I. Identification of antigenic regions of the human Ro 60 kDa protein using recombinant antigen and synthetic peptides. J Autoimmun. 1992;5(3):319–32.
44. Scofield RH, Dickey WD, Jackson KW, James JA, Harley JB. A common autoepitope near the carboxyl terminus of the 60-kD Ro ribonucleoprotein: sequence similarity with a viral protein. J Clin Immunol. 1991;11(6):378–88.
45. Scofield RH, Harley JB. Autoantigenicity of Ro/SSA antigen is related to a nucleocapsid protein of vesicular stomatitis virus. Proc Natl Acad Sci USA. 1991;88(8):3343–7.
46. Routsias JG, Sakarellos-Daitsiotis M, Detsikas E, Tzioufas AG, Sakarellos C, Moutsopoulos HM. Antibodies to EYRKK vesicular stomatitis virus-related peptide account only for a minority of anti-Ro60kD antibodies. Clin Exp Immunol. 1994;98(3):414–8.
47. Routsias JG, Tzioufas AG, Sakarellos-Daitsiotis M, Sakarellos C, Moutsopoulos HM. Epitope mapping of the Ro/SSA60KD autoantigen reveals disease-specific antibody-binding profiles. Eur J Clin Invest. 1996;26(6):514–21.
48. McClain HM, Heinlen LD, Dennis GJ, Roebuck J, Harley JB, James JA. Early events in lupus humoral autoimmunity suggest initiation through molecular mimicry. Nat Med. 2005;11(1):85–9.
49. Staikou EV, Routsias JG, Makri AA, et al. Calreticulin binds preferentially with B cell linear epitopes of Ro60 kD autoantigen, enhancing

recognition by anti-Ro60 kD autoantibodies. Clin Exp Immunol. 2003;134(1):143–50.
50. Routsiasv, Kosmopoulou A, Makri A, et al. Zinc ion dependent B-cell epitope, associated with primary Sjogren's syndrome, resides within the putative zinc finger domain of Ro60kD autoantigen: physical and immunologic properties. J Med Chem. 2004;47(17):4327–34.
51. Reed JH, Jackson MW, Gordon TP. A B cell apotope of Ro 60 in systemic lupus erythematosus. Arthritis Rheum. 2008;58(4):1125–9.
52. Scofield AN, Kurien BT, Gordon TP, Scofield RH. Can B cell epitopes of 60 kDa Ro distinguish systemic lupus erythematosus from Sjogren's syndrome? Lupus 2001;10(8):547–53.
53. Shimono Y, Murakami H, Hasegawa Y, Takahashi M. RET finger protein is a transcriptional repressor and interacts with enhancer of polycomb that has dual transcriptional functions. J Biol Chem. 2000;275(50):39411–9.
54. Borden KL. RING fingers and B-boxes: zinc-binding protein–protein interaction domains. Biochem Cell Biol. 1998;76(2–3):351–8.
55. Frank MB. Characterization of DNA binding properties and sequence specificity of the human 52 kDa Ro/SS-A (Ro52) zinc finger protein. Biochem Biophys Res Commun. 1999;259(3):665–70.
56. Wang D, Buyon JP, Yang Z, Di Donato F, Miranda-Carus ME, Chan EK. Leucine zipper domain of 52 kDa SS-A/Ro promotes protein dimer formation and inhibits in vitro transcription activity. Biochim Biophys Acta. 2001;1568(2): 155–61.
57. Blange I, Ringertz NR, Pettersson I. Identification of antigenic regions of the human 52 kD Ro/SS-A protein recognized by patient sera. J Autoimmun. 1994;7(2):263–74.
58. Dorner T, Feist E, Wagenmann A, et al. Anti-52 kDa Ro(SSA) autoantibodies in different autoimmune diseases preferentially recognize epitopes on the central region of the antigen. J Rheumatol. 1996;23(3):462–8.
59. Kato T, Sasakawa H, Suzuki S, et al. Autoepitopes of the 52-kd SS-A/Ro molecule. Arthritis Rheum. 1995;38(7):990–8.
60. Salomonsson S, Dorner T, Theander E, Bremme K, Larsson P, Wahren-Herlenius M. A serologic marker for fetal risk of congenital heart block. Arthritis Rheum. 2002;46(5):1233–41.
61. Strandberg L, Winqvist O, Sonesson SE, et al. Antibodies to amino acid 200–239 (p200) of Ro52 as serological markers for the risk of developing congenital heart block. Clin Exp Immunol. 2008;154(1):30–7.
62. Salomonsson S, Sonessonv SE, Ottosson L, et al. Ro/SSA autoantibodies directly bind cardiomyocytes, disturb calcium homeostasis, and mediate congenital heart block. J Exp Med. 2005;201(1): 11–7.
63. Michalak M, Corbett EF, Mesaeli N, Nakamura K, Opas M. Calreticulin: one protein, one gene, many functions. Biochem J. 1999;344(Pt 2):281–92.
64. Eggleton P, Ward FJ, Johnson S, et al. Fine specificity of autoantibodies to calreticulin: epitope mapping and characterization. Clin Exp Immunol. 2000;120(2):384–91.
65. Routsias JG, Tzioufas AG, Sakarellos-Daitsiotis M, Sakarellos C, Moutsopoulos HM. Calreticulin synthetic peptide analogues: anti-peptide antibodies in autoimmune rheumatic diseases. Clin Exp Immunol. 1993;91(3):437–41.
66. Kinoshita G, Keech CL, Sontheimer RD, Purcell A, McCluskey J, Gordon TP. Spreading of the immune response from 52 kDaRo and 60 kDaRo to calreticulin in experimental autoimmunity. Lupus 1998;7(1):7–11.
67. Jerne NK. Towards a network theory of the immune system. Ann Immunol. 1974;125C(1–2):373–89.
68. Jerne NK, Roland J, Cazenave PA. Recurrent idiotopes and internal images. EMBO J. 1982; (2):243–7.
69. Blalock JE. Complementarity of peptides specified by 'sense' and 'antisense' strands of DNA. Trends Biotechnol. 1990;8(6):140–4.
70. Weathington NM, Blalock JE. Rational design of peptide vaccines for autoimmune disease: harnessing molecular recognition to fix a broken network. Expert Rev Vaccines. 2003;2(1):61–73.
71. Pendergraft WF 3rd, Presslerv, Jennette JC, Falk RJ, Preston GA. Autoantigen complementarity: a new theory implicating complementary proteins as initiators of autoimmune disease. J Mol Med. 2005;83(1):12–25.
72. WF Pendergraft WF 3rd, Preston GA, Shah RR, et al. Autoimmunity is triggered by cPR-3(105-201), a protein complementary to human autoantigen proteinase-3. Nat Med. 2004; 10(1):72–9.
73. Routsias JG, Touloupi E, Dotsika E, et al. Unmasking the anti-La/SSB response in sera from patients with Sjogren's syndrome by specific blocking of anti-idiotypic antibodies to La/SSB antigenic determinants. Mol Med. 2002;8(6): 293–305.
74. Routsias JG, Dotsika E, Touloupi E, et al. Idiotype–anti-idiotype circuit in non-autoimmune mice after immunization with the epitope and complementary epitope 289–308aa of La/SSB: implications for the maintenance and perpetuation of the anti-La/SSB response. J Autoimmun. 2003;21(1):17–26.
75. Stea EA, Routsiasv, Clancy RM, Buyon JP, Moutsopoulosv HM, Tzioufas AG. Anti-La/SSB antiidiotypic antibodies in maternal serum: a marker of low risk for neonatal lupus in an offspring. Arthritis Rheum. 2006;54(7):2228–34.
76. Arbuckle MR, McClain MT, Rubertone MV, et al. Development of autoantibodies before the clinical onset of systemic lupus erythematosus. N Engl J Med. 2003;349(16):1526–33.

77. Lehmann PV, Forsthuber T, Miller A, Sercarz EE. Spreading of T-cell autoimmunity to cryptic determinants of an autoantigen. Nature 1992;358(6382):155–7.
78. Yiannaki E, Vlachoyiannopoulos PG, Manoussakis MN, et al. Study of antibody and T cell responses in rabbits immunized with synthetic human B cell epitope analogues of La (SSB) autoantigen. Clin Exp Immunol. 2000;121(3):551–6.
79. Monneaux F, Muller S. Key sequences involved in the spreading of the systemic autoimmune response to spliceosomal proteins. Scand J Immunol. 2001;54(1v2):45–54.
80. Monneaux F, Muller S. Epitope spreading in systemic lupus erythematosus: identification of triggering peptide sequences. Arthritis Rheum. 2002;46(6):1430–8.
81. Monneaux F, Dumortier H, Steiner G, Briand JP, Muller S. Murine models of systemic lupus erythematosus: B and T cell responses to spliceosomal ribonucleoproteins in MRL/Fas(lpr) and (NZB × NZW)F(1) lupus mice. Int Immunol. 2001;13(9):1155–63.
82. James JA, Harley JB. Peptide autoantigenicity of the small nuclear ribonucleoprotein C. Clin Exp Rheumatol. 1995;13(3):299–305.
83. Brahms H, Meheus L, de Brabandere V, Fischer U, Luhrmann R. Symmetrical dimethylation of arginine residues in spliceosomal Sm protein B/B′ and the Sm-like protein LSm4, and their interaction with the SMN protein. RNA 2001;7(11): 1531–42.
84. Pettersson I. Methods of epitope mapping. Mol Biol Rep. 1992; 16(3):149–53.
85. Mahler M, Fritzler MJ, Bluthner M. Identification of a SmD3 epitope with a single symmetrical dimethylation of an arginine residue as a specific target of a subpopulation of anti-Sm antibodies. Arthritis Res Ther. 2005;7(1):R19–29.
86. Miranda TB, Khusialv, Cook JR, et al. Spliceosome Sm proteins D1, D3, and B/B′ are asymmetrically dimethylated at arginine residues in the nucleus. Biochem Biophys Res Commun. 2004;323(2): 382–7.
87. Vossenaar ER, Nijenhuis S, Helsen MM, et al. Citrullination of synovial proteins in murine models of rheumatoid arthritis. Arthritis Rheum. 2003;48(9):2489–500.
88. Terzoglou AG, Routsias JG, Moutsopoulos HM, Tzioufas AG. Post-translational modifications of the major linear epitope 169–190aa of Ro60 kDa autoantigen alter the autoantibody binding. Clin Exp Immunol. 2006;146(1):60–5.
89. Intine RV, Tenenbaum SA, Sakulich AL, Keene JD, Maraia RJ. Differential phosphorylation and subcellular localization of La RNPs associated with precursor tRNAs and translation-related mRNAs. Mol Cell. 2003;12(5):1301–7.
90. Stea EA, Routsias JG, Samiotaki M, et al. Analysis of parotid glands of primary Sjogren's syndrome patients using proteomic technology reveals altered autoantigen composition and novel antigenic targets. Clin Exp Immunol. 2007;147(1): 81–9.
91. Terzoglou AG, Routsias JG, Avrameas S, Moutsopoulos HM, Tzioufas AG. Preferential recognition of the phosphorylated major linear B-cell epitope of La/SSB 349–368 aa by anti-La/SSB autoantibodies from patients with systemic autoimmune diseases. Clin Exp Immunol. 2006;144(3):432–9.
92. Robinson WH, DiGennaro C, Hueber W, et al. Autoantigen microarrays for multiplex characterization of autoantibody responses. Nat Med. 2002; 8(3):295–301.
93. Haaheim LR, Halse AK, Kvakestad R, Stern B, Normann O, Jonsson R. Serum antibodies from patients with primary Sjogren's syndrome and systemic lupus erythematosus recognize multiple epitopes on the La(SS-B) autoantigen resembling viral protein sequences. Scand J Immunol. 1996;43(1):115–21.
94. Kohsaka H, Yamamoto K, Fujii H, et al. Fine epitope mapping of the human SS-B/La protein. Identification of a distinct autoepitope homologous to a viral gag polyprotein. J Clin Invest. 1990;85(5):1566–74.
95. Huang SC, Yu H, Scofield RH, Harley JB. Human anti-Ro autoantibodies bind peptides accessible to the surface of the native Ro autoantigen. Scand J Immunol. 1995;41(3):220–8.
96. James JA, Scofield RH, Harley JB. Lupus humoral autoimmunity after short peptide immunization. Annl NY Acad Sci. 1997;815:124–7.
97. Scofield RH, Henry WE, Kurien BT, James JA, Harley JB. Immunization with short peptides from the sequence of the systemic lupus erythematosus-associated 60-kDa Ro autoantigen results in anti-Ro ribonucleoprotein autoimmunity. J Immunol. 1996;156(10):4059–66.
98. Veldhoven CH, Pruijn GJ, Meilof JF, et al. Characterization of murine monoclonal antibodies against 60-kD Ro/SS-A and La/SS-B autoantigens. Clin Exp Immunol. 1995;101(1): 45–54.
99. Ricchiuti V, Briand JP, Meyer O, Isenberg DA, Pruijn G, Muller S. Epitope mapping with synthetic peptides of 52-kD SSA/Ro protein reveals heterogeneous antibody profiles in human autoimmune sera. Clin Exp Immunol. 1994;95(3): 397–407.
100. Buyon JP, Slade SG, Reveille JD, Hamel JC, Chan EK. Autoantibody responses to the "native" 52-kDa SS-A/Ro protein in neonatal lupus syndromes, systemic lupus erythematosus, and Sjogren's syndrome. J Immunol. 1994;152(7):3675–84.

101. Bozic B, Pruijn GJ, Rozman B, van Venrooij WJ. Sera from patients with rheumatic diseases recognize different epitope regions on the 52-kD Ro/SS-A protein. Clin Exp Immunol. 1993;94(2):227–35.
102. Dorner T, Feist E, Held C, Conrad K, Burmester GR, Hiepe F. Differential recognition of the 52-kd Ro(SS-A) antigen by sera from patients with primary biliary cirrhosis and primary Sjogren's syndrome. Hepatology 1996;24(6):1404–7.
103. Frank MB, Itoh K, McCubbin V. Epitope mapping of the 52-kD Ro/SSA autoantigen. Clin Exp Immunol. 1994;95(3):390–6.

Neurobiology and Hormonal Control of Lacrimal and Salivary Gland Function

11

Yrjö T. Konttinen, Alberto Vivó Porcar, Pauliina Porola, Katja Koskenpato, María Lorés Rodriguez, Raimo Pöllänen, Vasily Stegaev, Liisa Virkki, Michelle Spaan, and Beata D. Przybyla

Abstract

Sjögren's syndrome (SS) is characterized by diminished production of secretes from exocrine glands and sicca complex, which occur in an autoimmune context; 90% of patients are women, usually developing the disease when they are 40–50 years old. This characterization comprises several neuroimmunoendocrine aspects. The sympathetic, parasympathetic, vascular, acinar, and myoepithelial systems normally work in a co-ordinated fashion in two phases, resting and stimulated phases, corresponding to the secretion of resting and stimulated saliva. Stimulation of the exocrine flow with acetylcholine is coupled with a proportional local release of acinotrophic vasoactive intestinal peptide (VIP) from post-ganglionic parasympathetic nerve terminals, which helps to recover and repair the acinar cell during the "resting" (recovery) phase. Lost (dead and detached) acinar cells are replaced by remodeling based on an asymmetric division of the intercalated duct progenitor cells, which as a result are able to maintain their unipotent stemness and at the same time able to replace the lost acinar cells. This remodeling is maintained by dehydroepiandrosterone (DHEA) produced in the reticular zone of the endocrine adrenal gland in an endocrine process, but is locally in exocrine glands converted to dihydrotestosterone (DHT) in an intracrine process. SS is characterized by deranged intracrine enzymatic machinery and impaired DHEA-to-DHT conversion. This impairment leads particularly in women to acinar cell atrophy/loss and a reciprocal ductal cell hyperplasia. Men are protected because they feed the intracrine machinery also with testosterone, only one step away from DHT. Abnormally processed self antigens are released from dying

Y.T. Konttinen (✉)
Department of Medicine, Biomedicum Helsinki, Helsinki University Central Hospital, Helsinki, Finland; ORTON Orthopaedic Hospital of the ORTON Foundation, Helsinki, Finland; COXA Hospital for the Joint Replacement, Tampere, Finland
e-mail: yrjo.konttinen@helsinki.fi

R.I. Fox, C.M. Fox (eds.), *Sjögren's Syndrome*, DOI 10.1007/978-1-60327-957-4_11,

cells and break the immunologic tolerance so that autoantibodies are formed against previously hidden endotopes. Immune inflammation leads to synthesis and release of tumor necrosis factor-α, interleukin-1ß, and other cytokines, which impair signal transduction in acinar cells and add to the burden of the inflammatory *functio laesa*.

Keywords
Sjögren's syndrome • Salivary glands • Acinus • Acetylcholine • Neuropeptide • DHEA • Cytokines

11.1 Introduction to Sjögren's Syndrome

Sjögren's syndrome (SS), originally mostly defined according to the Copenhagen criteria [1], is nowadays usually defined using the European–American inclusion and exclusion criteria and classification rules [2], although this praxis can in the clinical setting also be questioned [3]. Emphasis is on lacrimal and salivary gland dysfunction and mucosal membrane drying, which, however, must occur in an autoimmune setting. Half of the patients have circulating SS-A/Ro and/or SS-B/La autoantibodies, in the rest focal adenitis is often the clue. Basically all known causes for somewhat similar histopathology and/or clinical manifestations form exclusions, "pseudo-Sjögren's syndromes." The "true" syndromes occur as "primary Sjögren's syndrome" (pSS) or develop to complicate some underlying disease, like rheumatoid arthritis ("secondary Sjögren's syndrome," sSS). Because its cause and even pathomechanisms are largely unknown, creation of such relatively widely accepted diagnostic classification criteria can be considered as a major policy achievement. At the same time, these widely cited criteria represent nothing but our consensus what we believe, without actually knowing, is SS.

SS is also characterized by non-ocular and non-oral sicca symptoms, general symptoms, and visceral manifestations and complications, all nicely described in the so-called wheel of Oxholm [4]. Apart from keratoconjunctivitis sicca and xerostomia, also nose, throat, vagina, and skin are dry. General symptoms comprise fatigue, often in patient-centered studies experienced as the most difficult individual disease manifestation, arthralgia/arthritis, myalgia/myositis, lymphadenopathy, and Raynaud's phenomenon. Internal organ changes include involvement of the central and peripheral nervous systems, thyroiditis, interstitial lung disease, chronic atrophic gastritis, celiac disease, primary biliary cirrhosis and other liver manifestations, interstitial nephritis, lymphocytic and collagen colitis, and interstitial cystitis. Complications include caries, candidiasis, middle ear infections, dry cough and bronchoconstriction, respiratory tract, and other infections associated with the sicca syndrome, congenital heart conduction abnormalities, and neonatal subacute lupus as a result of SS antibodies (transferred via the placenta from the mother to the developing fetus) and, last but not least, lymphoma associated with the B-cell hyperreactivity [5]. These lymphomas are usually extranodal, mucosal-associated lymphatic tissue tumors (MALTomas) [6, 7] often developing in pre-existing lymphocyte infiltrates in lacrimal, salivary, or thyroid gland, interstitial lung tissue, or chronic atrophic gastritis lesions. They can present as "premalignant lesions," myoepithelial sialadenitis (MESA) or lymphoepithelial sialadenitis (LESA), characterized by clustered B cells interdigitating with ductal epithelial cells, epimyoepithelial islands [8].

Women represent close to 90% of all patients, so relatively few patients are men [9]. This gender aspect remains unexplained. A recent overview of the published studies did not find any consistent differences between female and male SS. Individual studies showed statistically highly significant differences in some characteristics, but other studies could show differences quite in the opposite direction [10]. This is probably due to selection bias. This similarity of SS in women and men is consistent with the current praxis to use the same set of diagnostic criteria for both women and men.

SS typically starts at 40–50 years. Patients with atypical presentation, such as a 9-year-old boy presenting with SS-like condition, should be carefully analyzed for a "pseudo-SS," some but not all of which are mentioned in the current European–American criteria. If such a patient finally is shown to suffer from pSS, he probably has some very important individual factor(s) predisposing him to this disease, because it precipitates it against the odds and in spite of barriers, which normally prevent its development in such a setting. The story could be unraveled from both of these two ends, the typical or the atypical. However, as it is easier to define the typical than atypical, the starting point of the present chapter is the typical patient with SS. Some reasons, which might explain the targeting of the exocrine glands of middle aged women for SS, are discussed below.

11.2 Acinar Cell

Primary secrete of exocrine glands is produced by acinar cells. SS is characterized by, diminished secretion of in particular resting tear and salivary fluid, secretory cell failure. If causes and mechanisms are looked for SS, the secretory acinar cell should be in focus.

Acinar cells function in part spontaneously to provide resting (non-stimulated) basal secretion, which does not vary much over time. However, this does not necessarily mean fully resting, but only refers to lack of any major stimulus (see below for more). In contrast, secretion triggered by a stimulus leads to stimulated secretion over and above secretion provided by the resting flow. The effector arm of this reflex arch is formed by the sympathetic and parasympathetic nerve fibers.

From the point of view of the sympathetic nervous system the exocrine gland function can be divided into two distinct phases. During the resting phase, arteriolar blood flows via metarterioles directly to post-capillary venules, bypassing the peri-acinar capillary network. This together with some spontaneous background activity typical for the autonomic nervous system might explain the continuous and relatively stable (non-regulated) flow of resting saliva. This two-phase organization can possibly also be based on parallel organization of the acinar and intralobular capillary networks [11].

During the stimulation phase sympathetic nerve endings release norepinephrine (noradrenaline), which relaxes the precapillary sphincters and redirects arteriolar blood flow to peri-acinar capillary network. The increased hydrostatic capillary pressure causes formation of transudate fluid. This transudate forms bulk of the watery flow drawn into the acinar lumen as a result of osmosis generated by the action of the parasympathetic nervous system (see below). Acinar cells do not have the capacity to store much fluid although they contain some mucins. Instead, they produce it from plasma. It was earlier thought that sympathetic stimulation diminishes salivary flow, but this conclusion was based on an artifact observed in early salivary gland studies in which supra-physiological concentrations of epinephrine were used. Concentrations used were so high that they caused a general vasoconstriction of arterioles and prevented almost totally flow of blood through (met)arterioles and capillaries and, thus, also the subsequent formation of watery saliva.

Activity of the sympathetic nervous system needs to occur in a topologically and timely coordinated fashion together with the acetylcholine-mediated (Fig. 11.1) parasympathetic stimulation of the acinar cells (Fig. 11.2). Therefore, logically also from the point of view of the

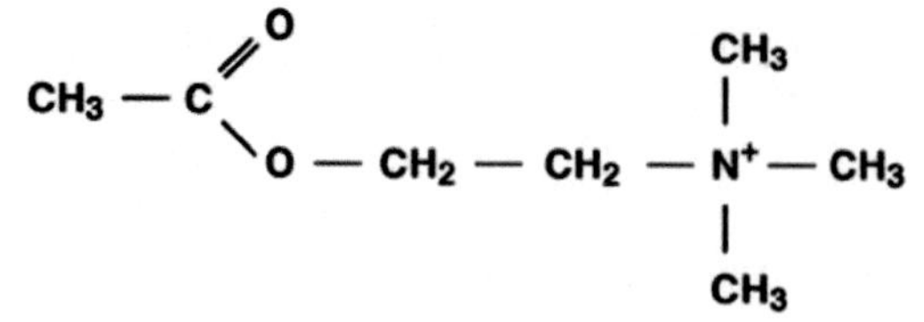

```
         10         20         30
MDTRNKAQLL VLLTLLSVLF SQTSAWPLYR
         40         50         60
APSALRLGDR IPFEGANEPD QVSLKEDIDM
         70         80         90
LQNALAENDT PYYDVSRNAR HADGVFTSDF
        100        110        120
SKLLGQLSAK KYLESLMGKR VSSNISEDPV
        130        140        150
PVKRHSDAVF TDNYTRLRKQ MAVKKYLNSI
        160        170
LNGKRSSEGE SPDFPEELEK
```

Fig. 11.1 On the top of the figure is acetylcholine, which is the classical neurotransmitter released from the small clear vesicles of the post-ganglionic parasympathetic nerve terminals. Below it is vasoactive intestinal peptide (VIP), which is a non-cholinergic, non-adrenergic (NANC), non-conventional peptide transmitter released from the large dense-core vesicles of the post-ganglionic parasympathetic nerve terminals. Their release occurs concomitantly, which leads to a coupling between (1) the rapidly occurring acetylcholine-induced ion channel opening and production of watery secrete during the stimulation phase and (2) a prolonged VIP-induced, gene transcription-mediated restoration during the recovery phase. This figure shows the first isoform of the prepropolypeptide, which is bioprocessed into a signal peptide (1–20), propeptide (21–79), intestinal peptide PHV-42 (81–122), intestinal peptide PHM-27 (81–107), vasoactive intestinal peptide (VIP) (125–152, *darker shading* in the figure), and a propeptide (156–170). In the other slightly different pre-propolypeptide precursor the same mature VIP peptide forms the residues 124–151

parasympathetic nervous system the exocrine gland function can be divided into two distinct phases. During the resting phase the acinar cell is loaded with $Cl^-$and K^+. During the stimulation phase acetylcholine leads to a discharge of the osmotic potential by opening two ion channels, which leads to secrete flow and helps to maintain the prolonged secretory phase of the acinar cell (Fig. 11.3). To this fluid the sympathetic nervous system, by its direct action on acinar cells, adds a protein-rich and mucin-rich viscous component. Interestingly, anti-cholinergic medication is today among list of exclusions in the diagnostic criteria and, vice versa, cholinergic agonists, sialogogues, pilocarpine, and cevimeline are used to stimulate salivary flow.

Two to three myoepithelial cells surround individual acini. Naturally also their function is divided into two distinct phases. During the resting phase they provide dynamic structural support for the underlying acini, which become swollen due to filling with mucin hydrogel or secretory protein-rich granules. In sialosis in diabetic, anorectic, or alcoholic patients the volume of individual cells and the size of the whole gland increase. Filling phases are extended, because the acinar cells are not properly and regularly emptied due to an autonomic neuropathy, lack of stimuli, or "liquid" alcohol diet. Upon autonomic nervous system stimulation in healthy individuals myoepithelial cells receive a dual stimulus from sympathetic and parasympathetic branches, which acts synergistically to promote outflow of saliva and salivary mucins. This phenomenon, a short-term improvement of salivary flow, has been also observed in patients with pSS [12].

In addition to its function as a secretagogue, acetylcholine and its α7-nicotinic acetylcholine receptor form the central component in "the cholinergic anti-inflammatory pathway" [13].

11.3 Neuropeptides

11.3.1 Acinotrophic Neurogenic Stimuli

Although the two phases of the sympathetic, parasympathetic, vascular, acinar, and myoepithelial cell function are often referred to as resting and stimulated phases, probably because it is commonplace to refer to measurement of resting (particularly from the minor and submandibular glands) and stimulated (particularly from the major salivary glands) flow, "rest" is by no means total rest for the main player of this review and this enigmatic syndrome, the acinar cell. As a matter of fact, right after the reflex secretory flow has stopped, follows a very feverous period in the life cycle of the secretory acinar cell because it has to recover from stimulated emptying and

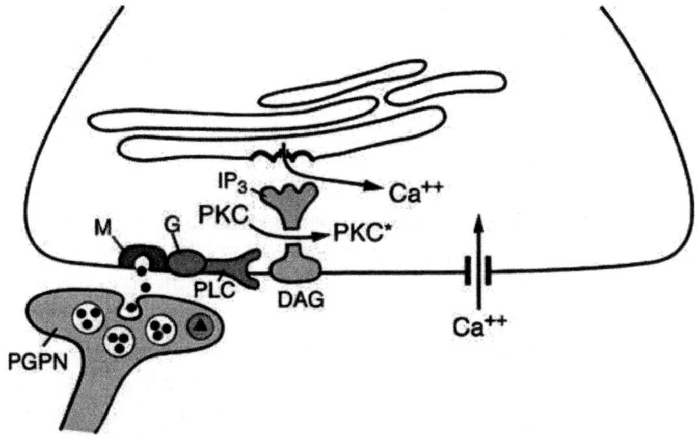

Fig. 11.2 Acetylcholine (*black circles*) released from the post-ganglionic parasympathetic nerve (PGPN) terminals binds to post-synaptic muscarinic (M3 and M1) receptor. It is via a G-protein coupled to activation of phospholipase C (PLC), which has just cleaved phosphatidyl inositol bisphosphate (PIP_2) in the cell membrane to cell membrane-bound diacyl glycerol (DAG) and inositol 1,4,5-trisphosphate (IP3), which has been released into the cytoplasm. IP3 binds to its receptors in the endoplasmic reticulum, which leads to rapid cytoplasmic calcium increase (or coupled with re-uptake, to oscillations) via release of Ca^{2+} through these IP3 receptors. This triggers Ca^{2+} influx from the extracellular space along its 10,000-fold concentration gradient through store-operated Ca^{++} SOC channels. Intracellular Ca^{2+} together with DAG activates in the figure the conventional protein kinase C (PKC) molecule into its active counterpart (marked with ∗). Increase in intracellular Ca^{2+} activates two ion channels, which lead to production of primary secrete. Notice that at the same time when acetylcholine is released, also VIP (*white triangles*) is concomitantly released

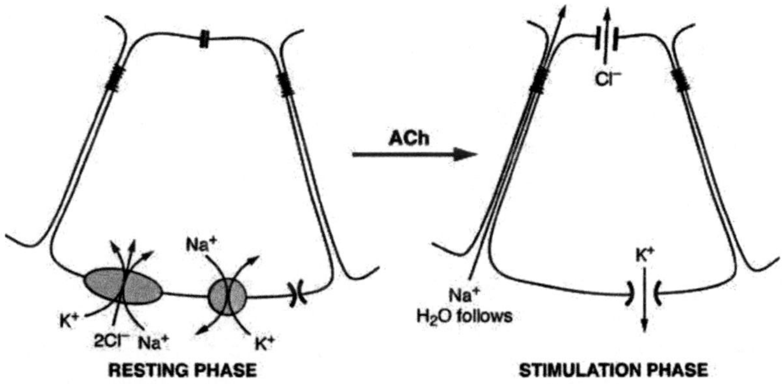

Fig. 11.3 During the resting phase $Na^+/K^+/2Cl^-$ co-transporter and Na^+/K^+-ATPase load (charge) the acinar cell with potassium and chloride. As a result of acetylcholine–muscarinic receptor interaction, the acinar cell is stimulated and during stimulation phase it discharges its osmotic potential via opening of the apical Cl^- channel allowing chloride to flow into the acinar lumen. Sodium follows due to the electrical charge and water due to the osmotic gradient. Opening of the basolateral K^+ channel and secretion of K^+ into the extracellular space lead to improved function of the $Na^+/K^+/2Cl^-$ co-transporter, which stimulates Na^+/K^+-ATPase so maintaining and increasing the effective secretory process

eventual cellular damage inflicted by forceful secretory activity burst, to be prepared for the next activity cycle. Because reflectory flow is stimulated by post-ganglionic parasympathetic nerve fibers, it would be reasonable to expect that there is a coupling between the extent of stimulation (secretory work) of the acinar cells and their subsequent recovery, which is mediated by some neuronal stimulus released concomitantly with acetylcholine.

According to the classic view one type of nerve was considered to use only one type of transmitter in its synapses, e.g., the post-ganglionic parasympathetic nerve terminals release acetylcholine (Figs. 11.1 and 11.2). This view has long been challenged by discovery of neuropeptides, excitatory and inhibitory amino acids, purines, nitric oxide, carbon oxide, and other "non-adrenergic, non-cholinergic" (NANC) transmitters in nerve cells and terminals containing conventional neurotransmitters. In exocrine gland function vasoactive intestinal peptide (VIP), released from the very same post-ganglionic parasympathetic nerve terminals which release acetylcholine, raises particular interest (Fig. 11.2) [14, 15, 16].

The importance of the nervous system for the exocrine glands is illustrated by the effect of surgical, chemical, or functional parasympathectomy, the last mentioned being accomplished by feeding rats with only liquid food instead of solid pellets, which in the long term leads to glandular disuse atrophy. Similar atrophy was not induced upon prolonged treatment with antimuscarinic agents and parasympathetic muscarin receptor agonists did not prevent it, so it is hardly due to acetylcholine deprivation. In contrast, if VIP was administered, the atrophic effect of parasympathectomy was prevented and acinar cells become enlarged, indicating an acinotrophic effect for VIP.

Physiological local VIP release as a result of stimulation of the post-ganglionic parasympathetic nerves may help to maintain acinar cells and promote their recovery [17]. These basic neurophysiological experiments suggest that acinotrophic neurogenic stimuli are released at the same time when also acetylcholine is released, during neuronal stimulation of the glands. They are released in the immediate vicinity of the putative acinar target cells and in proportion to the parasympathetic stimulation. Thus, the multiplicity of neurotransmitters in the post-ganglionic neurons could reflect their complex function, coupling functional stimulation of the secretory target cells with the long-term maintenance of these very same cells (the proportional response principle). The problem with this type of coupling of acetylcholine and NANCs release is that it can lead to inflammation and depletion.

11.3.2 Neurogenic Inflammation

Inflammation is often in clinical medicine seen as a pathological condition, which needs to be symptomatically treated, in increasing order of potency, with non-steroidal, steroidal, or biological anti-inflammatory drugs. If inflammation is immunologically driven, immunomodulatory or disease-modifying drugs are used. In contrast, in wound healing inflammation is envisioned as an early and necessary phase of subsequent repair. Necrotic tissues need to be phagocytosed and degraded and microbes killed, blood flow needs to increase to improve oxygenation and provision of nutrients, which are in increased demand, and local cytokines must be produced to orchestrate the complicated healing cascades. It is therefore, perhaps, not so surprising that neuropeptides with trophic effects, supporting repair, also have pro(and anti-)inflammatory actions; those dealt with in this chapter are shown in Table 11.1. Neurogenic inflammation was first realized as a wheal and flare response evoked by an axon reflex, but understanding of the sophistication of this potential has since increased tremendously. Neuropeptides can be considered as extravascular, intra-axonal potent "neuronal cytokines," which are delivered close to the effector cells via a special mechanism of delivery, release from the nerve terminal.

Apart from the molecular coupling of the nervous system and inflammation with each other, the nervous and the immune systems are anatomically coupled through the autonomic nervous system [47]. There are rich autonomic neural connections with lymphoid tissue, including thymus, bone marrow, lymph nodes, spleen, and gut-associated lymphatic tissue [71, 72, 26].

Substance P is a short, 11-amino acid long neuropeptide belonging to the tachykinin family [73], widely distributed throughout the nervous system, including salivary glands [74]. Neuropeptides are synthesized through gene transcription and translation, not enzymatically, and

Table 11.1 Examples of effects of neuropeptides (substance P, calcitonin gene-related peptide, neuropeptide Y, and vasoactive intestinal peptide)

Substance P	Calcitonin gene-related peptide	Neuropeptide Y	Vasoactive intestinal peptide
Release of NO, vasodilatation [18, 19]	Vasodilatation [39]	Vasoconstriction [51]	Involved in the nervous control of ovum transportation [60]
Histamine release [20]	Inhibition of bone resorption [40, 41]	Modulation of myocardial contractility [52]	Sexual arousal [60]
Mitogenic to smooth muscle cells [21], fibroblasts [22], endothelial cells [23], and synoviocytes [24]	Modulation of carbohydrate metabolism [42]	Modulation of neurotransmitter release from sensory and postganglionic sympathetic (PGS) neurons [53]	Smooth muscle cell relaxation [61, 62]
Neovascularization in vivo [25]	Mitogenic to endothelial cells [43]	Inhibition of adrenaline-induced platelet aggregation [54]	Coronary vasodilation [63]
IL-1, IL-6, and TNF-α release from monocytes [26, 27]	Muscle trophic factor [44, 45]	Trophic effects on non-neuronal cells [55, 56]	Regulation of prolactin secretion [64]
LTB4, PGE2, and TXB2 release from macrophages [28, 29, 30]	Potentiates neutrophil accumulation and IL-1, IL-6, TNF-α, and SP effects [46, 47, 48]	Up-regulation of adhesiveness of endothelial cells for leukocytes [57]	Dilation of peripheral blood vessels [65]
Stimulation of monocyte chemotaxis [31]	Chemotactic to T lymphocytes [49]	Mitogenic to mesangial cells [58]	Stimulation of pancreatic bicarbonate secretion [66, 67]
Enhancement of phagocytosis [32]	Enhancement of neutrophil adherence to endothelial cells [34]	Mediates proliferation, adhesion, and differentiation of T lymphocytes toward Th2 cells [59]	Stimulation of pepsinogen secretion by chief cells [68]
Enhancement of B-lymphocyte IgA and IgM production [33]	Inhibition of natural killer cell activity [50]	Stimulates leukocyte trafficking [59]	Communication between individual brain cells within suprachiasmatic nucleus (SCN) [69]
Enhancement of neutrophil adherence to endothelial cells [34]		Up-regulation of adhesiveness of endothelial cells for leukocytes [57]	Synchronizing the timing of SCN function with the environmental light–dark cycle [69]
PGE2 and MMP-1 release from fibroblasts and synoviocytes [24, 35, 36, 37, 38]		Stimulates antibody production from B-lymphocytes [59]	Reduces production of pro-inflammatory cytokines such as IL-2 and IFN-γ [70]
			Increases production of anti-inflammatory cytokines IL-10, IL-1Ra, and TGF-β1 [70]
			Inhibits expression of co-stimulatory molecules CD80 (B7-1) and CD86 (B7-2) on APCs surface [70]
			Promotes Th2-cell response and reduces Th1-cell response [70]

thus differently from the classic neurotransmitters [29]. Preproneuropeptide synthesis occurs in the neuronal cell body far away from the site of neuropeptide storage and release, the nerve terminal, or site of action [75]. From the perinuclear region the newly synthesized neuropeptide precursors are transported (and simultaneously processed, maturation) in vesicles in the extravascular, intra-axonal space along microtubules to the nerve terminals [76]. If coupling of the synthesis and fast intra-axonal transport (5–40 cm/day) or "delivery" does not meet neuropeptide demand, neuropeptide depletion follows. This happens rarely with enzymatically and locally synthesized classical neurotransmitters, which can be recycled and form a much easier replenishable transmitter pool. This has some potentially important consequences [32].

In peripheral tissues substance P is released from unmyelinated polymodal nociceptors. Apart from reflexes substance P release can be directly induced by molecules, like capsaicin from paprika. Substance P acts via endogenous neurokinin (NK) 1 receptor [77, 78, 79]. The NK1 receptor is widely distributed in the central and peripheral nervous systems [80, 81] and in nonneuronal structures [82, 31]. High levels of mRNA for NK1 are expressed in the salivary glands of rats [83]. Substance P up-regulates aromatase [84]. Although it is not very likely, substance P might play a role in focal adenitis or substance P depletion might protect from excessive host responses [82, 28, 31].

Calcitonin gene-related peptide (CGRP) is mainly produced in the nervous tissue and its receptor CALCR is expressed throughout the body [46]. CGRP is the most potent endogenous neurogenic vasodilator and a likely participant in the migraine development [48]. Although many earlier papers suggested a role for CGRP in neurogenic inflammation, more recent studies suggest that CGRP does not induce neurogenic inflammation in humans or rodents but only causes a neurogenic vasodilatation by acting via CALCR and cAMP on vascular smooth muscles [85]. It is not known if this potent vasodilator plays a role in the SS-related vascular phenomena, like the various phases of the Raynaud's phenomenon or the regulation of the precapillary sphincters of the metarterioles, which forms as an essential component in the regulation of salivary flow at rest and upon stimulation.

Neuropeptide Y (NPY) is in the central nervous system secreted by the hypothalamus. NPY receptors (Y1R–Y5R) are widely present in many different cells and tissues [86]. NPY is ubiquitous in sympathetic nervous terminals, including those of resistance blood vessels [87]. As a matter of fact, one of the first effects of NPY reported in the literature was its sympathetic vasoconstrictor effect resistant to α-adrenoceptor blockade [88], which although not strong by itself alone, greatly enhanced the effects of noradrenaline released from the same post-ganglionic sympathetic nerve terminals [89]. It is unknown if NPY perhaps directly mediates vasoconstriction or indirectly potentiates the vasoconstrictor effects of noradrenaline in the precapillary sphincters of the metarterioles. It could turn them "off" (or in case of ceased release turn them "on"). NPY could also participate in the regulation of the myoepithelial cells.

NPY is involved in the innervation of lymphatic organs and in immune cell functions. NPY receptors are expressed by leukocytes [90]. NPY mediates proliferation, adhesion, and differentiation of T lymphocytes toward Th2 cells, but vice versa, in a typical bidirectional communication also many immune-inflammatory molecules regulate NPY synthesis and/or release [91]. NPY stimulates leukocyte trafficking and B lymphocytes, including their immunoglobulin production [59], but it is not known if these effects play a role for the autoantibody production in SS.

Perhaps the most interesting neuropeptide from the SS point of view is vasoactive intestinal peptide (VIP), due to its potential as an acinotrophic factor. It might play a role for the autoimmune aspects of the syndrome. Acinar cell, which is not properly maintained, undergoes apoptosis or even necrosis and its molecular components can be abnormally degraded. This could lead to a local release, processing, and presentation of hidden or "unforeseen" epitopes (or actually endotopes) instead of the dominant epitopes, which are produced under "business as usual" type of apoptosis and against which the host therefore has developed immunologic self-tolerance [92, 93, 94]. It is proposed that such hidden epitopes are presented to lymphocytes in the secondary lymphatic organs and maybe also ectopically in the inflamed glands because tubuloacinar glandular HLA-DR-positive cells themselves may act as aberrant antigen-presenting cells [95, 96, 8, 6]. Co-operative T-cell and B-cell responses develop against such molecules, their nature being revealed in the specificities of the autoantibodies produced, which in SS include ribonucleosomal bodies [97, 98, 99, 100], cell cytoskeleton [101], and muscarinic acetylcholine receptor [102].

VIP, although called a neuropeptide, is like many other "neuropeptides," also synthesized by non-neuronal cells, mainly Th2 $CD4^+$ and type 2 $CD8^+$ cells. VIP has been identified as a potent anti-inflammatory factor [70, 33]. It participates in the regulation of DHEA and testosterone production [103], probably via gene transcription fine-tuning steroidogenic enzymes. VIP activated directly androgen receptors via VIP receptor in an androgen-independent and protein kinase A-dependent manner [104]. On the other hand, low 17β-estradiol levels lead to an increased expression of VIP receptors [105]. Depletion of VIP from post-ganglionic, parasympathetic nerve fibers could result from excessive stimulation in a dry mouth patient or muscarinic acetylcholine receptor autoantibodies [106], which might deprive the acinar cell from its acinotrophic support. VIP as a target for therapy has raised great interest, but attempts have been hampered by poor metabolic stability and poor penetration to targets [107]. These problems hint to a high potency of VIP. These difficulties are in the human body circumvented by delivery from the protected environment of the nerve terminal.

11.4 Sex Steroids

11.4.1 Steroidogenesis in Adrenal Glands

In primates sex steroids are not only synthesized in gonads, but also locally from adrenal prohormones in peripheral tissues. Adrenal gland-derived DHEA, DHEA-S, and androstenedione serve as substrates for the peripheral synthesis of active androgens and estrogens, like testosterone, dihydrotestosterone (DHT), and 17β-estradiol (17β-E2). Adrenal glands consist of two compartments which differ both structurally and functionally, medulla and cortex (constitutes 90% of the weight of the gland).

Catecholamines, epinephrine and norepinephrine, are produced in medulla, a specialized ganglion of the sympathetic nervous system. It is innervated by cholinergic post-ganglionic sympathetic nerves. Medullary neuroendocrine cells contain post-synaptic cholinergic receptors. Upon stimulation these chromaffin cells secrete (nor)epinephrine, which is exocytosed directly into the bloodstream [108].

The cortex of the adrenal gland is organized into three morphologically distinct layers. The superficial glomerular zone represents 15% of the weight of the cortex, the intermediate fasciculate zone 65%, and the innermost reticular zone 20%. Their phenotypic differences reflect their specialized functions: glomerular zone produces mineralocorticoids (aldosterone), fasciculate zone glucocorticoids (such as cortisol), and reticular zone DHEA prohormones. Reticular zone is unique to primates and does not exist in non-primates, like in mice or rats often used as models for SS [109].

During their lifespan the cells of the cortex migrate from the outer parts of the cortex centripetally toward the inner parts, undergoing successive transformations from glomerular to fasciculate and finally to reticular zone cells, apparently guided by the changing composition of the basement membrane laminin chains [110]. Glomerular zone cells divide fast, whereas cells in the inner parts of the cortex in the reticular zone have a slow division rate. Conversely, reticular zone cells die more rapidly than in other cortical cells. Cells are forced from the superficial zone toward the deeper zones. These events regulate the cell turnover in the cortex [109].

Corticosteroids refer to hormones produced in the adrenal cortex. The metabolic pathway from cholesterol substrate to DHEA and DHEA-S involves three and four steps, respectively (Fig. 11.4) [111, 112]. DHEA-S concentration

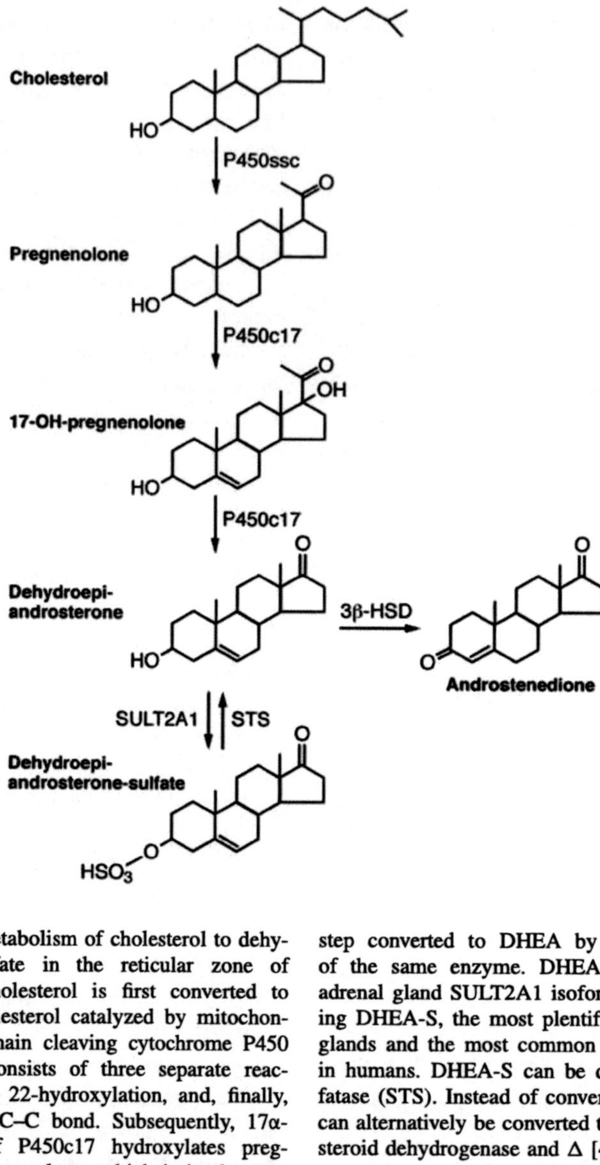

Fig. 11.4 Endocrine metabolism of cholesterol to dehydroepiandrosterone sulfate in the reticular zone of the adrenal cortex. Cholesterol is first converted to pregnenolone from cholesterol catalyzed by mitochondrial cholesterol side chain cleaving cytochrome P450 (P450ssc). This step consists of three separate reactions: 20-hydroxylation, 22-hydroxylation, and, finally, breakage of the 20,22 C–C bond. Subsequently, 17α-hydroxylase activity of P450c17 hydroxylates pregnenolone to 17-OH-pregnenolone, which is in the next step converted to DHEA by the 17,20-lyase activity of the same enzyme. DHEA sulfotransferase (in the adrenal gland SULT2A1 isoform) sulfates DHEA yielding DHEA-S, the most plentiful product of the adrenal glands and the most common steroid in the circulation in humans. DHEA-S can be desulfated by steroid sulfatase (STS). Instead of conversion to DHEA-S, DHEA can alternatively be converted to androstenedione by 3β-steroid dehydrogenase and Δ [4, 5]-isomerase (3β-SDH)

is approximately 300-fold higher than that of DHEA. Actually, adrenal glands are almost solely responsible for the production of DHEA and DHEA-S so that 90% of DHEA and 98% of DHEA-S in the human body is produced in the cortex.

The synthesis of mineralocorticosteroids continues from pregnenolone to progesterone and then to deoxycorticosterone and corticosterone in reactions catalyzed by 3β-SDH, P450c21, and P450c11, respectively. Reaction catalyzed by aldosterone synthase finally yields aldosterone. The synthesis of glucocorticosteroids from pregnenolone involves 3β-SDH, P450c21, and P450c11 following the route 17-OH-pregnenolone → 17-OH-progesterone → 17-OH-deoxycortisol → cortisol.

Conversion of cholesterol to pregnenolone by P450scc is the rate-limiting step in corticosteroid synthesis. In contrast, P450c17 determines the direction of the synthesis. When this enzyme is not present (glomerular zone), C-21 17-deoxysteroids, like aldosterone, are produced. On the other hand, when the 17α-hydroxylase activity of P450c17 is present, C-21 17-hydroxysteroids, like cortisol, are produced. Finally, in the presence of both 17α-hydroxylase and 17,20-lyase C-19 steroid DHEA(-S) is synthesized [112].

11.4.2 Regulation of the Adrenal Steroidogenesis

Corticosteroid synthesis in the cortex is regulated by the hypothalamus–pituitary–adrenal (HPA) axis. Corticotropin-releasing hormone (CRH) and corticotropin (adrenocorticotrophic hormone, ACTH) regulate synthesis of all corticosteroids. CRH released by hypothalamic neuroendocrine cells binds to its CRH-R1 receptor in the pituitary gland, which stimulates secretion of pro-opiomelanocortin (POMC). POMC is a precursor polypeptide, which is processed in a tissue-specific manner to various hormonal peptides, in the pituitary gland by pituitary prohormone convertases to a large extent to ACTH, which is released into circulation. In adrenal cortex ACTH stimulates secretion of glucocorticosteroids, aldosterone, and sex steroid precursors [111]. Cortisol exerts negative feedback on the hypothalamus (CRH secretion) and pituitary gland (ACTH secretion).

Although in part regulated by ACTH, the primary regulators of aldosterone synthesis are angiotensin II and extracellular potassium. Adipocyte-derived factors, adrenaline, serotonin, and VIP, also increase production of corticosteroids, especially aldosterone [113, 114, 115]. Synthesis of cortisol is stimulated by high concentrations of potassium, T-cell-derived glucosteroid response-modifying factor (GRMF), and IL-1. Other systemic factors regulating DHEA(-S) synthesis include estrogens, insulin, and growth hormone [116, 117, 118].

Apart from systemic factors, intra-adrenal factors regulate corticosteroids independently from ACTH so that serum DHEA(-S) levels are low in chronic inflammation in spite of normal ACTH levels [119]. Both immune and the adrenal cells themselves are potential sources [120]. Macrophages infiltrate adrenal glands, especially the reticular zone, in healthy people [121]. These cells secrete cytokines, e.g., IL-1, IL-6, and tumor necrosis factor-α (TNF-α), which influence the function of the adrenal cortex. Lymphocyte infiltrates are present in the adrenal glands, in particular in the reticular zone of elderly people, making lymphocyte-derived ACTH a potential regulator of DHEA(-S) synthesis [122].

Adrenocortical cells can themselves secrete cytokines. Glomerular zone cells secrete IL-6 and TNF-α, fasciculate zone cells TNF-α and IL-18, and reticular zone cells IL-1, IL-6, and IL-18 [120]. The effects of these cytokines on the adrenal glands are variable. IL-1 enhances glucocorticosteroids and inhibits aldosterone production. IL-6 stimulates release of cortisol and DHEA from the fasciculate and reticular zones, respectively. TNF-α induces a shift from cortisol to DHEA production in humans. Furthermore, corticosteroid-producing cells are regulated by nerve endings in contact with them [123].

Aging affects DHEA(-S) production (Fig. 11.5) [124]. The fetal adrenal cortex consists of two layers, the fetal zone, which produces high concentrations of DHEA(-S), and neocortex. Glomerular zone and fasciculate zone later develop from the neocortex, whereas the fetal zone atrophies. The focal development of the reticular zone begins first around the age of 3 and a continuous reticular zone has developed by filled 6 years. In addition to these morphological zonation changes, adrenarche involves changes in the expression of steroidogenic enzymes. Cytochrome *b*5 (CYB5) and steroid sulfotransferase (which are regulators of the 17,20-lyase activity of P450c17 and of the enzyme converting DHEA to DHEA-S, respectively) increase in the enlarging reticular zone [125] concomitantly with a decrease of 3β-SDH, which competes with P450c17 for substrate [126].

After adrenarche, circulating concentrations of DHEA(-S) increase and reach their adult peak levels at 20–30 years. Thereafter, their concentrations start to decline due to adrenopause

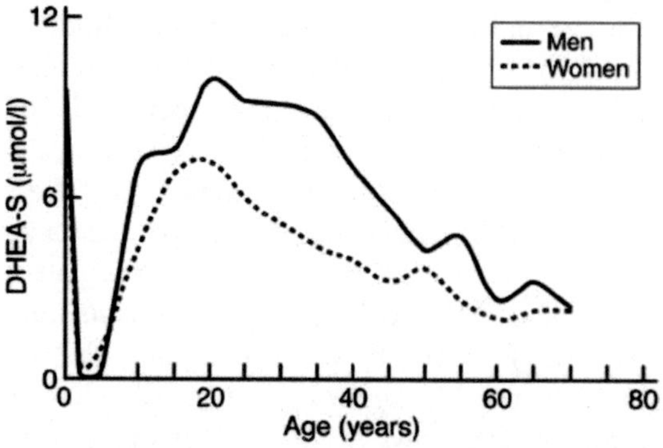

Fig. 11.5 Effect of aging on DHEA-S concentration. Fetal adrenal glands produce great quantities of DHEA-S so that its concentration is very high in newborns. DHEA-S concentrations fall rapidly after birth and stay low for a few years upon regeression of the fetal zone. Between the ages of 6 and 8 the adrenal glands undergo changes in the expression of steroidogenic enzymes and morphology in a process called adrenarche, which leads to formation of the reticular zone and to a rise in the systemic concentration of DHEA-S to high levels between the ages of 20 and 30. Thereafter, DHEA-S concentrations start to decline due to adrenopause and regression of the reticular zone and by the ages of 70–80 the DHEA-S levels are only 20 and 30% of the peak concentrations in men and women, respectively

[111, 123]. Reticular zone decreases in thickness and zonal irregularity develops [109]. The exact mechanisms behind these changes are still obscure. Cell deaths caused by infarcts, telomere shortening, or mutations could disrupt the architecture of the adrenal cortex. Cytokines and enzymes related to senescence could contribute [109]. A decrease in the 17,20-lyase activity could explain diminished DHEA(-S) production [127]. Finally, a decrease in the DHEA response of the adrenal cortex to CRH has been observed in aging people, with no change in ACTH or cortisol [128].

Adrenal synthesis of so-called prohormones DHEA(-S) plays a remarkable role in primates for the peripheral synthesis of sex steroids.

11.4.3 Adrenal Function in Sjögren's Syndrome

During long-lasting inflammatory diseases secretion of the adrenal prohormones decreases [129], probably as the result of the abovementioned neuroimmunoendocrine dysregulation. Accordingly, patients with both pSS and sSS have decreased DHEA-S concentrations [130, 131, 132], probably due to decreased production in the adrenal glands. However, the ultimate reason behind this diminished production might differ in pSS and sSS.

Low systemic levels of DHEA in pSS may ensue from premature and deeper-than-usual adrenopause [109] as a result of primary adrenal gland failure. There are no differences in the concentrations of ACTH or cortisol between patients with pSS and healthy controls [130], suggesting changes in the reticular zone.

Patients with sSS have an underlying autoimmune rheumatic disease, which precedes its development. This underlying disease causes alterations in the entire cytokine and cellular environment of the patient's body [133, 134]. In the short term, inflammatory cytokines acutely stimulate CRH and ACTH secretion and thus stimulate production of corticosteroid "stress" hormones. However, during chronic inflammation the responsiveness of the HPA axis becomes blunted. This is especially noticeable for DHEA(-S), which is decreased and remains decreased even after stimulation with ACTH. Chronic inflammation leads to a secondary adrenal gland failure. There are contradictory findings about the levels of cortisol secreted in chronic inflammation, but cortisol levels seem inappropriately low considering the disease-related stress.

Cytokines, especially IL-1β, IL-2, IL-3, IL-6, and TNF-α, directly decrease DHEA(-S) synthesis [119], causing a shift from production of DHEA toward cortisol [135, 136]. Primary SS is characterized by lower concentrations of cortisol than sSS [137]. Thus, production of DHEA is perhaps decreased for a different reason in pSS and sSS. Naturally, the cytokine-mediated down-regulation also develops in pSS, in addition to the primary failure of the adrenal glands in pSS. We will later see how this diminution of the endocrine DHEA(-S) production can unmask the peripheral intracrine DHEA-to-DHT conversion defect in the exocrine glands.

11.4.4 Peripheral Intracrine Synthesis of Sex Steroids

In addition to the synthesis in the gonads, primates are unique in synthesizing active sex steroids also locally in peripheral tissues. Unlike other mammals, the cortex of the adrenal glands of the primates secretes large amounts of prohormones. These precursors constitute a large reservoir of substrate and can be further processed into active sex steroid extragonadally. This allows tailor-making according to local tissue needs, enables similar function of "unisex" organs (organs, which work similarly in men and women in spite of the systemic differences in the sex steroid milieu), and provides a buffering system against changes over time in the systemic sex steroid levels. This local intracrine sex steroid production acts as a buffer with regards to circadian, menstrual, pregnancy, and lifelong chronobiological changes in systemic hormone levels. This field of the study of the local synthesis of active sex steroids from precursor hormones produced in adrenal glands is called intracrinology [138]. Sex steroids produced have usually but not always an intracrine mode of action [139, 132, 140]. Classical intracrine tissues include prostate, uterus, and mammary glands. However, many other tissues have been shown to produce sex steroids locally, adipose tissue and bone being among them [141].

Steroidogenic intracrine enzymes catalyze the peripheral synthesis of active androgens or estrogens from DHEA (Fig. 11.6) [142]. Approximately 50% of total androgens in the prostate of an adult man and 75% and nearly 100% of peripheral estrogens in premenopausal and post-menopausal women, respectively, are synthesized locally [138, 143]. It would be interesting to know the corresponding figures in exocrine glands. The higher the figure, the more dependent the exocrine glands are on their local intracrine enzymatic machinery.

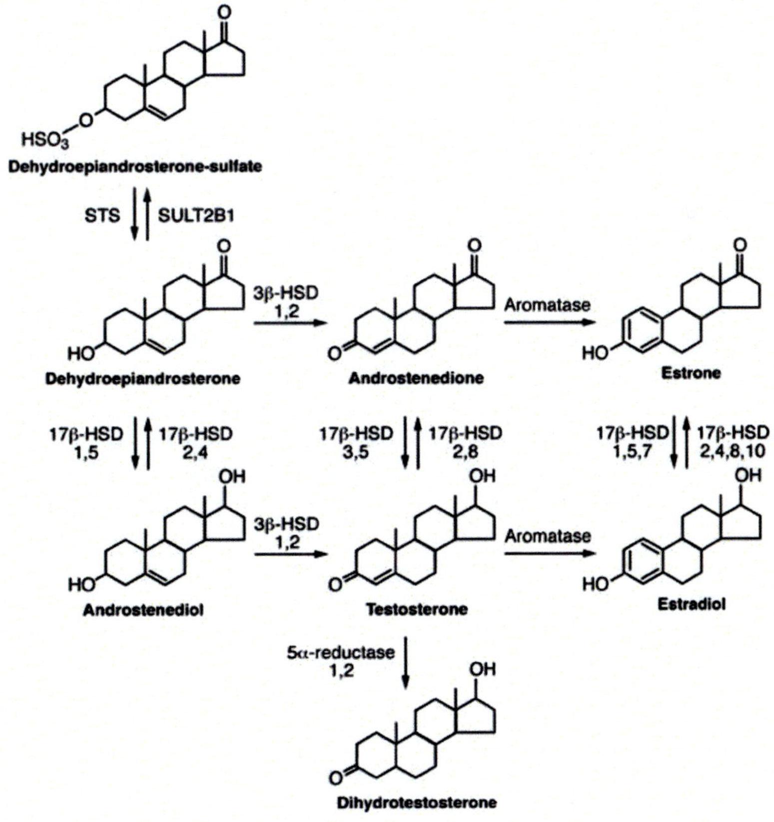

Fig. 11.6 Intracrine metabolism of DHEA-S in exocrine glands. DHEA-S is first desulfated by steroid sulfatase (STS), although conversion back to DHEA-S by steroid sulfotransferase isoform SULT2B1 is possible. DHEA is processed further by 17β-hydroxysteroid dehydrogenase (17β-HSD) and 3β-SHD yielding testosterone, which can be further converted either to 17β-estradiol or dihydrotestosterone by the action of aromatase or 5α-reductase, respectively. Notice that some of these enzymes have different isoforms, indicated by numbers, which can catalyze some of the reactions either forward or backward

11.4.5 Intracrine Sex Steroids Production in pSS and sSS

In the periphery cytokines, e.g., TNF, IL-1, and IL-6, are generally considered to increase the activity of aromatase and to shift the production of active sex steroid toward estrogens, at the cost of androgens [144, 145]. The function of 17β-HSD is stimulated by epidermal growth factor (EGF), IFN-γ, TGF-α, and TGF-β and that of 5α-reductase by TGF-β1 and TGF-β2 [119]. Additionally, TNF-α has been shown to inhibit the conversion of DHEA-S to DHEA in rheumatoid arthritis synovial cells leading to decreased local concentrations of DHEA in the diseased joints [146].

The effect of sex steroids on the production of cytokines is double-faced: androgens tend to inhibit the synthesis of pro-inflammatory cytokines, whereas estrogens have an opposite role [147]. Testosterone decreases secretion of pro-inflammatory cytokines by macrophages and epithelial cells of the lacrimal glands. Androgens enhance production of anti-inflammatory cytokines in the lacrimal gland [148, 149].

Intracrine conversion of DHEA to DHT is impaired in the exocrine glands in pSS [132, 140, 150]. If this is the primary underlying defect, then as long as there is enough prohormone input from the adrenal glands to the intracrine enzymatic machinery, the exocrine glands could produce enough DHT for their needs (for acinar cell remodeling). If such a SS-prone person happens to be genetically programmed to an early and/or deep adrenopause, this "tolerance" or "stress" test would unmask the primary, peripheral intracrine defect and lead to a local DHT deficiency in the glandular tissues. Adrenopause could explain the peak age of incidence of new SS cases. In this scenario pSS is associated with an inherent intracrine defect, which is aggravated by adrenopause. In sSS inflammation-associated changes impair adrenal gland function and when this has continued for 10–20 years such a systemic DHEA deficiency might finally damage the glands and provoke an immune attack. Thus, pSS would be mainly provoked by a primary intracrine (local) DHEA deficiency, whereas sSS would be provoked by a secondary deficiency caused solely by endocrine (systemic) DHEA failure.

11.4.6 Sex Steroids in Female and Male Sjögren's Syndrome

The above-mentioned paradigm has an additional advantage. It is not known why SS is so heavily dominated by women. The reason might be that the DHT demand in exocrine glands in women has to be totally satisfied by the local intracrine conversion from DHEA-S. This requires co-ordinated function of at least four enzymes, which in addition can go astray due to the many crossroads in the intracrine metabolic pathways. Men have similar intracrine machinery, but are less vulnerable to its local malfunction because they also feed this system directly with testosterone, only one step away from DHT. This could secure men against SS and could explain the female dominance.

11.4.7 Putative Mechanism of Action of the Intracrine Processing Defect

The acinotrophic VIP may play an important role in the maintenance of acini. Acinar remodeling also means that apoptotic and/or necrotic (lost) acinar cells have to be replaced. Progenitor cells residing in the intercalated ducts have the capacity to undergo asymmetric cellular divisions. This way they retain their stemness, but one of the two daughter cells can *trans*-differentiate to an acinar cell, to replace the lost one. This progenitor capacity has been confirmed by cellular cloning [151, 152].

It is not known what initiates the asymmetric division of the progenitor cell(s), but loss of confluence of the cells on the tubuloalveolar basement membrane upon death and detachment of one or more acinar cells might trigger it. The intercalated duct progenitor cell destined to become an acinar cell has first to transmigrate from the duct to the acinar space. Second, it needs to receive a site-specific or acinus-specific differentiation signal. It seems that these two functions are fulfilled by the extracellular basement membrane matrix read by cellular integrin receptors. Indeed, similar to the cloned intercalated duct cells, human submandibular gland HSG intercalated duct cell line [153], when cultured on laminin α1 (laminin-α1β1γ1 or simply laminin-111) containing basement membrane (Matrigel), *trans*-differentiate into acinar cells and start to produce acinar cell markers, such as salivary amylase and cystatin C [154, 155]. They form acinus-like clusters, where cells in the middle, not in contact with laminin-111, undergo apoptosis creating an acinar lumen-like structure. Matrigel membranes used in such experiments are growth and differentiation factors depleted to avoid confounding factors. It seems that laminin-111 is necessary for the *trans*-differentiation.

Progenitor cells migrate on basement membrane using laminin-111-binding integrin receptors. The acinus-specific differentiation signal responsible for the outside–inside signaling and *trans*-differentiation is also read using these α1β1 and α2β1 integrins [156]. Their level of expression is greatly increased by DHEA treatment, 5.6-fold and 11.7-fold in ductal cells and 3-fold and 5-fold in acinar cells [157]. Thus, in DHEA deficiency the progenitor cells have probably a much decreased capability to migrate to the acinus and, in particular, to *trans*-differentiate there to a secretory acinar cell. SS is characterized by low levels or loss of acinar-specific (not found in the salivary ducts) laminin-111 [158] and of the corresponding epithelial cell integrins α1β1 and α2β1 [156]. In advanced SS acini disappear, which is associated with a reciprocal ductal cell hyperplasia [159], as if the ductal cells had filled the acinar spaces without being able to *trans*-differentiate into secretory acinar cells, probably due to deprivation of the laminin-111/Int α1β1 and α2β1 signaling.

11.5 Inflammatory Cells and Cytokines

11.5.1 General Histopathology

Impairment of the quantity and/or quality of the secretory acinar cells not only leads to a compensatory increased stimulation of acetylcholine secretion, but also to a depletion of the acinotrophic VIP. In this speculative scenario immune attack would be secondarily activated against altered self and further impair the structure and function of the exocrine glands.

At early stages of involvement of the adaptive immune system, lymphocytes start to accumulate in exocrine glands via tethering, rolling, adhesion, and migration through the high endothelial cell venules (homing). If some recirculating lymphocytes happen to get into contact with altered self, they become activated. The process continues to be facilitated by amplification and chemokines. Apoptosis of the infiltrating cells is inhibited by cytokines IL-2, IL-10, TNF-α, and others.

This leads to the characteristic histopathological finding, formation of focal, periductal lymphoplasmacytoid infiltrates, which is the single best criterion of the salivary gland involvement and syndrome.

The infiltrating cells are not only predominantly mature T lymphocytes (80%), mostly $CD4^+$ cells, but also $CD8^+$ cells, with the remaining 20% being composed of B lymphocytes and plasma cells. Infiltrates are first dominated by T lymphocytes, but the proportion of B lymphocytes and in particular plasma cells increases over time. Monocytes or NK cells are rare, but macrophages and dendritic cells appear when germinal centers are formed [160].

Some salivary ducts become slightly dilated. With increasing severity of disease, there is an increase in the number of lymphocyte foci and a progressive loss of acini. At the end stage, ducts undergo hyperplasia and only a few acini remain in a confluent mass of lymphocytoid cells [6].

11.5.2 T Lymphocytes

The majority of the infiltrating $CD4^+$ and some $CD8^+$ cells secrete IL-17 and are actually Th17 cells [161]. TGF-β, IL-6, and IL-18 induce IL-17 production [162]. IL-17, in co-operation with IL-18, stimulates secretion of IL-6 and IL-8 by salivary epithelial cells, which may be important for the recruitment of immigrant inflammatory cells. The majority of the $CD4^+$ cells are $CD45RO^+$ with αβ TCR (T-cell receptor), with perhaps a low frequency of T cells expressing TCRs with Vβ 7.2 in SS patients producing autoantibodies [163]. Adhesion and co-stimulatory molecules may lead to perpetuation and they secrete IFN-γ, which induces ectopic HLA-DR expression of the ductal epithelial cells.

$CD8^+$ T cells expressing αEβ7 (CD103) integrin localize around acinar epithelial cells, which express E-cadherin. However, the number of apoptotic acinar cells is not much increased in SS [164].

11.5.3 B Lymphocytes

Altered proportions of Bm1–5 subpopulations with a relatively high percentage of circulating activated B cells have been observed in SS. A diminished percentage of peripheral memory B cells, with accumulation of such cells and plasma cells in the parotid glands, suggest disturbances in B-cell trafficking.

IgG is the predominant isotope expressed in the infiltrating B cells, whereas IgA dominates in normal glands [164]. A substantial number of the B cells infiltrating salivary glands are potentially self-reactive $CD5^+$ B-1 plasma cells. Ectopic germinal center-like structures are frequently found in pSS, reflecting antigen-driven, T-cell-dependent, B-cell-mediated immune responses. Histologically they in their fully developed stage contain follicular dendritic cells and comprise a central (*dark*) zone of proliferating B-cells (centroblasts) surrounded by a light zone of B cells (centrocytes) now undergoing selection for high affinity surface antibody expression to generate memory cells or plasma cells. Germinal center is surrounded by a mantle zone containing small B cells.

Primary SS is characterized by a disturbed B-cell maturation with abnormal selection, defects in editing Ig receptors, and abnormal mutational targeting. Disturbances in the B-cell maturation during early B-cell development and in germinal centers might play a role in the autoimmune/lymphoproliferative syndrome [165]. B cell may play a much more important role in SS than has been previously appreciated and, accordingly, B-cell ablative treatment seems to work quite well in SS [166].

IL-12 or IL-18 might play a role in lymphoma development in pSS and excessive BAFF might result in inappropriate maturation of B-cell subsets, paired with an increased survival of mature cells. Constitutive activation of activation-induced cytidine deaminase (AID) promoting illegitimate DNA recombinations and somatic mutations could result in neoplastic transformations [167].

11.5.4 Chemokines

The role of chemokines attracting lymphocytes to exocrine glands in SS has generated a lot of interest. CXCL13 (B-cell attracting chemokine 1), CXCL12 (stromal cell-derived factor-1), CCL19 (EBV-induced molecule 1 ligand chemokine), and CCL21 (secondary lymphoid tissue chemokine) all contribute to lymphoid cell homing and to the persistence of chronic inflammation in pSS. Regarding B lymphocytes, ectopic expression of CXCL13 was found on endothelial cells and germinal center-like structures and CXCL12 was strongly expressed by ductal epithelial cells. CXCL9 (monokine induced by IFN-γ) and CXCL10 (IFN-γ inducible protein-10) and impaired function of their epithelial receptor CXCR3 or "chemokine scavenger" are involved in the accumulation of T lymphocytes [168]. The CXCL13 receptor CXCR5 on infiltrating mononuclear cells contributes to recruitment of B cells and activated T cells. B lymphocyte attracting chemokines contributes to local microenvironment supportive of germinal center [169, 165].

11.5.5 Adhesion Molecules

In SS molecules in charge of the endothelial cells–leukocyte interactions are necessary for the homing and affect the composition of the cellular infiltrates. Adhesion molecules are controlled in a paracrine manner by locally produced pro-inflammatory cytokines. Intercellular adhesion molecule-1 (ICAM-1), vascular cell adhesion molecule (VCAM-1), and E-selectin are not normally expressed on endothelium, but are significantly up-regulated by a number of cytokines, including TNF-α, IL-4, and IFN-γ. Activation of endothelial cells is important for the recruitment of T cells, which express CD45RO, L-selectin, and MHC class II, because they migrate preferentially into the lesional tissue [6].

ICAM-1 and E-selectin are increased on endothelium and ICAM-1 on epithelium associated with a strong expression of LFA-1 (integrin $\alpha_L\beta_2$) and Mac-1 ($\alpha_M\beta_2$) on the infiltrating lymphocytes and monocytes. This finding suggests a role in the pathogenesis of SS.

11.5.6 Cytokines

Cytokines control the trafficking and interactions of cellular components of the immune system, in pSS mostly IL-1, IL-6, IL-10, IL-17, TGF-β, IFN-γ, IFN-α/β, and TNF-α. Reduced levels of TGF-β1 (regarded as an anti-inflammatory cytokine) in SS glands with intense lymphocytic infiltrates have not only been reported but also refuted [170]. IFN-α/β system is activated in pSS and IFN-α/β is produced by plasmacytoid dendritic cells (pDCs) in tissues [171]. In an already established disease IFN-α/β production by the natural IFN-producing cells is stimulated by intake of anti-SS-A-RNP immune complexes, which are endocytosed by pDC via FcγRIIa. This way the ssRNA hY-RNA molecules get access to Toll-like receptor 7, which stimulates production of IFN-α/β. This is important because hY-RNA is an adjuvant or a danger signal, whereas the 52 and 60 kDa SS-A protein components can act as autoantigens. It is interesting to study if perhaps membrane-bound microparticles and apoptotic bodies formed from activated and/or apoptotic tubuloacinar epithelial cells can be endocytosed by pDCs already during the early disease stages, before SS autoantibodies have been formed. This could break the autotolerance, stimulate IFN-α/β production, and produce the interferon signature so typical for fully developed salivary glands in SS. Curiously, low-dose oral IFN-α increased production of salivary and diminished the focus score values [172], which may provide a hint that pDCs are not necessarily autoimmune aggressors, but might, for example, via indoleamine 2,3-dioxygenase (IDO) exert immunosuppressive effects. Although effective in many rheumatic diseases, TNF-blocker infliximab was inefficient in a controlled clinical trial in pSS [173] and also effects of rituximab seem to be minor. A more directed use of these drugs might be possible if we could better identify pathogenic subgroups among the patients with SS.

Cytokines have been studied in pSS at three different levels: circulating Th1/Th2 cytokines, cytokine mRNA and proteins in glands, and genetic polymorphism of cytokine genes. Peripherally pSS patients are characterized by a Th2 response, with high levels of circulating IL-6 and IL-10 and cells secreting them. IL-10 levels correlated with IgG_1 levels and salivary IL-6 levels have a positive correlation with the focus score. On the other hand, Th1/Th2 cytokines in the SS salivary glands suggest an opposite pattern, with a predominant local Th1 response, although this may have to be revised in favor of Th17 cells (see below) [161]. Therefore, the Th1/Th2 balance shifts in favor of Th1 in exocrine tissues. This shift is most remarkable in glands with the highest focus (infiltrate) scores. Th1 cytokines IL-2, IL-6, IL-10, TGF-β, and IFN-γ might induce and/or maintain pSS, whereas Th2 cytokines, detected in B and plasma cell-rich cases, might be involved in the progression of the disease [169, 165].

Cytokines can impair secretory function by impairing acetylcholine release [174, 175] and structural maintenance by stimulating matrix metalloproteinase-mediated destruction of the tubuloalveolar basement membrane [176, 177, 178, 179, 180, 181].

Three cytokines have recently raised interest, IL-18, IL-17, and B-cell-activating factor BAFF. The crucial role for IL-18 in the development of Th1 immune responses has been established since its identification as a major IFN-γ-inducing factor. IL-18 directly stimulates TNF-α production in macrophages, $CD4^+$, and NK cells, with subsequent release of IL-1β and IL-8, leading to up-regulation of CC and CXC chemokines and adhesion molecules [182].

IL-18, not found in healthy labial salivary glands, is in SS secreted by acinar cells that stimulate them in an autocrine and paracrine mode [182, 183]. IL-18 in periductal infiltrates was confined to $CD68^+$ macrophages [161, 184] being not present in the diffuse cellular infiltrates, suggesting that a "critical mass" is required for IL-18 expression and that it amplifies chronic inflammation [182]. IL-17 was found in ductal epithelial cells, also in healthy controls, and in SS in the infiltrating T cells [161]. Human parotid gland HSY and salivary acinar AZA3 cell lines express IL-18R and IL-17R on their surface. IL-18, together with IL-17, may activate salivary gland cells and form potential therapeutic targets in SS [161].

IL-17-producing $CD4^+$ T cells are called Th17 cells, which contribute critically to autoimmune diseases. TGF-β induces differentiation of Th17 cells and regulatory T cells from naive T cells, whereas IL-6 and IL-2 act as switch factors for the development of Th17 and regulatory T cells, respectively [161].

Neither IL-17 nor IL-23 (produced by activated antigen-presenting cells) was detected in the submandibular glands of young C57BL/6. NODAec1Aec2 mice, prior to lymphocytic infiltration, but both were detected in adult mice corresponding to the presence of lymphocyte foci. These cytokines were not observed in SS-non-susceptible C57BL/6 J mice even when leukocyte infiltrates were present [162]. BAFF (or B-lymphocyte stimulator BLyS) is a transmembrane protein on cell surface of several cell types [185] and can be proteolytically solubilized. BAFF plays a role in survival, proliferation, and differentiation of B cells. BAFF levels are elevated in systemic autoimmune diseases characterized by autoreactive B cells [5].

The three receptors for BAFF are B-cell maturation antigen (BCMA), BAFF-R, and transmembrane activator and calcium modulator and cyclophilin ligand interactor (TACI). BCMA and BAFF-R are predominantly expressed on B lymphocytes, whereas TACI is mostly found on memory B cells and activated T cells [167].

Increased serum BAFF has been reported in pSS, in some studies associated with increased autoantibody and immunoglobulin levels. BAFF is increased in labial salivary glands, especially among infiltrating T lymphocytes and increases upon stimulation with IFN-α and IFN-γ [185]. BAFF-mediated survival signals might compromise the ability of autoreactive B cells to die via apoptosis (impaired negative selection). BAFF is required for maintenance, but not initiation of the germinal centers [167].

Two classes of human BAFF antagonist have been developed. BAFF neutralizing fully humanized (human) antibody (belimumab, LymphoStat-B®), which binds soluble human BAFF and prevents its interaction with the BAFF receptors, is currently in clinical trials in systemic lupus erythematosus and rheumatoid arthritis [186]. BAFF-neutralizing soluble decoy receptor, a fusion protein of TACI with immunoglobulin IgG_1-Fc, TACI-Ig (atacicept), is in trials for systemic lupus erythematosus, lupus nephritis, rheumatoid arthritis, multiple sclerosis, and several B-cell malignancies [187]. Finally, intervenous immunoglobulin contains anti-BAFF and anti-APRIL antibodies indicating that BAFF is also one of the targets of IVIg therapy [188].

It is an open question if SS is either characterized by improperly functioning lymphocytes attacking innocent acinar targets or, vice versa, by damaged acini attracting an immune aggression mediated by properly functioning lymphocytes [189]. This chapter was written to highlight the last-mentioned side of the coin.

Aknowledgments This study was supported by grants from the Academy of Finland, Finska Läkaresällskapet, evo-funds, Invalid Foundation, the Finnish Dental Society Apollonia, CIMO, Orion-Farmos Research Foundation, and Helsinki University. Michelle Spaan was during her fellowship supported by ErasmusMC-Scholarship from Erasmus University and by the Erasmus-Scholarship from the European Union. Maria Lores-Rodriquez and Alberto Vivó were supported by FaroGlobal.

References

1. Manthorpe R, Oxholm P, Prause JU, Schiødt. The Copenhagen criteria for Sjögren's syndrome. Scand J Rheumatol Suppl. 1986;61:19–21.
2. Vitali CS, Bombardieri R, Jonsson R, et al. Classification criteria for Sjögren's syndrome: a revised version of the European criteria proposed by the American–European Consensus Group. Ann Rheum Dis. 2002;61:554–8.
3. Locht H, Pelck R, Manthorpe R. Clinical manifestations correlated to the prevalence of autoantibodies in a large ($n = 321$) cohort of patients with primary Sjögren's syndrome: a comparison of patients initially diagnosed according to the Copenhagen classification criteria with the American–European consensus criteria. Autoimmun Rev. 2005;4: 276–81.
4. Oxholm P, Asmussen K. Classification of disease manifestations in primary Sjögren's syndrome: present status and a new proposal. Clin Rheumatol. 1995;14 Suppl 1:3–7.
5. Mariette X. Therapeutic potential for B-cell modulation in Sjögren's syndrome. Rheum Dis Clin North Am. 2008;34:1025–33.
6. Fox PC, Speight PM. Current concepts of autoimmune exocrinopathy: immunologic mechanisms in the salivary pathology of Sjogren's syndrome. Crit Rev Oral Biol Med. 1996;7:144–58.
7. Fox PC. Autoimmune diseases and Sjögren's syndrome: an autoimmune exocrinopathy. Ann NY Acad Sci. 2006;1098:15–21.
8. Amft N, Bowman SJ. Chemokines and cell trafficking in Sjögren's syndrome. Scand J Immunol. 2001;54:62–9.
9. Horvath IF, Szodoray P, Zeher M. Primary Sjögren's syndrome in men: clinical and immunological characteristic based on a large cohort of Hungarian patients. Clin Rheumatol. 2008;27:1479–83.
10. Konttinen YT, Spaan M, Stegaev V, Porola P, Lorés M, Vivó A, Koskenpato K, Przybyla BD. Female dominance in Sjögren's syndrome – a paradox and a new paradigm. In: Zeher M, Szodoray P, editors. Sjögren's syndrome and associated disorders. Kerala, India: Transworld Research Network; 2009, pp. 59–77.
11. Fraser PA, Smaje LH. The organization of the salivary gland microcirculation. J Physiol. 1977;272;121–36.
12. Peen E, Haga HJ, Haugen AJ, Kahrs GE, Haugen M. The effect of a liquid diet on salivary flow in primary Sjögren's syndrome. Scand J Rheumatol. 2008;37:236–7.
13. Gallowitsch-Puerta M, Pavlov VA. Neuro-immune interactions via the cholinergic anti-inflammatory pathways. Life Sci. 2007;80:2325–9.
14. Tsukada T, Horovitch SJ, Montminy MR, Mandel G, Goodman RH. Structure of the human vasoactive intestinal polypeptide gene. DNA 1985 4: 293–300.
15. Konttinen YT, Sorsa T, Hukkanen M, et al. Topology of innervation of labial salivary glands by protein gene product 9.5- and synaptophysin-immunoreactive nerves in patients with Sjögren's syndrome. J Rheumatol. 1992;19:30–7.
16. Konttinen YT, Hukkanen M, Kemppinen P, et al. Peptide-containing nerves in labial salivary glands in Sjögren's syndrome. Arthritis Rheum. 1992;35:815–30.
17. Månsson B, Nilsson BO, Ekström J. Effects of repeated infusions of substance P and vasoactive intestinal peptide on the weight of salivary glands subjected to atrophying influence in rats. Br J Pharmacol. 1990;101:853–8.
18. Tagawa T, Mohri M, Tagawa H, et al. Role of nitric oxide in substance P-induced vasodilation differs between the coronary and forearm circulation in humans. J Cardiovasc Pharmacol. 1997;29:546–5.
19. O'Shaughnessy MC, Vetsika EK, Inglis JJ, et al. The effect of substance P on nitric oxide release in a rheumatoid arthritis model. Inflamm Res. 2006;55:236–4.
20. Heaney LG, Cross LJ, Stanford CF, Ennis M. Substance P induces histamine release from human pulmonary mast cells. Clin Exp Allergy. 1995;25:179–8.
21. Payan DG. Receptor-mediated mitogenic effects of substance P on cultured smooth muscle cells. Biochem Biophys Res Commun. 1985;130: 104–9.
22. Kumaran C, Shivakumar K. Calcium- and superoxide anion-mediated mitogenic action of substance P on cardiac fibroblasts. Am J Physiol Heart Circ Physiol. 2002;282:H1855–6.
23. Villablanca AC, Murphy CJ, Reid TW. Growth-promoting effects of substance P on endothelial cells in vitro. Synergism with calcitonin gene-related peptide, insulin, and plasma factors. Circ Res. 1994;75:1113–2.
24. Lotz M, Carson DA, Vaughan JH. Substance P activation of rheumatoid synoviocytes: neural pathway in pathogenesis of arthritis. Science 1987;20;235:893–5.
25. Ziche M, Morbidelli L, Pacini M, Geppetti P, Alessandri G, Maggi CA. Substance P stimulates

neovascularization in vivo and proliferation of cultured endothelial cells. Microvasc Res. 1990;40:264–78.
26. Lotz M, Vaughan JH, Carson DA. Effect of neuropeptides on production of inflammatory cytokines by human monocytes. Science 1988;241:1218–21.
27. Laurenzi MA, Persson MA, Dalsgaard CJ, Haegerstrand A. The neuropeptide substance P stimulates production of interleukin 1 in human blood monocytes: activated cells are preferentially influenced by the neuropeptide. Scand J Immunol. 1990;31:529–33.
28. Hartung HP, Wolters K, Toyka KV. Substance P: binding properties and studies on cellular responses in guinea pig macrophages. J Immunol. 1986;136:3856–63.
29. Hartung HP, Toyka KV. Activation of macrophages by substance P: induction of oxidative burst and thromboxane release. Eur J Pharmacol. 1983;89:301–5.
30. Murris-Espin M, Pinelli E, Pipy B, Leophonte P, Didier A. Substance P and alveolar macrophages: effects on oxidative metabolism and eicosanoid production. Allergy 1995;50:334–9.
31. Ruff MR, Wahl SM, Pert CB. Substance P receptor-mediated chemotaxis of human monocytes. Peptides 1985;6 Suppl 2:107–11.
32. Bar-Shavit Z, Goldman R, Stabinsky Y, et al. Enhancement of phagocytosis—a newly found activity of substance P residing in its N-terminal tetrapeptide sequence. Biochem Biophys Res Commun. 1980;94:1445–51.
33. Stanisz AM, Befus D, Bienenstock J. Differential effects of vasoactive intestinal peptide, substance P, and somatostatin on immunoglobulin synthesis and proliferations by lymphocytes from Peyer's patches, mesenteric lymph nodes, and spleen. J Immunol. 1986;136:152–6.
34. Zimmerman BJ, Anderson DC, Granger DN. Neuropeptides promote neutrophil adherence to endothelial cell monolayers. Am J Physiol. 1992;263:G678–82.
35. Qian Y, Zeng BF, Zhang XL, Jiang Y. Substance P augments PGE2 and IL-6 production in titanium particles-stimulated fibroblasts from hip periprosthetic membrane. J Biomed Mater Res A. 2007;83:401–6.
36. Cury PR, Canavez F, de Araújo VC, Furuse C, de Araújo NS. Substance P regulates the expression of matrix metalloproteinases and tissue inhibitors of metalloproteinase in cultured human gingival fibroblasts. J Periodontal Res. 2008;43:255–60.
37. Hecker-Kia A, Kolkenbrock H, Orgel D, Zimmermann B, Sparmann M, Ulbrich N. Substance P induces the secretion of gelatinase A from human synovial fibroblasts. Eur J Clin Chem Clin Biochem. 1997;35:655–60.
38. Ramos C, Montaño M, Cisneros J, Sommer B, Delgado J, Gonzalez-Avila G. Substance P up-regulates matrix metalloproteinase-1 and down-regulates collagen in human lung fibroblast. Exp Lung Res. 2007;33:151–67.
39. McCormack DG, Mak JC, Coupe MO, Barnes PJ. Calcitonin gene-related peptide vasodilation of human pulmonary vessels. J Appl Physiol. 1989;67:1265–70.
40. Zhang WZ, Yu SF, Zheng LF. Effects of calcitonin gene-related peptide on bone resorption mediated by interleukin-1. Chin Med J (Engl). 1994;107: 351–4.
41. Zaidi M, Fuller K, Bevis PJ, GainesDas RE, Chambers TJ, MacIntyre I. Calcitonin gene-related peptide inhibits osteoclastic bone resorption: a comparative study. Calcif Tissue Int. 1987;40:149–54.
42. Leighton B, Foot EA. The role of the sensory peptide calcitonin-gene-related peptide(s) in skeletal muscle carbohydrate metabolism: effects of capsaicin and resiniferatoxin. Biochem J. 1995;307:707–12.
43. Haegerstrand A, Dalsgaard CJ, Jonzon B, Larsson O, Nilsson J. Calcitonin gene-related peptide stimulates proliferation of human endothelial cells. Proc Natl Acad Sci USA. 1990;87:3299–303.
44. Sarasa M, Terrado J, Mengod G, Climent S, Muniesa P, Palacios JM. Differential expression of alpha-CGRP and beta-CGRP genes within hypoglossal motoneurons in response to axotomy. Brain Res Mol Brain Res. 1996;35:269–77.
45. Hashimoto K, Uchida S, Yoshida H. Effects of calcitonin gene-related peptide on the adenylate cyclase system in cultured rat skeletal muscle cells. Life Sci. 1989;45:2183–92.
46. Buckley TL, Brain SD, Rampart M, Williams TJ. Time-dependent synergistic interactions between the vasodilator neuropeptide, calcitonin gene-related peptide (CGRP) and mediators of inflammation. Br J Pharmacol. 1991;103:1515–9.
47. Hernanz A, Medina S, de Miguel E, Martín-Mola E. Effect of calcitonin gene-related peptide, neuropeptide Y, substance P, and vasoactive intestinal peptide on interleukin-1beta, interleukin-6 and tumor necrosis factor-alpha production by peripheral whole blood cells from rheumatoid arthritis and osteoarthritis patients. Regul Pept. 2003;115:19–24.
48. Brokaw JJ, White GW. Calcitonin gene-related peptide potentiates substance P-induced plasma extravasation in the rat trachea. Lung 1992;170: 85–93.
49. Foster CA, Mandak B, Kromer E, Rot A. Calcitonin gene-related peptide is chemotactic for human T lymphocytes. Ann NY Acad Sci. 1992;657: 397–404.
50. Umeda Y, Arisawa M. Inhibition of natural killer activity by calcitonin gene-related peptide. Immunopharmacol Immunotoxicol. 1989;11: 309–20.
51. Komaru T, Ashikawa K, Kanatsuka H, Sekiguchi N, Suzuki T, Takishima T. Neuropeptide Y

modulates vasoconstriction in coronary microvessels in the beating canine heart. Circ Res. 1990;67:1142–51.
52. Awad SJ, Einstein R, Potter EK, Richardson DP. The effects of neuropeptide Y on myocardial contractility and coronary blood flow. Br J Pharmacol. 1991;104:195–201.
53. Walker MW, Ewald DA, Perney TM, Miller RJ. Neuropeptide Y modulates neurotransmitter release and Ca^{2+} currents in rat sensory neurons. J Neurosci. 1988;8:2438–4.
54. Dewar HA, Zar MA, Oxley A. Neuropeptide Y and platelet aggregation by adrenaline. Life Sci. 1989;45:367–70.
55. Ubink R, Calza L, Hökfelt T. 'Neuro'-peptides in glia: focus on NPY and galanin. Trends Neurosci. 2003;26:604–9.
56. Hansel DE, Eipper BA, Ronnett GV. Neuropeptide Y functions as a neuroproliferative factor. Nature 2001;410:940–4.
57. Sung CP, Arleth AJ, Feuerstein GZ. Neuropeptide Y upregulates the adhesiveness of human endothelial cells for leukocytes. Circ Res. 1991;68:314–8.
58. Ganz MB, Perfetto MC, Boron WF. Effects of mitogens and other agents on rat mesangial cell proliferation, pH, and Ca^{2+}. Am J Physiol. 1990;259:F269–78.
59. Bedoui S, Kawamura N, Straub RH, et al. Relevance of neuropeptide Y for the immune crosstalk. J Neuroimmunol. 2003;134:1–11.
60. Fahrenkrug J. Gut/brain peptides in the genital tract: VIP and PACAP. Scand J Clin Lab Invest Suppl. 2001;234:35–9.
61. Rekik M, Delvaux M, Tack I, Frexinos J, Bueno L. VIP-induced relaxation of guinea-pig intestinal smooth muscle cells: sequential involvement of cyclic AMP and nitric oxide. Br J Pharmacol. 1996;118:477–84.
62. Gu ZF, Jensen RT, Maton PN. A primary role for protein kinase A in smooth muscle relaxation induced by adrenergic agonists and neuropeptides. Am J Physiol. 1992;263:G360–4.
63. Sawmiller DR, Henning RJ, Cuevas J, Dehaven WI, Vesely DL. Coronary vascular effects of vasoactive intestinal peptide in the isolated perfused rat heart. Neuropeptides 2004;38:289–97.
64. el Halawani ME, Pitts GR, Sun S, Silsby JL, Sivanandan V. Active immunization against vasoactive intestinal peptide prevents photo-induced prolactin secretion in turkeys. Gen Comp Endocrinol. 1996;104:76–83.
65. Ito H, Matsuda K, Sato A, Tohgi H. Cholinergic and VIPergic vasodilator actions of parasympathetic nerves on the thyroid blood flow in rats. Jpn J Physiol. 1987;37:1005–17.
66. Fahrenkrug J, Schaffalitzky de Muckadell OB, Holst JJ, Jensen SL. Vasoactive intestinal polypeptide in vagally mediated pancreatic secretion of fluid and HCO_3. Am J Physiol. 1979;237:E535–40.
67. Konturek SJ, Domschke S, Domschke W, Wünsch E, Demling L. Comparison of pancreatic responses to portal and systemic secretin and VIP in cats. Am J Physiol. 1977;232:E156–8.
68. Felley CP, Qian JM, Mantey S, Pradhan T, Jensen RT. Chief cells possess a receptor with high affinity for PACAP and VIP that stimulates pepsinogen release. Am J Physiol. 1992;263:G901–7.
69. Bechtold DA, Brown TM, Luckman SM, Piggins HD. Metabolic rhythm abnormalities in mice lacking VIP-VPAC2 signaling. Am J Physiol Regul Integr Comp Physiol. 2008;294:R344–51.
70. Gonzalez-Rey E, Delgado M. Role of vasoactive intestinal peptide in inflammation and autoimmunity. Curr Opin Investig Drugs. 2005;6:1116–23.
71. Felten SY, Felten DL, Bellinger DL, et al. Noradrenergic sympathetic innervation of lymphoid organs. Prog Allergy. 1998;43:14–36.
72. Livnat S, Felten SY, Carlson SL, Bellinger DL, Felten DL. Involvement of peripheral and central catecholamine systems in neuroimmune interactions. J Neuroimmunol. 1985;10:5–30.
73. Harrison S, Geppetti P. Substance P. Int J Biochem Cell Biol. 2001;33:555–76.
74. Sabbadini E, Berczi I. The submandibular gland: a key organ in the neuro-immuno-regulatory network?. Neuroimmunomodulation 1995;2:184–202.
75. Hokfelt T, Kuteeva E. Substance P: a neuropeptide. Am J Psychiatry. 2006;163:578.
76. Nelson DA, Bost KL. Non-neuronal mammalian tachykinin expression. Front Biosci. 2004;9:2166–76.
77. Gerard NP, Garraway LA, Eddy RL, et al. Human substance P receptor (NK-1): organization of the gene, chromosome localization, and functional expression of cDNA clones. Biochemistry 1991;30:10640–6.
78. Hokfelt T, Kuteeva E. Substance P: a neuropeptide. Am J Psychiatry. 2006;163:578.
79. Van der Kleij HP, Ma D, Redegeld FA, Kraneveld AD, Nijkamp FP, Bienenstock J. Functional expression of neurokinin 1 receptors on mast cells induced by IL-4 and stem cell factor. J Immunol. 2003;171:2074–9.
80. Maggi CA. The mammalian tachykinin receptors. Gen Pharmacol. 1995;26:911–44.
81. Mcbillis P, Mitsuhashi M, Payan DG. Immunomodulation by tachykinin neuropeptides. Ann NY Acad Sci. 1990;594:85–94.
82. Daniel A, Nelson, Kenneth L Bost. Non-neuronal mammalian tachykinin expression. Front Biosci. 2004;9:2166–76.
83. Hershey AD, Dykema PE, Krause JE. Organization, structure, and expression of the gene encoding the rat substance P receptor. J Biol Chem. 1991;266:4366–74.

84. Abe-Dohmae S, Takagi Y, Harada N. Autonomous expression of aromatase during development of mouse brain is modulated by neurotransmitters. J Steroid Biochem Mol Biol. 1997;61:299–306.
85. Peroutka SJ. Neurogenic inflammation and migraine: implications for the therapeutics. Mol Interv. 2005;5:304–11.
86. Ericsson A, Schalling M, McIntyre KR, et al. Detection of neuropeptide Y and its mRNA in megakaryocytes: enhanced levels in certain autoimmune mice. Proc Natl Acad Sci USA. 1987;84:5585–9.
87. Ericsson A, Hemsen A, Lundberg JM, Persson H. Detection of neuropeptide Y-like immunoreactivity and messenger RNA in rat platelets: the effects of vinblastine, reserpine, and dexamethasone on NPY expression in blood cells. Exp Cell Res. 1991;192:604–11.
88. Lundberg JM, Tatemoto K. Pancreatic polypeptide family (APP, BPP, NPY and PYY) in relation to sympathetic vasoconstriction resistant to alpha-adrenoceptor blockade. Acta Physiol Scand. 1982;116:393–402.
89. Ekblad E, Edvinsson L, Wahlestedt C, Uddman R, Håkanson R, Sundler F. Neuropeptide Y co-exists and co-operates with noradrenaline in perivascular nerve fibers. Regul Pept. 1984;8:225–35.
90. Wheway J, Mackay CR, Newton RA, et al. A fundamental bimodal role for neuropeptide Y1 receptor in the immune system. J Exp Med. 2005;202:1527–38.
91. Barbany G, Friedman WJ, Persson H. Lymphocyte-mediated regulation of neurotransmitter gene expression in rat sympathetic ganglia. J Neuroimmunol. 1991;32:97–104.
92. Duan-Porter WD, Casciola-Rosen L, Rosen A. Autoantigens: the critical partner in initiating and propagating systemic autoimmunity. Ann NY Acad Sci. 2005;1062:127–36.
93. Lanzavecchia A. How can cryptic epitopes trigger autoimmunity? J Exp Med. 1995;181:1945–8.
94. Humphreys-Beher MG, Peck AB, Dang H, Talal N. The role of apoptosis in the initiation of the autoimmune response in Sjögren's syndrome. Clin Exp Immunol. 1999;16:383–7.
95. Mircheff AK, Gierow JP, Lee LM, Lambert RW, Akashi RH, Hofman FM. Class II antigen expression by lacrimal epithelial cells. An updated working hypothesis for antigen presentation by epithelial cells. Invest Ophthalmol Vis Sci. 1991;32:2302–10.
96. Nakamura S, Hiroki A, Shinohara M. Aberrant expression of HLA-DR antigens on acinar and ductal epithelial cells of salivary glands in Sjögren's syndrome. Nippon Rinsho. 1995;53:2407–11.
97. Yewdell JW, Anton LC, Bennink JR. Defective ribosomal products (DRiPs): a major source of antigenic peptides for MHC class I molecules? J Immunol. 1996;157:1823–6.
98. Yewdell JW. Serendipity strikes twice: the discovery and rediscovery of defective ribosomal products (DRiPS). Cell Mol Biol. 2005;51:635–41.
99. Schubert U, Antón LC, Gibbs J, Norbury CC, Yewdell JW, Bennink JR. Rapid degradation of a large fraction of newly synthesized proteins by proteasomes. Nature 2000;404:770–4.
100. von Muhlen CA, Tan EM. Tan. Autoantibodies in the diagnosis of systemic rheumatic diseases. Sem Arthritis Rheum. 1995;24:323–58.
101. Watanabe T, Tsuchida T, Kanda N, Mori K, Hayashi Y, Tamaki K. Anti-alpha-fodrin antibodies in Sjögren syndrome and lupus erythematosus. Arch Dermatol. 1999;135:535–9.
102. Bacman S, Berra A, Sterin-Borda L, Borda E. Muscarinic acetylcholine receptor antibodies as a new marker of dry eye Sjögren syndrome. Invest Ophthalmol Vis Sci. 2001;42:321–7.
103. El-Gehani F, Tena-Sempere M, Huhtaniemi I. Vasoactive intestinal peptide stimulates testosterone production by cultured fetal rat testicular cells. Mol Cell Endocrinol. 1998;140:175–8.
104. Xie Y, Wolff DW, Lin MF, Tu Y. Vasoactive intestinal peptide transactivates the androgen receptor through a protein kinase A-dependent extracellular signal-regulated kinase pathway in prostate cancer LNCaP cells. Mol Pharmacol. 2007;72: 73–85.
105. Degerman A, Chun D, Nguyen TB, et al. Local action of estrogen and thyroid hormone on vasoactive intestinal peptide (VIP) and galanin gene expression in the rat anterior pituitary. Neuropeptides 2002;36:50–7.
106. Törnwall J, Konttinen YT, Tuominen RK, Törnwall M. Protein kinase C expression in salivary gland acinar epithelial cells in Sjögren's syndrome. Lancet 1997;349:1814–5.
107. Onoue S, Misaka S, Yamada S. Structure–activity relationship of vasoactive intestinal peptide (VIP): potent agonists and potential clinical applications. Naunyn-Schmiedeberg's Arch Pharmacol. 2008;377:579–90.
108. Aunis D, Langley K. Physiological aspects of exocytosis in chromaffin cells of the adrenal medulla. Acta Physiol Scand. 1999;167:89–97.
109. Hornsby PJ. Aging of the human adrenal cortex. Sci Aging Knowledge Environ. 2004;35:re6.
110. Virtanen I, Korhonen M, Petäjäniemi N, et al. Laminin isoforms in fetal and adult human adrenal cortex. J Clin Endocrinol Metab. 2003;88:4960–6.
111. Kroboth PD, Salek FS, Pittenger AL, Fabian TJ, Frye RF. DHEA and DHEA-S: a review. J Clin Pharmacol. 1999;39:327–48.
112. Miller WL. Androgen biosynthesis from cholesterol to DHEA. Mol Cell Endocrinol. 2002;198:7–14.
113. Bornstein SR, Haidan A, Ehrhart-Bornstein M. Cellular communication in the neuro-adrenocortical axis: role of vasoactive intestinal polypeptide (VIP). Endocr Res. 1996;22:819–29.
114. Connell JM, Davies E. The new biology of aldosterone. J Endocrinol. 2005;186:1–20.
115. Schinner S, Willenberg HS, Krause D, et al. Adipocyte-derived products induce the transcription

of the StAR promoter and stimulate aldosterone and cortisol secretion from adrenocortical cells through the Wnt-signaling pathway. Int J Obes (Lond). 2007;31:864–70.
116. Gell JS, Oh J, Rainey WE, Carr BR. Effect of estradiol on DHEAS production in the human adrenocortical cell line, H295R. J Soc Gynecol Investig. 1998;5:144–8.
117. Kristiansen SB, Endoh A, Casson PR, Buster JE, Hornsby PJ. Induction of steroidogenic enzyme genes by insulin and IGF-I in cultured adult human adrenocortical cells. Steroids. 1997;62:258–65.
118. Brown TJ, Ginz B, Oakey RE. Effects of polypeptide hormone preparations on steroid production by the human foetal adrenal gland during superfusion. J Endocrinol. 1978;79:60–1.
119. Herrmann M, Scholmerich J, Straub RH. Influence of cytokines and growth factors on distinct steroidogenic enzymes in vitro: a short tabular data collection. Ann NY Acad Sci. 2002;966: 166–86.
120. Ehrhart-Bornstein M, Hinson JP, Bornstein SR, et al. Intraadrenal interactions in the regulation of adrenocortical steroidogenesis. Endocr Rev. 1998;19:101–43.
121. González-Hernández JA, Bornstein SR, Ehrhart-Bornstein M, Geschwend JE, Adler G, Scherbaum WA. Macrophages within the human adrenal gland. Cell Tissue Res. 1994;278:201–5.
122. Hayashi Y, Hiyoshi T, Takemura T, Kurashima C, Hirokawa K. Focal lymphocytic infiltration in the adrenal cortex of the elderly: immunohistological analysis of infiltrating lymphocytes. Clin Exp Immunol. 1989;77:101–5.
123. Alesci S, Koch CA, Bornstein SR, Pacak K. Adrenal androgens regulation and adrenopause. Endocr Regul. 2001;35:95–100.
124. Nakamura Y, Gang HX, Suzuki T, Sasano H, Rainey WE. Adrenal changes associated with adrenarche. Rev Endocr Metab Disord. 2008.
125. Suzuki T, Sasano H, Takeyama J, et al. Developmental changes in steroidogenic enzymes in human postnatal adrenal cortex: immunohistochemical studies. Clin Endocrinol. 2000;53:739–47.
126. Gell JS, Carr BR, Sasano H, et al. Adrenarche results from development of a 3beta-hydroxysteroid dehydrogenase-deficient adrenal reticularis. J Clin Endocrinol Metab. 1998;83:3695–701.
127. Liu CH, Laughlin GA, Fischer UG, Yen SS. Marked attenuation of ultradian and circadian rhythms of dehydroepiandrosterone in postmenopausal women: evidence for a reduced 17,20-desmolase enzymatic activity. J Clin Endocrinol Metab. 1990;71:900–6.
128. Pavlov EP, Harman SM, Chrousos GP, Loriaux DL, Blackman MR. Responses of plasma adrenocorticotropin, cortisol, and dehydroepiandrosterone to ovine corticotropin-releasing hormone in healthy aging men. J Clin Endocrinol Metab. 1986;62: 767–72.
129. Straub RH, Besedovsky HO. Integrated evolutionary, immunological, and neuroendocrine framework for the pathogenesis of chronic disabling inflammatory diseases. FASEB J. 2003;17: 2176–83.
130. Valtysdóttir ST, Wide L, Hällgren R. Low serum dehydroepiandrosterone sulfate in women with primary Sjögren's syndrome as an isolated sign of impaired HPA axis function. J Rheumatol. 2001;28:1259–65.
131. Sullivan DA, Bélanger A, Cermak JM, et al. Are women with Sjögren's syndrome androgen-deficient? J Rheumatol. 2003;30:2413–9.
132. Porola P, Virkki L, Przybyla BD, et al. Androgen deficiency and defective intracrine processing of dehydroepiandrosterone in salivary glands in Sjögren's syndrome. J Rheumatol. 2008;35: 2229–35.
133. Brennan FM, Maini RN, Feldmann M. Role of pro-inflammatory cytokines in rheumatoid arthritis. Springer Semin Immunopathol. 1998;20: 133–47.
134. Aringer M, Smolen JS. Tumour necrosis factor and other proinflammatory cytokines in systemic lupus erythematosus: a rationale for therapeutic intervention. Lupus 2004;13:344–7.
135. Straub RH, Glück T, Cutolo M, et al. The adrenal steroid status in relation to inflammatory cytokines (interleukin-6 and tumour necrosis factor) in polymyalgia rheumatica. Rheum Ox. 2000;39:624–31.
136. Zietz B, Reber T, Oertel M, Glück T, Schölmerich J, Straub RH. Altered function of the hypothalamic stress axes in patients with moderately active systemic lupus erythematosus. II. Dissociation between androstenedione, cortisol, or dehydroepiandrosterone and interleukin 6 or tumor necrosis factor. J Rheumatol. 2000;27:911–8.
137. Johnson EO, Kostandi M, Moutsopoulos HM. Hypothalamic–pituitary–adrenal axis function in Sjögren's syndrome: mechanisms of neuroendocrine and immune system homeostasis. Ann NY Acad Sci. 2006;1088: 41–51.
138. Labrie F. Intracrinology. Mol Cell Endocrinol. 1991;78:113–8.
139. Nestler JE, Barlascini CO, Clore JN, Blackard WG. Dehydroepiandrosterone reduces serum low density lipoprotein levels and body fat but does not alter insulin sensitivity in normal men. J Clin Endocrinol Metab. 1988;66:57–61.
140. Spaan M, Porola P, Laine M, Rozman B, Azuma M, Konttinen YT. Healthy human salivary glands contain a DHEA-S processing intracrine machinery, which is deranged in primary Sjögren's syndrome. J Cell Mol Med. 2009;13: 1261–70.

141. Simpson ER. Sources of estrogen and their importance. J Steroid Biochem Mol Biol. 2003;86: 225–30.
142. Labrie F. Extragonadal synthesis of sex steroids: intracrinology. Ann Endocrinol. 2003 Apr;64: 95–107.
143. Bélanger A, Brochu M, Cliche J. Levels of plasma steroid glucuronides in intact and castrated men with prostatic cancer. J Clin Endocrinol Metab. 1986;62:812–5.
144. Macdiarmid F, Wang D, Duncan LJ, Purohit A, Ghilchick MW, Reed MJ. Stimulation of aromatase activity in breast fibroblasts by tumor necrosis factor alpha. Mol Cell Endocrinol. 1994;106:17–21.
145. Purohit A, Ghilchik MW, Duncan L, et al. Aromatase activity and interleukin-6 production by normal and malignant breast tissues. J Clin Endocrinol Metab. 1995;80:3052–8.
146. Weidler C, Struharova S, Schmidt M, Ugele B, Schölmerich J, Straub RH. Tumor necrosis factor inhibits conversion of dehydroepiandrosterone sulfate (DHEAS) to DHEA in rheumatoid arthritis synovial cells: a prerequisite for local androgen deficiency. Arthritis Rheum. 2005;52: 1721–9.
147. Janele D, Lang T, Capellino S, Cutolo M, Da Silva JA, Straub RH. Effects of testosterone, 17beta-estradiol, and downstream estrogens on cytokine secretion from human leukocytes in the presence and absence of cortisol. Ann NY Acad Sci. 2006;1069:168–82.
148. Cutolo M, Accardo S, Villaggio B, et al. Androgen metabolism and inhibition of interleukin-1 synthesis in primary cultured human synovial macrophages. Mediators Inflamm. 1995;4:138–43.
149. Zoukhri D. Effect of inflammation on lacrimal gland function. Exp Eye Res. 2006;82:885–98.
150. Laine M, Porola P, Udby L, et al. Low salivary dehydroepiandrosterone and androgen-regulated cysteine-rich secretory protein 3 in Sjögren's syndrome. Arthritis Rheum. 2007;56:2575–84.
151. Sato M, Azuma M, Hayashi Y, Yoshida H, Yanagawa T, Yura Y. 5-Azacytidine induction of stable myoepithelial and acinar cells from a human salivary intercalated duct cell clone. Cancer Res. 1987;47:4453–9.
152. Man YG, Ball WD, Marchetti L, Hand AR. Contributions of intercalated duct cells to the normal parenchyma of submandibular glands of adult rats. Anat Rec. 2001;263:202–14.
153. Shirasuna K, Sato M, Miyazaki T. A neoplastic epithelial duct cell line established from an irradiated human salivary gland. Cancer. 1981;48: 745–52.
154. Royce LS, Kibbey MC, Mertz P, Kleinman HK, Baum BJ. Human neoplastic submandibular intercalated duct cells express an acinar phenotype when cultured on a basement membrane matrix. Differentiation 1993;52:247–55.
155. Hoffman MP, Kibbey MC, Letterio JJ, Kleinman HK. Role of laminin-1 and TGF-β3 in acinar differentiation of a human submandibular gland cell line (HSG). J Cell Sci. 1996;109:2013–21.
156. Laine M, Virtanen I, Porola P, et al. Acinar epithelial cell laminin-receptors in labial salivary glands in Sjögren's syndrome. Clin Exp Rheumatol. 2008;26:807–13.
157. Porola P, Laine M, Virtanen I, Pöllänen R, Przybyla BD, Konttinen YT. Androgens and integrins in salivary glands in Sjogren's syndrome. J Rheumatol. 2010;37(6):1181–7.
158. Laine M, Virtanen I, Salo T, Konttinen YT. Segment-specific but pathologic laminin isoform profiles in human labial salivary glands of patients with Sjögren's syndrome. Arthritis Rheum. 2004;50:3968–73.
159. Poduval P, Sillat T, Virtanen I, Porola P, Konttinen YT. Abnormal basement membrane type IV collagen alpha chain composition in labial salivary glands in Sjögren's syndrome. Arthritis Rheum. 2009;60:938–45.
160. Katsifis GE, Moutsopoulos NM, Wahl SM. T lymphocytes in Sjögren's syndrome: contributors to and regulators of pathophysiology. Clin Rev Allergy Immunol. 2007;32:252–64.
161. Sakai A, Sugawara Y, Kuroishi T, Sasano T, Sugawara S. Identification of IL-18 and Th17 cells in salivary glands of patients with Sjögren's syndrome, and amplification of IL-17-mediated secretion of inflammatory cytokines from salivary gland cells by IL-18. J Immunol. 2008;181: 2898–906.
162. Nguyen CQ, Hu MH, Li Y, Stewart C, Peck AB. Salivary gland tissue expression of interleukin-23 and interleukin-17 in Sjögren's syndrome: findings in humans and mice. Arthritis Rheum. 2008;58:734–43.
163. Manavalan SJ, Valiando JR, Reeves WH, et al. Genomic absence of the gene encoding T cell receptor Vbeta7.2 is linked to the presence of autoantibodies in Sjögren's syndrome. Arthritis Rheum. 2004;50:187–98.
164. Yamamoto K. Pathogenesis of Sjögren's syndrome. Autoimmun Rev. 2003;2:13–8.
165. Ramos-Casals M, Font J. Primary Sjögren's syndrome: current and emergent aetiopathogenic concepts. Rheumatology (Oxford) 2005;44: 1354–67.
166. Youinou P, Devauchelle V, Hutin P, Le Berre R, Saraux A, Pers JO. A conspicuous role for B cells in Sjögren's syndrome. Clin Rev Allergy Immunol. 2007;32:231–7.
167. Szodoray P, Jonsson R. The BAFF/APRIL system in systemic autoimmune diseases with a special emphasis on Sjögren's syndrome. Scand J Immunol. 2005;62:421–8.
168. Sfriso P, Oliviero F, Calabrese F, et al. Epithelial CXCR3-B regulates chemokines bioavailability in

normal, but not in Sjögren's syndrome, salivary glands. J Immunol. 2006;176:2581–89.

169. Dörner T, Lipsky PE. Abnormalities of B cell phenotype, immunoglobulin gene expression and the emergence of autoimmunity in Sjögren's syndrome. Arthritis Res. 2002;4:360–71.

170. Koski H, Konttinen YT, Xu-Hong G, Hietanen J, Malmström M. Transforming growth factor β2 in labial salivary glands in Sjögren's syndrome. Ann Rheum Dis. 1995;54:744–7.

171. Båve U, Nordmark G, Lövgren T, et al. Activation of the type I interferon system in primary Sjögren's syndrome: a possible etiopathogenic mechanism. Arthritis Rheum. 2005;52:1185–95.

172. Shiozawa S, Tanaka Y, Shiozawa K. Single-blinded controlled trial of low-dose oral IFN-alpha for the treatment of xerostomia in patients with Sjögren's syndrome. J Interferon Cytokine Res. 1998;18: 255–62.

173. Mariette X, Ravaud P, Steinfeld S, et al. Inefficacy of infliximab in primary Sjögren's syndrome: results of the randomized, controlled trial of remicade in primary Sjögren's syndrome (TRIPSS). Arthritis Rheum. 2004;50:1270–6.

174. Main C, Blennerhassett P, Collins SM. Human recombinant interleukin 1 beta suppresses acetylcholine release from rat myenteric plexus. Gastroenterology 1993;104:1648–54.

175. Cao W, Cheng L, Behar J, Fiocchi C, Biancani P, Harnett KM. Proinflammatory cytokines alter/reduce esophageal circular muscle contraction in experimental cat esophagitis. Am J Physiol Gastrointest Liver Physiol. 2004;287:G1131–9.

176. Azuma M, Motegi K, Aota K, Hayashi Y, Sato M. Role of cytokines in the destruction of acinar structure in Sjögren's syndrome salivary glands. Lab Invest. 1997;77:269–80.

177. Azuma M, Ashida Y, Tamatani T, et al. Cepharanthin, a biscoclaurine alkaloid, prevents destruction of acinar tissues in murine Sjögren's syndrome. J Rheumatol. 2006;33:912–20.

178. Hanemaaijer R, Visser H, Konttinen YT, Koolwijk P, Verheijen J. A novel and simple immunocapture assay for determination of gelatinase-B (MMP-9) activities in biological fluids: saliva from patients with Sjögren's syndrome contain increased latent and active gelatinase-B levels. Matrix Biol. 1998;17:657–65.

179. Konttinen YT, Halinen S, Hanemaaijer R, et al. Matrix metalloproteinase (MMP)-9 type IV collagenase/gelatinase implicated in the pathogenesis of Sjögren's syndrome. Matrix Biol. 1998;17: 335–47.

180. Pérez P, Goicovich E, Alliende C, Aguilera S, Leyton C, Molina C, Pinto R, Romo R, Martinez B, González. Differential expression of matrix metalloproteinases in labial salivary glands of patients with primary Sjögren's syndrome. Arthritis Rheum. 2000;43:2807–17.

181. Goicovich E, Molina C, Pérez P, et al. Enhanced degradation of proteins of the basal lamina and stroma by matrix metalloproteinases from the salivary glands of Sjögren's syndrome patients: correlation with reduced structural integrity of acini and ducts. Arthritis Rheum. 2003;48: 2573–84.

182. Bombardieri M, Barone F, Pittoni V, et al. Increased circulating levels and salivary gland expression of interleukin-18 in patients with Sjögren's syndrome: relationship with autoantibody production and lymphoid organization of the periductal inflammatory infiltrate. Arthritis Res. 2004;6:447–56.

183. Eriksson P, Andersson C, Ekerfelt C, Ernerudh J, Skogh T. Relationship between serum levels of IL-18 and IgG1 in patients with primary Sjögren's syndrome, rheumatoid arthritis and healthy controls. Clin Exp Immunol. 2004;137: 617–20.

184. Manoussakis MN, Boiu S, Korkolopoulou P, et al. Rates of infiltration by macrophages and dendritic cells and expression of interleukin-18 and interleukin-12 in the chronic inflammatory lesions of Sjögren's syndrome: correlation with certain features of immune hyperactivity and factors associated with high risk of lymphoma development. Arthritis Rheum. 2007;56: 3977–88.

185. Lavie F, Miceli-Richard C, Ittah M, Sellam J, Gottenberg JE, Mariette X. B-cell activating factor of the tumour necrosis factor family expression in blood monocytes and T cells from patients with primary Sjögren's syndrome. Scand J Immunol. 2008;67:185–92.

186. Ding C. Belimumab, an anti-BLyS human monoclonal antibody for potential treatment of inflammatory autoimmune diseases. Expert Opin Biol Ther. 2008;8:1805–14.

187. Gatto B. Atacicept, a homodimeric fusion protein for the potential treatment of diseases triggered by plasma cells. Curr Opin Investig Drugs. 2008;9:1216–27.

188. Le Pottier L, Bendaoud B, Dueymes M, et al. BAFF, a new target for intravenous immunoglobulin in autoimmunity and cancer. J Clin Immunol. 2007;27:257–65.

189. Robinson CP, Yamamoto H, Peck AB, Humphreys-Beher MG. Genetically programmed development of salivary gland abnormalities in the NOD (nonobese diabetic)-scid mouse in the absence of detectable lymphocytic infiltration: a potential trigger for sialoadenitis of NOD mice. Clin Immunol Immunopathol. 1996;79:50–9.

Part IV
Clinical and Therapeutic Considerations

Overview of Management of Dry Eye Associated with Sjögren's Syndrome

12

Paul E. Michelson and Robert I. Fox

Abstract

This initial discussion of dry eye in the patient with primary Sjögren's syndrome (SS) is provided primarily for the non-ophthalmologist who will, hopefully, find useful the explanations of common diagnostic tests and therapeutic interventions employed in treating dry eye patients. A more detailed description of lacrimal gland and tear film physiology is presented in the chapter by Stern and Pflugfellder. In particular, the authors of this chapter have collaborated during the past 25 years on patients with dry eyes referred for evaluation and treatment of their SS. This chapter summarizes many of the *common problems* that the primary physician may refer to the rheumatologist and the "daily practical" questions from the SS patient that are not generally covered in academic reviews of dry eye care.

Keywords

Sjögren's syndrome • Keratoconjunctivitis sicca • Blepharitis • Herpetic keratitis • Uveitis • Aqueous tear deficiency • Neuroparalytic or neurotrophic keratitis • Schirmer's test • Rose Bengal • Lissamine Green • Artificial tear • Artificial lubricant • Ocular ointment • Ocular gel • corneal topography • Punctal occlusion • Punctal plugs • Moisture shields • Lacrimal gland pathology • Tear surface physiology

12.1 Background

Patients seeking relief for their dry eyes associated with Sjögren's syndrome (SS) often see a variety of specialists and use both prescription and over-the-counter medications. Many of the medications used for other medical conditions (i.e., antihistamines, antihypertensives, antidepressants, hypnotics, and analgesics) may exacerbate ocular and oral dryness. Although evaluation and treatment of dry eyes is truly in the domain of the ophthalmologist, it is common for the SS patient to direct their questions to their rheumatologist.

It is important to emphasize that *a rheumatologist, armed with an ophthalmoscope and a bottle*

P.E. Michelson (✉)
Eye Care of La Jolla, Scripps Memorial Hospital, La Jolla, CA, USA; UCSD School of Medicine, La Jolla, CA, USA
e-mail: pmichel2@san.rr.com

R.I. Fox, C.M. Fox (eds.), *Sjögren's Syndrome*, DOI 10.1007/978-1-60327-957-4_12,

of Rose Bengal, Fluorescein, or Lissamine Green diagnostic agents, is not a substitute for an ophthalmologist who is highly skilled in the use of a slit lamp and experienced in treating dry eyes.

In this chapter, we will present some of the more *common questions* that may be directed to the rheumatologist by the patient including

- How should I choose one or more artificial tear products from the great variety of branded and generic (preserved and non-preserved) tears that are available?
- How should I compare the components of generic and brand name tears?
- What are guidelines to use of mixing and matching different types of artificial tears?
- What are some suggestions and hints to preserve eye moisture?
- What are most prominent environmental and lifestyle factors that contribute to dryness, and how can they be minimized?
- What incidental iatrogenic factors, including prescription medicines and over-the-counter remedies, contribute to dryness?
- What are surgical iatrogenic factors, including cosmetic surgery or LASIK surgery, that may contribute to dryness and subsequent corneal erosions?
- What are the precautions for the patient undergoing surgery to prevent exacerbation of the eye symptoms?
- Are *cosmetic eye procedures* such as LASIK and blepharoplasty therapeutically contraindicated for the patient with dry eye?

In a world of managed care, medical–legal considerations, and fixed resources, rheumatologists must decide *if the patient needs to be seen and evaluated the same day, the same week, or at the next available scheduled appointment that may be weeks or months away.*

12.2 Incidence, Symptomatic Presentation, and Impact on Quality of Life

There is a generally high level of dissatisfaction on the part of both the treating physician as well as the patient with respect to the medical care and management for dry eyes [1, 2], largely due to three factors:

1. The complex difficulty in managing a chronic, variable, and problematic condition;
2. The inadequate appreciation by clinicians of the true impact on patients' lifestyles; and
3. The extensive time and resources required to educate and treat patients appropriate to their individual needs [3].

The International Task Force and Delphi panel [4], among others, were assembled to address these issues, and their recommendations have been addressed elsewhere in this chapter and incorporated in this discussion [5–7].

While dry eye associated with SS represents a very small subset of the increasingly better recognized large group of our general population suffering from dry eyes, the Sjögren's population is disproportionately skewed to the more severe and problematic.

Estimates of the *incidence of dry eye syndrome* in general depend on selection and diagnostic criteria.

Reports vary from:

- *17% of females and 11% males*, increasing with age, to a *more recent study suggesting*
- *7% in females and 3% in males* in their sixth to seventh decade of life, increasing to
- *10–12% of females and 4–5% of males in the eighth decade* [8, 9].

There are *a minimum of several million people in the United States* alone who, by any reasonable diagnostic criteria, suffer from significant dry eye disorders.

Of course, it is also reasonable to say that virtually 100% of us experience some symptoms of dry eyes under extreme conditions, endogenous and exogenous, such as

- dehydration,
- profound illness and debility,
- a dry, windy day outdoors, and
- a long airplane ride where the humidity is notoriously low.

It is important to be mindful as treating physicians of the extent to which even mild-to-moderate dry eyes affect the lifestyle and visual functioning of our patients. When patients do not present in the most extreme and obvious distress, it is too easy to dismiss even moderate dry eyes as a relatively minor inconvenience, remedied quite easily with over-the-counter artificial tears [10].

A fairly recent study attempting to assess the actual impact of this condition on the patient's lifestyle and activities of daily living, the so-called utility value, found that patients with moderate dry eyes literally equate their dry eyes with the effects of moderate angina [11].

Reinforcing this surprising assessment, other studies and industry surveys have shown that close to half the patients said mild-to-moderate dry eyes affect their life "a lot," with more than 40% relating a detrimental effect on their reading ability, and about a third on their use of computers [5]—indeed, *intently staring at monitors can unknowingly reduce blink rate by up to 90%*, thereby *dramatically exacerbating* dry eye problems.

Thus, we suggest that the Sjögren's patient select a dependable means of *reminding himself/herself to consciously blink* while at the computer.

In clinical practice, we must remain receptive to our patients' concerns and appraisals of the disease impact as well as our own knowledge of its threat to the patient's well-being.

The diagnosis of dry eyes in association with Sjögren's syndrome may literally be painfully apparent to both patient and clinician. Indeed, patients are often sent to an ophthalmologist with the established diagnosis of autoimmune disease, dry mouth, and obvious ocular inflammation. The eyes often look dry, and the patient may even complain of dryness. Of course, other more common and less obvious presentations require some diagnostic acumen.

While patients with Sjögren's syndrome often exhibit more severe disease, they do include the entire spectrum from subclinical to extreme/acute threat to vision.

When asked to assess a patient with mild-to-moderate symptoms suggesting dry eyes or a patient who has not articulated symptoms but is suspect, given other systemic features of possible Sjögren's syndrome, the array of signs and symptoms must be considered.

It has long been a great frustration to those of us attempting to investigate various diagnostic and treatment approaches to note the often profound disconnect between patients' signs and symptoms. Recent basic science and clinical studies have led to an epiphany, suggesting an explanation for this seeming disconnect.

We now better understand that the chronic inflammation attending the vicious cycle of dry eye disease, also called "dysfunctional tear disorder," causes the release of cytokines and other inflammatory by-products that are neurotoxic and desensitizing.

Also, the role of mucins in maintaining the viscosity of the tear film is increasingly important. When the patient describes increased discomfort in their eyes, they may be referring to an increased friction as the upper lid traverses the orbit.

On the other hand, the patient's symptoms may be much less severe than the observation of disrupted tear film and corneal surface. Thus, a neuroparalytic or neurotrophic keratitis (a rare degenerative corneal disease caused by an impairment of trigeminal corneal innervation, leading to a decrease or absence of corneal sensation) can reduce, if not eliminate, corneal sensitivity. This adaptation may allow a remarkable degree of corneal disruption in patients otherwise expected to be quite symptomatic.

The possibility of significantly diminished corneal sensitivity in the presence of chronic dry eye disease is important to keep in mind when trying to assess the range of signs and symptoms. For example, chronic contact lens wear may lead to corneal desensitization, and thus, the normal pain mechanism may not alert the patient in time to prevent corneal damage.

Another basic concept to keep in mind is the distinction between:

- *Basal tear production* (the more or less steady-state lubrication produced largely by tear glands located in the cul-de-sacs), and

- *Reflex tear production* (largely from the lacrimal gland seated in the upper outer portion of the orbit; more responsive to external irritation, neuro-endocrine stimuli, and emotion).

Basal tear production is largely the result of small glands that reside in the inner portion of the lids.

Medications with anticholinergic/drying side effects, including antihistamines (including Tylenol PM), tricyclic antidepressants (TCAs), also selective serotonin reuptake inhibitor (SSRI) antidepressants, birth control pills (due to hormone changes), antihypertensives, diuretics, angiotensin-converting enzyme (ACE) inhibitors, isotretinoin-type drugs (for acne), and opiates *taken at bedtime* will have much more drying effect than if taken at other times when tearing stimulation is higher.

While patients may complain of chronic or episodic redness, signs of ocular inflammation are neither not always present nor not always obvious to the patient in mild-to-moderate cases.

The five most common complaints voiced by the patient related to dry eye include

1. "There seems to be something foreign or 'gritty' in my eye that keeps my eye irritated most all the time."

   Probably the most common and characteristic complaint of dry eye patients is *chronic foreign body sensation, or grittiness,* which, along with other symptoms of dry eyes, tend to increase as the day progresses, as demanding visual tasks are undertaken, and as potentially drying environmental conditions are encountered for long periods.

   Some patients describe *burning, stinging, and varying degrees of pain.*

   While many practitioners believe the *sensation of itching* to be almost pathognomonic of allergy, it is occasionally related as a symptom of dry eye. Of course, the reduced tear volume and flow, allowing irritants and allergens for more prolonged contact with the ocular surface, may initiate or exacerbate co-existing allergy.

2. "My eye seems to keep tearing up for no (apparent) reason." One of the seemingly paradoxical symptoms of dry eye disease is *excessive tearing* (*epiphora*).

   Generally, this excess tearing will occur under conditions of increased ocular exposure and drying; for example, prolonged computer use or reading (when the blink rate is usually unknowingly significantly reduced), or outdoors during windy and/or dry conditions. Typically, golfers will complain of annoying and exuberant tearing while out on the course. While some of these complaints may be within normal limits, they may reflect underlying mild-to-moderate dry eye in which the basal tear secretion is deficient, stimulating excessive reflex tearing, that can result in significant overflow.

3. "I seem to be losing visual acuity in one or both eyes." Another frequent symptom of dry eye disease is *episodic and sometimes persistent, loss of best-corrected vision.* Disruption of the normally regular and clear optical surface of the eye can result in very annoying, if not disabling, visual disturbances.

   Even without visible surface disruption when examined by slit-lamp biomicroscopy, the reduced flow of abnormally constituted tears alternating with excessive reflex tearing can be the explanation of patients' vague visual complaints. Of course, more severe dry eye syndrome results in obvious surface disruption and irregularity with reduction in visual acuity.

4. "(Bright) light seems to be intolerable to my eyes, requiring me to lower the lights or keep sunglasses on." *Photophobia—abnormal light sensitivity*—is also a result of the abnormal ocular surface, causing optical light scattering. Significant changes in the ocular surface can cause disabling light sensitivity and pain.

5. "I seem to be waking up most mornings with lots of sticky 'gunk' in my eyes." Another subtle, sometimes chief, complaint of patients with mild-to-moderate dry eyes is tenacious *mucus found in the eyes upon awakening*. In the absence of infection, one explanation for this uniquely stringy mucus secretion may be that the goblet cell mucus production is undiluted by the aqueous component of the normal tear film.

12.3 Diagnostic Screening Examination

Examination of the eyes may reveal obvious injection, or the eyes may appear white and quiet. There is often some injection of the lid margins, in the absence of other evidence suggesting blepharitis such as collarettes about the lashes or scaling and crusting typical of staphylococcal and/or seborrheic involvement.

In more severe cases, the eyes actually *look dry*. The normal corneal luster is absent and no tear meniscus can be appreciated at the lid margin.

Examination with magnification, performed in the ophthalmology office with a slit lamp, will commonly reveal diminished or absent tear meniscus at the lid margin and variable disruption and irregularity of the ocular surface.

Diagnostic dyes can be placed in the eye to demonstrate abnormal and/or absent epithelium on the cornea and conjunctiva:

Fluorescein is an orange dye used, along with a cobalt-blue light, to detect foreign bodies in the eye or damage to the cornea. It is most commonly used either instilled as a drop or from a commercially available strip of paper impregnated with the dye. This paper strip is wetted and touched to the lid margin. Areas of absent epithelium on the cornea stain and may be seen as yellow-green areas of persistent dye, even after blinking.

- Staining areas are more obvious fluorescing under a cobalt-blue filtered light, an option built into most slit lamps.
- Mild-to-moderate cases exhibit punctate staining, while more severe cases may show confluent areas of abnormal and absent epithelium.
- These affected areas are characteristically located in the more exposed inferior portion of the cornea and the interpalpebral zones of the conjunctiva.

Rose Bengal is another dye used in the eye to reveal stained abnormal tissue and devitalized cells of the cornea in keratoconjunctivitis sicca. It can be instilled either in drop form or from an impregnated paper strip. It is more sensitive than fluorescein, staining abnormal epithelial cells (as opposed to absent, dead epithelium). In the case of dry eyes, it can be particularly obvious on the conjunctiva and/or cornea in the most exposed inferior and interpalpebral areas.

- Although the Rose Bengal is best done with a slit lamp by an ophthalmologist, it can also be performed by a rheumatologist using a simple ophthalmoscope (Fig. 12.1).
- Increased uptake in the exposure zone (between the eyelids) can be visualized by retained dye, after the initial Rose Bengal is removed by application of artificial tears.

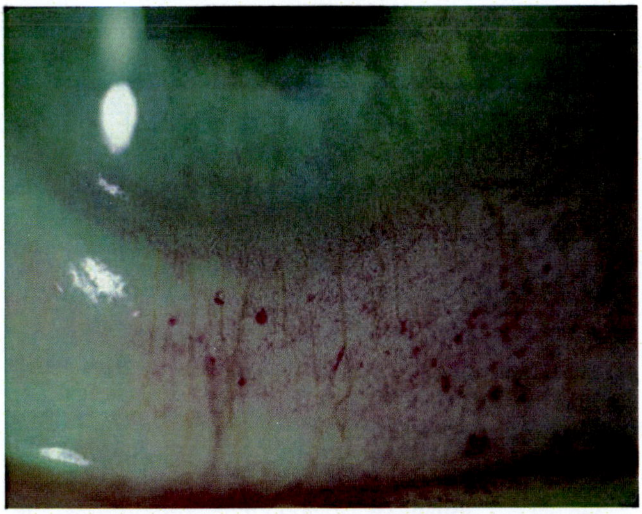

Fig. 12.1 Rose bengal (tetraiodofluorescein) stain of ocular surface in SS patient

- The extent of staining may provide clues to help determine if the patient's symptoms of dry eyes are commensurate with the objective findings on examination.

When the rheumatologist does Rose Bengal staining, topical anesthetic is not used.

Lissamine Green is used to detect damaged cells on the eye's surface, flagging them green under special lighting. It is an alternative to Rose Bengal that causes less stinging and less staining of the lid and facial skin if it overflows, thus, is more accommodating to the patient and the practitioner (and practitioner's white coat) alike. It must be stressed that positive staining with any of these dyes is seen in dry eye conditions but is not pathognomonic.

- Any disorder, infection, noxious exposure, or insult to the ocular surface can produce similar patterns of abnormal or denuded epithelium and staining.

  For those unfamiliar with the use of these dyes, it is advised to avoid flooding the eye or using any more than a *minimum* amount necessary to expose the complete surface after a blink. More dye can obscure subtle areas of actual stain and produce unflattering messiness.

  Ensure that a paper drape is provided to the patient for protection of garments prior to these potentially messy examination screenings.

  Tear film breakup time is another common test—actually observation—with fluorescein dye. In this test, the time is measured with the eye kept open after the instillation of dye and a blink until its dissipation into a characteristic breakup into darker dry areas within the otherwise uniform tear/dye film.

- This test can be quite variable and insensitive, but if the amount of dye placed in the eye and extent of exposure are controlled, a positive test can be a strong indication of dysfunctional tear disorder.
- The integrity of the outermost lipid layer of the three-part tear film, moderating evaporation of the underlying aqueous component, is necessary to prevent abnormal breakup, but the test is usually positive in non-specific dysfunctional tear syndrome and Sjögren's syndrome as well.
- It is most useful in less obvious cases, particularly in disorders of the meibomian glands (the lipid producers).

Two observations well known to ophthalmologists, relating to the tear film breakup, are worthy of mention.

1. A tear film breakup time shorter than the time interval between normal blinks for a given patient will result in symptoms.

   In fact, if a patient's eyes are kept open for more than a second after the tear film breakup, more than 70% of patients will report ocular awareness.

2. For the clinician questioning a diagnosis of dry eye, a supportive observation is simply having the patient stare and report the time at which ocular awareness or irritation develops.

   If the time from opening the lids to this sensation is less than 5 s, it is highly suggestive of an abnormal tear film. Normal response is greater than 5 s, with a mean of about 7 s.

   In the standard observation for breakup utilizing a slit lamp with copious fluorescein in the tear film, 10 s or more is considered a normal breakup time.

   Under more standardized and critical techniques applying only 5 μL of fluorescein, a positive test is considered less than 5 s.

The *Schirmer's test* is probably *the most common diagnostic test* used by ophthalmologist and non-ophthalmologist alike to diagnose dry eye syndrome. It is used to determine whether the eye produces enough tears to keep it adequately moist.

In this test, a small strip of filter paper is placed over the lid margin, usually at the junction of the mid and lateral thirds, and the amount of wetting observed after 5 min.

There is no unanimous agreement on the best way to perform this test; however, it can be done with or without topical anesthesia, yielding different results depending upon the patient and conditions.

Obviously, with adequate topical anesthesia, one attempts to eliminate the foreign body irritation and reflex component to the tearing; thus, a better approximation of basal tear production can be obtained.

In our experience, we find it most useful to perform the test *with topical anesthesia*, being certain enough applications of topical anesthetic have been given to eliminate the irritation of the filter strip.

Care must be taken to wick away (gently, without irritation) any reservoir of tears or fluid in the inferior cul-de-sac that will immediately wet the test strip and invalidate the results.

The eyes may be closed or kept open with normal blinking, whichever the patient prefers and causes minimal or no sensation.

A *positive Schirmer's test* of less than 5 mm of wetting is always a positive indication of inadequate tear production. Between 5 and 10 mm of wetting is suspect.

A *negative Schirmer's test* with copious wetting, however, indicates only that adequate innervation to the lacrimal system exists to produce reflex tearing. It does not rule out mild-to-moderate disease and diminished basal secretion, but does suggest a more favorable, more easily managed course.

It is worth noting that *there is a very poor correlation between symptoms and Schirmer's test results*. One explanation for this difference is that the Schirmer's test is predominantly a measurement of water flow, while the patient's symptoms may be correlated with mucin content and stability of the tear film that allow the upper lid to glide over the ocular surface.

It is important to recognize this difference not only in the review of outside records, but also in publications describing studies that compare eye treatments, as they may use different methods (with and without topical anesthetic) in their patients in evaluating treatments.

Corneal topography—a non-invasive medical imaging technique for mapping the surface curvature of the cornea (the outer structure of the eye)—often produces images that are highly suggestive, if not diagnostic, of dysfunctional tear conditions.

Rather than the nice regular optical contour maps seen in a normal eye, areas of irregularity and distortion, which change frequently after blinking, can be observed. Even without such sophisticated instrumentation, this same phenomenon may be observed utilizing an ophthalmoscope focused on the surface of the eye (high plus lenses) and observing the regularity and quality of the red reflex through the pupil. Such observations may corroborate patients' symptoms of fluctuating acuity and episodically blurred or distorted vision.

Other tests exist to clarify the diagnosis of dry eye and/or "dysfunctional" tear disorders, but they often require more expensive and elaborate equipment, represent investigational procedures and have yet to be standardized, or are simply impractical. One such test is *measurements of tear film osmolarity* that demonstrates

- *The hyperosmolar nature of the abnormal tear film* (when not subjected to an excessively evaporative environment),
- *The decrease in the concentration of normal tear components* such as lactoferrin, fibronectin, epidermal growth factor and dinucleotide adenosine polyphosphate (AP4A)
- *The increased concentration of inflammatory by-products* such as cytokines, proteases, and even white blood cells.

They have all been documented and provide important insights into the pathophysiology of the disease. But they are not widely used in clinical practice.

12.4 Overview of Dry Eye Management

12.4.1 Dry Eyes Deserve Respect and Careful Monitoring

Once a diagnosis of dry eye has been entertained and supported by any of the above signs, symptoms, and tests, it must still be borne in mind that many of the other disorders considered in the general differential diagnosis of the red eye and ocular irritation may, and in fact often do, co-exist!

For the rheumatologist, *it is important to look for medications with anticholinergic side effects*.

Indeed, more than 50% of the 100 most commonly used prescription medications list ocular and oral dryness as a significant adverse effect.

- *The most common troublesome drugs are amitriptyline (given for fibromyalgia) or blood pressure medications (such as clonidine).*
- Other choices of medications can be suggested with less anticholinergic side effect. However, the list of medications with significant anticholinergic side effects is quite extensive, ranging from *antidepressants* to *antiseizure* medications as well as *cardiac medications.*

Reduced tear flow may render a susceptible dry eye patient more prone to complaints of ocular irritants and allergies. Irritants—topical and airborne—will also be less tolerated and more likely to exacerbate symptoms.

The reduced concentrations of tear-borne antibodies and other protective elements render the eye more susceptible to infection. Especially common with dry eye is co-existent *blepharitis*, which by itself can alter the tear film and create the dysfunctional evaporative state that leads to symptomatic dry eye.

Also common is the patient currently under treatment with one or more topical *antibiotics*, *antihistamines*, or other medications, including *glaucoma drops*, all of which may be exacerbating an underlying dry eye condition.

In fact, one of the most common presentations of the dry eye patient is conjunctivitis *medicamentosa*, the persisting red eye unresponsive to prior therapies, actually aggravated by pharmacologic inhibition, preservatives, and/or other toxic ingredients of the drops currently in use.

Contact lens use deserves mention, as chronic contact lens wear (even with soft lenses) results in a reduction in corneal sensitivity.

- As noted before and elsewhere in this chapter, a significant component of the cycle of dry eye disease is the reduced corneal sensitivity from inflammatory by-products.
- Similar reduction in corneal sensitivity from contact lens use may also result in an impaired feedback loop and dry eye and will certainly exacerbate a dry eye associated with Sjögren's disease.

Last, but certainly not least, it must be mentioned that the *Sjögren's syndrome patients, disproportionately represented in the most severe category of dry eye*, may develop some of the most serious consequences of this disorder, namely *trophic corneal thinning* and *melt.*

While, as mentioned, *these patients are more susceptible to infection and thus corneal ulcers*, the corneal ulcers usually present as painful, red eyes with evident corneal infiltrates or opacities.

- The trophic melting and thinning may be more *insidious* and sometimes occur in an otherwise white eye.
- *The patient may note a sudden change in vision*, and the clinician may see some definite irregularity to the cornea, even without magnification.

If a suspicion of corneal thinning, melt, or ulceration exists, an emergency consultation should be obtained. The patient is at risk of losing the eye from perforation and/or endophthalmitis, and extension of infection from the eye to the CNS and/or sepsis is possible.

While these dreadful problems are quite rare, if not kept in mind and detected by the clinician at a treatable stage, disaster ensues.

Treatment for dry eye is generally calibrated to the level of symptoms and signs. It merits emphasis again that *signs and symptoms do not always correlate*, presumably because of the co-existent neuropathy of chronic dry eye, which renders some eyes less sensitive to surface insult than would otherwise be expected.

Thus, *the primary symptom in some of these patients is simply reduced or fluctuating vision. We must assess both subjective and objective findings* as we seek the most appropriate course of action.

12.4.2 Four Levels of Severity Differentiation

12.4.2.1 Level 1

1. Patients with the *minimal levels of dysfunctional tear syndrome*, so-called Level 1, exhibit *mild-to-moderate symptoms* as described above but have no corneal signs of surface disruption or abnormality.
2. There may be *mild–to-moderate conjunctival injection* or staining with the vital dyes Rose Bengal and/or Lissamine Green.

3. These patients should be educated about the nature of their disease, how it often waxes and wanes symptomatically but can be directly affected by adverse environmental conditions, general physical well-being, and some topical and systemic medications (which may be blocking agents or inhibitory to lacrimal secretion).
4. Attention should always be paid to co-existent problems such as allergy, blepharitis, and lid disorders; these disorders should be treated aggressively and appropriately to avoid exacerbation of the underlying dry eye condition.
5. Over-the-counter preserved artificial teardrops (Tables 12.1 and 12.2) are available in 5 mL and larger bottles and can be used as needed to relieve or prevent symptoms.
5. Prophylactic use of teardrops before and during activities such as prolonged computer use, reading, or outdoor exposure can be very helpful in preventing symptomatic bouts.

12.4.2.2 Level 2

Level 2 consists of *moderate-to-severe symptoms* with signs of an abnormal tear film, complaints or evidence of fluctuating or impaired vision, and mild corneal punctate staining along with conjunctival staining.

These patients are best treated with non-preserved artificial teardrops, as they should be using the drops three or more times per day, a dosage at which the preservatives can become toxic and create an epitheliopathy, regardless of how mild they are reputed to be. The following are helpful to bear in mind to optimize artificial tear therapy.

1. Non-preserved tears come in unit-dose containers with the implication they are for single-use only.
2. In our years of experience with these drops in many patients, we have not encountered any definite infection from contamination after multiple uses, as long as the ampule is kept clean, upright, covered, and discarded at the end of first day's use.
3. Patients report considerable savings by obtaining three or more daily applications of drops from each ampule.

None of the artificial tears, however viscous, provide as long-lasting lubrication as gels and ointments. *A dramatic improvement can be obtained in many patients by adding gels or ointments prior to sleep*. Generally, the gels and ointments will dissipate by morning and thus will not represent any significant visual blurring or discomfort.

4. Patients who awaken frequently at night should be forewarned, however, that their vision may be slightly blurred if residue of the gel or ointment is present when they awaken.
5. Most commercial over-the-counter *ointments* do not contain preservatives, and few contain lanolin, which on rare occasions excites an allergic response.
6. Most *gels* are non-preserved or contain a peroxide or perborate preservative, which dissipates on exposure to air, rarely causing some irritation. The ointments are more viscous, lasting and effective than the gels if this level of lubrication is preferred or required.

12.4.2.3 Level 3

We term the patient's disease at Level 3 if:

1. The aforementioned measures are not adequate for good control, or
2. The frequent applications of tears and other lubricants are incompatible with the patient's lifestyle.

Anti-inflammatory agents such as Cyclosporin A and mild topical steroids may be considered.

Cyclosporine-A, available commercially as prescription *Restasis*, has been proven effective for a significant percentage of patients [12–18].

It is a drop taken twice daily, and, as noted elsewhere, suppresses the T-cell immune response and the inflammation attending dry eyes. It may take several months to achieve full effect.

The vehicle in which the active ingredient is suspended is also available as a non-prescription artificial tear called *Endura* and has proved, in our experience, to be a particularly effective, well-tolerated artificial tear for moderate-to-severe cases.

Table 12.1 Preserved and non-preserved artificial tears for mild-to-moderate dry eyes

Product	Active ingredient(s)	Preservative
Advanced Eye Relief "Environmental"	1.0% Propylene glycol, 0.3% glycerin	BAK
Advanced Eye Relief "Rejuvenation"	0.95% Propylene glycol	BAK
Advanced Eye Relief "Rejuvenation"	0.95% Propylene glycol	None (PF)
Advanced Eye Relief Night Time® (formerly Moisture Eyes PM)	White petrolatum, mineral oil	None (PF)
Bion Tears	0.3% HPMC, 0.1% Dextran 70	None (PF)
Blink		
Clarymist	Soy lecithin 1.0%	Phenoxyethanol 0.5%
Dakrina	2.7% Blended PVAs, 2% povidone	Polixetonium
Dwelle	2.7% Blended PVAs, 2% povidone	Polixetonium
Freshkote		
GenTeal Mild	0.2% HPMC	GenAqua
GenTeal Moderate to Severe	0.3% HPMC, 0.25% CMC	GenAqua
GenTeal Gel	0.3% HPMC, Carbopol 980	GenAqua
GenTeal PM	White petrolatum, mineral oil	None (PF)
Hypotears	1.0% PVA, 1.0% polyethylene glycol	BAK; but also comes in unpreserved unit dose
Lacrilube	White petrolatum, mineral oil	Chlorobutanol
Lacrisert		
Moisture Eyes	See "Advanced Eye Relief" (this product line was recently re-named)	
Nature's Tears Eye Mist		None
NutraTear (1)	0.4% PVA (99% hydrolyzed), 0.2% PVA (87% hydrolyzed)	Polixetonium
Quintess Qusome Eyelid Spray	TBA	TBA
Oasis Tears	0.2% Glycerin (15%)	None (PF)
Oasis Tears Plus	0.2% Glycerin (30%)	None (PF)
Optive Lubricant Eye Drops	0.5% CMC, 0.9% glycerin	Purite
Refresh Lubricant Eye Drops	1.6% PVA, 0.4% povidone	None (PF)
Refresh Tears	0.5% CMC	Purite
Refresh Plus	0.5% CMC	None (PF)
Refresh Celluvisc	1.0% CMC	None (PF)
Refresh Endura	Glycerin 1.0%, polysorbate 80 1.0%	None (PF)
Refresh Liquigel	1.0% CMC	Purite
Refresh PM	White petrolatum, mineral oil	None (PF)
Similasan	Homeopathic mercurius sublimatus 6×, belladonna 6×, euphrasia 6×	Silver sulfate
Soothe	Light mineral oil, mineral oil	Polyhexamethylene biguanide
Systane	0.4% Polyethylene glycol 400, 0.3% polyethylene glycol	Polyquad

Table 12.1 (continued)

Product	Active ingredient(s)	Preservative
Systane	0.4% Polyethylene glycol 400, 0.3% polyethylene glycol	None (PF)
Systane Free	0.4% Polyethylene glycol 400, 0.3% polyethylene glycol	"Preservative-free in the eye"
Tears Again liposome spray	TBA	TBA
Tears Naturale Forte	0.3% HPMC, 0.1% Dextran 70, 0.2% glycerin	Polyquad
Tears Naturale II	0.3% HPMC, 0.1% Dextran 70	Polyquad
Tears Naturale Free	0.3% HPMC, 0.1% Dextran 70	None (PF)
Tears Naturale PM	White petrolatum, mineral oil	None (PF)
Thera Tears	0.25% CMC	Sodium perborate
Thera Tears single-use vials	0.25% CMC	None (PF)
Thera Tears Liquigel	1.0% CMC	None (PF)
Visine Tears	0.2% HPMC, 0.2% glycerin, 1% polyethylene glycol 400	BAK
Visine Pure Tears Portables	0.2% HPMC, 0.2% glycerin, 1% polyethylene glycol 400	None (PF)
Visine Pure Tears Single Drop Dispenser	0.2% HPMC, 0.2% glycerin, 1% polyethylene glycol 400	
Viva Drops	Polysorbate 80	None

In fact, it is been our belief that those patients responding almost instantaneously to Restasis are in fact responding to the Endura and may not need an expensive prescription drug.

It may seem counterintuitive, but in our present day medical care system, some patients may not appreciate substituting an over-the-counter, equally effective medication for the prescription-only drops, which may be covered under their insurance plan, when over-the-counter medicines are paid for out-of-pocket, and thus cost them more.

Nonetheless, Restasis has proven to be quite effective and is an exciting new approach targeting the pathophysiology of the disease rather than simple palliation of symptoms. Many patients who previously had been using multiple drops, requiring pockets or handbags full in anticipation of aggravating conditions on the golf course, for extended work on a computer, in an air-conditioned or heated environment, etc., have been able to eliminate most or all of their ancillary drops and their apprehensions with the use of twice-daily Restasis.

While the FDA studies elicited no serious side effects from topical use, we should remain mindful that we do not at present have any long-term data exceeding that of the FDA study.

Also, patients with herpes simplex keratitis, and other potential chronic recurrent infections, were not included in the study and should not be treated with Restasis unless fully informed of potential risks and followed with extreme care.

An interesting observation in some patients using Restasis is the recurrence of irritation or awareness after several weeks or more of use. Such new corneal sensitivity may in fact represent an indication of recovery of the heretofore impaired corneal nerves, and the patient should be encouraged to persist through this transient phenomenon as a positive development.

Obviously, for those patients experiencing increasing symptoms that do not abate after several days or a week, true intolerance or allergy

Table 12.2 Artificial tears, grouped by type and ingredient

Product	Active ingredient(s)	Preservative
Artificial tears and liquigels: methylcellulose		
Bion Tears	0.3% HPMC, 0.1% Dextran 70	None (PF)
GenTeal Mild	0.2% HPMC	GenAqua
GenTeal Moderate to Severe	0.3% HPMC, 0.25% CMC	GenAqua
Optive	0.5% CMC 0.9% Glycerin	Purite?
Refresh Tears	0.5% CMC	Purite
Refresh Plus	0.5% CMC	None (PF)
Refresh Celluvisc	1.0% CMC	None (PF)
Refresh Endura	Glycerin 1.0%, polysorbate 80 1.0%	None (PF)
Refresh Liquigel	1.0% CMC	Purite
Tears Naturale Forte	0.3% HPMC, 0.1% Dextran 70, 0.2% glycerin	Polyquad
Tears Naturale II	0.3% HPMC, 0.1% Dextran 70	Polyquad
Tears Naturale Free	0.3% HPMC, 0.1% Dextran 70	None (PF)
Thera Tears	0.25% CMC	Sodium perborate
Thera Tears single-use vials	0.25% CMC	None (PF)
Thera Tears Liquigel	1.0% CMC	None (PF)
Visine Tears	0.2% HPMC, 0.2% glycerin, 1% polyethylene glycol 400	BAK
Visine Pure Tears Portables	0.2% HPMC, 0.2% glycerin, 1% polyethylene glycol 400	None (PF)
Visine Pure Tears Single Drop Dispenser	0.2% HPMC, 0.2% glycerin, 1% polyethylene glycol 400	
Artificial tears: propylene glycol and/or glycerin		
Note: "Advanced Eye Relief" is the B&L product line formerly known as MoistureEyes		
Advanced Eye Relief "Environmental"	1.0% Propylene glycol, 0.3% glycerin	BAK!!!
Advanced Eye Relief "Rejuvenation"	0.95% Propylene glycol	BAK!!!
"Advanced Eye Relief "Rejuvenation"	0.95% Propylene glycol	None (PF)
Oasis Tears	0.2% Glycerin (15%)	None (PF)
Oasis Tears Plus	0.2% Glycerin (30%)	None (PF)
Optive	0.5% CMC 0.9% Glycerin	Purite
Systane	0.4% Polyethylene glycol 400, 0.3% polyethylene glycol	Polyquad
Systane	0.4% Polyethylene Glycol 400, 0.3% polyethylene glycol	None (PF)
Artificial tears: PVA, povidone		
Dwelle	2.7% Blended PVAs, 2% povidone	Polixetonium
Dakrina	2.7% Blended PVAs, 2% povidone	Polixetonium

Table 12.2 (continued)

Product	Active ingredient(s)	Preservative
Freshkote		
Hypotears	1% Polyvinyl alcohol, 1% polyethylene glycol 400	BAK But also available PF
NutraTear	0.4% PVA (99% hydrolyzed), 0.2% PVA (87% hydrolyzed)	Polixetonium
Refresh Lubricant Eye Drops	1.6% PVA, 0.4% povidone	None (PF)
NutraTear	0.4% PVA (99% hydrolyzed), 0.2% PVA (87% hydrolyzed)	Polixetonium
Emollients		
Soothe	Light mineral oil, mineral oil	Polyhexamethylene biguanide
Artificial tears: homeopathic		
Similasan	Homeopathic mercurius sublimatus 6×, belladonna 6×, euphrasia 6×	Silver sulfate
Gels, liquigels, and ointments		
Product	**Active ingredient(s)**	**Preservative**
GenTeal Gel	0.3% HPMC, Carbopol 980	GenAqua
Refresh Liquigel	1.0% CMC	Purite
Systane Free	0.4% Polyethylene glycol 400, 0.3% polyethylene glycol	"Preservative-free in the eye"
Thera Tears liquid gel	1.0% CMC	None (PF)
Ointments		
Advanced Eye Relief Night Time (formerly. Moisture Eyes PM)	White petrolatum, mineral oil	None (PF)
GenTeal PM	White petrolatum, mineral oil	None (PF)
Lacrilube	White petrolatum, mineral oil	Chlorobutanol
Refresh PM	White petrolatum, mineral oil	None (PF)
Tears Naturale PM	White petrolatum, mineral oil	None (PF)
Sprays/Mists		
Clarymist (UK)	Soy lecithin 1.0%	Phenoxyethanol 0.5%
Nature's Tears		None
Quintess Qusome Eyelid Spray	TBA (Note: As far as we know, this is NOT a liposome spray but some other kind of eyelid spray.)	TBA
Tears Again Liposome Spray	TBA (We understand this to be equivalent to the Clarymist liposome spray but there is very little information available about it.)	TBA
Specialty prescription-only lubricants		
FreshKote	2.7% Blended PVAs, 2% povidone	Polixetonium
Lacrisert		n/a

may have developed, and the medication should be discontinued.

While the *recommended dosage is one drop twice daily*, we have had patients who, for economic or other reasons, reported using one drop daily without any recurrence of symptoms. It is expected that at some point after discontinuation of the medication, or reduction to some subthreshold dosage, surface disruption, inflammation and the full cycle will recur, but reports of such long-term follow-up and experimentation are not yet available.

Similarly, whether the early introduction of Cyclosporine-A therapy in patients easily controlled without this medication will prevent progression represents an interesting question that should be addressed in future studies.

As already mentioned, dry eye syndrome in general, waxes and wanes over the years, clearly progresses in some, but the risk and rate of progression is not now predictable, as no controlled longitudinal studies have been reported. Sjögren's syndrome patients, with their documented autoimmunity, might represent an excellent cohort for such a controlled study.

12.4.2.4 Level 4

In Level 4 disease, *the symptoms are severe enough to create major changes and limitations in a patient's lifestyle and visual functioning*.

More severe signs and symptoms represent Level 4, characterized by marked punctate staining of the cornea, often involving the central area. *Filamentary keratitis* may also be noted in advanced and generally much more symptomatic cases. Filaments of desquamated epithelial cells are noted dangling on the cornea. Patients exhibiting these filaments usually have marked pain, chronic irritation, and photophobia.

At this level of disease, careful reconsideration of all possible co-existent and contributory eye disorders must be made.

A co-existent *blepharitis*, for example, should be treated aggressively with systemic tetracyclines as well as all topical measures including lid hygiene and compresses.

Punctal occlusion—One must also consider at this point *temporary or permanent punctal plugs*.

Generally, punctal occlusion is one of the most dramatic and helpful interventions in the treatment of moderate-to-severe dry eye in appropriate candidates.

By blocking the puncta and canaliculi, drainage of applied lubricantsand whatever natural tears occur can be reduced substantially, if not eliminated, providing significant and quick relief.

While it has been reported that punctal occlusion should not be performed prior to the initiation of Cyclosporine-A therapy topically for fear of accumulating a reservoir of toxic cytokines and inflammatory by-products that would exacerbate the condition, for generations, punctal occlusion has been carried out without benefit of this immunomodulator.

The concern of the rare initial exacerbation is rendered somewhat moot, as most clinicians prescribe topical Cyclosporine-A, plus or minus steroids, prior to punctal occlusion as part of the generally accepted escalation of therapy indicated by signs and symptoms.

When the extent of disease warrants the most aggressive intervention, all therapies, punctal occlusion, and the initiation of topical steroids with cyclosporine, along with ancillary daytime artificial tears and nighttime ointments, can be initiated and continued simultaneously.

Severe corneal staining, often widely confluent, associated with possible *erosions* and even some *conjunctival scarring* may be noted upon examination.

Treatment in such instances consists of adding to the aforementioned aggressive therapy serious consideration *of systemic anti-inflammatory and immunomodulatory agents* in co-operation with the treating rheumatologist.

More obvious and effective *ocular protection* such as

- *Snugly fitting moisture goggles*,
- The constant use of *humidifiers* in the patient's immediate environment
- *Partial tarsorrhaphy* (surgically closing the temporal and sometimes the medial portions of the eyelids to limit the exposed area) may now be acceptable to the patient, given the severity of symptoms and disability.

Be aware that some eye care professionals recommend *bandage contact lenses* for dry eye patients.

These soft contact lenses can—in theory—serve as a reservoir of lubricating fluid as well as a possible evaporation barrier.

In our experience—and we believe it conforms with general experience in ophthalmology practices unless the patients have quite mild dry eyes—these lenses easily dry themselves and may present more of an irritant and potential stimulus to infection.

A particular type of bandage lens called the *Boston Lens* is an expensive moisturizing lens that may be used in selected patients with severe corneal problems and must be carefully followed by an ophthalmologist skilled in their use.

Contact lenses in general must be used with extreme caution in dry eye patients. Even if well tolerated, corneal hypesthesia may be present and the risks of corneal erosions and increased susceptibility to serious corneal infection exist.

Again—last but not least—in the most extreme instances of dry eye syndrome, particularly in those with known vasculitis, as in Sjögren's syndrome or advanced rheumatoid disease, *a definite but fortunately remote risk of corneal melting and perforation exists.*

While a microperforation or an area of dangerous thinning might not be immediately apparent without biomicroscopy, if suspected based on a sudden change in symptoms or vision, or a reported leak or burst of fluid from the eye, or a shallow or absent anterior chamber, such a patient should be referred *immediately* to an ophthalmologist.

Sealing of perforations with ophthalmic glue and reinforcement of thin areas with autologous or donor cornea or sclera may be necessary as an emergency operative procedure to save an eye otherwise destined for blindness and a potential nidus of infection for systemic spread.

There are a variety of new compounds and approaches to therapy in the pipeline that we can hopefully anticipate adding to our arsenal in the future (studies currently in progress are listed on http://www.clinicaltrials.gov).

- *Topical picrolimus* (a drug similar to tacrilimus)
- *Topical Voclosporin* (LX214), a compound similar to cyclosporine)
- *Topical soft steroid eye drops* such as Lotemax, which are used for short duration
- An *adenosine A3 receptor agonist (CF101)*
- *Rebamipide topical drops*, an agent used previously to augment gastric mucin content
- *Diquafosol (INS 365)*, a purine P2Y2 agonist that reached late-stage clinical trial, which was designed to help transport water directly across the conjunctival membrane
- *Topical androgens* have been examined

However, while some preliminary studies and anecdotal reports suggest that these agents may be helpful, and in reasonable recommended doses seem harmless, the definitive evidence has yet to appear.

12.5 Practical Suggestions for the Selection of Artificial Tears

12.5.1 Types of Artificial Tears Available

Rheumatologists and ophthalmologists generally initiate therapy by reaching into their pharmaceuticals sample cabinet and seeing what samples of artificial tears that they have available. Alternatively, they initiate therapy by telling the patient to go to the local pharmacy or grocery store and pick up an assortment of artificial tears to try.

However, upon following our own suggestion, we were struck by the bewildering array of choices that confront the patient in the "eye care" aisle of the pharmacy or grocery store (Fig. 12.2). These products differ in terms of content and price.

A partial listing of artificial tears in alphabetical order is provided in Table 12.1. A partial listing of artificial tears based on the ingredient is provided in Table 12.2.

In addition to the wide variety of brands available, many of artificial tears with similar sounding names and descriptions come in mild,

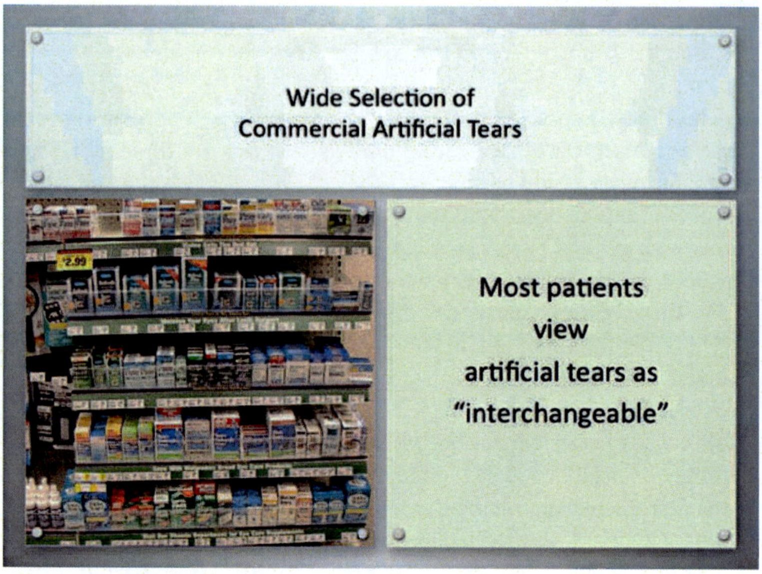

Fig. 12.2 Wide array of available artificial tears may lead to patient confusion

Table 12.3 Types of polymers used for dry eyes—useful in comparing generics with branded version of tears

Polymer	Properties
Cellulose esters (hypromellose, hydroxyethylcellulose, methylcellulose, carboxymethylcellulose)	Viscoelastic polysaccharides increase the viscosity of tears; large increase in viscosity when concentration is increased
Polyvinyl alcohol	Low viscosity, optimal wetting at 1.4%
Povidone (polyvinylpyrrolidone)	Wetting is improved when combined with polyvinyl alcohol
Carbomers (polyacrylic acid)	High molecular weight polymers of acrylic acid; high viscosity when eye is statin, the tear thickness dynamically changes during blinking to maximize the thickness and longer retention time than polyvinyl alcohol
Hyaluronic acid, autologous tears	Glycosaminoglycan biopolymers that exhibit long retention times. However, expense prohibits these as usual alternatives

CMD methylcellulose, *HPMC* hydroxypropylmethylcellulose, *EDTA* ethylenediaminetetra acetic acid

moderate, and severe or intensive formulations—terms that refer to the *relative viscosity* of each preparation. Also, tears may come in branded form that are more expensive than the generic or store brand. However, it is extremely difficult to compare the brand versus the generic. Thus, Table 12.3 lists the basic components of artificial tears.

The polymer component determines the viscosity of the tear, which the patient may describe as how long the tear lasts. The preservative in the tears may also contribute to the tolerability of the tear.

A literature search reveals relatively few crossover studies that compare different artificial tear preparations, and most of these trials are short-term trials.

12.5.2 General Guidelines for the Dry Eye Patient

We generally start with a selection of branded artificial tears that patients have told us are tolerated (Table 12.4). As guidelines listed in Table 12.5, we emphasize to patients that:

- Treatment is a trade-off between preserved tears (that are cheaper) and non-preserved

Table 12.4 Poll of artificial tear preference

Refresh (any kind)	75
Thera Tears (any kind)	52
Systane	57
GenTeal (any kind)	62
Bion Tears	17
Muro-128	9
Saline	14
Soothe	18

tears that can be used more frequently (as they lack preservative).

- Another trade-off is the viscosity of the tear that makes it last longer but may lead to transient blurred vision.
- The patient must be prepared to mix and match the frequency and type of tear to match their symptoms and environment.
- An additional point is that nighttime use of gels and ointments may prove very helpful so that the patient does not arise in the morning with a severely diminished tear film and already compromised ocular surface.
- *Artificial tears containing preservatives should not be used more than four times a day*; preserved tear products contain substances that can lead to ocular surface epithelial toxicity.
- Even if we use preservative-free artificial tears in our dry eye patients, patients may still be receiving other eye drops (such as treatment for glaucoma or infection) that may contain a preservative. Thus, we have to consider the entire cumulative effect of preservatives on the eye.
- Gels may not be as effective as ointments, but the gel produces less blurring and dissipates faster. However, some people do not tolerate gels, perhaps due to the preservatives. We often suggest an initial trial of Refresh PM (ointment), GenTeal gel (may have preservative), or Lacrilube (ointment).
- It is important not to overuse the gels or ointments, as they may leave a residue on the lashes. A small amount (such as 1/8 inch or less) should be used.

12.6 Additional Types of Therapy

Lacriserts are solid pellets of hydroxymethylcellulose that are placed under the lower lid. The pellet is dissolved slowly in patients who retain sufficient tear flow to dissolve the pellet. We have found that some patients with mild dryness can obtain benefit. The patient must have good dexterity to insert the pellets and avoid corneal abrasion. Also, a decrease in tear flow, even transiently as weather conditions or concurrent medications change, these pellets may not be adequately dissolved and the patient experiences irritation and blurring.

Mild topical steroids (such as *Lotemax*) have also been used to alleviate symptoms of dry eye disease. They are remarkably effective at rapidly reducing or eliminating the inflammatory component and breaking the vicious cycle.

Even mild topical steroids, however, entail the risks of secondary glaucoma, cataract induction, increased susceptibility to infection, and dependence. Some patients really do become physiologically dependent upon the soothing effect of topical eye steroids (not unlike dependence upon lip balm that temporarily soothes chapped lips), and it may be difficult to wean-off after prolonged use.

For all these reasons, most ophthalmologists use steroids only for limited periods of time to help patients through severe symptomatic episodes. Topical steroids can also be used temporarily for more rapid relief in conjunction with the institution of topical Cyclosporine-A until the latter's pharmacologic effect develops sufficiently.

Another remarkably effective topical therapy is the use of *autologous serum tears*. Patients unresponsive to other intensive treatment often show remarkable subjective and objective improvement with the use of teardrops made from their own serum, which most likely contains many essential and restorative components.

Our own positive experience with autologous serum tears [19] has been corroborated by numerous reports in the literature [20–23]. Elsewhere in this book, a chapter by Saito and Tsubota of Japan

Table 12.5 General rules for the dry eye patient

Artificial tears
A list showing a wide selection of artificial tear, gels, and lubricants (including their active agent and preservatives) is available on http://www.dryeyezone.com.
An initial selection of preserved or unpreserved tears for the patient might include Refresh, GenTeal, Systane, Thera Tears, or their non-preserved counterpart.
These recommendations for a starting selection are based on a poll of "patient preference" available on http://www.dryeyezone.com as double-blind studies for comparison are not available.
Be prepared to "mix and match" different types of tears.
The patient must be flexible in balancing the frequency of artificial tear use and viscosity to the conditions of the environment and concurrent medications.
Artificial tear use must also balance the cost of preserved versus non-preserved tear as well as brand name versus generic.
Be aware that some generic artificial tears (or tears for other conditions) may contain preservatives, especially benzalkonium chloride or thimerosal that are poorly tolerated in the dry eye patient.
Start increasing treatment to "build" the tear film 2–3 days before the "challenge" to the eyes, as it can take several days to build the tear film and about half an hour for it to get damaged.
Avoid the use of preserved tears for more than *four times per day*.
Be aware that drops for other conditions (glaucoma, etc.) contain preservatives and these must be included in the four times preserved tear/day rule.
When using generic artificial tears, be sure to carefully compare the ingredients.
Gels and ointments
Gels are best for nighttime use. They are thicker than artificial tears—though liquid gels may be somewhere in between.
Gels may not be as effective as ointments, but less transient blurring.
Some people do not tolerate gels, perhaps due to preservatives.
Do not use excessive amounts of ointment or gel, as only a tiny amount is required (1/8″).
An initial selection of ointments and gels may include Refresh PM (ointment), GenTeal Gel (may have preservative), and Lacrilube (ointment), based on user's poll (http://www.dryeyezone.com).
Identification of medications (including over-the-counter cold and sleep remedies) and nutritional supplements/herbs with anticholinergic side effects may help minimize dryness.
Recognize that other conditions cause a dry and painful eye—ranging from corneal abrasions to infections and require immediate referral to emergency room or ophthalmology (in case the patient calls or is seen by the rheumatologist with suggestive signs and symptoms).
Recognize that blepharitis (infection of the lids) may mimic a dry eye flare.
Providing patients with written information and suggestions (including by email) will help education and compliance.
Patients with dry eyes may have other causes for a sudden increase in symptoms ranging from corneal abrasions to infections (both bacterial and viral).

relate their experience and method for preparing autologous serum tears.

For the motivated patient in distress, the logistics involved in preparing and using serum tears are certainly worth the effort. The use of tears made from umbilical cord blood, or simply the use of a dilution of commercially available gammaglobulin (IV-Ig), has also been reported [23].

In the United States, enlisting a co-operative laboratory can be complicated by concerns over liability due to potential contamination of these preparations.

The topical use of *secretagogues*, usually acetylcholine or its analogs, have been tried but generally have intolerable side effects, such as miosis and accommodative spasm, and minimal or evanescent increased tearing.

In glaucoma patients with dry eyes, however, *pilocarpine*, an old but effective glaucoma treatment, may provide help for both conditions in patients who tolerate the small pupil and are old enough to avoid accommodative visual change.

12.7 Moisture Preservation and Oral Medications

12.7.1 Moisture Chambers, Humidifiers, and Contact Lenses

The basic idea behind so-called moisture chambers is to enclose the eye so that evaporative loss of tears is minimized. Since *approximately 25% of tears are lost by way of evaporation*, this strategy will preserve tears in the eye for a longer time by limiting evaporation. These devices range from a wrap-around sunglass design to side shields adapted to regular eyeglasses. Sunglasses may be adapted with sponge-like lining to help retard evaporation.

During prolonged exposure in dry environments, such as airline trips, devices such as *ecco-eye shields* with moisturizing sponges may prove helpful. A selection of these adjuncts may be found on a website http://www.dryeyezone.com.

For those patients experiencing moderate or severe episodic or chronic dry eye, the use of *humidifiers* is also suggested. The preference for the newer ultrasonic *cold air humidifiers* over the older warm air humidifiers (which are more prone to spread potential infection on larger droplets) is noted.

For those individuals with pets or who live in areas with particulate smog, the use of *air filters* such as those with *hepa filters* may prove very helpful.

The patient is asked to remain mindful of *environmental conditions, indoors and outside, changes in their own physical sense of well-being, stamina, and health, and any changes in systemic medications* that would indicate the need for either self-adjustment or consultation for change in management.

12.7.2 Punctal Plugs

The use of punctal plugs can be an effective step in treating moderate-to-severe dry eye that is unresponsive to artificial teardrops and ointments. *The tears drain into the nose via the tear ducts, and blocking this outflow is a reasonable strategy to keep the tears in the eye for a longer time.*

Punctual plugs increase the comfort level in the eyes and lower the frequency of the need for artificial tears in most dry eye patients. The decreased artificial tear use may be economically beneficial, considering the high cost of preservative-free artificial tears.

It is emphasized that choices regarding punctal occlusion are the domain of the experienced ophthalmologist.

Temporary punctal occlusion with collagen implants may be considered to ascertain if the punctal blockage will help reduce dry eye symptoms and also to rule out excessive tearing due to such blockage. However, a failure to respond to a temporary trial with these plugs is difficult to interpret. In many patients, they do not provide sufficient occlusion to make any conclusion about the benefit of more definitive punctal occlusion.

There are a variety of punctal plugs available. Most *silicone punctal plugs* are umbrella-shaped, and the top part of the punctal plug rests on the eyelid surface.

A different type of punctal plug (*Herrick plug*) is completely embedded within the tear ducts (the canaliculi).

Another type of punctal plug is made of a *thermosensitive, hydrophobic acrylic polymer* that changes from a rigid solid to a soft, cohesive gel when its temperature changes from room temperature to body temperature.

About 40% of punctal plugs are lost within 6 months of insertion, usually within the initial month's post-insertion, mostly due to spontaneous extrusion.

In addition, *about 10% of patients may complain of local discomfort at the plug site or excessive tearing* (especially if both upper and lower puncta are blocked), and the punctal plug may need to be removed in these patients. Patients who have lost the initial plug are twice as likely to lose the replacement plug.

12.8 Oral Medications and Supplements

12.8.1 Dietary Fatty acids (Flaxseed Oil) and Dry Eyes

Our diet contains two types of fat (saturated and unsaturated). Recent research has shown that *oral therapy with polyunsaturated fatty acids reduces ocular surface inflammation and improves dry eye symptoms.*

Americans obtain an excess of linoleic acid (omega-6 fatty acid) through their consumption of beef, dairy, vegetable cooking oils, and vegetable shortenings (i.e., cookies, potato chips, and snacks). However, the American diet is deficient in gamma-linolenic acid (omega-3 fatty acid). The two best sources of omega-3 fatty acid are fish oil and flaxseed oil. Although supplements containing omega-6 fatty acid may help dry eye patients, there is a possibility that they may not be good for patients with macular degeneration.

12.8.2 Oral Medications

Systemic secretagogues (such as pilocarpine or cevimeline) have been shown to increase tear flow slightly but not to a level sufficient for them to gain FDA approval as therapy for dry eyes.

Preparations of time-release pilocarpine or cevimeline have been proposed to yield a more linear pharmacokinetic release of drug, resulting in improved patient tolerance, reduced the systemic side effects and may prove useful in the future for both tear and saliva production [24, 25]. Although discussed for the last decade, they are not yet currently available or listed as currently in clinical trial.

Past reports of bromhexine, a mucolytic agent used in the past in many parts of the world, were reported to have proved helpful in improving dry eye [26–28]. However, this medication was relatively expensive at the doses required, was never available in the United States, and has disappeared from the market in most countries.

A role of *androgens*, either topically or orally, has been suggested based on animal studies [29]. Although a series of trials have been conducted, clear recommendations have not yet been made. Research reports have suggested that patients may prefer artificial tears supplemented with DHEA, while oral administration of DHEA showed less impressive results [30].

Other reports have suggested benefit from non-preserved steroid (methylprednisolone hemisuccinate) [31, 32], although there is a risk of glaucoma and ocular hypertension after a short duration of use [33].

Obviously, dry eye in general, and certainly the dry eyes accompanying Sjögren's syndrome, represents a chronic and potentially serious, debilitating, even vision-threatening disorder. Satisfactory management requires a partnership between an educated patient, empowered to alter his or her management within reasonable parameters, and a patient and dedicated clinician.

12.9 Complications Associated with Ophthalmologic Cosmetic Procedures

Cosmetic surgery such as *blepharoplasty* may disrupt the function of tear glands. Another side effect of cosmetic surgery (or thyroid exophthalmia) is that the lids may not have adequate closure at night and result in an area of increased corneal exposure with resulting evaporative loss. The problem of tear loss at night is particularly important since basal tear rates show important diurnal variation with the lowest rate being during sleep.

Many patients seeking *LASIK* and refractive surgery are contact lens intolerant as a result of dry eyes. Contact lens wear can be an excellent provocative test for otherwise subclinical dry eyes!

LASIK refractive surgery is therapeutically and categorically controversial and potentially dangerousfor a dry eye patient!

These patients must be extremely cautious when considering this cosmetic surgery [34], which results in actual cutting of about 90% of the corneal sensory nerves.

A significant percentage of *normal* eyes suffer from dryness for months after LASIK surgery, until the corneal nerves regenerate; others, who may have had a pre-existing mild or asymptomatic dry eye, may develop a significant and persistent dry eye.

LASIK vision-corrective surgery may lead to a relative denervation of the corneal surface, as this procedure uses a microtome to create a flap, i.e., cut across the corneal surface and also cuts across some of the sensory nerves that innervate the cornea.

We thus feel patients with Sjögren's syndrome and other immune disorders or vasculitis should probably not consider themselves candidates for LASIK surgery.

Other refractive surgeries *that spare the corneal nerves* may be considered, but so-called photorefractive keratectomy (PRK) (which avoids creating the flap that severs the nerves) removes the surface epithelium, which depends upon an adequate tear film for recovery and sustenance.

Aggressive pre-treatment and post-treatment in some mild-to-moderate dry eyes may allow a successful result.

12.10 Summary

It is essential for the rheumatologist, ophthalmologist, and patient to establish good working relationships to optimize continuity of care.

Additionally, if the rheumatologist provides written information to the patient as well as referring physician (and/or ophthalmologist), it will aid in effective management of dry eye and help minimize its negative effects on patient quality of life.

Therapy of dry eye in Sjögren's syndrome (aqueous tear deficiency or lacrimal keratoconjunctivitis sicca—KCS) requires a multi-pronged approach aimed at

- Eliminating exacerbating factors,
- Supporting tear-producing glands,
- Hydrating the ocular surface,
  - Restoring normal tear film osmolarity,
  - Stabilizing the tear film, and
- Inhibiting the production of inflammatory mediators and proteases.

Take home points for tear selection include

1. *Be prepared to mix and match different tear preparations.* This includes recognition of mild (i.e., hypotonic and less viscous) to moderate and more extreme higher severe/intensive concentration polymers (more viscous and consequently longer action tears).
2. *Do not use preserved tears more than four times a day.*
3. *There is no basic incompatibility in the various lubricants.* For example, for patients concerned about cost but are using drops more than four times per day, they can still use less expensive preserved drops more or less equally spaced and then supplement with the non-preserved tears in-between.
4. *Patients who really need the more viscous but transiently blurring drops should use less viscous, non-blurring drops while driving or doing other visually demanding activities.* Then use the more viscous drops at other times where safety and critical vision is not at issue.
5. *Read the ingredient label content on packages of generic (as well as branded) tears carefully,* as some still contain older more toxic preservatives, including benzalkonium chloride or thimerosal.
6. *The judicious use of ointments and/or gels may be very effective in breaking the cycle of periodic surface disruption.*
7. *Involve the patient in the treatment planning and decision-making process* and recognize the role of medications and environments that increase dryness.
8. *Rheumatologists are not ophthalmologists and should not oversee or try to take over the*

management of dry eyes. Treatment of these special patients should always be a joint/collaborative effort on the part of both the rheumatologist and ophthalmologist.

However, patients will ask their rheumatologist about the initial choice of artificial tears and expect some knowledge about the choice of tears (more than simply reaching into the sample cabinet to see what is available).

Successful treatment with artificial tears is a lot more than just "add water (and stir)" and there is more to the successful management of dry eye disorders than artificial tears.

References

1. Lemp MA. Tear film: new concepts and implications for the management of the dry eye. Trans New Orleans Acad Ophthalmol. 1987;35:53–64.
2. Pflugfelder SC, Solomon A, Stern ME. The diagnosis and management of dry eye: a twenty-five-year review. Cornea 2000;19(5):644–9.
3. Comment E. 2005 Gallup Study of dry eye sufferers: summary. Gallup Poll Summary. 2005. 2005:1–160.
4. The definition and classification of dry eye disease: report of the Definition and Classification Subcommittee of the International Dry Eye WorkShop (2007). Ocul Surf. 2007;5(2):75–92.
5. Behrens A, Doyle JJ, Stern L, et al. Dysfunctional tear syndrome: a Delphi approach to treatment recommendations. Cornea 2006;25(8):900–7.
6. Lemp MA. Epidemiology and classification of dry eye. Adv Exp Med Biol. 1998;438:791–803.
7. Oden NL, Lilienfeld DE, Lemp MA, Nelson JD, Ederer F. Sensitivity and specificity of a screening questionnaire for dry eye. Adv Exp Med Biol. 1998;438:807–20.
8. Moss S, Klein R, Klein B. Prevalence of and risk factors for dry eye syndrome. Arch Ophthalmol. 2000;118(9):1264.
9. Schaumberg DA, Sullivan DA, Buring JE, Dana MR. Prevalence of dry eye syndrome among US women. Am J Ophthalmol. 2003;136(2):318–26.
10. Schiffman RM, Christianson MD, Jacobsen G, Hirsch JD, Reis BL. Reliability and validity of the ocular surface disease index. Arch Ophthalmol. 2000;118(5):615–21.
11. Schiffman RM, Walt JG, Jacobsen G, Doyle JJ, Lebovics G, Sumner W. Utility assessment among patients with dry eye disease. Ophthalmology 2003;110(7):1412–9.
12. Thanou-Stavraki A, James JA. Primary Sjögren's syndrome: current and prospective therapies. Semin Arthritis Rheum. 2008;37(5):273–92.
13. Jain AK, Sukhija J, Dwedi S, Sood A. Effect of topical cyclosporine on tear functions in tear-deficient dry eyes. Ann Ophthalmol (Skokie). 2007;39(1): 19–25.
14. Strong B, Farley W, Stern ME, Pflugfelder SC. Topical cyclosporine inhibits conjunctival epithelial apoptosis in experimental murine keratoconjunctivitis sicca. Cornea 2005;24(1):80–5.
15. O'Brien PD, Collum LM. Dry eye: diagnosis and current treatment strategies. Curr Allergy Asthma Rep. 2004;4(4):314–19.
16. Tsubota K, Fujita H, Tadano K, et al. Improvement of lacrimal function by topical application of CyA in murine models of Sjögren's syndrome. Invest Ophthalmol Vis Sci. 2001;42(1):101–10.
17. Avunduk AM, Avunduk MC, Erdol H, Kapicioglu Z, Akyol N. Cyclosporine effects on clinical findings and impression cytology specimens in severe vernal keratoconjunctivitis. Ophthalmologica 2001;215(4):290–3.
18. Stern ME, Beuerman RW, Fox RI, Gao J, Mircheff AK, Pflugfelder SC. The pathology of dry eye: the interaction between the ocular surface and lacrimal glands. Cornea 1998;17(6):584–9.
19. Fox RI, Chan R, Michelson JB, Belmont JB, Michelson PE. Beneficial effect of artificial tears made with autologous serum in patients with keratoconjunctivitis sicca. Arthritis Rheum. 1984;27: 459–61.
20. Kojima T, Ishida R, Dogru M, et al. The effect of autologous serum eyedrops in the treatment of severe dry eye disease: a prospective randomized case–control study. Am J Ophthalmol. 2005;139(2):242–6.
21. Tsubota K. Tear dynamics and dry eye. Prog Retin Eye Res. 1998;17(4):565–96.
22. Tsubota K, Goto E, Fujita H, et al. Treatment of dry eye by autologous serum application in Sjögren's syndrome [see comments]. Br J Ophthalmol. 1999;83(4):390–5.
23. Yoon KC, Heo H, Im SK, You IC, Kim YH, Park YG. Comparison of autologous serum and umbilical cord serum eye drops for dry eye syndrome. Am J Ophthalmol. 2007;144(1):86–92.
24. Lockhart PB, Fox PC, Gentry AC, et al. Pilot study of controlled-release pilocarpine in normal subjects. Oral Surg, Oral Med, Oral Pathol, Oral Radiol and Endodontol. 1996;82(5):517–24.
25. Scholz OA, Wolff A, Schumacher A, et al. Drug delivery from the oral cavity: focus on a novel mechatronic delivery device. Drug Disc Today. 2008;13 (5–6):247–53.
26. Frost-Larsen K, Isager H, Manthorpe, R. Sjogren syndrome treated with Bromhexine: a randomized clinical study. Br Med J. 1978(1):1579–84.
27. Manthorpe R, Frost-Larsen K, Hoj L, Isager H, Prause JU. Bromhexine treatment of Sjögren's syndrome: effect on lacrimal and salivary secretion, and on proteins in tear fluid and saliva. Scand J Rheumatol. 1981;10:177–80.

28. Misawa M, Ohmori S, Yanaura S. Effects of bromhexine on the secretions of saliva and tears. J Pharmacol. 1985;39:241–50.
29. Azzarolo AM, Mircheff AK, Kaswan RL, et al. Androgen support of lacrimal gland function. Endocrine 1997;6(1):39–45.
30. Pillemer SR, Brennan MT, Sankar V, et al. Pilot clinical trial of dehydroepiandrosterone (DHEA) versus placebo for Sjögren's syndrome. Arthritis Rheum. 2004;51(4):601–4.
31. Avunduk AM, Avunduk MC, Varnell ED, Kaufman HE. The comparison of efficacies of topical corticosteroids and nonsteroidal anti-inflammatory drops on dry eye patients: a clinical and immunocytochemical study. Am J Ophthalmol. 2003;136(4):593–602.
32. Marsh P, Pflugfelder SC. Topical nonpreserved methylprednisolone therapy for keratoconjunctivitis sicca in Sjogren syndrome. Ophthalmology 1999;106(4):811–6.
33. Ponte F, Giuffre G, Giammanco R, Dardanoni G. Risk factors of ocular hypertension and glaucoma. The Casteldaccia Eye Study. Doc Ophthalmol. 1994;85(3):203–10.
34. Albietz JM, Lenton LM, McLennan SG. Dry eye after LASIK: comparison of outcomes for Asian and Caucasian eyes. Clin Exp Optom. 2005;88(2):89–96.

Pathogenesis: Emphasis on Dry Eye and the Role of the Lacrimal Functional Unit in Sjögren's Syndrome

13

Michael E. Stern and Stephen C. Pflugfelder

Abstract

Sjögren's syndrome lacrimal keratoconjunctivitis is a chronic autoimmune disease that has a significant impact on the quality of patient's lives throughout the world. Current evidence suggests that dysfunction of the complex *lacrimal function unit* (LFU: cornea, conjunctiva, lacrimal glands, and meibomian glands) results in unstable tear film and chronic inflammation. Inflammatory cell (e.g., $CD4^+$ T cells) infiltration, elevated pro-inflammatory cytokine levels, increased epithelial cell apoptosis, and diminished goblet cell numbers within the LFU, coupled with decreased tear production, are hallmark features of Sjögren's syndrome. The inability of lacrimal glands to adequately respond to signals of ocular surface dryness, an early feature of Sjögren's syndrome, is hypothesized to perpetuate chronic inflammation. The cycle of autoimmunity during Sjögren's syndrome is simplified into two main stages: (1) the afferent arm, in which desiccating stress on the ocular surface elicits the initial immune response and (2) an efferent arm, which describes activation and homing of autoreactive $CD4^+$ T cells to the ocular surface that contribute to local tissue remodeling and destruction. Indeed, early inflammatory intervention can restore secretory function within the LFU; however, if left untreated, chronic inflammation may irreversibly impact the function of the lacrimal glands and/or conjunctival goblet cells. Current research is focused on gaining a better understanding of the mechanisms that contribute to the immunopathogenesis of Sjögren's syndrome with the goals of developing sensitive diagnostics and superior therapeutics.

Keywords

Sjögren's syndrome • Lacrimal keratoconjunctivitis • Ocular surface • Lacrimal functional unit • Autoimmunity • Inflammation • T cells

13.1 Introduction

Sjögren's syndrome is a systemic autoimmune disease predominantly seen in women (90%) of perimenopausal and postmenopausal age. The

M.E. Stern (✉)
Inflammation Research Program, Allergan, Inc., Irvine, CA, USA
e-mail: stern_michael@allergan.com

R.I. Fox, C.M. Fox (eds.), *Sjögren's Syndrome*, DOI 10.1007/978-1-60327-957-4_13,

signature symptoms are xerostomia and xerophthalmia, although due to the mucosal nature of this inflammatory disease, periodic flare-ups can occur in the lungs, gut, and vagina. Diagnosis of this disease is commonly made by identifying dryness of the mouth and eyes and the presence of circulating (serum) antibodies [anti-ro, anti-la (SSA, SSB)]. In some cases a labial biopsy of a minor salivary gland is taken to look for lymphocytic foci.

13.2 The Lacrimal Functional Unit (LFU)

The ophthalmic pathology seen in Sjögren's syndrome surrounds an immune-based inflammatory disruption of the lacrimal functional unit (LFU). The LFU is composed of the ocular surface (cornea, conjunctiva, conjunctival blood vessels), eyelids, the lacrimal glands (main and accessory [Wolfring and Krauss]), and the interconnecting innervation (V, VII) [1]. This tear-secreting reflex is also modulated with input from hormonal and immune factors. The role of the LFU is to secrete a tear film of specific composition in order to maintain a trophic (i.e., homeostatic) environment around the epithelial cells of the ocular surface.

13.3 The General Role of the LFU in Normal and Pathological Situation

The important purpose of the ocular surface is to preserve corneal clarity and vision. The main and accessory lacrimal glands, the corneal limbus, and the meibomian glands provide a vital supportive function to protect the sensitive epithelial surfaces of the conjunctival and corneal tissues from injury, which could result in loss of vision. The main function of the LFU is secretion of tear constituents that help to sustain a stable, defensive, and supportive tear layer that is essential for the optics of the eye to function at optimal levels [1]. Bioelectric energy emanating from ocular surface sensory nerves supplies continuous input into CNS pathways, which connect changes in the ocular surface milieu with tear secretory activity by these specialized support tissues.

13.4 Innervation of the Lacrimal Functional Unit

Normal tears are secreted when the highly innervated corneal nerves are subconsciously stimulated. This can occur from a variety of stresses; however, environmentally induced "dry spot" formation is thought to be a normal stimulus. Through evolution the cornea has become the most densely sensory nerve innervated epithelial surface in the body. Myelinated and unmyelinated nerves end in the cornea, limbus, and conjunctiva epithelium and are associated with conduction of pain. The neural receptors in the cornea are free nerve endings which terminate in the wing cell layer of the corneal epithelium. These nerve ending are protected from direct irritation by zonula occludens in and tear mucin gel adherent to the apical corneal epithelial cells [2, 3]. Afferent nerve traffic through the ophthalmic branch of the trigeminal nerve (V) enters the central nervous system in the area of the pons (midbrain) and the para-spinal sympathetic tract. These signals are integrated with cortical and other inputs and trigger efferent secretomotor impulses to stimulate secretion of the components of the tear film.

13.5 Efferent Structures

13.5.1 Lacrimal Glands

Tear secretion by the lacrimal gland occurs in response to neural stimulation [4]. The acni, ducts, and blood vessels of the lacrimal gland are innervated by parasympathetic, sympathetic, and sensory nerves. Signaling pathways are initiated by parasympathetic cholinergic nerves releasing acetylcholine, which then binds to M_3 acetylcholine receptors on the basolateral cell membrane of secretory epithelia [5, 6], and vasoactive intestinal peptide (VIP) binds to

VIPergic receptors [7]. Norepinephrine, a sympathetic neurotransmitter, binds to α_1-adrenergic and β-adrenergic receptors. A neural innervation of the accessory lacrimal glands has been reported [8–10]. Fibers found to be positive for calcitonin gene-related peptide (CGRP) and substance P were associated with secretory tubules, interlobular and excretory ducts, and blood vessels. However, the degree of neural influence over accessory lacrimal glands has not been as clearly proven as it has for orbital lacrimal glands.

13.5.2 Goblet Cells

Sensory, sympathetic, and parasympathetic neuropeptides are present in the conjunctiva [11]. Conjunctival goblet cells have a secretory response to the parasympathetic cholinergic muscarinic output from the pterygopalatine ganglion. Goblet cells express M_3-muscarinic receptors on their membranes. M_1 and M_2 receptors are located all through the conjunctiva [12]. α(alpha)$_{1A}$-adrenergic and β(beta)$_3$-adrenergic receptors are found on conjunctival goblet cells, suggesting the presence of sympathetic nerves.

13.5.3 Meibomian Glands

Transmission electron microscopy of meibomian glands has demonstrated the presence of unmyelinated axons with granular and agranular vesicles. Substance P-positive and CGRP-positive axons have been identified [13, 14], but their functions are uncertain because these neurological peptides would be expected to conduct information to the CNS. It is likely that parasympathetic fibers innervating the meibomian glands are present at higher levels. Parasympathetic neurotransmitters, neuropeptide Y and VIP, have been found around the meibomian glands, as well as tyrosine hydroxylase in sympathetic axons, implicating that both types of autonomic nerves may play a role in stimulating lipid secretion onto the ocular surface.

Patients with lacrimal keratoconjunctivitis commonly complain of constant corneal sensations, normally described as gritty, sandy, or itchy. These complaints are usually accompanied by pathophysiological changes including a chronic inflammation and a dysfunctional tear film composition. Infiltrating inflammatory cells onto the ocular surface have been reported in dry eye [15–17]. These inflammatory cells, in addition to antibodies to gangliosides and other neural proteins, could result in regional degeneration of small diameter axons and their terminals. Chronic dysfunction of the lacrimal functional unit results in a shift toward inflammation and more persistent psychological distress.

13.6 Maintenance of the Lacrimal Functional Unit

13.6.1 Hormonal

The LFU is maintained through the activities of the endocrine and immune systems. Initial data indicated that the presence of androgen hormones provided an anti-inflammatory environment over the ocular surface essentially acting as physiological steroids. Androgenic hormones provide an immunosuppressive umbrella to help protect the secretory immune function of the lacrimal glands and the meibomian glands [18–20]. Perimenopausal and postmenopausal women have relative androgen deficiency, which may be a cause for the higher prevalence of dry eye in women. Interestingly, Sjögren's syndrome keratoconjunctivitis sicca (KCS) arises almost exclusively in women [21]. There is also a body of data that indicates that estrogens can be anti-inflammatory and help protect the ocular surface. In most probability, the balance between the two is the key hormonal factor, and it is currently well known that there is a redundant series of cells, both circulating and resident in the ocular surface, which provides a strong immunosuppressive environment in order to prevent the formation of chronic inflammatory disease.

13.6.2 Immunological

Several types of immunoregulatory cells are present at the ocular surface to restrain activation and infiltration of autoreactive lymphocytes to the ocular surface in an acute inflammatory event. The ocular surface is constantly being surveyed by immunovigilant T cells. These immunovigilant T cells undergo apoptosis if no threat is detected. $CD4^+CD25^+FoxP3^+$ regulatory T cells have recently been shown to modulate dry eye disease in an experimental mouse model of dry eye [16, 22]. The exact mechanisms by which $CD4^+CD25^+FoxP3^+$ regulatory T cells and resident intraepithelial lymphocytes (including γδ(gamma/delta)-T cells, natural killer cells, and $CD8^+$ T cells) contribute to the anti-inflammatory environment remain to be determined. $CD8^+$ Tregs in secondary lymphoid organs are crucial for ablating Th1 and Th2-mediated phlogistic responses and have been extensively studied using models of anterior chamber-associated immune deviation (ACAID) [23, 24]. The role of efferent $CD8^+$ Tregs following direct ocular surface injury has not been elucidated.

13.7 Conjunctival-Associated Lymphoid Tissue (CALT)

Exogenous antigen comes into contact with mucosal surfaces, such as the conjunctiva, and encounters both the innate and adaptive defensive immune systems. In the conjunctiva, the adaptive immune system includes the conjunctival-associated lymphoid tissue (CALT) [25, 26]. The CALT contains lymphoid cells within and beneath the conjunctival epithelium. This mucosal defensive system is also present in the tear drainage system and the lacrimal glands [27]. Knop and Knop [146] have proposed that the mucosal-associated lymphoid tissue of the ocular surface exists as a whole defense unit, the eye-associated lymphoid tissue.

13.8 The Normal Ocular Surface Environment

The ocular surface environment is regulated in large part by tears. The tear film serves four important functions: maintenance of a smooth high-quality optical surface, maintenance of ocular surface comfort, protection from environmental and infectious insults, and maintenance of epithelial cell health.

First, the tear film is a critical component of the eye's optical system. It and the anterior surface of the cornea combine to provide approximately 80% of the refractive power for the eye's focusing mechanism [28]. Even a small change in tear film stability and volume will significantly change the quality of vision (primarily contrast sensitivity) [29, 30]. The lens and its controlling anatomy "fine-tune" this refractive power. Tear film breakup causes optical aberrations that can degrade the quality of images focused on the retina [31]. Accordingly, the irregular preocular tear film of patients with Sjögren's syndrome lacrimal keratoconjunctivitis may be responsible for symptoms of visual fatigue and photophobia [32–34].

Second, the tear film helps maintain ocular surface comfort by continuously lubricating the ocular surface. The normal tear film is subjected to a shear force of about 150 dynes/cm^2 by the superior lid margin traversing the ocular surface during a normal blink cycle [28, 35]. Non-Newtonian properties of the tear film's mucin layer decrease this shear force, which would otherwise be exerted on the ocular surface epithelium, to a negligible level [36]. In lacrimal keratoconjunctivitis, alterations of the mucin layer render the ocular surface epithelial cell membranes more susceptible to this shear force, resulting in increased epithelial desquamation and induction of pathological apoptosis [37].

Third, the tear film protects the ocular surface from environmental and infective intrusions. The ocular surface is the most environmentally exposed mucosal surface of the body. It continually encounters temperature extremes, low humidity, wind, UV irradiation, allergens, and irritants, such as pollutants and particulate matter. The tear film must have sufficient stability to buffer the ocular surface microenvironment against these challenges. Protective components of the tear film, such as immunoglobulin A, lactoferrin, lysozyme, and peroxidase, resist bacterial or viral infections. The surface lipid layer minimizes evaporation of the aqueous component of the tear film in adverse environments. Additionally, tear production may be stimulated to help wash out particulates, irritants, and allergens.

Fourth, the tear film provides a trophic environment for the corneal epithelium. Because it lacks vasculature, the corneal epithelium depends on the tear film for growth factors and for certain nutritional support. The electrolyte and oxygen supply of the corneal epithelium is provided by the tear film. While most of the glucose utilized by the corneal epithelium is supplied by diffusion from the aqueous humor, tears contain about 25 μg/mL glucose, roughly 4% of the glucose concentration in blood [38], a sufficient concentration to support non-muscular tissue. Tear film anti-oxidants help maintain a reducing environment and scavenge free radicals. The tear film also contains a plethora of growth factors, important for the constant regeneration of the corneal epithelium and for wound healing.

13.9 The Makeup of the Tear Film

The tear film is currently viewed as a hydrated mucin gel that contains fluid, electrolytes, and proteins that are secreted by the lacrimal glands and ocular surface epithelium. The surface is covered with a lipid layer that is produced by the meibomian glands.

13.9.1 Hydrated Mucin Gel

The mucin layer functions as a surfactant for the ocular surface, facilitating even spread of tears over the hydrophobic epithelium. It maintains tear film viscosity and protects against the shear force of blinking that would otherwise cause irritation, inflammation, and accelerated sloughing of surface epithelial cells. The mucin layer also helps to maintain optical clarity and smoothness of the cornea [39].

At first glance the mucin layer appears loosely organized and amorphous, although recent findings have demonstrated that it is highly organized in a manner that facilitates its function. The ocular surface epithelia express transmembrane mucins 1, 2, 4, and 16, which form the glycocalyx and anchor the mucin layer to the hydrophobic epithelial cell surface [40–43]. The membrane-spanning domain of MUC1 anchors it to epithelial cells, and its extracellular domain extends 200–500 nm into the glycocalyx [44]. MUC4, expressed by the stratified conjunctival epithelium [45], forms a sialomucin complex on the surfaces of corneal and conjunctival epithelial cells and can also be shed into tear fluid as a soluble mucin [46]. Conjunctival goblet cells secrete the soluble mucin MUC5AC [47], which interacts with the membrane-bound mucins and the aqueous layer to form a water-trapping gel. Lacrimal glands secrete MUC7 into the tear fluid [48, 49]. MUC1 and MUC4 have been shown to prevent inflammatory cell adhesion [50, 51], suggesting that the mucin layer may function, in general, to prevent adherence to or repel inflammatory cells, bacteria, or debris from the ocular surface [43, 47]. In summary, the chemical interactions between membrane and soluble mucins create a stable tear film that coats the ocular surface epithelium and facilitate tear film spreading and ocular surface wetting. An intact and hydrated mucin gel helps protect the epithelium from environmental insult and minimizes shear forces during blinking [35, 39, 52].

13.9.2 Lipid Profile

The lipid layer, secreted by the meibomian glands whose ducts exit just anterior to the mucocutaneous junction of the lids, functions to facilitate tear film spreading over the corneal surface and minimize tear evaporation [35, 39, 52, 53]. In addition, the lipid layer prevents skin lipids on the lid margins from entering and disrupting the tear film [35, 39, 52, 54].

The lipid layer varies in composition. Polar lipids such as phospholipids, sphingomyelin, ceramides, and cerebrosides are found adjacent to the aqueous phase of the tear film [35, 39, 52, 55], while non-polar lipids, including wax and cholesterol esters, triglycerides, and free fatty acids, associate with the polar lipids and form the lipid–air interface [35, 39, 52, 56]. Even spreading of the lipid layer is important because accumulation of lipid in thick patches, especially the non-polar oils, may contaminate the mucin layer, rendering it unwettable [57, 58]. Blinking helps spread the lipid layer evenly over the tear film surface [59]. Uniform tear film spreading is also facilitated by the low surface tension of the lipid–air interface, about half that of an aqueous–air interface [60].

13.9.3 Aqueous Components

The aqueous layer of the tear film, or the more aqueous portion of the mucin gel, contains dissolved oxygen, electrolytes, and numerous proteins, including growth factors that help maintain a trophic and protective environment for the ocular surface epithelium. The health of ocular surface epithelial tissues depends on growth factors, such as EGF [61, 62], HGF, and KGF [63, 64]. Immunoglobulins and other proteins such as lactoferrin [65], lysozyme [66], defensins [67], and immunoglobulin A [68] protect the ocular surface from infection by bacteria and viruses. Still other proteins, such as TGF-β(beta) and interleukin-1 receptor antagonist, help minimize ocular surface inflammation [69–71].

Tear film electrolytes, such as Na^+, K^+, Cl^-, Ca^{2+}, and others, present in concentrations similar to those found in serum, result in a normal tear osmolarity of about 300 mOsm/L [72, 73], which helps maintain normal epithelial cell volume. Ions help solubilize proteins, and in some cases, are essential for enzymatic activity. Proper osmolarity is also required for maintenance of normal corneal nerve membrane potential and for cellular homeostasis and secretory function.

The roles of the main and accessory lacrimal glands in tear secretion and the pathogenesis of dry eye disease remain unresolved. Most of the normal daily tear flow comes from the accessory lacrimal glands (the glands of Wolfring and Krause) located in the superior conjunctival fornix and in the upper lid just superior to the meibomian glands. The main lacrimal gland is thought to function primarily as a reservoir supplying the ocular surface with copious amounts of fluid to wash out infectious or irritating particles that threaten epithelial integrity [74]. Removal of the main lacrimal glands from squirrel monkeys resulted in no damage to the cornea, conjunctiva, or eyelid, indicating that accessory lacrimal gland function was sufficient to maintain a healthy ocular surface [75]. The same procedure performed in cats and humans led to signs of KCS [76], suggesting an important role for the main lacrimal glands in maintaining ocular surface health in these species [77].

Most tear secretion by the LFU is driven by stimulation of the afferent sensory nerves on the ocular surface. These signals are integrated in the central nervous system and may be modified or altered by cortical functions such as emotion. Tear production decreases by as much as 66% following topical anesthesia of the ocular surface [4] or to below detectable levels under general anesthesia when all emotional and afferent sensory stimulus for tear secretion is removed [78]. Anesthesia of the nasal mucosa decreased tear secretion in the ipsilateral eye by about 34% [79]. The effects of anesthesia underscore the importance of neuronal control for normal tear production.

13.10 The Pathophysiology of Dry Eye

13.10.1 Loss of Hormonal Support

Both the lacrimal and meibomian glands are androgen responsive tissues. Androgens have been found to suppress inflammation in the lacrimal glands [18–20]. Relative androgen deficiency might explain the greater prevalence of dry eye in women. Consistent with this, Sjögren's syndrome KCS occurs almost exclusively in women [80]. Androgen levels decrease with age in both sexes and may be responsible in part for the age-related deterioration in tear secretion. Hormone replacement therapy in postmenopausal women may also be associated with dry eye. Women taking estrogen replacement therapy are at a greater risk for developing dry eye than women taking a combination of estrogen and progesterone [81]. It has not been established whether oral contraceptives alter aqueous tear production [82].

13.10.2 Ocular Surface Inflammatory Cycle in Sjögren's Syndrome

The immune response on the ocular surface is designed to respond efficiently to stress and/or microbial insults and, paradoxically, may contribute to autoimmunity. The exact mechanism by which Sjögren's syndrome lacrimal keratoconjunctivitis develops has not been established; however, our research suggests that an autoimmune cycle in the LFU (Fig. 13.1) may be triggered by ocular surface desiccation; perhaps due to inability of the lacrimal glands to adequately respond to signals of ocular surface dryness, which is an early feature of Sjögren's syndrome [83, 84]. This cycle consists of an afferent arm, where desiccating stress on the ocular surface elicits an immune response, and an efferent arm, where activated $CD4^+$ T cells home to the ocular surface and modulate epithelial differentiation.

13.10.2.1 Afferent Arm

The afferent arm of the dry eye immune reaction is initiated by a stress response of the ocular surface epithelial cells to desiccation and/or increased tear osmolarity. Increased tear osmolarity in dry eye has been recognized for decades [85]. Clinical studies have reported increases in mean tear osmolarity of about 10–20% in tear samples collected from the inferior tear meniscus [85]; however, ocular surface epithelial cells underlying areas of marked thinning or frank breakup of the tear layer may be subjected to much greater osmotic stress [86]. This is supported by a study that found a doubling of tear osmolarity in an experimental murine model of dry eye using sodium ion concentration in tear washings collected from the entire ocular surface to measure tear osmolarity [87].

Osmotic stress activates signaling pathways in a variety of cell types, including the ocular surface epithelia [88]. We have reported that exposure to increased osmolarity in vivo or in vitro activates mitogen-activated protein kinase (MAPK) pathways, particularly p38 and c-Jun N-terminal kinases, and nuclear factor (NF)-κB in the ocular surface epithelia [89, 90]. These pathways regulate transcription of a wide variety of genes involved in the inflammatory/immune response. We have found that desiccating and osmotic stress, by MAPK activation, stimulates production of a variety of inflammatory mediators by the corneal epithelium, including interleukin (IL)-1β(beta), tumor necrosis factor (TNF)-α(alpha), IL-8, and a number of matrix metalloproteinases (MMPs; MMP-1, MMP-3, MMP-9, MMP-10, and MMP-13) [89–93].

Under homeostatic conditions, resident corneal dendritic cells are immature and have limited or no MHC class II antigen membrane expression [94]. Following ocular surface desiccating challenge, immune-mediated inflammation is initiated by release of inflammatory cytokines (IL-1, TNF-α(alpha), and IL-6) by the stressed ocular surface epithelial cells. These cytokines activate immature dendritic cells and increase their expression of CC chemokine receptor 7 (CCR7) and major histocompatibility complex class II antigen [94, 95]. Dendritic cells uptake and process antigen, travel to the lymph nodes via the lymphatic system, and activate antigen-specific naïve T cells. Following activation and differentiation within these secondary lymphoid organs, effector T cells home to the ocular surface.

Dry eye also leads to a decrease in the number of conjunctival goblet cells, which produce and secrete the immunoregulatory molecule transforming growth factor-β2 that has been reported to suppress activation of dendritic cells on the ocular surface [16, 96, 97]. Desiccating stress

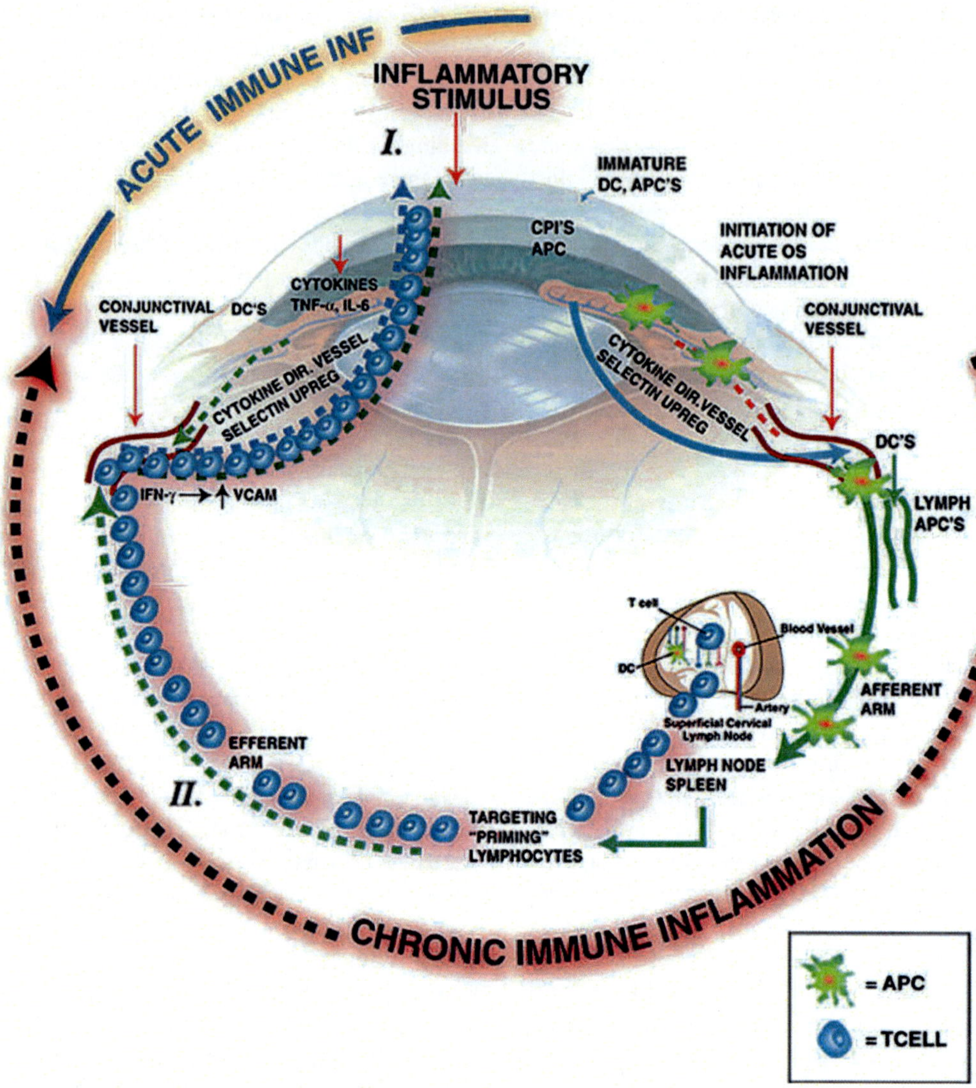

Fig. 13.1 Autoimmune cycle in the lacrimal functional unit (LFU) in Sjögren's syndrome. *Afferent arm*: environmental stimulus initiates an acute immune inflammation on the ocular surface, activating epithelial, dendritic, and endothelial cells. Activated dendritic cells process autoantigen and traffic to the regional lymph nodes where they present antigen to naïve $CD4^+$ T cells. *Efferent arm*: primed and targeted $CD4^+$ T cells travel via the circulation to the LFU where they diapedise into the local tissues, releasing pro-inflammatory cytokines which promote chronic inflammatory disease and secretory dysfunction

may also expose autoantigens by the ocular surface and lacrimal gland epithelia. For example, kallikrein 13, an EGF-binding protein, has been implicated as an autoantigen [98]. Our group has found that kallikrein 13 production by the ocular surface epithelia is increased following desiccating stress. Furthermore, decreased EGF production by the lacrimal glands in Sjögren's syndrome results in less kallikrein 13 binding and greater exposure of the unbound of kallikrein 13 to antigen-presenting cells.

Adoptive transfer models indicate that antigen-loaded antigen-presenting cells migrate from the ocular surface to regional lymph nodes where they present antigen to $CD4^+$ T cells capable of reacting to ocular surface antigens.

$CD4^+$ T cells isolated from spleen and superficial cervical lymph nodes of mice subjected to desiccating stress have been shown to induce severe autoimmune lacrimal keratoconjunctivitis when they are adoptively transferred to nude mouse recipients [16]. These findings suggest that ocular surface epithelial cells play a key role in the innate immune/inflammatory response to desiccating stress that facilitates the development of an adaptive immune response.

13.10.2.2 Efferent Arm

In the efferent arm of the immune cycle of dry eye activated $CD4^+$ T cells migrate from the lymph nodes to the ocular surface and lacrimal glands, where if conditions are favorable, they are recruited to the epithelium where the putative lacrimal keratoconjunctivitis-inducing autoantigen is located. In normal immunocompetent individuals, experimental evidence indicates that this process is inhibited by T-regulatory cells in the regional lymph nodes and in the conjunctival epithelium [16]. We have observed that dry eye decreases the numbers of $CD8^+$ and $CD103^+$ conjunctival intraepithelial T cells that may serve as a barrier to migration of pathogenic autoreactive $CD4^+$ T cells into the conjunctival epithelium [99, 100]. T-cell recruitment to and retention in the ocular surface tissues may be facilitated by cytokines and chemokines that are produced by activated epithelia that alter the local immune milieu by increasing the expression of adhesion molecules by vascular endothelial cells and ocular surface epithelial cells [89, 101]. Increased production of MMPs by the ocular surface epithelia also facilitates migration of T cells through the epithelial basement membrane into the epithelium [91]. Dry eye also appears to decrease levels of Fas ligand by the ocular surface epithelia, which has been found to play a role in immune privilege by stimulating apoptosis of Fas-expressing T cells [102]. Cytokines released by the infiltrating $CD4^+$ T cells are capable of altering conjunctival epithelial homeostasis. IL-17 alone or in conjunction with interferon (IFN)-γ(gamma) or TNF-α(alpha) has been found to stimulate the production of inflammatory mediators by mucosal epithelial cells [103–110].

We have reported that IFN-γ(gamma) decreases goblet cell differentiation and increases expression of cornified envelope precursor proteins such as involucrin and small proline-rich protein-2 [111]. The relationship between T-cell infiltration of the conjunctiva and loss of goblet cells has been observed in other inflammatory models. Chronic activation of NF-κB signaling in IKBζ knockout mice has been observed to induce $CD4^+$ T-cell migration into the conjunctiva and marked goblet cell loss [112].

These findings are consistent with the clinical features of human dry eye disease. Decreased conjunctival goblet cell density is recognized as a sine qua non of Sjögren's syndrome-associated conjunctival disease [113]. Furthermore, increased expression of cornified envelope precursor proteins and crosslinking transglutaminase-1 enzyme in the conjunctival epithelium has been observed in Sjögren's syndrome [114]. Finally, epithelial stress pathways activated by osmotic stress and T-cell cytokines such as IFN-γ(gamma) and TNF-α(alpha) may contribute to the increased conjunctival epithelial apoptosis that has been observed in human and murine dry eye [115, 116].

13.11 Loss of Ocular Surface Homeostasis

13.11.1 Alterations of the Mucin, Lipid, and Aqueous Composition

Inflammation on the ocular surface can alter the tear film function resulting in visual disturbance and irritation, pathological inflammation, and infection. As previously discussed, the cornea is the most densely innervated tissue of the body. Constant irritation of the ocular surface stimulates ocular surface sensory nerve endings to release substance P and CGRP that induce neurogenic inflammation. This neurogenic component of lacrimal keratoconjunctivitis is thought to be a critical factor in the disease pathogenesis. If the environmental stimulation of the ocular surface is not inhibited, the surface shear forces will cause more irritation, abnormal sloughing of the ocular surface epithelium, and hyperemia of conjunctival vessels. Inflammation is instigated by blood proteins and immune cells diapedising from the vessels into the substantia propria of the conjunctiva. Constant irritation and the resulting chronic inflammation of the ocular surface trigger genes responsible for epithelial differentiation, such as cornified envelope precursors. Cornification of the corneal and conjunctival epithelia consequently changes the ocular surface into a poorly lubricated and non-wettable surface [117, 118], thereby increasing the circle of inflammation and further diminishing tear production.

The composition of the tears that are produced when the lacrimal functional unit is inflamed is significantly altered. These include a rise in osmolarity, reduced concentration of protective factors (i.e., mucins, lipids, proteins), and increased levels of pro-inflammatory cytokines and proteases. Destabilization of the tear film can be caused by loss or deterioration of lacrimal gland, conjunctival goblet cell, or meibomian gland secretions.

13.11.2 Mucins

Studies of dry eye patients have demonstrated that there are alterations in the amount and biochemical characteristics of the tear mucins. Consistent with the loss of conjunctival goblet cells and decreased production of the goblet cell mucin MUC5AC, the level of this mucin in the tear film was found to be decreased in dry eye patients as compared to age and gender-matched healthy individuals [119]. In a different study, Sjögren's syndrome patients had significantly reduced levels of MUC5AC in their tear fluid and MUC5AC mRNA transcripts in their conjunctival epithelium [120]. Levels of the gel-forming mucin MUC19 have also been found to be reduced in the conjunctival epithelium in Sjögren's syndrome [121].

Mucin synthesis in canine KCS has been reported to have altered mucin glycosylation and changes in mucin subunit linkage [122]. These changes in mucin glycosylation may be due in part to altered expression of polypeptide GalNAc-transferases (GalNAc-Ts) that have been detected in conjunctival squamous metaplasia [123]. Polypeptide GalNAc-transferases add *N*-acetyl galactosamine (GalNAc) to serine and threonine residues as the first step in O-glycosylation of mucin. Reduced sulfation of mucin due to metalloproteinase-induced disorganization of the basal lamina of secretory cells has also been reported [124].

13.11.3 Lipids

Meibomian gland dysfunction is a common finding in Sjögren's syndrome [125]. The lipid composition of meibomian gland secretions in healthy eyes and those with blepharitis has been investigated [126, 127]; however, there is little known regarding the biochemical changes in lipid composition in dry eye conditions that alter the tear film. Minimal levels of the phospholipids, phosphatidylethanolamine and sphingomyelin, in meibomian gland secretions were significantly linked with the progression of corneal epithelial disease in KCS [128]. There are two possibilities for these abnormalities. The first could be diminished lipid secretion. The second possibility is degradation of lipids by phospholipases. Phospholipase A_2 (PLA_2) was increased in the tear fluid of dry eye patients [129]. Pro-inflammatory cytokines including IL-1 and TNF-α stimulate the production of this phospholipase. The concentration of tear secretory phospholipase A_2 was found to increase in the tear film of KCS patients as Schirmer's test values decreased.

13.11.4 Pro-inflammatory Aqueous Component

Disruption of the LFU in Sjögren's syndrome can result in dysfunction or death of lacrimal gland secretory acini. Lacrimal gland damage decreases fluid, electrolyte, and protein secretion. Patients with lacrimal gland disease have been reported to have reduced levels of protective and supportive lacrimal proteins in their tears. These reduced protective factors include lysozyme [130, 131], lactoferrin, and EGF [132]. Reduced lactoferrin and EGF are found in patients with Sjögren's syndrome [71, 131] and correlate with irritation symptoms, Schirmer's test results, and tear breakup time in severe keratoconjunctivitis sicca patients [133].

A reduction in aqueous tear production and tear clearance has been correlated with elevated levels of pro-inflammatory cytokines such as IL-1(α and β) and IL-6 in the tear fluid [71, 134]. Among patients with dysfunctional tears, the highest levels of inflammatory cytokines in the tears were found in patients with Sjögren's syndrome. [135]. Additionally, the ratio of IL-1α to IL-1RA was reduced in tears of Sjögren's syndrome patients [71]. The cytokines, IL-1 and TNF-α, can amplify inflammation on the ocular surface by inducing adhesion molecule expression on surface epithelial and vascular endothelial cells. Accompanying the increased cytokine production are increased levels of matrix metalloproteinases (MMP-2, MMP-3, and MMP-9), which can destabilize tears by degrading tear and extracellular matrix proteins and activating latent cytokines and proteases [71, 136–141]. MMP-9 is key factor in corneal epithelial barrier disruption that is evident in dry eye. Compared with wild-type mice, MMP-9 knockout mice had significantly less disruption of the corneal epithelial barrier function in reaction to experimental dry eye. Topical application of MMP-9 on the ocular surface of MMP-9 knockout mice significantly enhanced corneal epithelial permeability.

Chemokines promote homing of autoreactive T cells to the ocular surface during an inflammatory event. In the experimental dry eye mouse model, increased expression of the chemokine receptors CCR5 and CXCR3 was observed. The chemokine ligands, CCL3, CCL4, CCL5, CXCL9, and CXCL10, were present within the cornea and conjunctiva of mice with experimental dry eye [101]. Dry eye patients express CCR5 on cells within conjunctival epithelium [101] and CCL5 and CXCL10 were increased in human conjunctival epithelium cells after treatment with cytokines [142]. These results suggest that CCL5:CCR5 and CXCL9/CXCL10:CXCR3 signaling axes are involved in autoreactive T-cell infiltration of the ocular surface during dry eye disease.

In the mouse model of dry eye, the presence of $CD4^+$ T cells within the LFU correlated with increased cytokine tear levels of IFN-γ, IL-1β, TNF-α, and the matrix metalloproteinase, MMP-9, epithelial cell apoptosis, decreased goblet cell density, tear production, and turnover [16, 99]. $CD4^+$ T cells are also found in human dry eye patients [17]. IFN-γ increases expression of pro-inflammatory factors, including the trafficking molecules ICAM-1, CCL5, and CXCL10, and the pro-apoptotic proteins, Fas–FasL [143]. $CD4^+$ T-cell infiltration into the LFU was associated with elevated levels of IFN-γ in the tears of dry eye mice. The increase in IFN-γ was inversely related to goblet cell density and conjunctival squamous metaplasia [99]. These findings suggest that IFN-γ is a mediator of the ocular surface epithelial metaplasia that develops in Sjögren's syndrome lacrimal keratoconjunctivitis.

Chronic ocular surface inflammation leads to destabilization of the tear film due to altered secretion and accelerated degradation. The unstable, pro-inflammatory tear film composition can induce injury to the corneal surface that can result in blurred and fluctuating vision. Altered cornea epithelial barrier renders the cornea more susceptible to desiccating environmental stress, microbial infection, and leukocyte infiltration. Furthermore the free nerve endings in the cornea area subjected to chronic environmental stimulation that can lead to irritation, neurogenic inflammation from release of neuropeptides and eventually altered nerve morphology [144, 145].

13.12 The Ocular Surface Immunosuppressive Environment

Adoptive transfer of superficial cervical lymph node pathogenic $CD4^+$ T cells from euthymic mice exposed to desiccating stress into euthymic (wild-type) mice did not induce significant lacrimal keratoconjunctivitis, suggesting that $CD4^+CD25^+$ regulatory T cells are important for regulating inflammatory events at the ocular surface. Antibody-mediated depletion of $CD25^+$ T cells in euthymic mice preceding adoptively transfer of pathogenic $CD4^+$ T cells results in dry eye disease [16]. When T-cell-deficient nude mice are reconstituted with pathogenic $CD4^+$ T cells alone, autoimmune lacrimal keratoconjunctivitis develops, but when transferred with $CD4^+CD25^+Foxp3^+$ regulatory T cells, the ability to transfer disease is ablated [16]. These experiments demonstrated the importance of regulatory T cells in sustaining a homeostatic environment at the ocular surface. The critical role regulatory T cells play in repressing inappropriate inflammatory events has gained increasing recognition over the past several years. Regulatory T cells have been found to restrain a number of reactions, including $CD4^+$ T-cell responses in autoimmune disease. The function of regulatory T cells in the inflammatory disease dry eye has recently been studied. In addition to $CD4^+CD25^+$ natural regulatory T cells, a number of intraepithelial regulatory T cells including $CD8^+$ regulatory T cells, and γδ-T cells have been identified on the ocular surface. It is recognized that certain of these populations, such as $CD8^+$ cells, decrease in response to desiccating stress and this may render the ocular surface more susceptible to effector T cells [99]. Bolstering these natural immunoregulatory mechanisms is one potential therapeutic strategy for Sjögren's syndrome. It is likely that these cell populations help to suppress the inflammation induced by everyday environmental stresses the ocular surface is exposed to. Therefore, there must be a system that suppresses the initiation of inflammation that develops from dry eye. It has been published in numerous experimental models that the $CD4^+CD25^+Foxp3^+$ population of regulatory T cells can control immune responses. Regulatory cells are critical to provide homeostatic ocular surface environment and limit disease pathology.

13.13 Sjögren's Syndrome—A Multisystem Disease of the Lacrimal Functional Unit

Among dry eye conditions, Sjögren's syndrome is considered to be the most severe condition because it affects the LFU at multiple points. It directly affects the lacrimal glands as well as the meibomian glands and ocular surface epithelia. Furthermore, it disrupts the neural signaling between components of the LFU rendering the tear-secreting apparatus unable to respond to the demands of the ocular surface. It appears that treatment of inflammation is capable of restoring secretory function early in the course of the disease. As the disease advances and irreversible changes occur in the lacrimal glands and conjunctival goblet cells, the disease may be less responsive to therapy. Future use of sensitive biomarkers of LFU dysfunction may permit identification of Sjögren's syndrome lacrimal keratoconjunctivitis at a stage where interventional therapy may be instituted.

13.14 Late-Breaking Additions

Current discoveries have added insights into the mechanisms underlying the afferent and efferent immune responses during the immunopathogenesis of Sjögren's syndrome. While the specific initiating triggers of Sjögren's syndrome are still enigmatic, there is new evidence supporting an autoantigenic role for epitopes of the type 3 muscarinic acetylcholine receptor [147], and adoptive transfer of M3R reactive T cells into T-cell-deficient mice was sufficient to induce Sjögren's syndrome-like autoimmune sialoadenitis [148, 149]. Along these lines, we recently demonstrated that resident ocular surface antigen-presenting cells are necessary for the initiation and development of experimental autoimmune lacrimal keratoconjunctivitis, further supporting the paradigm that Sjögren's syndrome is initiated by self-antigens shared among LFU tissues (unpublished data). Chemokine receptor signaling coupled with lymphangiogenesis within the ocular surface tissues appears to facilitate the afferent response by directing trafficking of antigen-presenting cells bearing self-antigen from the ocular surface tissues to the draining lymph nodes [150, 151], where they mingle with autoreactive T cells, in turn driving the efferent response.

Among the efferent lymphocyte subsets described in Sjögren's syndrome (e.g., Th1 $CD4^+$ T cells and B cells), the collective data show that the relatively new subset of T helper cells, Th17 cells, also exert a pathogenic affect within the LFU tissues. For instance, Th17 cells and related cytokines were found in the salivary glands of patients and animal models of Sjögren's syndrome [152, 153]. Th17-polarizing cytokines are also secreted from ocular surface epithelium exposed to hyperosmotic, microbial, and inflammatory stimuli and were sufficient to induce Th17 differentiation from naive murine $CD4^+$ T cells [154]. Elevated IL-17 levels correlated with metalloproteinase production and corneal barrier dysfunction during experimental autoimmune lacrimal keratoconjunctivitis [155]. Indeed, Th17 cells suppressed Treg function in a mouse model of dry eye [156], providing evidence that Th17 cells directly impact immunoregulation and help autoreactive lymphocytes escape peripheral tolerance to self-antigens. Further, overexpression of IL-17 in mice that were otherwise not susceptible to Sjögren's syndrome-like disease induced inflammatory cell infiltration and salivary gland dysfunction [157], and by contrast, IL-17 blockade reduced Sjögren's syndrome-like disease in susceptible mice [158].

These recent findings highlight the complexity of immunopathogenic factors expressed during Sjögren's syndrome and add value with potential as new therapeutic targets for disease intervention. There appears to be differences between patients, not only in symptomatology but also with respect to the relative contribution of the prominent pathogenic subsets driving the disease. These differences may explain why some treatment paradigms, such as T-cell inhibition, work well in some patients, but not in others. In this respect, Th17 cells have gained notoriety as key players in infection and autoimmunity. Based on the collective data, it is interesting to speculate that targeting Th17 cells may be a viable approach to inhibit T-cell-mediated Sjögren's syndrome without compromising the protective peripheral immunoregulatory mechanisms designed to keep autoreactive lymphocytes in check.

References

1. Stern ME, Beuerman RW, Fox RI, Gao J, Mircheff AK, Pflugfelder SC. The pathology of dry eye: the interaction between the ocular surface and lacrimal glands. Cornea 1998;17(6):584–9.
2. Roza AJ, Beuerman RW. Density and organization of free nerve endings in the corneal epithelium of the rabbit. Pain 1982;4:105–20.
3. Schimmelpfenning A. Nerve structures in human central corneal epithelium. Graefes Arch Clin Exp Ophthalmol. 1982;218:14–20.
4. Jordan A, Baum J. Basic tear flow. Does it exist? Ophthalmology. 1980;87:920–30.
5. Dartt DA. Regulation of tear secretion. Adv Exp Med Biol 1994; 350:1–9.
6. Nakamura M, Tada Y, Akaishi T, Nakata K. M3 muscarinic receptor mediates regulation of protein secretion in rabbit lacrimal gland. Curr Eye Res. 1997;16:614–9.
7. Hodges RR, Zoukhri D, Sergheraert C, Zieske JD, Dartt DA. Identification of vasoactive intestinal peptide receptor subtypes in the lacrimal gland and their signal-transducing components. Invest Ophthalmol Vis Sci. 1997;38:610–9.
8. Seifert P, Stuppi S, Spitznas M. Distribution pattern of nervous tissue and peptidergic nerve fibers in accessory lacrimal glands. Curr Eye Res. 1997;16:298–302.
9. Seifert P, Spitznas M. Vasoactive intestinal polypeptide (VIP) innervation of the human eyelid glands. Exp Eye Res. 1999;68:685–92.
10. Beuerman RW, Maitchouk DY, Varnell RJ, Pedroza-Schmidt L. Interactions between lacrimal function and the ocular surface. Curr Opin Kyoto Cornea Club. 1998;2:1–10.
11. Simons E, Smith PG. Sensory and autonomic innervation of the rat eyelid: neuronal origins and peptide phenotypes. J Chem Neuroanat. 1994;7:35–47.
12. Diebold Y, Rios JD, Hodges RR, Rawe I, Dartt DA. Presence of nerves and their receptors in mouse and human conjunctival goblet cells. Invest Ophthalmol Vis Sci. 2001;42:2270–82.
13. Kirch W, Horneber M, Tamm ER. Characterization of meibomian gland innervation in the cynomolgus monkey (*Macaca fascicularis*). Anat Embryol.1996;193:365–75.

14. Chung CW, Tigges M, Stone RA. Peptidergic innervation of the primate meibomian gland. Invest Ophthalmol Vis Sci. 1996;37:238–45.
15. Kunert KS, Tisdale AS, Stern ME, Smith JA, Gipson IK. Analysis of topical cyclosporine treatment of patients with dry eye syndrome: effect on conjunctival lymphocytes. Arch Ophthalmol. 2000;118(11):1489–96.
16. Niederkorn JY, Stern ME, Pflugfelder SC, et al. Desiccating stress induces T cell-mediated Sjogren's syndrome-like lacrimal keratoconjunctivitis. J Immunol. 2006;176(7): 3950–7.
17. Stern ME, Gao J, Schwalb TA, et al. Conjunctival T-cell subpopulations in Sjogren's and non-Sjogren's patients with dry eye. Invest Ophthalmol Vis Sci. 2002;43(8):2609–14.
18. Sullivan DA, Wickham LA, Rocha EM, Kelleher RS, da Silveira LA, Toda I. Influence of gender, sex steroid hormones, and the hypothalamic-pituitary axis on the structure and function of the lacrimal gland. Adv Exp Med Biol. 1998;438:11–42.
19. Sullivan DA, Hann LE. Hormonal influence on the secretory immune system of the eye: endocrine impact on the lacrimal gland accumulation and secretion of IgA and IgG. J Steroid Biochem. 1989;34:253–62.
20. Sullivan DA, Sullivan BD, Ullman MD, et al. Androgen influence on the meibomian gland. Invest Ophthalmol Vis Sci. 2000;41:3732–42.
21. Murillo-Lopez F, Pflugfelder SC. Dry eye. In: Krachmer JH, Mannis MJ, Holland EJ, editors. The cornea. St. Louis: Mosby; 1996, pp. 663–86.
22. Siemasko KF, Gao J, Calder VL, et al. In vitro expanded $CD4^{+}CD25^{+}Foxp3^{+}$ regulatory T cells maintain a normal phenotype and suppress immune-mediated ocular surface inflammation. Invest Ophthalmol Vis Sci. 2008. 49(12):5434–40.
23. Streilein JW, Niederkorn JY. Characterization of the suppressor cell(s) responsible for anterior chamber-associated immune deviation (ACAID) induced in BALB/c mice by P815 cells. J Immunol. 1985;134:1381–7.
24. Wilbanks GA, Streilein JW. Characterization of suppressor cells in anterior chamber-associated immune deviation (ACAID) induced by soluble antigen. Evidence of two functionally and phenotypically distinct T-suppressor cell populations. Immunology. 1990;71:383–9.
25. Chandler JW, Gillette TE. Immunologic defense mechanisms of the ocular surface. Ophthalmology. 1983;90:585–91.
26. Knop N, Knop E. Conjunctiva-associated lymphoid tissue in the human eye. Invest Ophthalmol Vis Sci. 2000;41:1270–9.
27. Knop E, Knop N. Lacrimal drainage-associated lymphoid tissue (LDALT): a part of the human mucosal immune system. Invest Ophthalmol Vis Sci. 2001;42:566–74.
28. Rolando M, Zierhut M. The ocular surface and tear film and their dysfunction in dry eye disease. Surv Ophthalmol. 2001;45(Suppl 2):S203–10.
29. Rieger G. The importance of the precorneal tear film for the quality of optical imaging. Br J Ophthalmol. 1992;76:157–8.
30. Rolando M, Iester M, Macri A, Calabria G. Low spatial-contrast sensitivity in dry eyes. Cornea. 1998;17(4):376–9.
31. Tutt R, Bradley A, Begley C, Thibos LN. Optical and visual impact of tear break-up in human eyes. Invest Ophthalmol Vis Sci. 2000;41:4117–23.
32. de Paiva CS, Lindsey JL, Pflugfelder SC. Assessing the severity of keratitis sicca with videokeratoscopic indices. Ophthalmology. 2003;110(6): 1102–9.
33. de Paiva CS, Harris LD, Pflugfelder SC. Keratoconus-like topographic changes in keratoconjunctivitis sicca. Cornea. 2003;22:22–4.
34. Liu Z, Pflugfelder SC. Corneal surface regularity and the effect of artificial tears in aqueous tear deficiency. Ophthalmology. 1999;106(5): 939–43.
35. Doane MG. Interaction of eyelids and tears in corneal wetting and the dynamics of the normal human eyeblink. Am J Ophthalmol. 1980;89: 507–16.
36. Dilly PN. Structure and function of the tear film. Adv Exp Med Biol. 1994;350:239–47.
37. Ren H, Wilson G. Apoptosis in the corneal epithelium. Invest Ophthalmol Vis Sci. 1996;37: 1017–25.
38. R, Jin Z, Colon LA. Analysis of tear fluid by CE/LIF: a noninvasive approach for glucose monitoring. J Capillary Electrophor, 1996;3:243–8.
39. Tiffany JM. The viscosity of human tears. Int Ophthalmol. 1991;15:371–6.
40. Blalock TD, Spurr-Michaud SJ, Tisdale AS, et al. Functions of MUC16 in corneal epithelial cells. Invest Ophthalmol Vis Sci. 2007;48:4509–18.
41. Chao CC, Vergnes JP, Freeman IL, Brown SI. Biosynthesis and partial characterization of tear film glycoproteins. Incorporation of radioactive precursors by human lacrimal gland explants in vitro. Exp Eye Res. 1980;30:411–25.
42. Dilly PN. Contribution of the epithelium to the stability of the tear film. Trans Ophthalmol Soc UK. 1985;104:381–9.
43. Gipson IK, Inatomi T. Cellular origin of mucins of the ocular surface tear film. Adv Exp Med Biol. 1998;438:221–7.
44. Gendler SJ, Spicer AP. Epithelial mucin genes. Annu Rev Physiol. 1995;57:607–34.
45. Inatomi T, Spurr-Michaud SJ, Tisdale AS, Gipson IK. Human corneal and conjunctival epithelia express MUC1 mucin. Invest Ophthalmol Vis Sci. 1995;36:1818–27.
46. Pflugfelder SC, Liu Z, Monroy D, et al. Detection of sialomucin complex (MUC4) in human ocular

surface epithelium and tear fluid. Invest Ophthalmol Vis Sci. 2000;41(6):1316–26.
47. Inatomi T, Spurr-Michaud SJ, Tisdale AS, Zhan Q, Feldman ST, Gipson IK. Expression of secretory mucin genes by human conjunctival epithelia. Invest Ophthalmol Vis Sci. 1996;37:1684–92.
48. Jumblatt MM, McKenzie RW, Steele PS, Emberts CG, Jumblatt JE. MUC7 expression in the human lacrimal gland and conjunctiva. Cornea. 2003;22(1):41–5.
49. Watanabe H. Significance of mucin on the ocular surface. Cornea. 2002;21:S17–22.
50. Allen M, Wright P, Reid L. The human lacrimal gland. A histochemical and organ culture study of the secretory cells. Arch Ophthalmol. 1972;88: 493–7.
51. Komatsu M, Tatum L, Altman NH, Carothers Carraway CA, Carraway KL. Potentiation of metastasis by cell surface sialomucin complex (rat MUC4), a multifunctional anti-adhesive glycoprotein. Int J Cancer. 2000;87:480–6.
52. Danjo Y, Watanabe H, Tisdale AS, et al. Alteration of mucin in human conjunctival epithelia in dry eye. Invest Ophthalmol Vis Sci. 1998;39:2602–9.
53. Tsubota K. Tear dynamics and dry eye. Prog Retin Eye Res. 1998;17:565–96.
54. Tiffany JM. The role of meibomian secretion in the tears. Trans Ophthalmol Soc UK. 1985;104: 396–401.
55. Greiner JV, Glonek T, Korb DR, Booth R, Leahy CD. Phospholipids in meibomian gland secretion. Ophthmic Res. 1996;28:44–9.
56. McCulley JP, Shine W. A compositional based model for the tear film lipid layer. Trans Am Ophthalmol Soc. 1997;95:79–88.
57. Doane MG. Abnormalities of the structure of the superficial lipid layer on the in vivo dry-eye tear film. Adv Exp Med Biol. 1994;350:489–93.
58. Lemp MA, Hamill JR. Factors affecting tear film breakup in normal eyes. Arch Ophthalmol. 1973;89:103–5.
59. Korb DR, Baron DF, Herman JP, et al. Tear film lipid layer thickness as a function of blinking. Cornea. 1998;13:354–9.
60. Holly FJ. Formation and rupture of the tear film. Exp Eye Res. 1973;15:515–25.
61. Daniele S, Frati L, Fiore C, Santoni G. The effect of the epidermal growth factor (EGF) on the corneal epithelium in humans. Albrecht Von Graefes Arch Klin Exp Ophthalmol.1979;210:159–65.
62. Ohashi Y, Motokura M, Kinoshita Y. Presence of epidermal growth factor in human tears. Invest Ophthalmol Vis Sci. 1989;30:1879–82.
63. Wilson SE, Liang Q, Kim WJ. Lacrimal gland HGF, KGF, and EGF mRNA levels increase after corneal epithelial wounding. Invest Ophthalmol Vis Sci. 1999;40:2185–90.
64. Wilson SE, Chen L, Mohan RR, Liang Q, Liu J. Expression of HGF, KGF, EGF and receptor messenger RNAs following corneal epithelial wounding. Exp Eye Res. 1999;68: 377–97.
65. Gillette TE, Allansmith MR. Lactoferrin in human ocular tissues. Am J Ophthalmol. 1980;90:30–7.
66. Hankiewicz J, Swierczek E. Lysozyme in human body fluids. Clin Chim Acta. 1974;57: 205–9.
67. Haynes RJ, Tighe PJ, Dua HS. Antimicrobial defensin peptides of the human ocular surface. Br J Ophthalmol. 1999;83:737–41.
68. McClellan BH, Whitney CR, Newman LP, Allansmith MR. Immunoglobulins in tears. Am J Ophthalmol. 1973;76:89–101.
69. Arend WP. Interleukin-1 receptor antagonist. Adv Immunol. 1993;54:167–227.
70. Kennedy MC, Rosenbaum JT, Brown J, et al. Novel production of interleukin-1 receptor antagonist peptides in normal human cornea. J Clin Invest. 1995;95:82–8.
71. Solomon A, Dursun D, Liu Z, Xie Y, Macri A, Pflugfelder SC. Pro- and anti-inflammatory forms of interleukin-1 in the tear fluid and conjunctiva of patients with dry-eye disease. Invest Ophthalmol Vis Sci. 2001;42(10):2283–92.
72. Craig JP, Singh I, Tomlinson A, Morgan PB, Efron N. The role of tear physiology in ocular surface temperature. Eye 2000;14(Pt 4):635–41.
73. Gilbard JP. Human tear film electrolyte concentrations in health and dry-eye disease. Int Ophthalmol Clin. 1994;34:27–36.
74. Walcott B. The lacrimal gland and its veil of tears. News Physiol Sci. 1998;13:97–103.
75. Maitchouk DY, Beuerman RW, Ohta T, Stern M, Varnell RJ. Tear production after unilateral removal of the main lacrimal gland in squirrel monkeys. Arch Ophthalmol. 2000;118:246–52.
76. McLaughlin SA, Brightman AH, Helper LC, Primm ND, Brown MG, Greeley S. Effect of removal of lacrimal and third eyelid glands on Schirmer tear test results in cats. J Am Vet Med Assoc. 1988;193:820–2.
77. Scherz W, Dohlman CH. Is the lacrimal gland dispensable? Keratoconjunctivitis sicca after lacrimal gland removal. Arch Ophthalmol. 1975;93:281–3.
78. Krupin T, Cross DA, Becker B. Decreased basal tear production associated with general anesthesia. Arch Ophthalmol. 1977;95:107–8.
79. Gupta A, Heigle T, Pflugfelder SC. Nasolacrimal stimulation of aqueous tear production. Cornea 1997;16(6):645–8.
80. Pflugfelder SC. Dysfunction of the integrated functional unit—impact on tear film stability and composition. In: SC Pflugfelder MSaRB, editors. Dry eye and the ocular surface. New York, NY: Marcel Dekker; 2009. pp. 63–88.
81. Schaumberg DA, Buring JE, Sullivan DA, Dana MR. Hormone replacement therapy and dry eye syndrome. JAMA 2001;286:2114–9.

82. Frankel SH, Ellis PP. Effect of oral contraceptives on tear production. Ann Ophthalmol. 1978;10:1585–8.
83. Pflugfelder SC, de Paiva CS, Li DQ, Stern ME. Epithelial–immune cell interaction in dry eye. Cornea 2008;27(Suppl 1):S9–11.
84. Tsubota K. The importance of the Schirmer test with nasal stimulation. Am J Ophthalmol. 1991;111:106–8.
85. Gilbard JP, Farris RL, Santamaria J. Osmolarity of tear microvolumes in keratoconjunctivitis sicca. Arch Ophthalmol. 1978;96(4):677–81.
86. Nichols JJ, Mitchell GL, King-Smith PE. Thinning rate of the precorneal and prelens tear films. Invest Ophthalmol Vis Sci. 2005;46:2353–61.
87. Stewart P, Chen Z, Farley W, Olmos L, Pflugfelder SC. Effect of experimental dry eye on tear sodium concentration in the mouse. Eye Contact Lens. 2005;31(4):175–8.
88. Rosette C, Karin M. Ultraviolet light and osmotic stress: activation of the JNK cascade through multiple growth factor and cytokine receptors. Science 1996;274(5290):1194–7.
89. Luo L, Li DQ, Doshi A, Farley W, Corrales RM, Pflugfelder SC. Experimental dry eye stimulates production of inflammatory cytokines and MMP-9 and activates MAPK signaling pathways on the ocular surface. Invest Ophthalmol Vis Sci. 2004;45(12):4293–301.
90. Luo L, Li DQ, Corrales RM, Pflugfelder SC. Hyperosmolar saline is a proinflammatory stress on the mouse ocular surface. Eye and Contact Lens. 2005;31(5):186–93.
91. Corrales RM, Stern ME, de Paiva CS, Welch J, Li DQ, Pflugfelder SC. Desiccating stress stimulates expression of matrix metalloproteinases by the corneal epithelium. Invest Ophthalmol Vis Sci. 2006;47(8):3293–302.
92. Li DQ, Chen Z, Song XJ, Luo L, Pflugfelder SC. Stimulation of matrix metalloproteinases by hyperosmolarity via a JNK pathway in human corneal epithelial cells. Invest Ophthalmol Vis Sci. 2004;45(12):4302–11.
93. Li DQ, Luo L, Chen Z, Kim HS, Song XJ, Pflugfelder SC. JNK and ERK MAP kinases mediate induction of IL-1beta, TNF-alpha and IL-8 following hyperosmolar stress in human limbal epithelial cells. Exp Eye Res. 2006;82:588–96.
94. Hamrah P, Liu Y, Zhang Q, Dana MR. The corneal stroma is endowed with a significant number of resident dendritic cells. Invest Ophthalmol Vis Sci. 2003;44:581–9.
95. Hamrah P, Liu Y, Zhang Q, Dana MR. Alterations in corneal stromal dendritic cell phenotype and distribution in inflammation. Arch Ophthalmol. 2003;121:1132–40.
96. Pflugfelder SC, de Paiva CS, Villarreal AL, Stern ME. Effects of sequential artificial tear and cyclosporine emulsion therapy on conjunctival goblet cell density and transforming growth factor-beta2 production. Cornea 2008;27:64–9.
97. Shen L, Barabino S, Taylor AW, Dana MR. Effect of the ocular microenvironment in regulating corneal dendritic cell maturation. Arch Ophthalmol. 2007;125(7):908–15.
98. Takada K, Takiguchi M, Konno A, Inaba M. Autoimmunity against a tissue kallikrein in IQI/Jic mice: a model for Sjogren's syndrome. J Biol Chem. 2005;280:3982–88.
99. de Paiva CS, Villarreal AL, Corrales RM et al. Dry eye-induced conjunctival epithelial squamous metaplasia is modulated by interferon-{gamma}. Invest Ophthalmol Vis Sci. 2007; 48(6):2553–60.
100. Yoon KC, de Paiva CS, Qi H et al. Desiccating environmental stress exacerbates autoimmune lacrimal keratoconjunctivitis in non-obese diabetic mice. J Autoimmun. 2008;30:212–21.
101. Yoon KC, de Paiva CS, Qi H et al. Expression of th-1 chemokines and chemokine receptors on the ocular surface of C57BL/6 mice: effects of desiccating stress. Invest Ophthalmol Vis Sci. 2007;48(6):2561–9.
102. Hori J, Joyce N, Streilein JW. Epithelium-deficient corneal allografts display immune privilege beneath the kidney capsule. Invest Ophthalmol Vis Sci. 2000;41:443–52.
103. Kawaguchi M, Kokubu F, Kuga H, et al. [Effect of IL-17 on ICAM-1 expression of human bronchial epithelial cells, NCI-H 292]. Arerugi 1999;48:1184–7.
104. Jones CE, Chan K. Interleukin-17 stimulates the expression of interleukin-8, growth-related oncogene-alpha, and granulocyte-colony-stimulating factor by human airway epithelial cells. Am J Respir Cell Mol Biol. 2002;26: 748–53.
105. Park H, Li Z, Yang XO, et al. A distinct lineage of CD4 T cells regulates tissue inflammation by producing interleukin 17. Nat Immunol. 2005;6: 1133–41.
106. Wilson NJ, Boniface K, Chan JR, et al. Development, cytokine profile and function of human interleukin 17-producing helper T cells. Nat Immunol. 2007;8:950–7.
107. Kawaguchi M, Kokubu F, Huang SK, et al. The IL-17F signaling pathway is involved in the induction of IFN-gamma-inducible protein 10 in bronchial epithelial cells. J Allergy Clin Immunol. 2007;119:1408–14.
108. van den BA, Kuiper M, Snoek M, et al. Interleukin-17 induces hyperresponsive interleukin-8 and interleukin-6 production to tumor necrosis factor-alpha in structural lung cells. Am J Respir Cell Mol Biol. 2005;33:97–104.
109. Teunissen MB, Koomen CW, de Waal MR, Wierenga EA, Bos JD. Interleukin-17 and interferon-gamma synergize in the enhancement of proinflammatory cytokine production by

human keratinocytes. J Invest Dermatol. 1998;111: 645–9.
110. Liang SC, Tan XY, Luxenberg DP, et al. Interleukin (IL)-22 and IL-17 are coexpressed by Th17 cells and cooperatively enhance expression of antimicrobial peptides. J Exp Med. 2006;203:2271–9.
111. de Paiva CS, Villarreal AL, Corrales RM, et al. IFN-γ promotes goblet cell loss in response to desiccating ocular stress. Invest Ophthalmol Vis Sci. 2006;47:e-abstract 5579.
112. Ueta M, Hamuro J, Yamamoto M, Kaseda K, Akira S, Kinoshita S. Spontaneous ocular surface inflammation and goblet cell disappearance in I kappa B zeta gene-disrupted mice. Invest Ophthalmol Vis Sci. 2005;46:579–88.
113. Pflugfelder SC, Tseng SCG, Yoshino K, Monroy D, Felix C, Reis BL. Correlation of goblet cell density and mucosal epithelial membrane mucin expression with Rose Bengal staining in patients with ocular irritation. Ophthalmology 1997;104: 223–35.
114. Hirai N, Kawasaki S, Tanioka H, et al. Pathological keratinisation in the conjunctival epithelium of Sjogren's syndrome. Exp Eye Res. 2006;82:371–8.
115. Luo L, Li DQ, Pflugfelder SC. Hyperosmolarity-induced apoptosis in human corneal epithelial cells is mediated by cytochrome *c* and MAPK pathways. Cornea 2007;26:452–60.
116. Yeh S, Song XJ, Farley W, Li DQ, Stern ME, Pflugfelder SC. Apoptosis of ocular surface cells in experimentally induced dry eye. Invest Ophthalmol Vis Sci. 2003;44(1):124–9.
117. Tseng SC, Hatchell D, Tierney N, Huang AJ, Sun TT. Expression of specific keratin markers by rabbit corneal, conjunctival, and esophageal epithelia during vitamin A deficiency. J Cell Biol. 1984;99(6):2279–86.
118. Nakamura T, Nishida K, Dota A, Matsuki M, Yamanishi K, Kinoshita S. Elevated expression of transglutaminase 1 and keratinization-related proteins in conjunctiva in severe ocular surface disease. Invest Ophthalmol Vis Sci. 2001;42(3): 549–56.
119. Zhao H, Jumblatt JE, Wood TO, Jumblatt MM. Quantification of MUC5AC protein in human tears. Cornea 2001;20(8):873–7.
120. Argueso P, Balaram M, Spurr-Michaud S, Keutmann HT, Dana MR, Gipson IK. Decreased levels of the goblet cell mucin MUC5AC in tears of patients with Sjogren syndrome. Invest Ophthalmol Vis Sci. 2002;43:1004–11.
121. Yu DF, Chen Y, Han JM et al. MUC19 expression in human ocular surface and lacrimal gland and its alteration in Sjogren syndrome patients. Exp Eye Res. 2008;86:403–11.
122. Hicks SJ, Corfield AP, Kaswan RL et al. Biochemical analysis of ocular surface mucin abnormalities in dry eye: the canine model. Exp Eye Res. 1998;67(6):709–18.
123. Argueso P, Tisdale A, Mandel U, Letko E, Foster CS, Gipson IK. The cell-layer- and cell-type-specific distribution of GalNAc-transferases in the ocular surface epithelia is altered during keratinization. Invest Ophthalmol Vis Sci. 2003;44: 86–92.
124. Alliende C, Kwon YJ, Brito M, et al. Reduced sulfation of MUC5b is linked to xerostomia in patients with Sjogren syndrome. Ann Rheum Dis. 2008;67:1480–7.
125. Shimazaki J, Goto E, Ono M, Shimmura S, Tsubota K. Meibomian gland dysfunction in patients with Sjögren syndrome. Ophthalmology 1998;105:1485–8.
126. McCulley JP, Shine WE. The lipid layer: the outer surface of the ocular surface tear film. Biosci Rep. 2001;21:407–18.
127. Bron AJ, Tiffany JM. The meibomian glands and tear film lipids. Structure, function, and control. Adv Exp Med Biol. 1998;438:281–95.
128. Shine WE, McCulley JP. Keratoconjunctivitis sicca associated with meibomian secretion polar lipid abnormality. Arch Ophthalmol. 1998;116: 849–52.
129. Aho VV, Nevalainen TJ, Saari KM. Group IIA phospholipase A2 content of tears in patients with keratoconjunctivitis sicca. Graefes Arch Clin Exp Ophthalmol. 2002;240:521–3.
130. Henderson JW, Prough WA. Influence of age and sex on flow of tears. Arch Ophthal. 1950;43: 224–31.
131. McGill JI, Liakos GM, Goulding N, Seal DV. Normal tear protein profiles and age-related changes. Br J Ophthalmol. 1984;68: 316–20.
132. Nava A, Barton K, Monroy DC, Pflugfelder SC. The effects of age, gender, and fluid dynamics on the concentration of tear film epidermal growth factor. Cornea 1997;16(4):430–8.
133. Lucca JA, Nunez JN, Farris RL. A comparison of diagnostic tests for keratoconjunctivitis sicca: lactoplate, Schirmer, and tear osmolarity. CLAO J. 1990;16:109–12.
134. Tishler M, Yaron I, Geyer O, Shirazi I, Naftaliev E, Yaron M. Elevated tear interleukin-6 levels in patients with Sjogren syndrome. Ophthalmology 1998;105(12):2327–9.
135. Lam H, Bleiden L, de Paiva CS, Farley W, Stern ME, Pflugfelder SC. Tear cytokine profiles in dysfunctional tear syndrome. Am J Ophthalmol. 2009;147:198–205.
136. Virtanen T, Konttinen YT, Honkanen N, Harkonen M, Tervo T. Tear fluid plasmin activity of dry eye patients with Sjogren's syndrome. Acta Ophthalmol Scand. 1997;75(2):137–41.
137. Afonso AA, Sobrin L, Monroy DC, Selzer M, Lokeshwar B, Pflugfelder SC. Tear fluid gelatinase B activity correlates with IL-1alpha concentration and fluorescein clearance in ocular

rosacea. Invest Ophthalmol Vis Sci. 1999;40(11): 2506–12.

138. Sobrin L, Liu Z, Monroy DC, et al. Regulation of MMP-9 activity in human tear fluid and corneal epithelial culture supernatant. Invest Ophthalmol Vis Sci. 2000;41(7):1703–9.
139. Smith VA, Rishmawi H, Hussein H, Easty DL. Tear film MMP accumulation and corneal disease. Br J Ophthalmol. 2001;85(2):147–53.
140. Sack RA, Beaton A, Sathe S, Morris C, Willcox M, Bogart B. Towards a closed eye model of the pre-ocular tear layer. Prog Retin Eye Res. 2000;19(6):649–68.
141. Sternlicht MD, Werb Z. How matrix metalloproteinases regulate cell behavior. Annu Rev Cell Dev Biol. 2001;17:463–516.
142. Enriquez-de-Salamanca A, Calder V, Gao J, et al. Cytokine responses by conjunctival epithelial cells: an in vitro model of ocular inflammation. Cytokine 2008;44:160–7.
143. Schroder K, Hertzog PJ, Ravasi T, Hume DA. Interferon-gamma: an overview of signals, mechanisms and functions. J Leukoc Biol. 2004;75: 163–89.
144. de Paiva CS, Pflugfelder SC. Corneal epitheliopathy of dry eye induces hyperesthesia to mechanical air jet stimulation. Am J Ophthalmol. 2004;137(1):109–15.
145. Tuisku IS, Konttinen YT, Konttinen LM, Tervo TM. Alterations in corneal sensitivity and nerve morphology in patients with primary Sjogren's syndrome. Exp Eye Res. 2008;86:879–85.
146. Knop E, Knop N. 2005 Influence of the eye-associated lymphoid tissue (EALT) on inflammatory ocular surface disease. Ocul Surf. 3(4 Suppl):S180–6.
147. Tsuboi H, Matsumoto I, Wakamatsu E, Nakamura Y, Iizuka M, Hayashi T, Goto D, Ito S, Sumida T. New epitopes and function of anti-M3 muscarinic acetylcholine receptor antibodies in patients with Sjogren's syndrome. Clin Exp Immunol. 2010;162:53–61.
148. Sumida T, Tsuboi H, Iizuka M, Nakamura Y, Matsumoto I. Functional role of M3 muscarinic acetylcholine receptor (M3R) reactive T cells and anti-M3R autoantibodies in patients with Sjogren's syndrome. Autoimmun Rev. 2010;9: 615–17.
149. Iizuka M, Wakamatsu E, Tsuboi H, Nakamura Y, Hayashi T, Matsui M, Goto D, Ito S, Matsumoto I, Sumida T. Pathogenic role of immune response to M3 muscarinic acetylcholine receptor in Sjogren's syndrome-like sialoadenitis. J Autoimmun. 2010;35:383–89.
150. Goyal S, Chauhan SK, El AJ, Nallasamy N, Zhang Q, Dana R. Evidence of corneal lymphangiogenesis in dry eye disease: a potential link to adaptive immunity? Arch Ophthalmol. 2010;128:819–24.
151. Jin Y, Shen L, Chong EM, Hamrah P, Zhang Q, Chen L, Dana MR. The chemokine receptor CCR7 mediates corneal antigen-presenting cell trafficking. Mol Vis. 2007;13:626–34.
152. Nguyen CQ, Hu MH, Li Y, Stewart C, Peck AB. Salivary gland tissue expression of interleukin-23 and interleukin-17 in Sjogren's syndrome: findings in humans and mice. Arthritis Rheum. 2008;58:734–43.
153. Sakai A, Sugawara Y, Kuroishi T, Sasano T, Sugawara S. Identification of IL-18 and Th17 cells in salivary glands of patients with Sjogren's syndrome, and amplification of IL-17-mediated secretion of inflammatory cytokines from salivary gland cells by IL-18. J Immunol. 2008;181:2898–906.
154. Zheng X, Bian F, Ma P, de Paiva CS, Stern M, Pflugfelder SC, Li DQ. Induction of Th17 differentiation by corneal epithelial-derived cytokines. J Cell Physiol. 2010;222:95–102.
155. de Paiva CS, Chotikavanich S, Pangelinan SB, Pitcher JD, III, Fang B, Zheng X, Ma P, Farley WJ, Siemasko KF, Niederkorn JY, Stern ME, Li DQ, Pflugfelder SC. IL-17 disrupts corneal barrier following desiccating stress. Mucosal Immunol. 2009;2:243–53.
156. Chauhan SK, El AJ, Ecoiffier T, Goyal S, Zhang Q, Saban DR, Dana R. Autoimmunity in dry eye is due to resistance of Th17 to Treg suppression. J Immunol. 2009;182:1247–52.
157. Nguyen, CQ, Yin H, Lee BH, Carcamo WC, Chiorini JA, Peck AB. Pathogenic effect of interleukin-17A in induction of Sjogren's syndrome-like disease using adenovirus-mediated gene transfer. *Arthritis Res. Ther.* 2010;12:R220.
158. Nguyen, C. Q, Yin H, Lee BH, Chiorini JA, Peck AB. IL17: potential therapeutic target in Sjogren's syndrome using adenovirus-mediated gene transfer.*Lab Invest.* 2011;91:54–62.

Oral and Dental Manifestations of Sjögren's Syndrome: Current Approaches to Diagnostics and Therapy

14

Malin V. Jonsson, Nicolas Delaleu, Mihaela C. Marthinussen, and Roland Jonsson

Abstract

Saliva plays a detrimental role in oral health and disease. The quality and the quantity of saliva are determined by the glands it is secreted from, the sampling method, and whether secretion is stimulated or not (stimulated or resting saliva). Mucin-rich saliva lubricates the oral tissues, and lactoferrin, peroxidase, histatin, and a range of other substances provide anti-microbial, anti-viral, and anti-mycotic properties. Symptoms related to xerostomia as in Sjögren's syndrome (SS) are burning sensation of the oral mucosa and tongue, impaired taste, dry lips, oral soreness and ulcers, difficulties in speaking and chewing dry foods, and difficulties in wearing removable dentures. Clinically, the mucosa is dry and sticky and the examination mirror may adhere to the buccal mucosa. In addition depapillation of the tongue, explosive development of cavities (dental caries), and fungal/yeast infections (oral candidiasis) of the mouth and pharynx may occur. An objective measure of oral dryness can be achieved by sialometry of unstimulated and/or stimulated whole saliva. The possibility of using saliva as a fluid for biomarkers and its potential benefit in SS patient diagnosis and patient follow-up are elaborated. Finally, current approaches to relief of xerostomia and prevention/treatment of dry mouth-induced complications such as dental caries and oral candidiasis are presented.

Keywords

Anti-mycotics • Biofilm • Biomarker • *Candida albicans* • Caries • Chlorhexidine • Diagnostic fluid • Dryness • Fluorides • Hyposalivation • Oral cavity • Salivary stimulation • Salivary substitutes • Teeth • Xerostomia

M.V. Jonsson (✉)
Institute of Medicine - Section for Rheumatology,
University of Bergen, Bergen, Norway
e-mail: malin.jonsson@odont.uib.no

R.I. Fox, C.M. Fox (eds.), *Sjögren's Syndrome*, DOI 10.1007/978-1-60327-957-4_14,

14.1 Saliva in Oral Health and Disease

14.1.1 Saliva in Dental and Mucosal Defense

Saliva plays a detrimental role in oral health and disease. The fluid composition and specific components of saliva protect the dental soft and hard tissues by providing an effective set of systems for rinsing, transport of food, bacterial clearance, lubrication of dental surfaces and mucosa, neutralization of acid by buffering actions, maintenance of supersaturation of hydroxyapatite, participation in enamel pellicle formation, and antimicrobial defense [1]. Involving proteins such as mucins, lysozymes, albumin, and anti-proteases, active and passive mechanisms act as a protective shield against desiccation and environmental insult, penetration, ulceration, and potential carcinogens, reviewed in Ref. [2].

Saliva is produced by three paired major glands and numerous minor salivary glands. Over a 24-h period, the average person produces approximately 500–1000 mL of whole saliva. Depending on the demand or the current physiological status of the individual, the salivary flow rates vary considerably [3, 4]. The largest glands are the parotid glands, made up of mainly serous acini and secreting a thin, watery, and amylase-rich saliva. The parotid glands contribute to a little less than 50% of the stimulated whole saliva volume. In resting conditions their contribution is much lower. In absence of salivary gland stimulation two-thirds of the resting whole saliva is secreted by the submandibular glands. Although mainly serous, the submandibular glands comprise both serous and mucous acini, but in contrast to the parotid gland, the secretion is more viscous. The smallest of the major glands, the sublingual salivary glands, comprise mainly mucous gland acini and contribute very little to the volume of whole saliva.

The minor salivary glands are mixed glands and largely contain mucous acinar epithelial cells and are located in the oral mucosa and named accordingly; labial, buccal, palatine, lingual, and glossopharyngeal. In contrast to the low contribution to the volume of whole saliva, the minor glands secrete a large fraction of saliva protein important for lubrication [4].

The protein content and composition of saliva vary depending on from which gland it is secreted. Pure parotid saliva is serous, with approximately the same viscosity as water, whereas submandibular and sublingual saliva is mucous, with a more "ropy" viscosity due to its mucin content [4].

Together with the clearance effect, mucin and the enzymes lactoferrin, lysozyme, and peroxidase have been claimed to play an important role in the non-immune protection of the oral cavity. In addition, agglutinins, histatins, and proline-rich proteins, statherins, and cystatins are among the non-immunologic salivary protein components, reviewed in Refs. [5, 6]. Mucins are the principal organic constituents of mucus, the slimy, viscous material coating all mucosal surfaces and play a role in lubrication, tissue coating, digestion, and microbe–host interactions, reviewed in Ref. [7]. Lactoferrin is a protein mainly produced by the interductal cells of serous acini [8]. By binding iron, an important nutrient factor for different oral microorganisms, it displays bacteriostatic/bactericidal, antimycotic, and anti-viral effects, reviewed in Ref. [9]. Lysozyme can exert an anti-microbial function based on its muramidase activity. Lysozyme is a strongly cationic protein, which can activate bacterial autolysins, "suicide packages", that can destroy the bacterial cell walls [5].

Almost all salivary proteins are glycoproteins, i.e., have variable amounts of carbohydrates attached to a protein core. The glycoproteins are often classified according to their cellular origin, mucus and serous glycoproteins, respectively. Glycoproteins are then subclassed by their biological properties, for instance calcium-binding proteins such as statherin and proline-rich proteins, digestive enzymes such as amylase, anti-microbial proteins and peptides such as lysozyme, lactoferrin, and peroxidase systems, and agglutinins [1]. Polymorphism, or occurrence of a protein in multiple forms, is a characteristic feature of glycoproteins, having several functions and functional differences [10]. In addition, saliva contains secretory immunoglobulin A (sIgA), which can neutralize viruses and bacterial and enzyme toxins [6].

The oral cavity naturally harbors more than 500 different microbial species [11]. Among these, oral Streptococci, *Actinomyces* [12, 13], and *Candida* species [14] are the most frequent. Containing approximately 99.5% water and 0.5% organic and inorganic components such as electrolytes and proteins, saliva has the ability to modulate the oral microflora by favoring the attachment and proliferation of certain microorganisms and promoting the clearance of others [3]. Quantitative and qualitative changes of saliva can, thus, result in dental caries and erosion [15] and candidiasis [16].

Following intake of food containing fermentable carbohydrates such as sugar and starch, the pH in dental biofilm will drop and remain lowered until the carbohydrates are cleared from the mouth and the bacterial acid is buffered. The amount of acid produced by the bacteria and the saliva buffering capacity counteracting the decrease in pH determine the total decrease in pH. Demineralization of tooth enamel, the initial step in the caries process, occur when pH goes below a critical value; the pH at which saliva and biofilm cease to be saturated with respect to enamel mineral. Hence, it is crucial to reduce the amount of time that the pH stays below this value [4].

Saliva is buffered by three main systems, namely, the phosphate, the carbonate/bicarbonate, and the protein buffer system, reviewed in Refs. [1, 4]. Within the physiological pH range, hydrogen and dihydrogen phosphate are the dominant forms of phosphate. Unstimulated saliva mainly contains dihydrogen phosphate, whereas stimulated saliva contains mainly hydrogen phosphate. The total saliva phosphate concentration decreases with increasing flow rate. Consequently, the contribution of phosphate to the overall buffer capacity is reduced from 50% in resting saliva to approximately 10% in (highly) stimulated saliva [4].

The saliva bicarbonate concentrations vary from less than 1 mmol/L in resting saliva and up to 60 mmol/L in highly stimulated saliva [3]. Due to these variations, the contribution from the bicarbonate buffer system to the overall buffer capacity varies from a little less than half in resting saliva to more than 90% in stimulated saliva (at high flow rates). Hydration of carbon dioxide to carbonic acid is mediated by the enzyme carbonic anhydrase, which is present in the salivary glands as well as in saliva [4].

Last, several of the proteins in saliva can act as buffers. When the pH exceeds a protein's isoelectric point, the protein can release protons and accept protons when pH declines the isoelectric point. With their isoelectric point around pHs 5 and 9, many salivary proteins exhibit good buffering properties at alkaline, and especially at acidic pH values. The buffering effect of proteins is less than bicarbonate and phosphate in human saliva, but has its own niche in integuments on mucosa and teeth and become the predominant buffering substances at these sites. By increasing the viscosity of saliva when pH becomes acidic, some salivary proteins also contribute physically by forming a diffusion barrier that protects the teeth against acid load [4]. Buffering capacity of stimulated saliva is easily measured by use of commercially available test strips (Dentobuff® strip, Orion Diagnostica Oy, P.O. Box 83, FI-02101 Espoo, Finland).

14.1.2 Assessment of Oral Dryness

14.1.2.1 Subjective Symptoms—Xerostomia

Oral dryness creates an environment prone to development of disease in the oral cavity and associated tissues. In addition to protection against caries and other disease states in the oral cavity, such as bacterial and fungal infections, saliva is important for digestion, reviewed in Ref. [17].

The first step in assessing xerostomia and salivary gland hypofunction in the evaluation of SS must include a thorough interview of the patient, with the purpose of ruling out possible influence by medication, other chronic disease, and previous radiation therapy to the head and neck region. Of importance in the revised American–European criteria for SS [18] patient classification are also questions regarding symptoms of oral dryness, such as (1) daily feeling of dry mouth for at least 3 months, (2) recurrent feeling of swollen salivary glands as an adult, and (3) drinking liquids to help to wash down dry foods. In addition, the physician can ask whether the patient has less saliva than usual, if the dryness is more pronounced at night or day, and how much water he/she drinks during 1 day.

Dry mouth can influence patients' health, well-being, and overall quality of life [19], with impact on speech, changes in taste sensation, and swallowing difficulties. Patients' complaints may include burning sensation of the oral mucosa and tongue and impaired taste [20], dry lips, oral soreness, ulcers, difficulties in speaking, chewing dry foods, and difficulties in wearing removable dentures, reviewed in Ref. [21], summarized in Table 14.1. A recent study has also shown the economic impact of primary Sjögren's syndrome, manifested through increased oral health care costs. With careful management and use of appropriate preventive measures, many of the negative health consequences can be minimized [22].

When the mouth is examined, the oral mucosa and tongue may be dry and sticky and the intraoral examination mirror may stick to the buccal mucosa or tongue. An increase in facial mimics is often observed. In women, the "lipstick sign," where lipstick adheres to the front teeth, may be a useful indicator of xerostomia [23]. The cracker/wafer test has also been validated to identify individuals with xerostomia [24]. Lips may be cracked, peeling, and atrophic [25]. Clinical symptoms of dry mouth may include sensitive and depapillated tongue (Fig. 14.1a), explosive development of dental caries [25] at atypical sites (cervical, buccal, and incisal) (Fig. 14.1b), and fungal/yeast infections (candidiasis) of the mouth and pharynx [16]. In addition, pronounced tooth wear/dental erosion (Fig. 14.1c) may occur [26].

Table 14.1 Approximate frequency of oropharyngeal clinical manifestations in patients with Sjögren's syndrome. Adapted and modified from Rhodus [21]

Clinical manifestation	Prevalence (%)
Angular cheilitis	88
Glossitis	90
Mucositis	30
Candidiasis	83
Dental caries	100

The main reason for complaints and symptoms of oral dryness/xerostomia is a deficiency in the continuous secretion of mucin-rich resting saliva. Previous reports indicate that the submandibular and sublingual salivary glands are most severely affected in SS [27]. As a result, the lubricating saliva from these glands is the first that is lost, while the watery, protein-rich parotid saliva remains seemingly at first, unaffected. Although xerostomia most often is associated with low saliva flow rates, xerostomia may exist without the patient fulfilling criteria for the diagnosis of hyposalivation, and hyposalivation may be symptom less [20]. Most likely, the sensation of oral dryness is due to localized oral dryness, notably in the palate where the salivary film is the thinnest, and not a complete absence of oral fluids [28]. Consequently, total salivary secretion can therefore be within normal values, while unstimulated, resting saliva is affected, giving a low secretion rate.

14.1.2.2 Objective Measurements of Hyposalivation

Sialometry

Measuring of unstimulated and stimulated whole saliva are two simple screening tests for the salivary gland involvement in SS and should ideally be a routine part of any oral examination. Subjective reports of xerostomia are not sufficient when diagnosing SS [29, 30]. However, it is debated how objective and reliable the unstimulated salivary secretion measurements are and how the unstimulated secretion from the parotid gland compares to the submandibular and sublingual glands [27, 31, 32]. In any case, to obtain reproducible, valid, and comparable results, the test should be standardized to routinely be carried out in the morning or midmorning after the patient has been fasting overnight. In addition, cleaning of teeth, mouth rinsing, chewing gum,

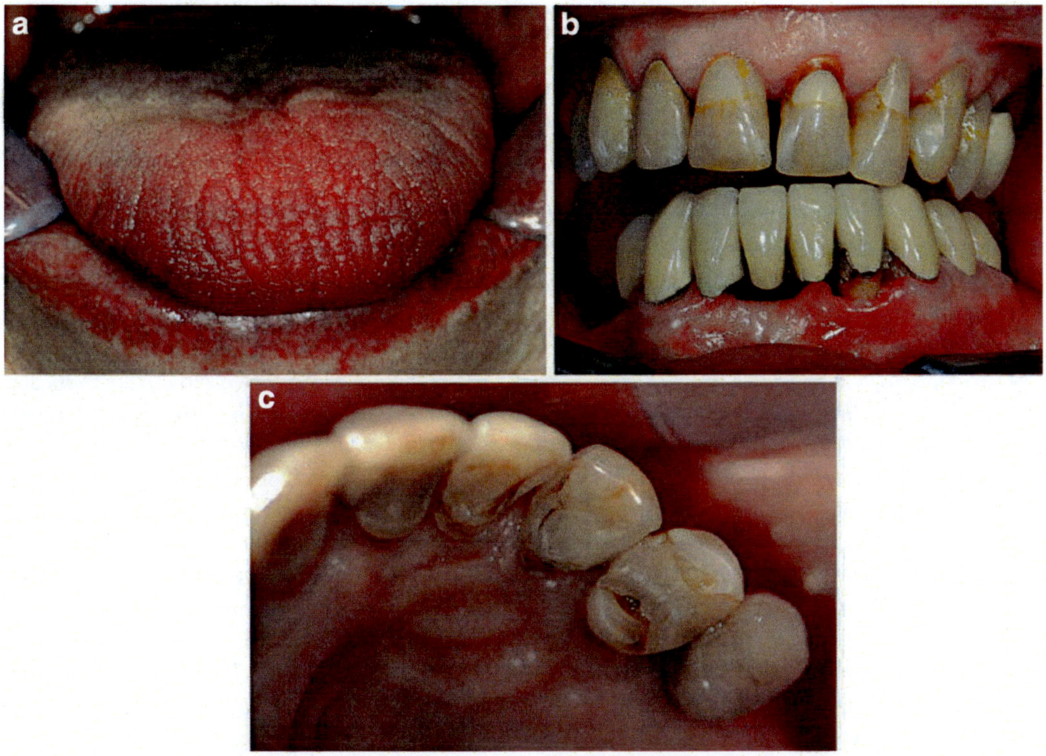

Fig. 14.1 Female patient with primary Sjögren's syndrome. (**a**) Sensitive, depapillated tongue with fungal/yeast infection (candidiasis). Note also dry, atrophic lower lip. (**b**) Extensive dental caries experience as indicated by fillings at atypical sites and abundant prosthetic restorations; buccal fillings in the upper jaw and a nine-unit bridge in the lower jaw. Recurrent cervical/root caries in the lower front indicate currently active caries disease. (**c**) Pronounced tooth wear/dental erosion on palatal and occlusal surfaces of the teeth

or smoking of tobacco should be avoided at least 2 h before the test is performed.

Tools required for measuring unstimulated and stimulated saliva are a timer and a 5 or 10-mL cylinder graded by 0.1 mL or, alternatively, a precision electronic weight balance with at least two digits and a plastic cup can be used to estimate the volume of saliva secreted. For stimulated saliva, 1 g paraffin may serve as an inert chewing material for masticatory stimulation of saliva secretion [4].

Unstimulated saliva is usually collected over 15 min and stimulated saliva collected over 5 min. Before collection of saliva starts, the patient should be seated in a chair and should relax for 10–15 min. The surrounding environment should be calm and relaxing.

Unstimulated saliva is collected without any masticatory or gustatory stimulus and is basically passive drooling of the saliva into the cylinder/cup. The patient should be seated in a relaxed position with elbows resting on the knees and the head tilted forward between the arms. Saliva is allowed to passively drain from the lower lip into a cylinder or pre-weighed container. Any movement in the tongue, cheeks, jaws, or lips should be avoided as this may stimulate secretion. Following an initial swallowing action, collection starts. After 15 min of drooling, the patient must empty all residual saliva into the collection device [4].

Stimulated saliva should be collected after the measurement of unstimulated salivary flow. It includes the same steps, except the application of an inert chewing stimulus and a shorter collection time of 5 min. Every time the mouth fills up with saliva, the patient is instructed to spit into the cylinder or pre-weighed container.

Flow rates can subsequently be calculated by reading the volume of saliva in the cylinder in milliliters and dividing by the number of minutes of saliva collection. Alternatively, saliva can be aspirated into a syringe and measured, or the cup of saliva can be weighed and after subtracting the weight of the container, salivary flow rate is calculated as g/min, considered equivalent to mL/min.

Unstimulated and stimulated whole saliva measurements are considered positive, i.e., decreased, when 1.5 mL/15 min or less, and 3.5 mL/5 min or less whole saliva is collected, unstimulated and stimulated saliva, respectively. Unstimulated saliva >0.1 mL/min was found to be sufficient to avoid the sensation of oral dryness [28]. A positive test for unstimulated saliva in patients with primary SS was found to be highly reproducible when repeated over a 1-year interval under standardized conditions [33].

The cut-off value for unstimulated whole salivary flow rate is ≤0.1 mL/min and that of paraffin-chewing stimulated whole saliva is ≤0.7 mL/min. These flow rates are significantly lower than "generally accepted" low levels; 0.3 and 1.5 mL/min, unstimulated and stimulated, respectively [34].

14.2 Saliva as a Diagnostic Fluid

Reliable diagnosis, assessment of a patient's individual risk, and the ability to monitor disease progression and treatment outcome are highly desirable goals in health care [35, 36]. In this context, oral fluids meet the need of an easy, non-invasive and inexpensive sampling method, which involves minimal discomfort for the patient [37, 38]. The use of saliva as a suggested diagnostic fluid allows repeated sample collection from large cohorts including risk groups such as aging individuals and young children. In most situations saliva can be collected in sufficient amounts, and such sampling does not expose patients or clinical personnel to additional health risks [37, 38]. Minimal sample processing, requirements before being able to analyze saliva for its constituents, further improves the applicability of saliva-based analyses in research and clinics [38, 39].

Saliva can be collected from an individual gland by using, for example, a Lashley cup, which adheres via mild suction to the duct orifice [38, 40]. Alternatively saliva can be sampled as whole saliva, which contains, compared to gland specific, more components that do not originate from the salivary glands specifically [38, 40–42]. Gland-specific saliva is primarily useful for the detection of pathological changes related to a specific gland, whereas whole saliva, due to its composition, is more prone to reflect both the state of all salivary glands and further the condition of an individual's systemic health [38, 40].

As already alluded to, whole saliva is a complex mixture that also includes, depending on the patient's oral status, a non-inflammatory serum transudate or inflammatory exudate derived from crevicular junctures around the teeth (i.e., gingival crevicular fluid), blood derivatives from oral ulcerations, and desquamated epithelial cells. Furthermore, exogenous components such as microorganisms, microbial products, and food debris are components of whole saliva [38, 40].

Gland specific or whole saliva can be collected with or without help of masticatory action, e.g., chewing on paraffin, or gustatory, e.g., application of citric acid, stimulation [38, 40]. For SS patient classification, the use of saliva to assess an individual's salivary gland involvement mandates the determination of the unstimulated whole salivary flow rate [18]. Importantly, stimulation of salivary flow does not only change the amount of saliva being secreted but also alters the relative volume of fluid contributed by the different types of glands to whole saliva. Furthermore, upon stimulation the molecular composition of saliva also changes according to the secreted proteins' biochemical properties [38, 43].

The quantity of saliva, however, is not only solely affected by the sampling method, but is also affected by other parameters such as hydration status, body position, exposure to light, circadian rhythms, circannual rhythms, food intake, smoking, and drugs [3]. Reliable measurement of secretion rate and valid diagnostic results critically depend on strict compliance with protocols for saliva collection controlling these factors [40, 43]. The most common methods for collecting whole saliva are the dripping/drooling method, in which saliva is allowed to passively drip/drain from the lower lip, and the spitting method, in which the individual actively disgorges the fluid into a collection tube [38, 40]; see also *Sialometry*. Handheld, microchip-based devices combining saliva collection and immediate analyses of multiple salivary protein or nucleic acid targets are further being explored for possible point-of-care diagnosis [44].

14.2.1 Biomarker Analyses in Saliva

Realization of the potential of saliva as a biofluid for health and disease discrimination and disease surveillance depends on three mainly factors: first, the ability of monitoring tissue-related changes in saliva relays on the paradigm that a specific tissue state is reflected in the spectrum and quantity of specific proteins liberated into certain biofluids [45]; second, the identification of specific biomarkers, which reliably indicate a specific condition [35, 45, 46]; and thirdly, the applicability of the proposed testing procedure in a clinical setting [35, 44].

In practice, a validated biomarker reduces the often ungraspable complexity behind the process it indicates to a rather simple measurement. In parallel, a high concentration of a certain protein in serum combines complexities related to factors, such as genetic background, metabolism, inflammation, and state of blood vessels walls, to an indicator of disease [47].

Today, most researchers anticipate that saliva principally reflects the entire spectrum of system states related with a patient's condition of health, irrespective of whether the disease involves the salivary gland or not [37–39, 45]. In addition, saliva is likely to reflect diseases involving the salivary glands more adequately than serum due to enrichment or unique presence of locally synthesized proteins in association with the disease process [37]. In this context, comprehensive efforts to catalogue the salivary transcriptome [42] and proteome [41] of healthy individuals are crucial to expand our general understanding of saliva and its composition.

One particular challenge when using saliva as a diagnostic fluid regards the notion that informative analytes are often present in significantly lower amounts in saliva compared to serum (see supplementary Table 2 of Ref. [48] for a selective overview). Indeed, molecules that are not produced by the glandular epithelium require to be translocated from the local vasculature into the salivary gland's interstitial space [39]. Subsequently, these constituents, together with molecules produced by tissues associated with the glandular epithelium, are transported by either the transcellular route (passive diffusion or active transport) or the paracellular route (ultrafiltration) into the lumen of the salivary glands where they become part of first, primary saliva and later, after traversing the ducts, final saliva [39].

The serum–saliva recovery rate depends on the biochemical properties of the molecule of interest [38]. This rather stable rate can, however, to a variable extent, be contaminated by serum components present in the gingival crevicular fluid or derived from oral ulcers [38]. At present, a few saliva-based diagnostic tests have been approved by the health authorities and are commercially available for screening purposes. Most notably, based on specific antibodies, saliva can be used to detect an HIV infection [49]. Considered as accurate as serological tests, these tests offer clinicians and patients a novel, simple, safe, and well-tolerated diagnostic method, which, in addition, improves the possibilities for epidemiological surveys. Interestingly, oral lesions did not seem to affect the results obtained by this method [49]. However, compared to exogenous factors, where this very factor, e.g., microorganism or drug component, largely defines the strategy for patient diagnosis and follow-up, the classification of other disease categories, such as cancer, cardiovascular, metabolic, neurological, and autoimmune disorders, often lacks such clear rational. The diagnosis of the latter is still largely based on clinical examination, often combined with histopathological evaluation of tissue biopsies and/or serological parameters.

The recent development of sophisticated, large-scale, and high-throughput genomic and proteomic platforms has created unprecedented possibilities to identify novel biomarker signatures for autoimmune diseases in a wide range of biofluids [35, 36, 45, 46, 50]. Improved sensitivity and the possibility of detecting multiple molecules simultaneously greatly aided saliva to become a biofluid recognized for its potential in biomarker discovery and subsequent use in a clinical setting. Technologies applied to biomarker discovery are either, at least theoretically, unbiased platforms such as microarrays covering the whole genome and mass spectrometry or biased technologies such as bead-based multiplex immunoassays, antigen arrays, or antibody arrays [35]. The inherent bias in the latter category is due to the use of existing capturing agents, e.g., purified proteins, peptides, or antibodies [35]. Which technology platform most accurately mirrors the true situation is often difficult to estimate, emphasizing the importance of appropriate and uniform guidelines for quality assurance and quality control [35]. One important task in the future also consists in the creation of bioinformatics tools for the analysis of disparate datasets such as mRNA profiles, protein profiles, and cell surface phenotypes [35, 51].

14.2.2 Exploration of Saliva as a Diagnostic Fluid in Sjögren's Syndrome

Compared with other systemic diseases that may secondarily affect the salivary glands, SS is a rheumatic disease, in which the exocrine glands are the principal target of an autoimmune reaction [52]. Histopathologically characterized by focal mononuclear cell infiltration in the salivary glands in the majority of patients, the disease significantly reduces salivary gland's secretory capacity through mechanisms that are not yet fully understood [52]. The degree of functional impairment, similar to the degree of inflammation, varies greatly among patients with SS and a direct correlation between these two parameters is not always obvious [53].

The actual diagnostic parameters, unfortunately, do not allow conclusions regarding underlying pathological processes, and a single marker or parameter specifically associated with all cases of SS has not been identified [18]. Also, the demand for an analytical test allowing detection of SS at an early stage has not yet been met.

Representing a less complex biofluid compared to blood, saliva has been suggested to contain disease-related molecules that reflect salivary gland pathology and conditions involving the oral cavity [38, 39, 41, 45]. Supporting such a notion, transcriptome-based diagnosis of oral cancers by analyzing saliva was shown to be slightly more accurate compared to blood-based analyses [54].

Salivary flow rates vary among patients with SS and salivary constituents have been subject to several biochemical studies in the field of SS since the early 1970s [39]. Sialochemistry consistently showed increased concentrations of sodium and chloride in saliva from patients with SS, whereas the levels of potassium and calcium appeared to be comparable with measurements obtained in saliva from healthy controls [15]. Other constituents altered in saliva from patients with SS included proteases such as lysozyme, kallikreins, MMP-2, and MMP-9 and members of the serine protease inhibitor family, e.g., cystatin C and cystatin S [39].

Elevated levels of total IgA and IgG together with the presence of autoantibodies against Ro/SSA and La/SSB have also been reported. Anti-La/SSB antibodies in saliva were primarily found in patients with especially low salivary flow rates and in some patients the antibody was detectable in saliva but not in serum or vice versa [55, 56]. Although anti-Ro/SSA and anti-La/SSB autoantibody levels in saliva and serum correlate significantly [56] and the number of antigen-specific antibody-producing cells in the salivary glands appears to be closely associated with Ro/SSA and La/SSB serology [57], the diagnostic value of these autoantibodies when measured in saliva remains to be determined.

By applying methods such as immunofluorescence and in situ hybridization, the presence and local production of several inflammatory mediators and autoantibodies in the salivary glands have been described (see supplementary Table 1 of Ref. [48] for a selective overview). The recent application of modern technology platforms to the field of SS allows for more comprehensive analyses of saliva collected from patients with SS and experimental animal models of SS [48, 58–60]. Although both frequencies of certain gene transcripts and specific proteins may represent valuable biomarkers, research based on specific proteins can rule out certain factors of uncertainty such as mRNA stability and correlation between mRNA copy numbers and levels of the corresponding protein. In addition, direct detection of proteins may facilitate conclusions regarding underlying molecular processes implicated in the pathogenesis of SS [60]. Indeed, a study combining global gene expression analyses with quantitative 2D gel electrophoresis-based mass spectrometry in pooled saliva obtained from SS patients revealed poor correlations between genomic and protein markers [58]. Interestingly, regarding the proteomic analyses, the panel of candidate peptide/protein markers for SS was clearly distinct from the panel described for oral cancer [54, 58], suggesting that the reported alterations in the salivary proteome may reflect rather specific conditions.

Using surface-enhanced laser desorption/ionization time-of-flight mass spectrometry and 2D gel electrophoresis-based mass spectrometry, Ryu et al. proposed to further explore lactoferrin, β(beta)-2-microglobulin, polymeric Ig receptor, lysozyme C, and carbonic anhydrase IV as potential diagnostic markers for SS [61]. These proteins, identified independently by both methods, were present in significantly different quantities in pooled parotid saliva from patients with SS when compared to non-SS controls with complaints of xerostomia. Subsequent mass spectrometry-based studies identified 24 and 42 proteins, which were significantly altered in pooled whole saliva from primary SS patients compared with healthy controls [58, 62]. Furthermore, pilocarpine administration partially restored levels or qualitative presence of several proteins identifiable by mass spectrometry to values comparable with measurements obtained in saliva from healthy controls [63]. Consistent in all studies, salivary proteomic profiles generated by mass spectrometry of primary SS saliva compared with profiles obtained from healthy controls indicated increased levels of proteins related to inflammation whereas amounts of acinar proteins were decreased. Interestingly, the profile associated with secondary SS resembled to some extent that of primary SS while in other aspects, being more similar to the profile of healthy subjects [59].

Nonetheless, mass spectrometry-based identification and quantification of immunological regulators, which operate at nanomolar to picomolar levels, still represent a great challenge, as abundant proteins might often mask relevant immunological modulators [50]. However, the technology is evolving at a fast pace and methods such as stable isotope protein tagging and subtractive proteomics may improve the number of less abundant and/or immune system-related proteins identified by mass spectrometry [50]. The gold standard for quantitative measurements is, however, still immunoassays due to the unmatched sensitivity provided by antibodies [36].

Applying comprehensive bead and antibody-based multiplex assays with the purpose to discriminate between mice presenting with SS-like disease and an SS unrelated strain, revealed besides 18 biomarkers in serum, 3 chemokines measured in saliva that had the potential to individually and reliably predict strain [48]. In a subsequent study applying the same technology, analyses revealed specific biomarker signatures, which, largely based on salivary proteins, could reliably predict treatment success regarding prevention of onset of hyposalivation as a result of immunization with heat shock protein 60 kDa (Hsp60) or Hsp60-derived peptide aa437–460 (Fig. 14.2a) [60]. Based on the same dataset, normal and impaired salivary secretion capacity, irrespective of strain and treatment group membership, could also accurately be predicted (Fig. 14.2b) [60].

Nevertheless, despite or due to significant technological advances and substantial research initiatives over the recent years, the reality of today is more than ever marked by an obvious gap between the large number of potential

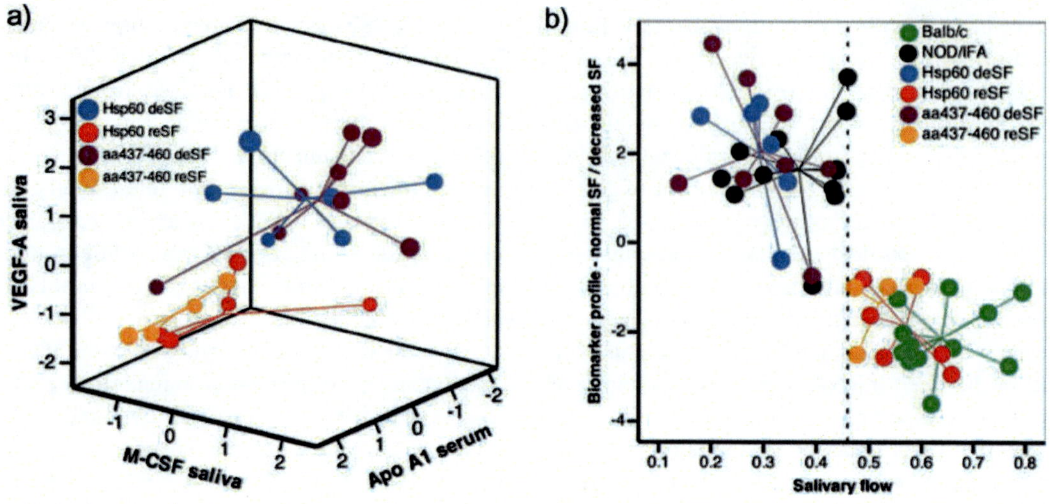

Fig. 14.2 Prediction of successful prevention of hyposalivation (**a**) as a result of treatment with Hsp60 or its derived peptide aa437–460 (hitrate: 95.8% cross-validated) and (**b**) normal and impaired salivary secretion capacity across strains and irrespective treatment group membership (hitrate: 93.8% cross-validated). Axes in (**a**): the discriminant score of the respective variables. In (**b**) The biomarker profile on the Y-axis comprises granulocyte chemotactic protein 2, myeloperoxidase, myoglobin, and macrophage inflammatory protein 3β(beta) in saliva and Il-1α(alpha) in serum. The X-axis indicates the salivary flow rate in μL/min/g. Untreated controls (*black*), mice treated with Hsp60 or aa437–460, in which the onset of hyposalivation could not be prevented (*blue and purple*, respectively), mice treated with Hsp60 or aa437–460 in which the onset of hyposalivation was successfully prevented (*red* and *orange*, respectively) and healthy controls (*green*). Figure adapted from Delaleu et al. [60]. deSF = treated mice with decreased salivary flow, reSF = treated mice with retained salivary flow

diagnostic markers proposed and the rare emergence of new, clinically applicable biomarkers [35, 36, 45]. As a significant core of knowledge attests saliva's great potential as a diagnostic fluid, significant efforts in identifying and especially validating salivary biomarkers remain to be undertaken. Consequently, we are likely to see increased utilization of saliva in research in general and biomarker discovery in particular.

14.3 Complications of Oral Dryness

14.3.1 Management of Xerostomia

Patients with reduced salivary function are predisposed to infections of the oral hard and soft tissues. To manage symptoms of oral dryness, it is imperative to identify the underlying cause [34]. In SS, the underlying cause of oral dryness is still a matter of speculation. Adequate symptomatic relief is possible with local palliative and systemic measures in many of the patients.

Nonetheless, the goal is to increase the amount of existing saliva or replace lost secretions in order to control the development of caries and, by specific measures, treat oral infections such as candidiasis (Table 14.2). There is not a definitive treatment for patients with SS, but treatment is rather directed toward local and systemic salivary gland stimulations, symptomatic relief, and prevention and treatment of local complications due to hyposalivation.

Clinical management of patients with SS demands an interdisciplinary collaboration between rheumatologists, ophthalmologists, oral medicine specialists, dentist, and dental hygienist. The physician does not necessarily need to handle all this information but has the possibility to, in relation to the patient, stress the meaning of preventive treatment in relation to oral and dental infections. Patients should be encouraged to daily carry out an oral self-examination for mucosal ulcers, lesions, or tooth decay, and report any unusual findings.

Table 14.2 Management of oral and dental complications of Sjögren's syndrome

Manifestation	Treatment
Xerostomia	Saliva stimulation
	Local
	Gustatory/masticatory stimulation with sugar-free/fluoride-containing tablets, xylitol-containing mints/lozenges, chewing gum
	Systemic
	Pilocarpine 5 mg × 4 times daily
	Cevimeline 30 mg × 3 times daily
	Acupuncture
	Saliva substitutes
	Artificial saliva, rinses, gels, sprays
	Use of bedside humidifier during sleeping hours
Caries	Fluorides
	Fluoride toothpaste applied twice daily
	One high fluoride application at home once a day
	or/and
	Weekly multiple applications using 1% NaF gel in custom-made tray
	Professional topical fluoride application of fluoride varnish; individual program relating to caries risk factors
	Salivary stimulation, and salivary substitutes, see above
	Oral hygiene
	Mechanical control of plaque formation
	Brushing with soft-bristled brush at least twice daily using low-abrasive fluoridated toothpaste or gel
	Daily flossing and/or interdental brush or toothpicks
	Anti-microbials
	0.2% chlorhexidine digluconat solution twice daily for 2–4 weeks
	1% chlorhexidine gel in individually fitted soft acrylic tray or used as toothpaste for 3 × 5 min for two consecutive days

Table 14.2 (continued)

Manifestation	Treatment
	Nutritional advice
	Analysis of food frequency; patients should complete a 5-day dietary record
	Reduce food intake to five meals daily; brush or rinse with water after every meal
	Drink lots of water
	Avoid sweet, soft, sticky, and spicy foods
	Dental care
	Caries recall
	2–4 times yearly to monitor caries risk, assess need for prophylactic and/or restorative therapy
	Dental plaque control and removal, motivation for oral hygiene
	Dietary instruction and advice (based on the patient's dietary history, see above)
	Topical application of fluorides
	Dental restorative therapy
	Avoid extensive dental prosthetic restorations unless caries cannot be controlled
Candidiasis	Topical
	Nystatin 3–4 times daily for 1 week
	Systemic
	Ketaconazole 200–400 mg tablets once or twice daily with food for 2 weeks, or
	Fluconazole 50–100 mg capsules once daily for 2–3 weeks, or
	Itraconazole 100 mg capsules daily, taken immediately after meals
Dentures	Denture adjustment
	Dentures should fit well
	Denture adhesives may be utilized when needed
	Denture hygiene
	Remove dentures at nighttime
	Clean dentures twice daily with dishwashing liquid
	Disinfect dentures periodically with sodium hypochlorite or chlorhexidine

Underlying systemic conditions must be eliminated and requires interdisciplinary collaboration between other health care providers

Findings such as an increase in caries activity, mucosal alterations, oral infections, and salivary gland enlargement may indicate salivary dysfunction. The dental team needs to explain the oral consequences of dry mouth in the patients' daily lives. Thus, patient education plays a central role. Early recognition will minimize damage and dysfunction and allow appropriate management to begin [25].

Dental caries is a multifactorial disease in which the simultaneous presence/occurrence of four main factors is detrimental: (1) host (teeth), (2) microorganisms (cariogenic bacteria), (3) substrate (fermentable carbohydrates), and (4) time [64]. In addition to these strictly biological factors, education, social class, income, knowledge, attitude and behavior, fluoride, and saliva will influence the development of carious lesions [65].

Caries lesions develop in so-called predilection sites where bacteria in biofilm are protected or difficult to remove, such as the occlusal surface, the approximal area between teeth, and cervically along the gingival border of the tooth. Important factors in the progression of caries are diet, fluorides, oral hygiene, and saliva [64]. In patients exhibiting alterations in saliva secretion capacity and saliva composition due to SS or other causes such as radiation to the head and neck region or xerogenic medication, atypical caries lesions such as incisal, cervical, buccal and lingual caries lesions, and rapidly progressing caries lesions are frequently observed [25]. In healthy individuals, caries on such "easy to clean" surfaces are uncommon and indicate a high caries activity [64], and studies have shown that unstimulated whole saliva composition was more important for caries development than stimulated whole saliva composition [66, 67].

Despite more thorough oral hygiene, patients with SS often present with more caries and fillings [15] and *Candida* infections [16]. Patients with SS and low stimulated salivary secretion were associated with *Candida* infection [68]. Fungal infections may be manifested as pseudomembranous or erythematous lesions in the mucosa, as median rhomboid glossitis and tongue fissuration, denture-associated stomatitis, or angular cheilitis, reviewed in Ref. [69].

14.3.2 Caries Preventive Measures

Caries preventive measures should aim to disrupt the four previously mentioned factors required for the formation and progression of caries. Early, non-cavitated caries lesions can be remineralized and, in theory, stopped from progressing by non-operative treatment. Manifest, cavitated lesions must be operatively treated, and further progression of the disease prevented to avoid secondary/recurrent caries and/or loss of restorations. Intensive caries preventive measures including an individually tailored prophylactic dental program are often needed [70]. The relation of saliva and dental caries is best documented in patients who have lost salivary function following tumoricidal radiation, and it is assumed that the same relationship exists in SS, reviewed in Ref. [71].

In a patient with dry mouth, key concepts of preventive dental care include measures to (1) increase the host factor resistance and quality, (2) modify the biofilm, (3) modify the substrate factor, and (4) affect the time factor. By this approach, individually adapted prophylaxis home programs including fluorides, hygiene measures, dietary advice, and salivary stimulation or substitution can be made for each patient, addressing each individuals' special needs.

14.3.2.1 Host Factors—Teeth and Saliva Fluorides

All patients with xerostomia should use some sort of supplemental fluoride in addition to fluoride toothpaste. The use of topical fluoride should be based on the severity of the patients' conditions as well as individual caries risk. The flour program should be made in collaboration with the dental team and the patient. A combination of in-office applied and at-home-based fluoride program is considered optimal.

Topical fluoridation may be effective for both prevention and possible remineralization of enamel. Supplements that contain sodium fluoride, acidulated phosphate fluoride, and sodium monofluorphosphate are present in different vehicles including gels, rinses, lozenges, and chewable tablets. Commercial fluoride varnish or lacquers, such as Duraphat® (2.26% F) or Fluor

Protector® (0.1% F), contain high levels of fluorides and are usually applied at intervals of 3–6 months in patients with hyposalivation/dry mouth.

For teeth, use of a fluoride-containing toothpaste with at least 1,500 parts per million (ppm) fluorides (F) is recommended. For high caries active patients recently introduced Duraphat® toothpaste from Colgate with 5,000 ppm F can be used either as an ordinary toothpaste or in an individually fitted tray. Non-foaming toothpaste with enzymes is seemingly milder to the dry oral mucosa and may be used instead of the conventional sodium lauryl sulfate (SLS)-containing toothpaste. SLS may disrupt the protective film of saliva on mucosa and, in an experimental model of oral mucosa, SLS induced epithelial shedding [72]. Available products are Salutem®, Sensodyne Proenamel®, and various Zendium® and Biotène® toothpastes.

In high caries active individuals, additional fluorides are warranted, for instance, provided by an individually fitted soft acrylic tray/spoon (Fig. 14.3) with 1% NaF gel used for 5 min/day [73]; custom-made fluoride carriers. This forces the fluoride into the interproximal areas and around the cervical margins. The combination of gels with 0.2% chlorhexidine and 0.05% fluoride may be beneficial by both suppressing oral bacteria and remineralizing the teeth [70].

Alternatively, in cases where gel treatment is not tolerated, patients can rinse their mouth with a 0.05 or 0.2% NaF solution for 1–2 min/day. Additional topical application of fluorides (see above) is then recommended. Patients with dry mouth should also be advised to avoid astringent products such as alcohol-containing or strong mint-flavored mouthwashes and strongly flavored toothpastes. It is also advised to use oral care products that have a neutral and alkaline pH, containing no sugar and with added lubricants.

In patients with low salivary flow, retention of fluoride is prolonged because of reduced oral clearance [4]. Systemic consequences of high-dose fluorides are critically discussed, but only very few randomized clinical trials on topical fluoride application are available, and a Cochrane review failed to present conclusive results regarding adverse effects of topical fluorides [74].

Stimulation

Local Salivary Stimulation

Patient's medication should always be checked for anti-cholinergic effects, and, if possible, changed to medication with fewer adverse effects. However, the systemic disease has a higher treatment priority compared to treatment of an oral condition and the necessary medication should not be changed for oral health reasons alone.

Gustatory and/or masticatory stimulation such as chewing food that requires more mastication, or regular use of sugar-free sweets or sugar-free chewing gum [75] are stimulants to increase the

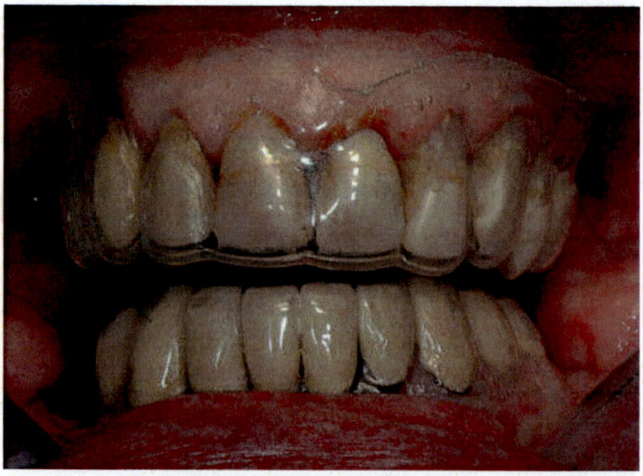

Fig. 14.3 Additional fluorides are recommended in high caries active individuals, for instance, 1% NaF gel used for 5 min/day in an individually fitted soft acrylic tray (custom-made fluoride carriers), forcing the fluoride into interproximal areas and around the cervical margins. Note buccal extension of tray to prevent leakage

secretion of saliva. Although patients may get the sensation that their mouth is drier following gum chewing, studies indicate that unstimulated salivary flow rate is not reduced even after prolonged gum chewing [76], and it was suggested that the sensation of dryness in such cases may be due to the excess of saliva during chewing.

Sucking on sugar-free saliva stimulating lozenges/tablets will increase salivary secretion through physiological stimulation of the taste buds. Ideally, tablets also contain low-dose fluorides; Xerodent® contains 0.25 mg F, malic acid, xylitol, and fluoride. According to the producer, this composition provides stimulation of saliva both by sucking on the tablet and by the buffered malic acid. Xylitol "protects" against caries and fluoride strengthens the tooth enamel. Such tablets can be ingested up to 12 times a day by patients with high caries activity. Sucking on regular fluoride tablets with concentration from 0.25 up to 1 mg F is also beneficial. In addition to fluorides, such tablets contain sorbitol and xylitol. However, it is important to remember that the use of tablet/lozenges will only be beneficiary if there is enough saliva to dissolve them. Another disadvantage of local saliva stimulants is limited effectiveness at nighttime when the symptoms are most severe.

Electrical stimulation of the salivary glands has been attempted. However, application is challenging and at best the results have been modest [77].

Systemic Salivary Stimulation

The Food and Drug Administration has approved two parasympathicomimetic medications, pilocarpine (Salagen®) and cevimeline (Evoxac®), for the relief of dry mouth symptoms [78–80]. Pilocarpine and cevimeline act via activation of muscarinic cholinergic receptors in the salivary gland tissue and may in patients with remaining functional salivary gland tissue lead to increased salivary secretion and ultimately improved subjective and objective symptoms. Common side effects of such systemic stimulants include extreme sweating, increased urinary frequency, flushing, and headache, reviewed in Ref. [34], and need to be prescribed in collaboration with the patient's physician to avoid possible unexpected side effects such as aggravation of heart disease or interactions with other medication. Parasympathicomimetics are contraindicated in patients with uncontrolled asthma, narrow angle glaucoma, and acute iritis and should be used with caution in patients with significant cardiovascular disease, Parkinson's disease, asthma, and chronic obstructive pulmonary disease, reviewed in Ref. [25].

The recommended dose of pilocarpine with minimal side effects is 5 mg four times a day (total 20 mg/day). An open, uncontrolled study evaluated the efficacy of a hydrogel polymer buccal insert as a controlled release delivery vehicle for pilocarpine in eight patients with SS [81]. The authors found that the insert delivered more than 85% of a 5-mg dose of pilocarpine hydrochloride with minimal side effects. The primary endpoint for the therapeutic efficacy is increased salivary flow. However, increased salivary flow does not necessarily give an improvement in subjective symptoms of dryness. In some cases it may require up to 4 weeks before the peak effect of pilocarpine is evident on salivary flow. Careful and frequent follow-up of the patient is important in order to assess clinical parameters as well as to determine adverse side effects and adjust dosage quantities and intervals. As long as the salivary flow continues to be stimulated and the patient does not suffer severe side effects, pilocarpine may be administered indefinitely. Pilocarpine may also be discontinued immediately and completely without adverse effects [78].

The recommended dose for cevimeline is 30 mg/day, given in three oral doses [79, 80]. Oral cevimeline was generally well tolerated in patients with SS [82]. Compared with pilocarpine, cevimeline has a 40-fold higher relative affinity for M3 receptors than for the M2 receptors found in cardiac muscle and a longer half-life in serum [83].

When saliva secretion can still be stimulated, a special type of acupuncture has been reported to provide some relief [84, 85], a possible alternative for patients who respond well to muscarinic agonists.

Systemic treatment with high doses of expectorant bromhexine have suggested a modest beneficial response in both tear and saliva flow, but controlled trials have failed to improve salivary output [86, 87].

Salivary Substitutes

Salivary substitutes and oral moisturizers intend to mimic the inorganic composition of natural saliva by containing calcium, phosphate, magnesium, and potassium and are the primary choices in initial, local treatment of xerostomia [88]. Depending on the degree of reduced salivary flow and xerostomia, artificial saliva can moisten and lubricate the mouth, but water may have the same beneficial effect. These agents attempt to replace essential salivary components with ingredients such as animal mucins, carboxymethylcellulose, polyglycerylmethacrylate, lactoperoxidase, glucose oxidase, lactoferrin, and lysozyme [19]. The substitute agents are formulated as solutions, sprays, or gels. However, viscosity, surface tension, and adsorption/desorption of saliva substitutes are different from the properties of whole saliva and may limit the duration and extent of their effects [89]. Preferentially, the pH is $\geq$6. Products containing anti-microbial proteins, such as peroxidase, lysozyme, and lactoferrins, are also available, with intent to compensate for the shortcomings of the host saliva. These products are most useful when used immediately before bedtime or speaking, but clinical studies on the efficacy of these products are still limited [70].

Small studies of over-the-counter oral moisturizers, e.g., Saliva Orthana®, Biotène®, and Oral Balance®, indicate that these agents can relieve oral discomfort [90–93]. There are few data to indicate superiority of any of the substitute products. Selection should therefore be based on availability and personal preference.

For instance, Saliva Orthana® contains natural mucin, namely, porcine gastric mucin and bovine mandibular mucin to simulate the viscoelastic properties of human saliva [94, 95]. At present, research is directed to saliva substitutes, which, besides wetting and purification, provide protection against microorganisms. Biotène® and Oral Balance® primarily contain three enzymes, namely, lactoperoxidase, lysozyme, and glucose oxidase, and the protein lactoferrin. The enzyme system penetrates the cell wall of plaque-forming bacteria, helping to maintain a healthy balance of oral flora [92].

Oral Balance® is a moisturizing gel that is applied toward the inside of the cheeks, lips, and on the tongue. The manufacturer claims that the gel quickly relieves dry mouth, protects against irritations and burning sensations for several hours, as well as promotes healing of inflammation. It is also recommended for use under dentures, reviewed in Ref. [96].

Biotène® is naturally sweetened with xylitol and provides a range of dry mouth products such as toothpaste, alcohol-free gentle mouthwash, and dry mouth chewing gum. The producer claims that Biotène® products are beneficial for patients with dry mouth. For the best results it is recommended to use Biotène® mouthwash in conjunction with Biotène® toothpaste, especially at bedtime [96].

Biotène® and Oral Balance® work by different mechanisms, and, therefore, using them in combination may be more effective [92].

Zendium® contains a composition of enzymes [97, 98]. According to the fabricant, the spray and saliva gel with fluoride can help patients with dry mouth by providing moisture. Both the gel and the spray can be used to supplement brushing.

Saliva substitutes based on polyacrylic acid and xanthan gum have also been developed and some studies have shown that they are effective for patients with extremely low salivary production rates [99]. Relief of symptoms may also be achieved by coating the lips and buccal mucosa with Vaseline®, oil, or glycerin swabs [70]. When at home the patient can hold ice chips in his or her mouth to provide moisture and hopefully relieve symptoms. For dry lips, a hydrating cream or ointment may reduce symptoms. Use of products with aloe vera or vitamin E may also be advised. In addition, several pseudopharmaceutical products and herbal supplements are available [25].

Smoking may be drying and irritating to the oral mucosa and should be avoided. An increase in environmental humidity is important. Patients, especially in the winter time often experience a worsening of their symptoms. Use of room humidifiers, particularly at night, may reduce discomfort [25].

14.3.2.2 Control of Plaque/Biofilm Formation

Dental caries is the clinical symptom of an infection with cariogenic bacteria. The most efficient way of treating caries is, therefore, to focus on removing the etiological factor, the bacteria in the biofilm, instead of merely treating symptoms by way of repairing cavities. Meticulous plaque control through excellent oral hygiene is important in prevention of dental caries. Patients should be instructed to brush their teeth at least twice per day using a soft bristled toothbrush and a low abrasive, highly fluoridated toothpaste or gel. Daily flossing is recommended. By simple measures, it is possible to measure levels of bacteria in the oral cavity, for instance, using stimulated saliva and the Dentocult® SM or Dentocult® LB (Orion Diagnostica Oy, P.O. Box 83, FI-02101 Espoo, Finland) for *Streptococcus mutans* and *Lactobacilli*, respectively. Elevated levels of cariogenic bacteria are found in the majority of patients with SS [100, 101]. High (>1,000,000 colony-forming units (CFU)/mL saliva) levels of lactobacillus may indicate a diet high in carbohydrates. For dietary advice, see below.

Not only the teeth, but the dental ful or partial prostheses require minute cleaning as well. Oral and dental prostheses are preferentially cleaned using a conventional dishwashing liquid as toothpaste may roughen up the surface making the prostheses more "available" to bacterial deposits. To reduce the number of bacteria, rigorous plaque control is of the essence; thorough cleaning of teeth, tongue, and oral cavity morning and night with non-abrasive toothpaste and an electric toothbrush and interdental brush, floss, or toothpicks [102]. Alternatively, rinsing with a 0.2% chlorhexidine digluconat solution can be employed on a daily basis for up to 4 weeks [103]. In patients with sensitive oral mucosa, chlorhexidine can be diluted 1:1 with water to a concentration of 0.1%. In cases where hygiene cannot be improved, 1% chlorhexidine gel can be used in an individually fitted soft acrylic tray or used as toothpaste. An application schedule of 3 × 5 min for 2 consecutive days is recommended. Cleaning and fluorides (see above) should be applied directly following meals.

14.3.2.3 Dietary Advice

Patients with salivary hypofunction have reduced oral clearance, causing increased retention of food and debris in the oral cavity [4]. Patients are therefore advised to reduce their food intake to a maximum of 5 meals/day, to drink a lot of water, and avoid soft and sticky food. Brushing with toothpaste after each meal or rinsing the mouth immediately after eating in order to remove food debris is advised. A recent study has shown that chewing sugar-free gum immediately after a meal may reduce the incidence of dental caries [75].

Liquid diets promote the formation of biofilm on teeth, and hot and spicy food can cause irritation or dry oral mucosa. Sugar, coffee, and alcohol also aggravate oral dryness. Patients should be encouraged to consume non-cariogenic foods and to maintain diets that enhance saliva secretion by proper chewing. Preferentially, patients should limit intake of foods and beverages that increase oral dryness, use sweeteners instead of sugar in coffee and tea, and avoid sweets and sugar-sweetened soft drinks. During meals, patients should be encouraged to sip water and rinse the mouth thoroughly with water following each meal [4]. Patients with SS should be encouraged to carry water with them at all times. Frequent sips of water will help to relieve dryness, ease swallowing, hydrate tissues, and cleanse the mouth [25]. In cases of nocturnal oral dryness, patients can be advised to let water rinse the mouth before swallowing.

Milk is a good source of protein containing all essential amino acids [104]. With cheese, milk is also one of the major sources of calcium in Western diets, although the amount of calcium, phosphates, and magnesium depends on the type of cheese and processing [105]. Cultured dairy products such as yogurt and buttermilk have a relatively low pH of 3.5–4.5. Nonetheless, due to the content of phosphate and calcium, the risk of erosive damage to teeth is low, and instead teeth are remineralized. In addition to calcium, phosphate, and proteins, milk contains lipids, all to which anti-cariogenic properties can be ascribed [104, 106, 107], and milk may be used for "sips" between meals.

The proteins in milk can be divided into caseins (80%) and whey proteins (20%) [104]. Casein phosphate peptides inhibit the growth of cariogenic bacteria such as *S. mutans*. In addition, they can form calcium phosphate on the tooth surface and provide a reservoir of calcium and phosphate ions, which buffer pH in plaque and provide ions that can remineralize the tooth [104]. Milk and dairy products can also affect and reduce bacterial adhesion to the tooth surface, change the composition of the biofilm, and improve the buffer capacity of the pellicle [104].

Patients should also be aware of the increased risk of tooth wear associated with hyposalivation or/and low buffering capacity [26, 108–110], and patients with low salivary flow should be aware not to consume acidic foods and beverages such as carbonated sodas in excess.

14.3.2.4 The Time Factor

Due to oral discomfort, tooth sensitivity, and mucositis, patients with SS may have problems with effective removal of dental plaque. With increasing awareness from the rheumatologist, dentist, and the patient, dry mouth patients can be diagnosed at an earlier time point and unnecessary destruction of dental hard and soft tissue be avoided.

Regular check ups every 3 months for follow-up at a dental clinic are recommended, with standardized control X-rays as often as every 6 months to monitor caries progression. Visits should contain dental plaque control and removal, dietary instruction, and advice, based on the patient's dietary history, as well as regular topical application of fluorides, e.g., Duraphat®, Fluor Protector®, or 2% NaF, to reduce caries activity and to help preserve the dentition.

Frequent appointments are necessary for regular topical fluoride application and control of and motivation for oral hygiene. Because caries at the gingival interproximal margins can progress quickly, patients with SS should also have frequent, high-quality bitewing radiographs. If caries cannot be controlled, extensive fixed prosthetic restorations are unwise and patients should be informed that former and present restorative work is susceptible to decay and may fail quickly [71].

14.3.3 Candida Infections—Prevention and Treatment

Candida albicans is part of the oral, commensal flora and will in stable health conditions colonize the oral cavity in small amounts. In situations where the immune system is suppressed or the anti-microbial effects of saliva are lacking as in SS, *C. albicans* may multiply and cause lesions in the soft tissue [68]. Patients with partial or full dentures with denture stomatitis often suffer from *C. albicans* infection, indicating suppression of the local immune system.

Infections with *C. albicans* may be asymptomatic, and lack of treatment is common. In patients with symptoms of oral candidiasis, an oral smear of the lesion is advisable. It is also possible to cultivate *Candida* from a chairside stimulated saliva sample by using for instance Dentocult® CA, which indicates excessive presence of *C. albicans* as brown colonies (Orion Diagnostica Oy, P.O. Box 83, FI-02101 Espoo, Finland).

Preferred treatment of oral candidal infections is topical application, as it allows the medication to be in direct contact with the tissues and the organism for a sufficient amount of time for control and elimination, reviewed in Soto-Rojas et al. [111].

Anti-fungal medications include nystatin, clotrimazole, and miconazole in the form of a gel, ointment, cream, suspension or vaginal tablets, to be used for weeks or months (Table 14.2). For mild cases of candidiasis, a suspension of nystatin (1,00,000 units) can be swished in the mouth following meals four times a day for 7 days, or a clotrimazole lozenge can be dissolved in the mouth. The corners of the mouth can be treated effectively with a nystatin ointment [69].

Oral rinses are useful for patients with dry mouth who may have difficulty in dissolving tablets. Unfortunately, some products intended for oral use are sweetened with sugar, thus predisposing dentate patients to dental caries. In more severe cases, ketoconazole or fluconazole may be administered for 7–10 days [69].

Poor oral hygiene predisposes individuals to *Candida* infections, hence dentures or oral prostheses should be removed at nighttime, thoroughly cleaned as previously described, and periodically disinfected using either sodium hypochlorite or chlorhexidine. Patients should also be encouraged to drink more water and use mouth moisturizers and saliva replacements, see *Section* 14.3.2 and Table 14.2 for recommendations. Consumption of sugar-free yogurt containing active yeast cultures may help to control oral fungal populations [25].

References

1. Van Nieuw Amerongen A, Bolscher JG, Veerman EC. Salivary proteins: protective and diagnostic value in cariology? Caries Res. 2004;38(3):247–53.
2. Dale BA, Fredericks LP. Antimicrobial peptides in the oral environment: expression and function in health and disease. Curr Issues Mol Biol. 2005;7(2):119–33.
3. Edgar MW, Dawes C, O'Mullane D. Saliva and oral health. 3rd ed. British Dental Association. London: BDJ Books; 2004.
4. Bardow A, Lagerlöf F, Nauntofte B, Tenuvuo J. The role of saliva. In: Fejerskov O, Kidd E, editors. Dental Caries. The Disease and Its Clinical Management. 2nd ed. Oxford: Blackwell Munksgaard; 2008, pp. 189–208.
5. Nieuw Amerongen AV, Ligtenberg AJ, Veerman EC. Implications for diagnostics in the biochemistry and physiology of saliva. Ann NY Acad Sci. 2007;1098:1–6.
6. de Almeida Pdel V, Gregio AM, Machado MA, de Lima AA, Azevedo LR. Saliva composition and functions: a comprehensive review. J Contemp Dent Pract. 2008;9(3):72–80.
7. Levine MJ, Reddy MS, Tabak LA, et al. Structural aspects of salivary glycoproteins. J Dent Res. 1987;66(2):436–41.
8. Reitamo S, Konttinen YT, Segerberg-Konttinen M. Distribution of lactoferrin in human salivary glands. Histochemistry. 1980;66(3):285–91.
9. Valenti P, Antonini G. Lactoferrin: an important host defence against microbial and viral attack. Cell Mol Life Sci. 2005;62(22):2576–87.
10. Levine MJ. Development of artificial salivas. Crit Rev Oral Biol Med. 1993;4(3–4):279–86.
11. Paster BJ, Boches SK, Galvin JL, et al. Bacterial diversity in human subgingival plaque. J Bacteriol. 2001;183(12):3770–83.
12. Beighton D. The complex oral microflora of high-risk individuals and groups and its role in the caries process. Community Dent Oral Epidemiol. 2005;33(4):248–55.
13. Aas JA, Paster BJ, Stokes LN, Olsen I, Dewhirst FE. Defining the normal bacterial flora of the oral cavity. J Clin Microbiol. 2005;43(11):5721–32.
14. Scully C, el-Kabir M, Samaranayake LP. Candida and oral candidosis: a review. Crit Rev Oral Biol Med. 1994;5(2):125–57.
15. Pedersen AM, Bardow A, Nauntofte B. Salivary changes and dental caries as potential oral markers of autoimmune salivary gland dysfunction in primary Sjögren's syndrome. BMC Clin Pathol. 2005;5(1):4.
16. Leung KC, McMillan AS, Cheung BP, Leung WK. Sjögren's syndrome sufferers have increased oral yeast levels despite regular dental care. Oral Dis. 2008;14(2):163–73.
17. Schenkels LC, Veerman EC, Nieuw Amerongen AV. Biochemical composition of human saliva in relation to other mucosal fluids. Crit Rev Oral Biol Med. 1995;6(2):161–75.
18. Vitali C, Bombardieri S, Jonsson R, et al. Classification criteria for Sjögren's syndrome: a revised version of the European criteria proposed by the American–European Consensus Group. Ann Rheum Dis. 2002;61(6):554–8.
19. Brosky ME. The role of saliva in oral health: strategies for prevention and management of xerostomia. J Support Oncol. 2007;5(5):215–25.
20. Bergdahl M. Salivary flow and oral complaints in adult dental patients. Community Dent Oral Epidemiol. 2000;28(1):59–66.
21. Rhodus NL. Sjögren's syndrome. Quintessence Int. 1999;30(10):689–99.
22. Fox PC, Bowman SJ, Segal B, et al. Oral involvement in primary Sjögren syndrome. J Am Dent Assoc. 2008;139(12):1592–601.
23. Scully C, Felix DH. Oral medicine—update for the dental practitioner: dry mouth and disorders of salivation. Br Dent J. 2005;199(7):423–7.
24. Sanchez-Guerrero J, Aguirre-Garcia E, Perez-Dosal MR, et al. The wafer test: a semi-quantitative test to screen for xerostomia. Rheumatology. 2002;41(4):381–9.
25. Fox PC. Xerostomia: recognition and management. Dent Assist. 2008;77(5):18,20,44–8; quiz 50–1.

26. Young W, Khan F, Brandt R, Savage N, Razek AA, Huang Q. Syndromes with salivary dysfunction predispose to tooth wear: case reports of congenital dysfunction of major salivary glands, Prader–Willi, congenital rubella, and Sjögren's syndromes. Oral Surg Oral Med Oral Pathol Oral Radiol Endod. 2001;92(1):38–48.
27. Lindvall AM, Jonsson R. The salivary gland component of Sjögren's syndrome: an evaluation of diagnostic methods. Oral Surg Oral Med Oral Pathol. 1986;62(1):32–42.
28. Dawes C. How much saliva is enough for avoidance of xerostomia? Caries Res. 2004;38(3):236–40.
29. Brun JG, Jacobsen H, Kloster R, et al. Use of sicca symptoms questionnaire for the identification of patients with Sjögren's syndrome in a heterogeneous hospital population with various rheumatic diseases. Clin Exp Rheumatol. 1994;12(6):649–52.
30. Brun JG, Madland TM, Gjesdal CB, Bertelsen LT. Sjögren's syndrome in an out-patient clinic: classification of patients according to the preliminary European criteria and the proposed modified European criteria. Rheumatology. 2002; 41(3):301–4.
31. Atkinson JC, Travis WD, Pillemer SR, Bermudez D, Wolff A, Fox PC. Major salivary gland function in primary Sjögren's syndrome and its relationship to clinical features. J Rheumatol. 1990;17(3):318–22.
32. Atkinson JC. The role of salivary measurements in the diagnosis of salivary autoimmune diseases. Ann NY Acad Sci. 1993;694:238–51.
33. Haldorsen K, Moen K, Jacobsen H, Jonsson R, Brun JG. Exocrine function in primary Sjögren syndrome: natural course and prognostic factors. Ann Rheum Dis. 2008;67(7):949–54.
34. Porter SR, Scully C, Hegarty AM. An update of the etiology and management of xerostomia. Oral Surg Oral Med Oral Pathol Oral Radiol Endod. 2004;97(1):28–46.
35. Balboni I, Chan SM, Kattah M, Tenenbaum JD, Butte AJ, Utz PJ. Multiplexed protein array platforms for analysis of autoimmune diseases. Annu Rev Immunol. 2006;24:391–418.
36. Lescuyer P, Hochstrasser D, Rabilloud T. How shall we use the proteomics toolbox for biomarker discovery? J Proteome Res. 2007;6(9):3371–6.
37. Wong DT. Salivary diagnostics powered by nanotechnologies, proteomics and genomics. J Am Dent Assoc. 2006;137(3):313–21.
38. Sahingur SE, Cohen RE. Analysis of host responses and risk for disease progression. Periodontol 2000. 2004;34:57–83.
39. Kaufman E, Lamster IB. The diagnostic applications of saliva—a review. Crit Rev Oral Biol Med. 2002;13(2):197–212.
40. Navazesh M. Methods for collecting saliva. Ann NY Acad Sci. 1993;694:72–7.
41. Denny P, Hagen FK, Hardt M, et al. The proteomes of human parotid and submandibular/sublingual gland salivas collected as the ductal secretions. J Proteome Res. 2008;7(5):1994–2006.
42. Li Y, Zhou X, St John MA, Wong DT. RNA profiling of cell-free saliva using microarray technology. J Dent Res. 2004;83(3):199–203.
43. Crouch DJ. Oral fluid collection: the neglected variable in oral fluid testing. Forensic Sci Int. 2005;150(2–3):165–73.
44. Gau V, Wong D. Oral fluid nanosensor test (OFNASET) with advanced electrochemical-based molecular analysis platform. Ann NY Acad Sci. 2007;1098:401–10.
45. Good DM, Thongboonkerd V, Novak J, et al. Body fluid proteomics for biomarker discovery: lessons from the past hold the key to success in the future. J Proteome Res. 2007;6(12):4549–55.
46. van der Greef J, Martin S, Juhasz P, et al. The art and practice of systems biology in medicine: mapping patterns of relationships. J Proteome Res. 2007 Apr;6(4):1540–59.
47. Lewington S, Whitlock G, Clarke R, et al. Blood cholesterol and vascular mortality by age, sex, and blood pressure: a meta-analysis of individual data from 61 prospective studies with 55,000 vascular deaths. Lancet. 2007;370(9602):1829–39.
48. Delaleu N, Immervoll H, Cornelius J, Jonsson R. Biomarker profiles in serum and saliva of experimental Sjögren's syndrome: associations with specific autoimmune manifestations. Arthritis Res Ther. 2008;10(1):R22.
49. Malamud D. Oral diagnostic testing for detecting human immunodeficiency virus-1 antibodies: a technology whose time has come. Am J Med. 1997;102(4A):9–14.
50. Veenstra TD. Global and targeted quantitative proteomics for biomarker discovery. J Chromatogr B Analyt Technol Biomed Life Sci. 2007;847(1):3–11.
51. Cline MS, Smoot M, Cerami E, et al. Integration of biological networks and gene expression data using cytoscape. Nat Protoc. 2007;2(10):2366–82.
52. Delaleu N, Jonsson R, Koller MM. Sjögren's syndrome. Eur J Oral Sci. 2005;113(2):101–13.
53. Dawson LJ, Fox PC, Smith PM. Sjögrens syndrome—the non-apoptotic model of glandular hypofunction. Rheumatology. 2006;45(7):792–8.
54. Li Y, St John MA, Zhou X, et al. Salivary transcriptome diagnostics for oral cancer detection. Clin Cancer Res. 2004;10(24):8442–850.
55. Horsfall AC, Rose LM, Maini RN. Autoantibody synthesis in salivary glands of Sjögren's syndrome patients. J Autoimmun. 1989;2(4):559–68.
56. Sreebny L, Zhu WX. Whole saliva and the diagnosis of Sjögren's syndrome: an evaluation of patients who complain of dry mouth and dry eyes. Part 2: immunologic findings. Gerodontology. 1996;13(1):44–8.

57. Tengner P, Halse AK, Haga HJ, Jonsson R, Wahren-Herlenius M. Detection of anti-Ro/SSA and anti-La/SSB autoantibody-producing cells in salivary glands from patients with Sjögren's syndrome. Arthritis Rheum. 1998;41(12):2238–48.
58. Hu S, Wang J, Meijer J, et al. Salivary proteomic and genomic biomarkers for primary Sjögren's syndrome. Arthritis Rheum. 2007;56(11):3588–600.
59. Baldini C, Giusti L, Bazzichi L, Lucacchini A, Bombardieri S. Proteomic analysis of the saliva: a clue for understanding primary from secondary Sjögren's syndrome? Autoimmun Rev. 2008;7(3):185–91.
60. Delaleu N, Madureira AC, Immervoll H, Jonsson R. Inhibition of experimental Sjögren's syndrome through immunization with HSP60 and its peptide amino acids 437–460. Arthritis Rheum. 2008;58(8):2318–28.
61. Ryu OH, Atkinson JC, Hoehn GT, Illei GG, Hart TC. Identification of parotid salivary biomarkers in Sjögren's syndrome by surface-enhanced laser desorption/ionization time-of-flight mass spectrometry and two-dimensional difference gel electrophoresis. Rheumatology. 2006;45(9):1077–86.
62. Giusti L, Baldini C, Bazzichi L, Ciregia F, Tonazzini I, Mascia G, et al. Proteome analysis of whole saliva: a new tool for rheumatic diseases—the example of Sjögren's syndrome. Proteomics. 2007;7(10):1634–43.
63. Peluso G, De Santis M, Inzitari R, et al. Proteomic study of salivary peptides and proteins in patients with Sjögren's syndrome before and after pilocarpine treatment. Arthritis Rheum. 2007;56(7):2216–22.
64. Fejerskov O, Nyvad B, Kidd EAM. Pathology of dental caries. In: Fejerskov O, Kidd E, editors. Dental caries. The disease and its clinical management. 2nd ed. Oxford: Blackwell Munksgaard; 2008, pp. 19–48.
65. Fejerskov O, Manji F. Reactor paper: risk assessment in dental caries. In: Bader JD, editor. Risk assessment in dentistry. Chapel Hill: University of North Carolina Dental Ecology; 1990, pp. 215–7.
66. Bardow A, Hofer E, Nyvad B, et al. Effect of saliva composition on experimental root caries. Caries Res. 2005;39(1):71–7.
67. Dawes C. A mathematical model of salivary clearance of sugar from the oral cavity. Caries Res. 1983;17(4):321–34.
68. Radfar L, Shea Y, Fischer SH, et al. Fungal load and candidiasis in Sjögren's syndrome. Oral Surg Oral Med Oral Pathol Oral Radiol Endod. 2003;96(3):283–7.
69. Ellepola AN, Samaranayake LP. Oral candidal infections and antimycotics. Crit Rev Oral Biol Med. 2000;11(2):172–98.
70. Kidd EAM, Nyvad B, Espelid I. Caries control for the individual patient. In: Fejerskov O, Kidd E, editors. Dental caries. The disease and its clinical management. 2nd ed. Oxford: Blackwell Munksgaard; 2008, pp. 487–504.
71. Atkinson JC, Fox PC. Sjögren's syndrome: oral and dental considerations. J Am Dent Assoc. 1993;124(3):74–6, 78–82, 84–6.
72. Neppelberg E, Costea DE, Vintermyr OK, Johannessen AC. Dual effects of sodium lauryl sulphate on human oral epithelial structure. Exp Dermatol. 2007;16(7):574–9.
73. Dreizen S, Brown LR, Daly TE, Drane JB. Prevention of xerostomia-related dental caries in irradiated cancer patients. J Dent Res. 1977;56(2):99–104.
74. Marinho VC, Higgins JP, Logan S, Sheiham A. Topical fluoride (toothpastes, mouthrinses, gels or varnishes) for preventing dental caries in children and adolescents. Cochrane Database Syst Rev. 2003(4):CD002782.
75. Stookey GK. The effect of saliva on dental caries. J Am Dent Assoc. 2008;139 (Suppl):11S–17S.
76. Dawes C. The unstimulated salivary flow rate after prolonged gum chewing. Arch Oral Biol. 2005;50(6):561–3.
77. Strietzel FP, Martin-Granizo R, Fedele S, et al. Electrostimulating device in the management of xerostomia. Oral Dis. 2007;13(2):206–13.
78. Vivino FB, Al-Hashimi I, Khan Z, et al. Pilocarpine tablets for the treatment of dry mouth and dry eye symptoms in patients with Sjögren syndrome: a randomized, placebo-controlled, fixed-dose, multicenter trial. P92-01 Study Group. Arch Intern Med. 1999;159(2):174–81.
79. Fife RS, Chase WF, Dore RK, et al. Cevimeline for the treatment of xerostomia in patients with Sjögren syndrome: a randomized trial. Arch Intern Med. 2002;162(11):1293–300.
80. Petrone D, Condemi JJ, Fife R, Gluck O, Cohen S, Dalgin P. A double-blind, randomized, placebo-controlled study of cevimeline in Sjögren's syndrome patients with xerostomia and keratoconjunctivitis sicca. Arthritis Rheum. 2002;46(3):748–54.
81. Gibson J, Halliday JA, Ewert K, Robertson S. A controlled release pilocarpine buccal insert in the treatment of Sjögren's syndrome. Br Dent J. 2007;202(7):E17; discussion 404–5.
82. Weber J, Keating GM. Cevimeline. Drugs. 2008;68(12):1691–8.
83. Fox RI. Use of cevimeline, a muscarinic M1 and M3 agonist, in the treatment of Sjögren's syndrome. Adv Exp Med Biol. 2002;506(Pt B):1107–16.
84. Blom M, Lundeberg T. Long-term follow-up of patients treated with acupuncture for xerostomia and the influence of additional treatment. Oral Dis. 2000;6(1):15–24.
85. Grisius MM. Salivary gland dysfunction: a review of systemic therapies. Oral Surg Oral Med Oral Pathol Oral Radiol Endod. 2001;92(2):156–62.
86. Frost-Larsen K, Isager H, Manthorpe R. Sjögren's syndrome treated with bromhexine: a randomised clinical study. Br Med J. 1978;1(6127):1579–81.

87. Prause JU, Frost-Larsen K, Hoj L, Isager H, Manthorpe R. Lacrimal and salivary secretion in Sjögren's syndrome: the effect of systemic treatment with bromhexine. Acta Ophthalmol. 1984;62(3):489–97.
88. von Bultzingslöven I, Sollecito TP, Fox PC, et al. Salivary dysfunction associated with systemic diseases: systematic review and clinical management recommendations. Oral Surg Oral Med Oral Pathol Oral Radiol Endod. 2007;103 (Suppl):S57 e1–e15.
89. Christersson CE, Lindh L, Arnebrant T. Film-forming properties and viscosities of saliva substitutes and human whole saliva. Eur J Oral Sci. 2000;108(5):418–25.
90. Guggenheimer J, Moore PA. Xerostomia: etiology, recognition and treatment. J Am Dent Assoc. 2003;134(1):61–9; quiz 118–9.
91. Rhodus NL, Bereuter J. Clinical evaluation of a commercially available oral moisturizer in relieving signs and symptoms of xerostomia in postirradiation head and neck cancer patients and patients with Sjögren's syndrome. J Otolaryngol. 2000;29(1): 28–34.
92. Warde P, Kroll B, O'Sullivan B, et al. A phase II study of Biotene in the treatment of postradiation xerostomia in patients with head and neck cancer. Support Care Cancer. 2000;8(3):203–8.
93. Epstein JB, Emerton S, Le ND, Stevenson-Moore P. A double-blind crossover trial of Oral Balance gel and Biotene toothpaste versus placebo in patients with xerostomia following radiation therapy. Oral Oncol. 1999;35(2):132–7.
94. Vissink A, Schaub RM, van Rijn LJ, Gravenmade EJ, Panders AK, Vermey A. The efficacy of mucin-containing artificial saliva in alleviating symptoms of xerostomia. Gerodontology. 1987;6(3): 95–101.
95. Davies AN. A comparison of artificial saliva and chewing gum in the management of xerostomia in patients with advanced cancer. Palliat Med. 2000;14(3):197–203.
96. Cassolato SF, Turnbull RS. Xerostomia: clinical aspects and treatment. Gerodontology. 2003;20(2):64–77.
97. Pedersen AM, Andersen TL, Reibel J, Holmstrup P, Nauntofte B. Oral findings in patients with primary Sjögren's syndrome and oral lichen planus—a preliminary study on the effects of bovine colostrum-containing oral hygiene products. Clin Oral Investig. 2002;6(1):11–20.
98. Nieuw Amerongen AV, Veerman EC. Current therapies for xerostomia and salivary gland hypofunction associated with cancer therapies. Support Care Cancer. 2003;11(4):226–31.
99. van der Reijden WA, van der Kwaak H, Vissink A, Veerman EC, Amerongen AV. Treatment of xerostomia with polymer-based saliva substitutes in patients with Sjögren's syndrome. Arthritis Rheum. 1996;39(1):57–63.
100. Almståhl A, Kroneld U, Tarkowski A, Wikström M. Oral microbial flora in Sjögren's syndrome. J Rheumatol. 1999;26(1):110–14.
101. Kolavic SA, Gibson G, al-Hashimi I, Guo IY. The level of cariogenic micro-organisms in patients with Sjögren's syndrome. Spec Care Dentist. 1997;17(2):65–9.
102. Nyvad B. Role of oral hygiene. In: Fejerskov O, Kidd E, eds. Dental Caries. The Disease and Its Clinical Management. 2nd ed. Oxford: Blackwell Munksgaard; 2008:257–64.
103. Scheie AA, Petersen FC. Antimicrobials in caries control. In: Fejerskov O, Kidd E, ed. Dental Caries. The Disease and Its Clinical Management. 2nd ed. Oxford: Blackwell Munksgaard; 2008:265–78.
104. Aimutis WR. Bioactive properties of milk proteins with particular focus on anticariogenesis. J Nutr. 2004 Apr;134(4):989S–95S.
105. Henning DR, Baer RJ, Hassan AN, Dave R. Major advances in concentrated and dry milk products, cheese, and milk fat-based spreads. J Dairy Sci. 2006;89(4):1179–88.
106. Shaw JH, Ensfield BJ, Wollman DH. Studies on the relation of dairy products to dental caries in caries-susceptible rats. J Nutr. 1959;67(2):253–73.
107. Harper DS, Osborn JC, Clayton R, Hefferren JJ. Modification of food cariogenicity in rats by mineral-rich concentrates from milk. J Dent Res. 1987;66(1):42–5.
108. Järvinen VK, Rytömaa, II, Heinonen OP. Risk factors in dental erosion. J Dent Res. 1991;70(6): 942–7.
109. Rytömaa I, Järvinen V, Kanerva R, Heinonen OP. Bulimia and tooth erosion. Acta Odontol Scand. 1998;56(1):36–40.
110. Lussi A, Schaffner M. Progression of and risk factors for dental erosion and wedge-shaped defects over a 6-year period. Caries Res. 2000;34(2):182–7.
111. Soto-Rojas AE, Kraus A. The oral side of Sjögren syndrome. Diagnosis and treatment. A review. Arch Med Res. 2002;33(2):95–106.

Etiology and Pathogenesis of Sjögren's Syndrome with Special Emphasis on the Salivary Glands

15

Nicolas Delaleu, Menelaos N. Manoussakis, Haralampos M. Moutsopoulos, and Roland Jonsson

Abstract

Pathogenesis from the Greek pathos, "disease," and genesis, "creation," is the process by which an etiological factor and subsequent downstream events cause disease. Although in Sjögren's syndrome (SS), alike for most other autoimmune diseases, the enigma leading to a pathogenic attack against self has not yet been solved, the disease must be mediated by specific immune reactions against somatic cells to qualify as an autoimmune disease. In SS the autoimmune response is greatly directed against the exocrine glands, which, as histopathological hallmark of the disease, display persistent focal mononuclear cell infiltrates. Clinically, the disease in most patients is manifested by two local severe symptoms: dryness of the mouth (xerostomia) and the eyes (keratoconjunctivitis sicca). A number of systemic features have also been described and the presence of autoantibodies against the ubiquitously expressed ribonucleoprotein particles Ro (SSA) and La (SSB) further underlines the systemic nature of SS. The original explanatory concept for the pathogenesis of SS proposed a specific, self-perpetuating, immune-mediated loss of acinar and ductal cells as the principal cause of salivary gland hypofunction. Although straightforward and plausible, the hypothesis, however, falls short of accommodating several SS-related phenomena and experimental findings. Consequently, researchers considered immune-mediated salivary gland dysfunction prior to glandular destruction and atrophy as potential molecular mechanisms underlying the symptoms of dryness in SS. Accordingly, apoptosis, fibrosis, and atrophy of the salivary glands would represent consequences of salivary gland hypofunction. This chapter will

R. Jonsson (✉)
Broegelmann Research Laboratory, The Gade Institute, University of Bergen, Bergen, Norway; Department of Rheumatology, Haukeland University Hospital, Bergen, Norway
e-mail: roland.jonsson@gades.uib.no

R.I. Fox, C.M. Fox (eds.), *Sjögren's Syndrome*, DOI 10.1007/978-1-60327-957-4_15,

also put into perspective research involving the etiology of SS by discussing the results in a broader context along lines drawn by the different basic concepts of immunity.

Keywords
Sjögren's syndrome • Etiology • Pathogenesis • Interferon • Toll-like receptors • B cells • Biomarkers

15.1 The Manifestation of Sjögren's Syndrome in the Salivary Glands

Primarily for diagnostic purposes, a salivary gland biopsy is evaluated for the presence and frequency of focal cellular aggregates, defined as clusters of at least 50 mononuclear cells [1]. Inflammatory foci tend to form around the ductal epithelium and infiltrates seem to subsequently expand and occupy at a later-stage acinar epithelium as well [2]. Analyses of gene expression profiles of salivary gland tissue from patients with SS confirmed the presence of many aspects of chronic inflammation [3–5]. The infiltrates in the salivary glands consist of T cells, B cells [6, 7], plasmacytoid dendritic cells (pDCs) [5], follicular DCs (FDC) [8], and macrophages [9]. Recent studies in rather large patient groups indicated that ultrasonography (US) and magnetic resonance imaging might be promising alternatives to the conventional invasive sampling of a lower lip biopsy [10, 11]. Whereas US takes the advantage as a diagnostic tool for routine examinations, both methods appear to correlate well with results obtained using histopathological evaluations [10, 11]. Such non-invasive imaging technologies have, however, not yet been applied to fields such as disease progression or prognosis and follow-up on treatment interventions in SS. These areas of study would most certainly benefit from a non-invasive method to access salivary gland pathology.

15.1.1 Endothelial Cells

Endothelial cells lining the lumina of blood vessels are involved in leukocyte extravasation as immune responses require the orchestrated movement of cells in particular directions to specific locations [12] (Fig. 15.1). Leukocytes thereby migrate in response to, and along concentration gradients of chemotactic factors such as chemokines [13]. Despite their uncontested potential as candidates for therapeutic intervention, and their involvement in angiogenesis, fibrosis, and malignancy [14], chemokines remain a rather poorly examined field of study in SS [15–19]. The growth of blood vessels from pre-existing vasculature, termed angiogenesis or neovascularization, contributes significantly to inflammatory cell migration and depends critically on the balance or imbalance between angiogenic mediators and inhibitors [20, 21]. Neovascularization is recognized as a pathogenic process in rheumatoid arthritis (RA) and key molecules in the molecular pathway of angiogenesis have been explored as targets for therapeutic intervention [22]. In the field of SS, conclusions derived from experimental studies argue for an interrelationship between neovascularization and impaired secretory function [19]. Additional research initiatives, however, need to clarify the exact role of neovascularization in the formation and perpetuation of the salivary gland pathology characteristic for SS.

Lymphocyte migration into the target tissue in SS is partly mediated by vascular cell adhesion molecule (VCAM)-1 and peripheral node addressin (PNAd) expressed on vascular endothelium (Fig. 15.1). Inhibition of these two molecules or their ligands (α4-integrin, L-selectin, and lymphocyte function-associated antigen-1 [LFA-1]) showed a nearly complete block of lymphocyte migration into the lacrimal glands of non-obese diabetic (NOD) mice [23], a strain accepted as a model of SS [24, 25].

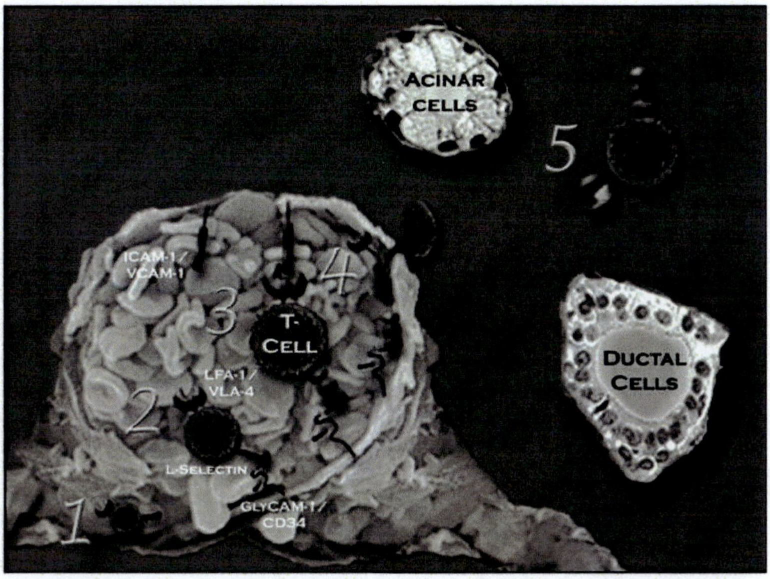

Fig. 15.1 Mechanisms involved in lymphocyte migration. An important feature in regulation of lymphocyte recirculation is the ability of lymphocytes to recognize and bind to the surface of endothelial cells before migrating through the vessel into surrounding tissue. (1) Circulating lymphocytes enter high endothelial venules. (2) *Initial transient tethering and rolling*: most lymphocyte adhesion molecules such as L-selectin are found on the tips of the lymphocytes microvilli where they can easily contact the endothelium by binding glycosylation-dependent cell adhesion molecule (GlyCAM)-1 or CD34. (3) *Appropriate activating factors*: chemokines such as CXCL13 encountered in the local environment render possible a first lymphocyte activation step which facilitates firm adhesion. Activated integrins, LFA-1 and VLA-4, on lymphocytes interact with ICAMs and VCAMs. (4) *Lymphocyte diapedesis*: migration through endothelium, from circulation to tissue, a process probably also directed by chemokines. (5) Migrated lymphocytes contribute to the local immune response. Figure adapted from Delaleu et al. [229]

In contrast, mucosal addressin cell adhesion molecule-1, E-selectin, or P-selectin did not seem to mediate monocyte migration into the target organs [23].

Besides guiding specific inflammatory cell populations to migrate through the vessel wall into surrounding tissues, endothelial cells are also crucial in the physiologic process of saliva secretion [26]. Upon parasympathetic nerve stimulation, vasodilatation and increased capillary blood pressure lead to increased filtration of fluid from glandular capillaries into the interstitial space of the salivary glands. Through this process acinar cells are provided with the fluid required for the secretion of primary saliva [27]. Reduced blood flow responses to parasympathetic stimuli have been reported in patients with SS and may contribute to the reduced salivary gland secretion [27, 28].

15.1.2 Epithelial Cells

Although being at the center of SS pathology and primary targets of the pathogenic autoimmune reaction, acinar and ductal epithelial cells in the past often took a back seat compared to cells of the immune system with respect to the extent of research conducted on different cell types [29] (Fig. 15.2).

The important role of the epithelial cells in the pathogenesis of SS is suggested by the occurrence of lesions in various epithelial tissues (described as autoimmune epithelitis) as well as the increased epithelial expression of several inflammatory proteins in the histopathological lesions of patients [29]. Although professional antigen-presenting cells (APCs), such as DCs, macrophages, and B cells, are present in states of chronic inflammation such as SS

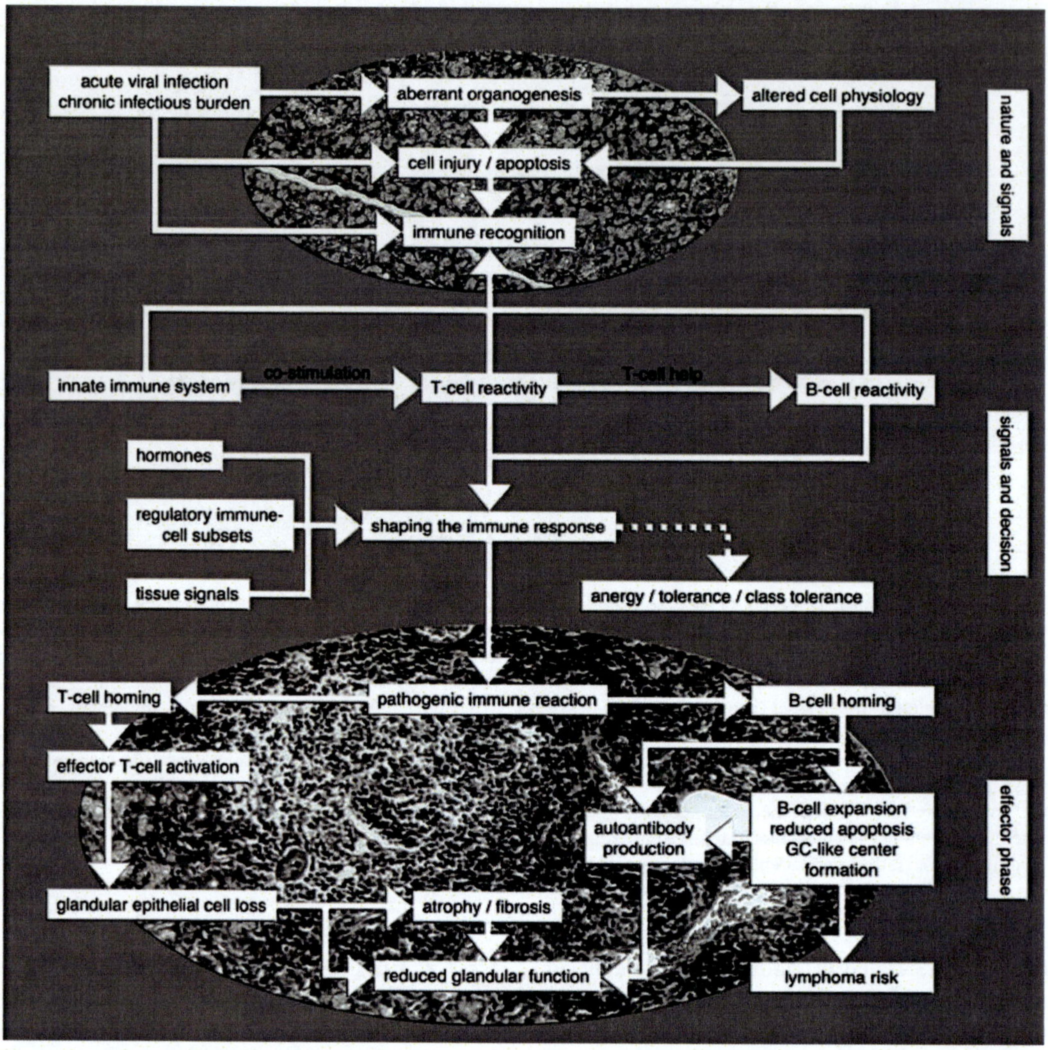

Fig. 15.2 Events related to etiology and pathogenesis of SS. Immune reactions to specific non-self or self-structures are initially determined by their nature. If recognized, the immune system's appropriate decision on quality and extent of the reaction meets the potential threat posed by the antigen. At the same time, it must consider tissue-specific requirements, spare healthy tissue, and subsequently ensure proper instauration of tissue homeostasis. Processes involved in mounting and shaping immune reactions are manifold and require co-operation of multiple immune-cell subsets. Such interactions also appear to expand the immune system's cognition from "self" and "non-self" to "how foreign" and probably also "how dangerous" the recognized entity is. In addition, specific immune-cell subsets appear to adequately regulate the ongoing effector phase of every immune reaction. Although, many of the processes described above are not entirely understood, different lines of evidence indicate that deficiencies in one or several of these complex processes may trigger or contribute to the pathogenesis manifested as SS. The exocrine glands in SS are characterized by distinct inflammatory foci, mainly consisting of T and B cells. Their distinct effector functions appear to specifically contribute to the pathogenesis of SS characterized by distinct exocrine gland inflammation and severe impairment of the affected glands' secretory capacity

[9], interestingly, epithelial cells have been proposed to contribute to the process of antigen presentation. Central for the testing of such a possibility was the establishment of methodology for the long-term cultivation of non-neoplastic salivary gland epithelial cell (SGEC) lines (of ductal type). These techniques have permitted the analysis of various aspects of phenotypic and functional properties of SGEC [30]. Two major concepts have emerged from these studies,

namely, the functional participation of SGEC in immune responses and the occurrence of "intrinsic activation" of salivary gland epithelial cells in SS patients [29].

The notion of epithelial cells acting as non-professional antigen-presenting cells in the salivary glands of SS is underpinned by the presence in vivo and functional analyses in vitro of several molecules representing the APC's side required for the formation of an immunological synapse [29] (Fig. 15.2). Major histocompatibility complex (MHC) class II molecules, HLA-DR/DP/DQ [31], on the epithelial cell's surface, provided the presence of immunogenic peptides, could enable the delivery of the primary activation signal to T cells. Furthermore, β-2 microglobulin, a principal component of the MHC class I molecule, has been localized on salivary gland epithelium [31].

Toll-like receptors (TLRs), whose signals are pivotal in either supressing or activating APCs, are expressed on epithelial cells from the salivary glands [32, 33]. Upon binding of pathogen-associated molecular patterns (PAMPs) [34] or specific endogenous factors [35], TLR ligation leads to significant cytokine production and upregulation of co-stimulatory and adhesion molecules [34, 35]. Indeed, co-stimulatory molecules such as cluster of differentiation (CD)80 (B7.1), CD86 (B7.2) [36], and CD40 [37], which mediate the second crucial signal for induction of an immune response, are expressed on epithelial cells and appear to be functional when tested in vitro [38]. Similar studies also suggested that CD86 on epithelial cells from patients might be more responsive to activation signals mediated via CD28 ligation compared to inhibitory signals provided by binding of cytotoxic T-lymphocyte-associated protein-4 (CTLA-4) [36]. The increased presence of adhesion molecules, VCAM-1, endothelial-leukocyte adhesion molecule (ELAM)-1, and more modestly of intercellular adhesion molecule (ICAM)-1, might further impact the outcome of non-professional APC/T-cell interactions [36, 37, 39].

Epithelial cells were also shown to produce several pro-inflammatory cytokines, e.g., interleukin (IL)-1, IL-6, and tumor necrosis factor (TNF)-α [40], and possibly contribute to the cellular composition and organization of glandular inflammation in SS through production of chemokines, such as C-X-C motif ligand (CXCL)13, CXCL12, C-C motif ligand (CCL)21, CCL19, and CCL18 [16, 41]. In NOD mice, however, injection of anti-CXCL12 antibodies was effective in preventing diabetes and insulitis but did not affect the SS-like disease in this strain [42]. By and large, these data strongly suggest the operation of intrinsic activation mechanisms in the epithelial cells of SS patients and provide support to the notion of active participation of epithelial cells in the pathogenesis of this inflammatory condition [29]. However, whether epithelial cell activation is an event closely linked to the initiation of SS or has to be considered as a secondary phenomenon of the ongoing immune response triggered and shaped by other cell types requires further investigation.

Epithelial cells express Fas and FasL together with B-cell lymphoma-2-associated X protein (Bax) [43, 44]. These and similar results led to the proposition of increased apoptosis as a major mechanism responsible for acinar cell destruction. However, despite aberrant expression of pro-apoptotic molecules apoptosis appears to be a rare event among acinar and ductal cells of patients with SS [45]. Researchers also suggested that increased matrix metalloproteinases (MMP) activity, e.g. MMP-2, MMP-3, and MMP-9, could be related to the dramatic changes in the structural organization in the basal lamina and apical surface of acini observed in patients with SS [46, 47].

15.1.3 T cells

The mononuclear cell infiltrate consists of up to 80% T cells representing a $CD4^+$ to $CD8^+$ T-cell ratio of more than 2 [6]. However, the proportion of different cell types within individual foci appears to vary significantly, possibly in association with the degree of lymphoid organization and disease progression [48]. Most $CD4^+$ T cells are of a primed memory phenotype ($CD45R0^+$)

and large shares express CD40L [49]. In context of T-cell activation, IL-2R has been found on a large fraction of infiltrating lymphocytes [31, 50]. Interestingly, circulating T cells showed only weak proliferation after exposition to anti-CD2 and anti-CD3 antibodies [51]. Furthermore, T-cell responses to stimulation with recombinant Ro and La in vitro seemed rather weak [52].

Analyses of T-cell receptors (TCRs) revealed that most T cells bear α/β TCRs [53] and the usage of the Vβ family repertoire was found to be relatively restricted. In addition, complementarity-determining region (CDR)3 analyses showed some conserved amino acid motifs suggesting a relatively limited number of recognized antigens [54]. Some T cells in the inflamed lesions expand clonally indicating an antigen-driven inflammation [55].

One form of how T cells and natural killer (NK) cells might contribute to the pathogenesis of SS is by epithelial cell death, induced by $CD8^+$ T cells, natural killer T cells, and NK cells [56] (Figs. 15.2 and 15.3). The different lymphocyte subsets involved in cytotoxic effector responses differ in the recognition process through which they identify infected or distressed somatic cells [12]. Cytotoxic lymphocytes use several pathways to induce target cell apoptosis, including Fas ligation and granule exocytosis of enzymes such as perforin and granzyme B [12].

High proportions of T cells within the salivary glands express *Fas* (CD95) and/or members of the B-cell lymphoma (*Bcl*) family [57]. Nevertheless, despite abundant expression of these pro-apoptotic molecules, neither Fas/FasL-induced apoptosis nor apoptosis implicating the Bax/Bcl-2 pathway seems to occur more often among infiltrating mononuclear cells in SS compared to control individuals [45, 58]. High expression of Bcl-2 compared to Bax in these cells may explain their resistance to apoptosis, a situation which might result in a prolonged production of pro-inflammatory mediators [58].

$CD4^+$ T cells, so-called T helper (T_H) cells, are involved in activating and directing other immune cells to meet the challenge posed by

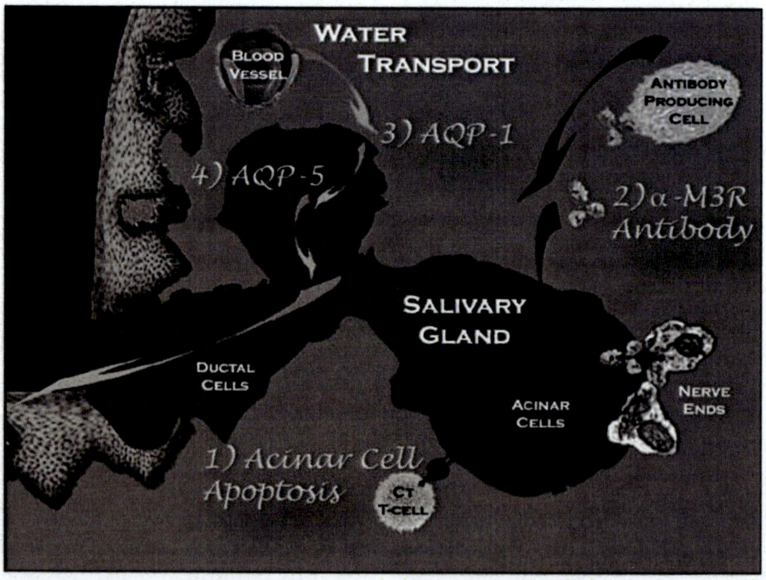

Fig. 15.3 Proposed mechanisms mediating glandular destruction and dysfunction in SS. (1) Altered apoptosis of glandular epithelial cells. (2) Antibodies targeting the M3R may directly be related to the impairment of the salivary glands by inhibiting neuronal innervation of acinar cells. (3 and 4) AQPs are suggested to play a major role in water transport through cell membranes. (3) AQP-1 expression was decreased in myoepithelial cells from patients with SS. (4) AQP-5 expression may be decreased in acinar cells from patients with SS. Figure adapted from Delaleu et al. [6]

antigens of different nature while, at the same time, considering tissue-specific requirements [59–62]. T_H cells are essential in determining B-cell antibody class switching, in the activation and growth of cytotoxic T cells, and in maximizing bactericidal activity of phagocytes such as macrophages. Based on the cytokines secreted, T_H cells are currently subdivided into three major and distinct functional effector subsets, termed T_H1, T_H2, and T_H17 [59–62].

These T cells differentiate from not yet committed T_H0 cells in response to exposure to specific cytokines [59–62]. Such stimuli are followed by the induction of independent patterns of gene transcription. T_H1 cells tend to be involved in host defense against intracellular pathogens and thought to perpetuate autoimmune responses [59, 61, 62]. T_H1 cell differentiation from T_H0 cells is dependent on interferon (IFN)-γ and IL-12. In their turn, T_H1 cells produce IL-2 and IFN-γ. T_H2 cells on the other hand tend to engage in immune responses, which depend on a substantial humoral component for the elimination of the pathogen [59, 61]. Key molecules of a T_H2-dominated immune response are IL-4, IL-5, and IL-13 [59, 61]. T_H1 and T_H2 cells counteract each other, mainly because their respective cytokines can exert inhibitory effects on the opposite T_H cell subset [59, 61].

An optimal scenario, before the emergence of T_H17 and regulatory T-cell (T_{reg}) subsets, seemed to consist of a well-balanced T_H1 and T_H2 responses, tailored in accordance with the encountered immunological challenge [59]. For example, protection from insulin-dependent diabetes mellitus (IDDM) in NOD mice has been associated with a shift from a T_H1 to a T_H2 cytokine expression profile in β-cell-specific autoreactive T cells, which was observed as a result of appropriate treatment intervention or genetic modification [63]. Subsequent studies indicated, however, that compartmentalization into disease-promoting T_H1 and protective T_H2 cytokines may represent an oversimplification, which cannot always be applied to the pathogenesis of IDDM or other autoimmune diseases [64]. Considering the limited knowledge about cytokines at the time the T_H1/T_H2 model was developed [59] and despite its flaws, the T_H1/T_H2 paradigm showed remarkable durability and still conserved some of its validity [65].

Cytokine profiles have been studied in blood and salivary gland tissues from patients with SS [17, 40, 66] and in mouse models for SS [18, 67]. However, because cytokines are characterized by redundancy, pleiotropism, synergism, and antagonism, the interpretation of results on cytokines is often challenging.

Applying the by-now expanded concept of T_H1/T_H2 cytokines and autoimmunity, it has been postulated that T_H2 cytokines may be predominant in an early phase of SS, while T_H1 cytokines would be associated with a later stage of the disease [68]. In opposition stands the proposed principle that the decrease in salivary flow, which is thought to follow the emergence of glandular inflammation [25, 69], might be associated with T_H2 cytokines [70–72]. The latter model is largely based on murine studies, in which crucial molecules involved in either T_H1 or T_H2 responses have been deleted. NOD *Ifn-γ*$^{-/-}$ and NOD *Ifn-γ R*$^{-/-}$ mice did not develop inflammation in the salivary glands and retained normal salivary secretion capacity, while, however, the inflammation within the lacrimal glands persisted [73]. In contrast, IL-4-[70, 71], alike signal transduction and activators of transcription (STAT)6-deficient [72] NOD or NOD-related strains retained salivary secretion rates similar to BALB/c mice. These genetically modified strains concomitantly failed to produce anti-muscarinic M3 receptor (M3R) antibodies of the IgG_1 isotype, despite the development of sialadenitis [70, 72].

The revision of the T_H1/T_H2 paradigm was caused by the emergence of a T-helper cell subset termed T_H17, producing IL-17 (IL-17A), IL-17F, and IL-22 [60]. A major role of IL-17 has been described in various models of immune-mediated tissue injury and autoimmune diseases, e.g., RA [60]. Recent results suggest that the T_H17/IL-23 system is activated in SS patients and C57BL/6.NOD-Aec1Aec2 mice during the overt disease state. Functional associations between IL-17/IL-23 levels and specific clinical manifestations have, however, not yet been identified [18, 74].

Analyses of circulating T_{reg} population showed inconsistent results [75–77], whereas in numbers they might be underrepresented in the salivary glands [76]. Their count was found to inversely correlate with the degree of glandular inflammation and certain risk factors for lymphoma development [77]. Regulatory mechanisms are discussed in Section 15.3.4.

15.1.4 B cells

Phenotypical analyses of B cells from patients with SS have revealed decreased numbers of circulating CD27$^+$ memory B cells [78, 79], which selectively overexpressed C-X-C motif receptors (CXCR)3 and CXCR4 [80]. In contrast, the fraction of CD27$^+$ memory B cells within the glands was enlarged [79]. Extensive analyses of mature B-cell subsets (Bm1–Bm5) in blood further showed altered proportions of most mature B-cell subsets in primary SS compared to healthy donors and patients with RA [81].

The percentage of B cells expressing mutated V(H) genes has been found to be significantly higher in B cells isolated from parotid glands compared to B cells in circulation [82]. Furthermore, V(L) gene analysis of B cells isolated from the glands revealed biased usage of V(L) chain genes [83]. However, if these alterations result from disturbed B-cell maturation and abnormal selection processes or if the biased repertoire reflects a normal antigen-driven local immune response is unclear. Polyclonal B-cell activation may develop into an oligoclonal or monoclonal B-cell expansion during disease progression. Such expansion may provide a basis for the initiation of a malignant lymphoproliferative disease [84, 85].

Patients with SS often present increased levels of polyclonal IgG in the serum [2]. Augmented production of IgM and IgG compared to IgA was further detected within labial salivary glands from patients with SS [86]. Autoantibodies specific for Ro and La are associated with SS and of major importance in SS diagnosis and patient classification [1]; 60–80% of the patients present anti-Ro and 40–60% present anti-La antibodies in the serum [2]. Even though the role of Ro and La in the pathogenesis of SS is still elusive, recent research efforts suggested new molecular mechanisms, by which Ro52 may directly contribute to the induction of autoimmune T cells and B cells in SS [87]. Rheumatoid factor (RF) is produced in approximately 60% of the patients [88], whereas anti-cyclic citrullinated peptide (CCP) antibodies are rarely found in patients with SS [89]. Other antibodies found in patients with SS are anti-α-fodrin [90, 91] and anti-phospholipid antibodies [92]. The latter antibody could not be associated with any of the typical clinical manifestations of SS [93] and anti-α-fodrin autoantibodies are a controversial issue [94], also since the original findings were difficult to verify [95]. Autoantibodies potentially inhibiting neuronal innervation of acinar cells are discussed in more detail in Section 15.2.1 and for more insight about autoantibodies in SS in general please see Chapter 9.

15.1.5 Lymphoid Organization and Germinal Center-Like Structure Formation

Histological and immunohistological investigations of minor salivary gland specimens identified germinal center (GC)-like structures, also known as tertiary lymphoid tissue, in approximately every fourth patient with primary SS [48]. Interestingly, generation of the SS patient's individual cytokine and chemokine profile revealed biomarker signatures in serum indicative for the presence of GC-like structures in the salivary glands [17]. Among 25 biomarkers B-cell-activating factor (BAFF), CCL11, and IFN-γ levels were found to discriminate best between patients with and without GC-like structure formation [17].

In secondary lymphoid tissues GCs develop dynamically after the activation of B cells by T-cell-dependent antigen [12]. Interestingly, within the salivary glands affected by SS T and B cell proportions vary significantly among different foci [48]. In GCs of the secondary lymphoid tissue B cells begin monoclonal expansion in close proximity to DCs. In a state of activated apoptosis B cells compete for survival signals from DCs that present antigen [12]. In the majority of cases, GC-like lesions in SS were marked by $CD21^+$ follicular dendritic cell networks [48] and signs of proliferation and apoptotic events were described in another study [9, 16]. B-cell fate in this process is believed to depend on the affinity of the surface antibody to the antigen and their responsiveness to anti-apoptotic signals [12]. B cells then have to interact with T_H cells, which provide final differentiation signals for an adaptive humoral immune response [12].

Interestingly, ectopic GC-like structure formation in SS was indeed paralleled with increased local production of antibodies against Ro and La [16]. Furthermore, patients presenting GC-like structures in the salivary glands presented higher degrees of glandular inflammation and elevated serum titers of RF, anti-Ro, anti-La, and total IgG [48, 96]. The formation of ectopic GC-like follicles in non-lymphoid organs might indeed participate in the pathogenesis of SS and indicate a more severe disease. The occurrence of GC-like structures in salivary glands has also been proposed as a potential predictor for the subsequent development of lymphoproliferative disorders [97] (Fig. 15.2). However, GC-like structures were not associated with salivary gland enlargement that is today defined as a principal risk factor for lymphoma in SS. In addition, similar signs of ectopic lymphoid tissue formation and lymphoid neogenesis also occur in RA synovia [98], in the thyroid gland of Hashimoto's thyroiditis [99], and chronic infectious reactions triggered by, for example, *Helicobacter pylori* in the gut mucosa [100]. To what extent ectopic GC-like structures in SS may overtake processes traditionally assigned to GC in secondary lymphoid organs and what molecules pave the way for their ectopic formation remain to be proven.

15.2 Mechanisms Mediating Salivary Gland Dysfunction

The original reasoning for the impairment in exocrine gland function in SS suggested loss of glandular epithelial cells as a result of lymphocyte-mediated cell death to be the main cause of hyoposalivation [101] (Figs. 15.2 and 15.3). Hence, loss of secretory capacity, degree of lymphoid infiltration, and production of specific autoantibodies have been anticipated to correlate with each other and indicate disease state and disease severity [102]. However, several SS-related observations and substantial experimental evidence could not be accommodated in such a model. Firstly, a lack of correlation between the amount of destroyed glandular tissue and the often disproportional decrease in salivary flow is often observed [103]. Secondly, glandular tissue isolated from patients with SS retained some functionality although appearing less sensitive to stimuli provided in in vitro systems [104]. Thirdly, administration of muscarinic receptor agonists (pilocarpine hydrochloride or cevimeline) significantly improved exocrine gland secretion capacity in many patients with SS [105]. A model of SS pathogenesis comprising mechanisms of glandular dysfunction is further supported by the observation that certain murine strains, which naturally [24] or as a result of genetic modification [70–72], retain full secretory function despite severe glandular inflammation. Furthermore, prevention of hyposalivation in NOD mice as a result of heat shock protein (Hsp)60 immunization was not paralleled by a greater decrease in salivary gland inflammation compared to mice in which the onset of hyposalivation could not be prevented [19]. Assuming that glandular destruction could be a result of inhibition of saliva secretion, and not hyposalivation to be the consequence of glandular destruction, led to the preposition of immune system-related processes, which appear to have the potential to mediate glandular dysfunction in SS [106] (Fig. 15.3).

15.2.1 Acinar Cell Innervation and Humoral Immunity

The secretion of water and electrolytes from acinar cells is directly induced by acetylcholine (ACh) and substance P released by the innervating parasympathic nerve ends [107]. In the salivary glands M1R and M3R are the predominant acetylcholine receptor subtypes, whereas

M3 is predominant in the lacrimal glands [108]. Experiments using knockout strains revealed a predominant role of the M3 subtype in triggering saliva secretion [109, 110]. In contrast to neuromuscular junctions the physical distance between nerve ends and acinar cells is rather long, which leaves the process of neuronal innervation of acinar cells susceptible to events such as degradation of ACh by acetylcholine esterase and antibodies to muscarinic receptors [106].

The importance of the latter was illustrated when studying NOD $Ig\mu^{null}$ mice, which lack functional B cells. Although T-cell-dominated focal inflammation was found in the salivary glands of NOD $Ig\mu^{null}$ mice, they retained salivary flow rates comparable to control strains [111]. Reversible induction of hyposalivation through serum transfer from old NOD mice and IgG fractions obtained from patients with SS in these mice [111] further supports the notion of a contribution of serum components to the pathogenesis of SS. Functional analyses demonstrated that IgG fractions from patients with primary SS reduced the carbachol-evoked increase in Ca^{2+} in murine and human acinar cells [112] as well as they had the potential to disturb muscarinic receptor-associated contraction of colon- [113] and bladder muscle cells [114]. Due to the laborious method, unfortunately, both tests described above are inadequate to screen large patient cohorts. The use of M3R transfectants in combination with flow cytometry [115], or the application of newly developed enzyme-linked immunosorbant assays (ELISAs) [116], may represent an alternative to further investigate the role and diagnostic value of anti-M3R antibodies in SS. However, studies also highlighted the apparent challenges when attempting detection of anti-muscarinic receptor antibodies by conventional immunochemical methods [117, 118]. Such difficulties continue to hamper the identification of the true incidence of anti-M3R antibodies in SS. In addition, antibodies inhibiting the function of M3R have also been shown to be present in some patients with scleroderma [113].

ACh ligation with M3R in vitro has been shown to mediate protection from apoptotic cell death [119]. Hence, inhibition of anti-apoptotic effects mediated through M3R signaling might potentially link functional quiescence with cellular destruction. However, chronic stimulation of membrane-bound M3R might also result in receptor desensitization over time [120].

In addition, it should be taken into account that mononuclear cells express muscarinic receptors, secrete ACh, and encode the synthesizing choline acetyltransferase and the degrading acetylcholine esterase [121], what adds to the complexity of how immune cells might affect the signaling mechanisms of saliva secretion [106].

15.2.2 Inflammatory Mediators

Results obtained in vitro have suggested that cytokines such as IL-1α and IL-1β may affect the process of saliva secretion by inhibiting the release of ACh from cholinergic nerves [122, 123]. Evidence against interferences of such kind was, however, presented when no relation between concanavalin A-induced cytokine production and Ach-evoked Ca^{2+} mobilization [124] was found.

Arguing against one aspect of the hypothesis involving MMP in the pathogenesis of SS [46, 125], namely, shedding M3R from the extracellular surface, is that, in contrast with murine models of SS, acini in the human labial salivary glands of patients with SS express significantly higher numbers of M3R compared to control individuals [126].

15.2.3 Fluid Movement in the Salivary Glands and Aquaporins

Obviously, the process of saliva secretion requires movement of fluid from the vasculature into the interstitial space of the salivary glands and ultimately into the ducts [26]. Water movement across the water permeable acini can occur either paracellularly or transcellularly [26]. Specific molecules conducting water in and out of cells, while preventing the passage of ions and other solutes critically, contribute to the process described above [127]. Termed aquaporins (AQPs), these transmembrane proteins form channels in the cell membrane and increase the water permeability of the lipid bilayer by up to a 100-fold [127]. Different isoforms exist and show specific cellular and subcellular distributions in salivary and lacrimal glands [128]. AQP-5 is located in the apical membrane of acinar cells, AQP-3 is present within the basal membrane of acinar cells and AQP-1 is expressed on myoepithelial cells [128]. Monoclonal anti-M3R antibodies had the potential to prevent translocation of AQPs to the plasma membrane [129]. Since then, AQPs have been suspected to contribute to the loss of exocrine gland secretory function in SS (Fig. 15.3). Mice deficient of AQP-5 exhibit an approximate decrease of 65% in salivary secretion capacity compared to wild-type mice [130] and AQP-5 has also been suggested to contribute to reduced saliva secretion observed in NOD mice [131]. However, analysis of AQP-5 distribution within the glandular tissue from patients with SS revealed controversial results [132, 133]. AQP-1 expression was decreased by 38% in salivary glands of patients with SS suggesting a possible insufficient AQP-1-dependent water flow across myoepithelial cells [134].

15.3 Concepts Thought to Underlay Immunity and Etiology of Autoimmune Diseases: A View on Sjögren's Syndrome

According to the paradigm of self versus non-self discrimination, the immune system, early in life, is taught to ignore or tolerate self, whereas it is supposed to recognize and attack foreign or non-self [12, 135, 136]. Ever since researchers studied the etiology of autoimmune diseases, the process of clonal deletion and spontaneous mutations of immune cells have been subjects of investigation in order to reveal at what level and by what process self versus non-self discrimination might have been compromised [12, 135, 137] (Fig. 15.2).

To a variable degree, depending on the autoimmune condition studied, an individual's genetic background defines a person's susceptibility for developing a certain autoimmune disease [138, 139]. A genetic predisposition for SS also seems to exist; a notion supported by reports about the accumulation of SS in certain families and among twins [140]. Subsequently, genes coding for immunorelevant molecules have been studied to identify certain genes, genotypes, and single-nucleotide polymorphisms, which might be associated with SS. A variant of the minor histocompatibility antigen HA-1 has been associated with reduced risk of primary SS [141], whereas another study indicated a significant association between primary SS and a specific interferon regulatory factor (IRF)5 allele [142]. In contrast, no association of SS with polymorphisms in *Fas* and *FasL* [143], *IL-10*, *TNF-α*, interleukin-1 receptor antagonist (*IL-1RA*) [144], *CTLA-4* [145], TNF-α receptor 2 [146], or *CCR7* [147] genes were observed. For more comprehensive discussion of genes and SS please see Chapter 8.

15.3.1 Environmental Factors

Environmental factors, most often sialotropic viruses, have been suspected to trigger the subsequent etiopathogenesis of SS through mechanisms of molecular mimicry in genetically susceptible individuals [148] (Fig. 15.2). Molecular mimicry is thereby defined as the possibility that sequence similarities and structural homology between foreign and self-peptides are sufficient to result in the cross-activation of autoreactive T or B cells by pathogen-derived peptides to mount pathogenic effector responses against self [149].

The infectious agents which have received most attention in the field of SS are Epstein–Barr virus [150], human T-cell leukemia virus-1 [151], and hepatitis C virus (HCV) [152]. Sialadenitis, now considered as an extrahepatic manifestation of chronic HCV infection, received attention in the newly proposed American–European Consensus Group criteria, in which HCV infection is listed as an illegibility criterion in clinical studies investigating SS [1].

To elaborate a possible viral etiology of SS, different murine strains were infected with murine cytomegalovirus (MCMV) [153].

Sialadenitis was observed as a result and in one particular strain anti-Ro and anti-La antibodies were observed [153]. Apoptotic cells, however, were solely detected during the acute, but not during the chronic phase of the inflammation and Fas and TNF-receptor I-mediated apoptosis seemed to be critical in clearing MCMV-infected cells from salivary glands [154]. As suggested by the authors, such defects may lead to a post-infectious, chronic inflammation resembling the histopathology of SS [154]. Significant reduction in both the number of inflammatory foci and extent of tissue destruction in salivary glands were observed as a result of local FasL gene transfer [154]. A more recent study identified a coxsackie virus as a potential agent involved in the induction or maintenance of SS in a Greek population [155]. However, the results could not be validated in a French patient cohort [156].

Although, associations between SS and all viral candidates yet investigated are rather weak, microarray-based investigation of the salivary gland transcriptome in patients with SS [3] and in congenic mouse models for SS [157, 158] indicated an activated type-I and type-II IFN system, which might originally have been triggerred by a viral infection. Critically promoting host defense against viruses, IFNs do directly affect multiple cell types and processes involved at an early stage of the immune reaction such as activation of NK cells and macrophages and may also facilitate antigen presentation to lymphocytes by pDC [159]. For more comprehensive discussion of viruses, genes, and SS please see Chapter 8.

15.3.2 Secondary Signals

Mounting an adaptive effector response requires the co-operation of at least two different cell types in each distinct phase of the immune response, e.g., APC/T-cell interaction and T-cell help delivery to B cells [12] (Fig. 15.2). Today's concept of immunity, besides the recognition of an assumingly foreign peptide, acknowledges the importance of secondary signals in the host's decision making process of self versus non-self discrimination [12]. These secondary signals are provided to B cells by T_H cells (T-cell help) and to T cells through APCs (co-stimulation) (Fig. 15.2). APCs in turn receive secondary signals via pattern recognition receptors (PRRs) such as TLRs [12]. PRRs are germline-encoded and received much of attention as they may expand the cognition of the immune system to discriminate between infectious non-self and non-infectious-self based on evolutionary distance between a host and the invading microorganism [34]. Due to their role in either supressing or activating APCs, TLRs have more recently received considerable attention in the field of autoimmunity [35]. Research has increasingly demonstrated that many of the same PRRs also recognize self-epitopes that either are released from dying or distressed cells or are present at the surface of apoptotic cells or apoptotic bodies [35].

Activated TLR3 and TLR7 pathways, prior to manifestation of the disease, have been described in the salivary glands in an experimental model of SS [158]. Furthermore, epithelial cells and macrophages within the salivary glands from patients with SS express TLRs [32, 33]. An interesting concept, involving the evolution of TLRs, revolves around the question of how the immune system is able to also take into consideration tissue-specific properties when shaping an efficient immune response [160, 161]. Considering recognition of endogenous danger signals to be recognized by PRR would attribute to the distressed tissue and its mediators a distinct role in the host's decision on immunological tolerance, immune activation, and qualitative aspects of the immune reaction [160, 161] (Fig. 15.2).

15.3.3 Apoptosis, Autoantigens, and Potential Danger Signals in the Salivary Glands

Asking the question why the salivary glands are often the primary target organ of a distinct pathogenic immune reaction, it has been speculated that due to their anatomical localization and their short excretory ducts exocrine glands should be considered as a *locus minoris resistentiae*, where apoptotic acinar cells cannot in the usual way be scavenged as they disintegrate

[162]. It is possible that acinar cells undergoing normal physiological death will be exposed to an immunologically active environment mounted for the purpose of host defense as they are extruded through the duct [162]. Such events might have a negative impact on the immune tolerance toward self-structures exposed during apoptosis as the border between non-self and self or harmful and harmless would be difficult to draw in such an environment [35]. Interestingly, autoantigens associated with SS become clustered and concentrated in the surface blebs of apoptotic cells [163]. Furthermore, their structure is altered during some types of cell death to generate structures not found during development and homeostasis [164]. The generation of unique potentially immunogenic fragments during granule exocytosis-mediated cell death has also been proposed for M3R and α-fodrin [165].

Recent reports suggested that SS autoantigen-associated RNAs, when encountering APCs such as pDCs, might be able to perpetuate IFN-α production even after a potential viral infection has been eliminated [4, 166]. These findings reanimate the discussion on Ro's role in the etiology and pathogenesis of SS and other autoimmune diseases characterized by autoantibodies against RNA-binding proteins [167].

Manifestation of several aspects of SS in an SS-unrelated murine strain was indeed observed after injection of peptides derived from Ro, emulsified in complete Freund's adjuvant and incomplete Freund's adjuvant [168]. The use of adjuvant, proven critical for the manifestation of the disease, might thereby deliver crucial secondary signals required to brake the tolerance against Ro [168]. Oral feeding of Ro or Ro peptides did, in contrast, diminish the susceptibility of the strain to the induction of SS through the immunization protocol described above [169]. Studies have also shown that reciprocal spreading to the Ro52, Ro60, and La polypeptides occurs following immunization with a single component [170, 171] and intermolecular epitope spreading suggests little tolerance to Ro and La in the B-cell and T-cell compartments [172, 173].

As a possible primary cause or secondary event to tissue injury involving environmental factors, researchers reported delayed organogenesis, aberrant proteolytic activity, and altered tissue homeostasis in the salivary glands from murine models of SS and their immune-compromised descendents (NOD-scid) [158, 174] (Fig. 15.2). Interestingly, similar morphogenic defects were no longer apparent in IFN-γ-deficient NOD-scid mice, further stressing the role of IFNs prior and independent from processes related to the adaptive immune system. SS-like disease manifestations in inhibitor of differentiation 3 (Id3)-deficient mice further support a possible relationship between defective T-cell development and altered vasculogenesis and initiation of pathological immune reaction targeting the salivary glands [175]. Interestingly, in the latter model, depletion of B cells ameliorated the SS-related symptoms [176]. However, glandular epithelium and T cells from patients with SS did not show altered Id3 expression compared to controls [177]. Furthermore, they did not differ in allele and genotype frequencies of Id3 single-nucleotide polymorphisms (SNPs) [177].

15.3.4 Immunoregulation

The immunological process of host defense requires an adequate balance between activation and suppression of effector cells in order to achieve an efficient immune response without damaging the host [12, 178] (Fig. 15.2). As an example, in diabetes, several lines of evidence indicate that progression from early insulitis to overt diabetes is promoted by the loss of immunoregulatory cells, such as T_{regs} and invariant NK T cells within the islets [63]. However, the mechanism, by which the different regulatory T-cell subsets (induced T_{regs}, Tr1 cells, and T_H3 cells and naturally occurring T_{reg} cells) limit effector responses in vivo, remains poorly understood. Crucial in this process seems their ability to control DCs in their capacity to activate T cells [179]. In addition, secretion of cytokines, such as transforming growth factor (TGF)-β and IL-10 by T_{regs}, are considered to exert anti-inflammatory effects [180, 181]. Animals homozygous for the mutated *Tgf-β1* allele present a syndrome marked by mixed inflammatory cell responses and tissue necrosis leading to organ failure and death. The syndrome also includes inflammation of the exocrine glands in about 50% of the animals [182]. With respect to IL-10, gene transfer of this particular cytokine into NOD mice partially suppressed the appearance of SS-like features [183]. However, C57BL/6 mice transgenic for IL-10 exhibit progressive histopathology and hyposalivation evocative of SS [184], indicating a dual role of *Il-10* in SS.

As alluded to previously, little is known about the exact role of regulatory cell subsets in the progression of SS. Nonetheless, the SS-like disease course in NOD mice deficient for E2f1, presenting a profound decrease in T_{regs}, was accelerated and aggravated [185]. By promoting growth and effectiveness of T_{regs}, IL-2 plays a crucial role in the maintenance of immunological self-tolerance [186]. IL-2 and IL-2Rα deficient C57BL/6 mice develop sialadenitis, hyposalivation, and histopathological manifestations related to other autoimmune diseases [187]. In addition, inhibition of circulating IL-2 led to the aggravation of diverse autoimmune manifestations in NOD mice [186]. Mice with a T-cell-specific loss of phosphoinositide 3-kinase class IA (PI3K Ia) develop inflammation resembling SS in addition to lymphoid infiltration in the lungs, liver, and intestines paralleled by reduced T_{reg} population in the periphery and increased anti-Ro and anti-La antibodies [188]. In summary, these findings indicate that in conditions with decreased regulatory cell populations the salivary glands are prone to exhibit autoimmune manifestations [77].

In the context of autoimmunity strong evidence suggests that every individual's immune system, healthy or diseased, consists of a relatively high number of autoreactive T and B cells specific for a relatively small number of immune, maintenance, and tissue molecules [189–191]. The recognition of these molecules seems to be crucial in the context of immunological tolerance and tissue homeostasis and has been termed physiological autoimmunity [192]. Based on this notion autoimmune diseases might be coined by insufficient anti-autoimmune regulation against key self-molecules [192] (Fig. 15.2). Indeed, administration of self-antigens such as heat shock proteins, taking into account dose, dose schedule, anatomical site, and context did prevent and in some cases induce remission of autoimmune diseases in murine models [63, 169, 193, 194]. In experimental SS, decreased salivary gland inflammation and prevention of hyposalivation as a result of Hsp60 administration were associated in part with strengthened immunoregulation [19]. The exact role of T_{regs} in the progression of SS is, however, still elusive [75, 76, 187]. Strengthening regulatory mechanisms may indeed lead to restoration of immunological tolerance and improvement of the clinical features of SS [180, 195], in absence of negative effects related to long-termed and generalized immunosuppression [196]. Even though T-cell populations have received most attention over the recent years, it is important to state that virtually all populations of cells, especially in close proximity of the inflammation, may contribute in one or another way to the outcome of the immune reaction [160, 161].

15.3.5 B-cell-Activating Factor

Investigation of BAFF, which is regulated by IFN-γ and is a member of the TNF superfamily, demonstrated the need of an obligate survival signal for both maturing and fully differentiated B cells [197]. Taken together, BAFF is suggested to lower the threshold required for B-cell survival, what may allow autoreactive B cells to escape from apoptosis and to exhibit their autoimmune potential [197].

BAFF has received considerable attention in the field of SS after it was reported that mice transgenic for BAFF develop a secondary pathology reminiscent of SS [198]. Major proportions of lymphocytes infiltrating the salivary glands were B cells displaying a marginal zone (MZ)-like phenotype. This specific B-cell subset was later on identified to be crucial for the development of the SS-like disease in this strain [199].

In patients with SS elevated levels of circulating BAFF were reported to correlate with increased autoantibody titers [200]. Increased

BAFF expression was furthermore observed within salivary glands of patients with SS [201, 202], together with a significantly lower rate of apoptosis among the BAFF-expressing cells [203]. BAFF levels also increased after the discontinuation of an anti-CD20 therapy what may promote the reemergence of autoreactive B cells [204]. Counteracting the BAFF-triggered repopulation of the periphery with pathogenic autoreactive B cells may therefore further improve the success of B-cell depletion in SS [205].

Experiments in mice indicate that the occurrence of glandular inflammation is not dependent on antigen presentation by B cells, whereas hyposalivation seems to be crucially dependent on B cells and autoantibodies [111]. The exact mechanisms of how B-cell effector responses are involved in the pathogenesis of SS in humans are still subject of current research efforts [112]. Nonetheless, depletion of patients' B cells, using anti-CD20 antibodies, has already been shown to ameliorate several manifestations of the disease [205]. For detailed discussion on biologics for the treatment of SS see Chapter 31.

15.3.6 Hormones

Female predominance and the late onset of SS directed the attention toward sex hormones and their possible role in the etiology of SS (Fig. 15.2). In general, androgenic hormones have been considered to protect from autoimmunity and it has been proposed that women with SS are androgen deficient [206]. Whereas neither estrogen receptor-α nor estrogen receptor-β-deficient mice develop SS, another model of estrogen deficiency, the aromatase-knockout mouse, develops a lymphoproliferative autoimmune disease resembling SS [207]. Alike BAFF, estrogen has the ability to promote naïve B-cell development in mice and to rescue B cells from B-cell receptor (BCR)-mediated apoptosis [208, 209] thereby affecting negative selection of autoreactive B cells. Indeed, non-autoimmune BALB/c mice, transgenic for the γ2b heavy chain of the R4A anti-double-stranded (ds)DNA antibody, failed to induce tolerance of high-affinity autoreactive anti-dsDNA B cells in the presence of estrogen [210]. As possible underlying mechanisms increased BCR co-receptor expression and increased Bcl-2 production have been suspected [208]. However, the relevance of such processes demonstrated in mice remains to be confirmed in humans.

15.3.7 Microchimerism

Microchimerism of fetal cells may play a role in generating an autoimmune potential in women who have been pregnant. Two studies detected Y chromosome-specific sequences in the minor salivary glands of approximately 50% of patients with SS [211, 212]. In contrast, another report suggests a role of microchimerism in systemic sclerosis, but found no evidence for microchimerism in SS [213]. Analyses of gene allele usage coding for autoantigens in SS may determine if there is a role of maternal graft-versus-host disease in generating an autoimmune potential. Age-dependent decrease in immune tolerance could then lead to a switch from a silent state of autoimmunity to an overt autoimmune disease.

15.4 Late-Breaking Additions

In the time period between submission of the initial manuscript in 2008 and the printing of this book in 2011, several exciting studies have been published pertaining to the etiology and pathogenesis of SS with special emphasis on the salivary glands. Therefore, we would like to use the occasion and refer to some of these studies in this section.

Analyses of global gene expression profiles obtained from salivary gland tissue of SS patients have recently been shown to have the capacity to predict a patient's response to therapeutic B-cell depletion triggered by anti-CD20. In addition, these profiles yielded further insight into potential processes underlying patient subgroup-specific manifestations of SS [214]. Applying similar technology, microRNA profiles have now been generated from salivary gland tissues and revealed encouraging results about the potential benefit of specific microRNA signatures in defining a patient's specific disease phenotype with respect to degree of salivary gland inflammation and remaining salivary gland function [215]. Several recently published studies have also contributed to a growing understanding of morphologic and molecular changes related to the integrity of the salivary gland tissue associated with SS [216, 217]. However, the chronological sequence of how these events relate to other manifestations of SS remains, in large parts, elusive. Nevertheless, although the lack of appropriate specimens obtained from humans renders the study of subclinical and preclinical stages difficult, recent work in murine models sheds some light on possible interrelationships between organogenesis, tissue homeostasis, tissue damage, the perpetuation of chronic inflammation, and overt disease [218]. With a subset of SS patients exhibiting type-I IFN signatures [3, 4], molecular pathways that may mediate continuous IFN production, e.g., involving TLR-dependent amplification and propagation of the immune response [219], these processes have over the recent years, been the most studied potential etiological factors in SS [220, 221]. More studies, however, are needed to estimate the contribution of specific gene variants to the regulation of this system [222–224].

Other research initiatives have contributed to a more detailed delineation of distinct populations of antigen-presenting cells, both in the target tissue and in circulation [225]. In order to better define the nature of the inflammatory lesions in the salivary glands, an increased number of distinct T-cell effector and T-cell regulatory subsets, in conjunction with more differentiated cytokine profiles, have been investigated [226, 227]. The different immune cell subsets' exact role in the pathogenesis of SS, however, often still remains to be clarified further.

The B cells residing in the salivary glands have also been assessed in more detail together with the inflammatory milieu that is thought to contribute to their fate and to the pathogenesis of SS [228]. Even though many questions about the role of the salivary gland in the etiology of the disease remain unanswered and the extent and specific workings of the immune system in the pathogenesis of SS remain, in part, elusive, there is currently a sense of optimism. New technologies will allow less biased study designs and may deliver on the promise of generating comprehensive datasets of exceptionally high quality also from target tissues of autoimmunity. Advances in systems biology and bioinformatics, in lockstep with the still ongoing revolution in information technology, have undoubtedly begun to revolutionize immunology and, thereby, autoimmune and SS-related research.

Acknowledgements We thank Dr. B. Delaleu-Justitz for careful revision of the manuscript. *Financial support*: The European Union (BMH4-CT96-0595; BMH4-CT98-3489; QLK2-1999-51079; QLK2-CT-2001-30115; MEST-CT-2004-514483, MEIF-CT-2007-041083), The Research Council of Norway's GLOBVAC program, The Strategic Research Program at Helse Bergen (regional health authorities of Western Norway), and The Broegelmann Foundation.

References

1. Vitali C, Bombardieri S, Jonsson R, et al. Classification criteria for Sjögren's syndrome: a revised version of the European criteria proposed by the American–European Consensus Group. Ann Rheum Dis. 2002;61:554–8.
2. Jonsson R, Bowman SJ, Gordon TP. Sjögren's syndrome. In: Koopman WJ, editor. Arthritis and allied conditions. 15th ed. Philadelphia: Lippincott Williams & Wilkins; 2005. pp. 1681–705.
3. Hjelmervik TO, Petersen K, Jonassen I, Jonsson R, Bolstad AI. Gene expression profiling of minor salivary glands clearly distinguishes primary Sjögren's syndrome patients from healthy control subjects. Arthritis Rheum. 2005;52:1534–44.
4. Båve U, Nordmark G, Lövgren T, et al. Activation of the type I interferon system in primary Sjögren's syndrome: a possible etiopathogenic mechanism. Arthritis Rheum. 2005;52:1185–95.
5. Gottenberg JE, Cagnard N, Lucchesi C, et al. Activation of IFN pathways and plasmacytoid dendritic cell recruitment in target organs of primary Sjögren's syndrome. Proc Natl Acad Sci USA. 2006;103:2770–5.
6. Delaleu N, Jonsson R, Koller MM. Sjögren's syndrome. Eur J Oral Sci. 2005;113:101–13.
7. Delaleu N, Jonsson MV, Appel S, Jonsson R. New concepts in the pathogenesis of Sjögren's syndrome. Rheum Dis Clin North Am. 2008;34:833–45, vii.
8. Aziz KE, McCluskey PJ, Wakefield D. Characterisation of follicular dendritic cells in labial

salivary glands of patients with primary Sjögren syndrome: comparison with tonsillar lymphoid follicles. Ann Rheum Dis. 1997;56:140–3.
9. Manoussakis MN, Boiu S, Korkolopoulou P, et al. Rates of infiltration by macrophages and dendritic cells and expression of interleukin-18 and interleukin-12 in the chronic inflammatory lesions of Sjögren's syndrome: correlation with certain features of immune hyperactivity and factors associated with high risk of lymphoma development. Arthritis Rheum. 2007;56:3977–88.
10. El Miedany YM, Ahmed I, Mourad HG, et al. Quantitative ultrasonography and magnetic resonance imaging of the parotid gland: can they replace the histopathologic studies in patients with Sjögren's syndrome? Joint Bone Spine. 2004;71:29–38.
11. Wernicke D, Hess H, Gromnica-Ihle E, Krause A, Schmidt WA. Ultrasonography of salivary glands—a highly specific imaging procedure for diagnosis of Sjögren's syndrome. J Rheumatol. 2008;35:285–93.
12. Janeway CA, Travers P, Walport M, Shlomchik M. Immunobiology: the immunesystem in health and disease. 6th ed. New York, NY: Garland Science Publishing; 2005.
13. Mantovani A, Bonecchi R, Locati M. Tuning inflammation and immunity by chemokine sequestration: decoys and more. Nat Rev Immunol. 2006;6:907–18.
14. Charo IF, Ransohoff RM. The many roles of chemokines and chemokine receptors in inflammation. N Engl J Med. 2006;354:610–21.
15. Amft N, Bowman SJ. Chemokines and cell trafficking in Sjögren's syndrome. Scand J Immunol. 2001;54:62–9.
16. Salomonsson S, Jonsson MV, Skarstein K, et al. Cellular basis of ectopic germinal center formation and autoantibody production in the target organ of patients with Sjögren's syndrome. Arthritis Rheum. 2003;48:3187–201.
17. Szodoray P, Alex P, Jonsson MV, et al. Distinct profiles of Sjögren's syndrome patients with ectopic salivary gland germinal centers revealed by serum cytokines and BAFF. Clin Immunol. 2005;117:168–76.
18. Delaleu N, Immervoll H, Cornelius J, Jonsson R. Biomarker profiles in serum and saliva of experimental Sjögren's syndrome: associations with specific autoimmune manifestations. Arthritis Res Ther. 2008;10:R22.
19. Delaleu N, Madureira AC, Immervoll H, Jonsson R. Inhibition of experimental Sjögren's syndrome through immunization with HSP60 and its peptide amino acids 437–460. Arthritis Rheum. 2008;58:2318–28.
20. Mehrad B, Keane MP, Strieter RM. Chemokines as mediators of angiogenesis. Thromb Haemost. 2007;97:755–62.
21. Holmes DI, Zachary I. The vascular endothelial growth factor (VEGF) family: angiogenic factors in health and disease. Genome Biol. 2005;6:209.
22. Szekanecz Z, Gaspar L, Koch AE. Angiogenesis in rheumatoid arthritis. Front Biosci. 2005;10:1739–53.
23. Mikulowska-Mennis A, Xu B, Berberian JM, Michie SA. Lymphocyte migration to inflamed lacrimal glands is mediated by vascular cell adhesion molecule-1/alpha(4)beta(1) integrin, peripheral node addressin/L-selectin, and lymphocyte function-associated antigen-1 adhesion pathways. Am J Pathol. 2001;159:671–81.
24. Jonsson MV, Delaleu N, Jonsson R. Animal models of Sjögren's syndrome. Clin Rev Allergy Immunol. 2007;32:215–24.
25. Cha S, Peck AB, Humphreys-Beher MG. Progress in understanding autoimmune exocrinopathy using the non-obese diabetic mouse: an update. Crit Rev Oral Biol Med. 2002;13:5–16.
26. Kaufman E, Lamster IB. The diagnostic applications of saliva—a review. Crit Rev Oral Biol Med. 2002;13:197–212.
27. Chikui T, Yonetsu K, Izumi M, Eguchi K, Nakamura T. Abnormal blood flow to the submandibular glands of patients with Sjögren's syndrome: Doppler waveform analysis. J Rheumatol. 2000;27:1222–8.
28. Berggreen E, Nylokken K, Delaleu N, Hajdaragic-Ibricevic H, Jonsson MV. Impaired vascular responses to parasympathetic nerve stimulation and muscarinic receptor activation in the submandibular gland in nonobese diabetic mice. Arthritis Res Ther. 2009;11:R18.
29. Mitsias DI, Kapsogeorgou EK, Moutsopoulos HM. Sjögren's syndrome: why autoimmune epithelitis? Oral Dis. 2006;12:523–32.
30. Dimitriou ID, Kapsogeorgou EK, Abu-Helu RF, Moutsopoulos HM, Manoussakis MN. Establishment of a convenient system for the long-term culture and study of non-neoplastic human salivary gland epithelial cells. Eur J Oral Sci. 2002;110:21–30.
31. Jonsson R, Klareskog L, Backman K, Tarkowski A. Expression of HLA-D-locus (DP, DQ, DR)-coded antigens, beta 2-microglobulin, and the interleukin 2 receptor in Sjögren's syndrome. Clin Immunol Immunopathol. 1987;45:235–43.
32. Spachidou MP, Bourazopoulou E, Maratheftis CI, et al. Expression of functional Toll-like receptors by salivary gland epithelial cells: increased mRNA expression in cells derived from patients with primary Sjögren's syndrome. Clin Exp Immunol. 2007;147:497–503.
33. Kawakami A, Nakashima K, Tamai M, et al. Toll-like receptor in salivary glands from patients with Sjögren's syndrome: functional analysis by human salivary gland cell line. J Rheumatol. 2007;34:1019–26.

34. Janeway CA, Jr., Medzhitov R. Innate immune recognition. Annu Rev Immunol. 2002;20:197–216.
35. Marshak-Rothstein A, Rifkin IR. Immunologically active autoantigens: the role of toll-like receptors in the development of chronic inflammatory disease. Annu Rev Immunol. 2007;25:419–41.
36. Kapsogeorgou EK, Moutsopoulos HM, Manoussakis MN. Functional expression of a costimulatory B7.2 (CD86) protein on human salivary gland epithelial cells that interacts with the CD28 receptor, but has reduced binding to CTLA4. J Immunol. 2001;166:3107–13.
37. Dimitriou ID, Kapsogeorgou EK, Moutsopoulos HM, Manoussakis MN. CD40 on salivary gland epithelial cells: high constitutive expression by cultured cells from Sjögren's syndrome patients indicating their intrinsic activation. Clin Exp Immunol. 2002;127:386–92.
38. Manoussakis MN, Dimitriou ID, Kapsogeorgou EK, et al. Expression of B7 costimulatory molecules by salivary gland epithelial cells in patients with Sjögren's syndrome. Arthritis Rheum. 1999;42:229–39.
39. Abu-Helu RF, Dimitriou ID, Kapsogeorgou EK, Moutsopoulos HM, Manoussakis MN. Induction of salivary gland epithelial cell injury in Sjögren's syndrome: in vitro assessment of T cell-derived cytokines and Fas protein expression. J Autoimmun. 2001;17:141–53.
40. Fox RI, Kang HI, Ando D, Abrams J, Pisa E. Cytokine mRNA expression in salivary gland biopsies of Sjögren's syndrome. J Immunol. 1994;152:5532–9.
41. Xanthou G, Polihronis M, Tzioufas AG, Paikos S, Sideras P, Moutsopoulos HM. "Lymphoid" chemokine messenger RNA expression by epithelial cells in the chronic inflammatory lesion of the salivary glands of Sjögren's syndrome patients: possible participation in lymphoid structure formation. Arthritis Rheum. 2001;44:408–18.
42. Matin K, Salam MA, Akhter J, Hanada N, Senpuku H. Role of stromal-cell derived factor-1 in the development of autoimmune diseases in non-obese diabetic mice. Immunology. 2002;107: 222–32.
43. Bolstad AI, Eiken HG, Rosenlund B, Alarcon-Riquelme ME, Jonsson R. Increased salivary gland tissue expression of Fas, Fas ligand, cytotoxic T lymphocyte-associated antigen 4, and programmed cell death 1 in primary Sjögren's syndrome. Arthritis Rheum. 2003;48:174–85.
44. Kong L, Ogawa N, McGuff HS, et al. Bcl-2 family expression in salivary glands from patients with primary Sjögren's syndrome: involvement of Bax in salivary gland destruction. Clin Immunol Immunopathol. 1998;88:133–41.
45. Ohlsson M, Skarstein K, Bolstad AI, Johannessen AC, Jonsson R. Fas-induced apoptosis is a rare event in Sjögren's syndrome. Lab Invest. 2001;81:95–105.
46. Goicovich E, Molina C, Perez P, et al. Enhanced degradation of proteins of the basal lamina and stroma by matrix metalloproteinases from the salivary glands of Sjögren's syndrome patients: correlation with reduced structural integrity of acini and ducts. Arthritis Rheum. 2003;48:2573–84.
47. Perez P, Goicovich E, Alliende C, et al. Differential expression of matrix metalloproteinases in labial salivary glands of patients with primary Sjögren's syndrome. Arthritis Rheum. 2000;43:2807–17.
48. Jonsson MV, Skarstein K, Jonsson R, Brun JG. Serological implications of germinal center-like structures in primary Sjögren's syndrome. J Rheumatol. 2007;34:2044–9.
49. Nakamura H, Kawakami A, Tominaga M, et al. Expression of CD40/CD40 ligand and Bcl-2 family proteins in labial salivary glands of patients with Sjögren's syndrome. Lab Invest. 1999;79:261–9.
50. Coll J, Tomas S, Vilella R, Corominas J. Interleukin-2 receptor expression in salivary glands of patients with Sjögren's syndrome. J Rheumatol. 1995;22:1488–91.
51. Gerli R, Bertotto A, Cernetti C, et al. Anti-CD3 and anti-CD2-induced T-cell activation in primary Sjögren's syndrome. Clin Exp Rheumatol. 1989;7 Suppl 3:S129–34.
52. Halse AK, Wahren M, Jonsson R. Peripheral blood in Sjögren's syndrome does not contain increased levels of T lymphocytes reactive with the recombinant Ro/SS-A 52 kD and La/SS-B 48 kD autoantigens. Autoimmunity 1996;23:25–34.
53. Skopouli FN, Fox PC, Galanopoulou V, Atkinson JC, Jaffe ES, Moutsopoulos HM. T cell subpopulations in the labial minor salivary gland histopathologic lesion of Sjögren's syndrome. J Rheumatol. 1991;18:210–4.
54. Ohyama Y, Nakamura S, Matsuzaki G, et al. T-cell receptor V alpha and V beta gene use by infiltrating T cells in labial glands of patients with Sjögren's syndrome. Oral Surg Oral Med Oral Pathol Oral Radiol Endod. 1995;79:730–7.
55. Sumida T. Sjögren's syndrome. Intern Med. 1999;38:165–8.
56. Ramos-Casals M, Font J. Primary Sjögren's syndrome: current and emergent aetiopathogenic concepts. Rheumatology (Oxford) 2005;44: 1354–67.
57. Kong L, Ogawa N, Nakabayashi T, et al. Fas and Fas ligand expression in the salivary glands of patients with primary Sjögren's syndrome. Arthritis Rheum. 1997;40:87–97.
58. Ohlsson M, Szodoray P, Loro LL, Johannessen AC, Jonsson R. CD40, CD154, Bax and Bcl-2 expression in Sjögren's syndrome salivary glands: a putative anti-apoptotic role during its effector phases. Scand J Immunol. 2002;56:561–71.
59. Mosmann TR, Coffman RL. TH1 and TH2 cells: different patterns of lymphokine secretion lead to different functional properties. Annu Rev Immunol. 1989;7:145–73.

60. Weaver CT, Hatton RD, Mangan PR, Harrington LE. IL-17 family cytokines and the expanding diversity of effector T cell lineages. Annu Rev Immunol. 2007;25:821–52.
61. Steinman L. A brief history of T(H)17, the first major revision in the T(H)1/T(H)2 hypothesis of T cell-mediated tissue damage. Nat Med. 2007;13:139–45.
62. Bettelli E, Oukka M, Kuchroo VK. T(H)-17 cells in the circle of immunity and autoimmunity. Nat Immunol. 2007;8:345–50.
63. Shoda LK, Young DL, Ramanujan S, et al. A comprehensive review of interventions in the NOD mouse and implications for translation. Immunity 2005;23:115–26.
64. Serreze DV, Chapman HD, Post CM, Johnson EA, Suarez-Pinzon WL, Rabinovitch A. Th1 to Th2 cytokine shifts in nonobese diabetic mice: sometimes an outcome, rather than the cause, of diabetes resistance elicited by immunostimulation. J Immunol. 2001;166:1352–9.
65. Wynn TA. Fibrotic disease and the T(H)1/T(H)2 paradigm. Nat Rev Immunol. 2004;4:583–94.
66. Konttinen YT, Kemppinen P, Koski H, et al. T(H)1 cytokines are produced in labial salivary glands in Sjögren's syndrome, but also in healthy individuals. Scand J Rheumatol. 1999;28:106–12.
67. van Blokland SC, Versnel MA. Pathogenesis of Sjögren's syndrome: characteristics of different mouse models for autoimmune exocrinopathy. Clin Immunol. 2002;103:111–24.
68. Mitsias DI, Tzioufas AG, Veiopoulou C, et al. The Th1/Th2 cytokine balance changes with the progress of the immunopathological lesion of Sjögren's syndrome. Clin Exp Immunol. 2002;128:562–8.
69. Jonsson MV, Delaleu N, Brokstad KA, Berggreen E, Skarstein K. Impaired salivary gland function in NOD mice: association with changes in cytokine profile but not with histopathologic changes in the salivary gland. Arthritis Rheum. 2006;54:2300–5.
70. Gao J, Killedar S, Cornelius JG, Nguyen C, Cha S, Peck AB. Sjögren's syndrome in the NOD mouse model is an interleukin-4 time-dependent, antibody isotype-specific autoimmune disease. J Autoimmun. 2006;26:90–103.
71. Brayer JB, Cha S, Nagashima H, et al. IL-4-dependent effector phase in autoimmune exocrinopathy as defined by the NOD. IL-4-gene knockout mouse model of Sjögren's syndrome. Scand J Immunol. 2001;54:133–40.
72. Nguyen CQ, Gao JH, Kim H, Saban DR, Cornelius JG, Peck AB. IL-4-STAT6 signal transduction-dependent induction of the clinical phase of Sjögren's syndrome-like disease of the nonobese diabetic mouse. J Immunol. 2007;179:382–90.
73. Cha S, Brayer J, Gao J, et al. A dual role for interferon-gamma in the pathogenesis of Sjögren's syndrome-like autoimmune exocrinopathy in the nonobese diabetic mouse. Scand J Immunol. 2004;60:552–65.
74. Nguyen CQ, Hu MH, Li Y, Stewart C, Peck AB. Salivary gland tissue expression of interleukin-23 and interleukin-17 in Sjögren's syndrome: findings in humans and mice. Arthritis Rheum. 2008;58:734–43.
75. Gottenberg JE, Lavie F, Abbed K, et al. CD4 CD25high regulatory T cells are not impaired in patients with primary Sjögren's syndrome. J Autoimmun. 2005;24:235–42.
76. Li X, Li X, Qian L, et al. T regulatory cells are markedly diminished in diseased salivary glands of patients with primary Sjögren's syndrome. J Rheumatol. 2007;34:2438–45.
77. Christodoulou MI, Kapsogeorgou EK, Moutsopoulos NM, Moutsopoulos HM. $Foxp^{3+}$ T-regulatory cells in Sjögren's syndrome: correlation with the grade of the autoimmune lesion and certain adverse prognostic factors. Am J Pathol. 2008;173:1389–96.
78. Bohnhorst JO, Bjorgan MB, Thoen JE, Jonsson R, Natvig JB, Thompson KM. Abnormal B cell differentiation in primary Sjögren's syndrome results in a depressed percentage of circulating memory B cells and elevated levels of soluble CD27 that correlate with serum IgG concentration. Clin Immunol. 2002;103:79–88.
79. Hansen A, Odendahl M, Reiter K, et al. Diminished peripheral blood memory B cells and accumulation of memory B cells in the salivary glands of patients with Sjögren's syndrome. Arthritis Rheum. 2002;46:2160–71.
80. Hansen A, Reiter K, Ziprian T, et al. Dysregulation of chemokine receptor expression and function by B cells of patients with primary Sjögren's syndrome. Arthritis Rheum. 2005;52:2109–19.
81. Bohnhorst JO, Bjørgan MB, Thoen JE, Natvig JB, Thompson KM. Bm1–Bm5 classification of peripheral blood B cells reveals circulating germinal center founder cells in healthy individuals and disturbance in the B cell subpopulations in patients with primary Sjögren's syndrome. J Immunol. 2001;167:3610–8.
82. Hansen A, Jacobi A, Pruss A, et al. Comparison of immunoglobulin heavy chain rearrangements between peripheral and glandular B cells in a patient with primary Sjögren's syndrome. Scand J Immunol. 2003;57:470–9.
83. Dorner T, Hansen A, Jacobi A, Lipsky PE. Immunoglobulin repertoire analysis provides new insights into the immunopathogenesis of Sjögren's syndrome. Autoimmun Rev. 2002;1:119–24.
84. Gottenberg JE, Aucouturier F, Goetz J, et al. Serum immunoglobulin free light chain assessment in rheumatoid arthritis and primary Sjögren's syndrome. Ann Rheum Dis. 2007;66:23–7.
85. Bahler DW, Swerdlow SH. Clonal salivary gland infiltrates associated with myoepithelial

sialadenitis (Sjögren's syndrome) begin as non-malignant antigen-selected expansions. Blood 1998;91:1864–72.
86. Speight PM, Cruchley A, Williams DM. Quantification of plasma cells in labial salivary glands: increased expression of IgM in Sjögren's syndrome. J Oral Pathol Med. 1990;19:126–30.
87. Espinosa A, Zhou W, Ek M, et al. The Sjögren's syndrome-associated autoantigen Ro52 is an E3 ligase that regulates proliferation and cell death. J Immunol. 2006;176:6277–85.
88. Muller K, Manthorpe R, Permin H, Hoier-Madsen M, Oxholm P. Circulating IgM rheumatoid factors in patients with primary Sjögren's syndrome. Scand J Rheumatol Suppl. 1988;75:265–8.
89. Gottenberg JE, Mignot S, Nicaise-Rolland P, et al. Prevalence of anti-cyclic citrullinated peptide and anti-keratin antibodies in patients with primary Sjögren's syndrome. Ann Rheum Dis. 2005;64:114–7.
90. Haneji N, Nakamura T, Takio K, et al. Identification of alpha-fodrin as a candidate autoantigen in primary Sjögren's syndrome. Science 1997;276:604–7.
91. Watanabe T, Tsuchida T, Kanda N, Mori K, Hayashi Y, Tamaki K. Anti-alpha-fodrin antibodies in Sjögren syndrome and lupus erythematosus. Arch Dermatol. 1999;135:535–9.
92. Asherson RA, Fei HM, Staub HL, Khamashta MA, Hughes GR, Fox RI. Antiphospholipid antibodies and HLA associations in primary Sjögren's syndrome. Ann Rheum Dis. 1992;51:495–8.
93. Cervera R, Garcia-Carrasco M, Font J, et al. Antiphospholipid antibodies in primary Sjögren's syndrome: prevalence and clinical significance in a series of 80 patients. Clin Exp Rheumatol. 1997;15:361–5.
94. Delaleu N, Jonsson R. Altered fractalkine cleavage results in an organ-specific 17 kDa fractalkine fragment in salivary glands of NOD mice. Arthritis Res Ther. 2008;10:114.
95. Zandbelt MM, Vogelzangs J, Van De Putte LB, Van Venrooij WJ, Van Den Hoogen FH. Anti-alpha-fodrin antibodies do not add much to the diagnosis of Sjögren's syndrome. Arthritis Res Ther. 2004;6:R33–R8.
96. Jonsson MV, Szodoray P, Jellestad S, Jonsson R, Skarstein K. Association between circulating levels of the novel TNF family members APRIL and BAFF and lymphoid organization in primary Sjögren's syndrome. J Clin Immunol. 2005;25:189–201.
97. Ioannidis JP, Vassiliou VA, Moutsopoulos HM. Long-term risk of mortality and lymphoproliferative disease and predictive classification of primary Sjögren's syndrome. Arthritis Rheum. 2002;46:741–7.
98. Takemura S, Braun A, Crowson C, et al. Lymphoid neogenesis in rheumatoid synovitis. J Immunol. 2001;167:1072–80.
99. Armengol MP, Juan M, Lucas-Martin A, et al. Thyroid autoimmune disease: demonstration of thyroid antigen-specific B cells and recombination-activating gene expression in chemokine-containing active intrathyroidal germinal centers. Am J Pathol. 2001;159:861–73.
100. Mazzucchelli L, Blaser A, Kappeler A, et al. BCA-1 is highly expressed in *Helicobacter pylori*-induced mucosa-associated lymphoid tissue and gastric lymphoma. J Clin Invest. 1999;104:R49–54.
101. Humphreys-Beher MG, Brayer J, Yamachika S, Peck AB, Jonsson R. An alternative perspective to the immune response in autoimmune exocrinopathy: induction of functional quiescence rather than destructive autoaggression. Scand J Immunol. 1999;49:7–10.
102. Delaleu N. The autonomy of different aspects of sjögren's syndrome and their treatment in an experimental model. Bergen: University of Bergen; 2008.
103. Jonsson R, Kroneld U, Backman K, Magnusson B, Tarkowski A. Progression of sialadenitis in Sjögren's syndrome. Br J Rheumatol. 1993;32:578–81.
104. Dawson LJ, Field EA, Harmer AR, Smith PM. Acetylcholine-evoked calcium mobilization and ion channel activation in human labial gland acinar cells from patients with primary Sjögren's syndrome. Clin Exp Immunol. 2001;124:480–5.
105. Tsifetaki N, Kitsos G, Paschides CA, et al. Oral pilocarpine for the treatment of ocular symptoms in patients with Sjögren's syndrome: a randomised 12 week controlled study. Ann Rheum Dis. 2003;62:1204–7.
106. Dawson LJ, Fox PC, Smith PM. Sjögrens syndrome—the non-apoptotic model of glandular hypofunction. Rheumatology (Oxford) 2006;45:792–8.
107. Baum BJ, Dai Y, Hiramatsu Y, Horn VJ, Ambudkar IS. Signaling mechanisms that regulate saliva formation. Crit Rev Oral Biol Med. 1993;4:379–84.
108. Luo W, Latchney LR, Culp DJ. G protein coupling to M1 and M3 muscarinic receptors in sublingual glands. Am J Physiol Cell Physiol. 2001;280:C884–96.
109. Bymaster FP, McKinzie DL, Felder CC, Wess J. Use of M1–M5 muscarinic receptor knockout mice as novel tools to delineate the physiological roles of the muscarinic cholinergic system. Neurochem Res. 2003;28:437–42.
110. Yamada M, Miyakawa T, Duttaroy A, et al. Mice lacking the M3 muscarinic acetylcholine receptor are hypophagic and lean. Nature. 2001;410:207–12.
111. Robinson CP, Brayer J, Yamachika S, et al. Transfer of human serum IgG to nonobese diabetic Igmu null mice reveals a role for autoantibodies in the loss of secretory function of exocrine tissues in Sjögren's syndrome. Proc Natl Acad Sci USA. 1998;95:7538–43.
112. Dawson LJ, Stanbury J, Venn N, Hasdimir B, Rogers SN, Smith PM. Antimuscarinic antibodies

in primary Sjögren's syndrome reversibly inhibit the mechanism of fluid secretion by human submandibular salivary acinar cells. Arthritis Rheum. 2006;54:1165–73.

113. Goldblatt F, Gordon TP, Waterman SA. Antibody-mediated gastrointestinal dysmotility in scleroderma. Gastroenterology 2002;123:1144–50.
114. Waterman SA, Gordon TP, Rischmueller M. Inhibitory effects of muscarinic receptor autoantibodies on parasympathetic neurotransmission in Sjögren's syndrome. Arthritis Rheum. 2000;43:1647–54.
115. Gao J, Cha S, Jonsson R, Opalko J, Peck AB. Detection of anti-type 3 muscarinic acetylcholine receptor autoantibodies in the sera of Sjögren's syndrome patients by use of a transfected cell line assay. Arthritis Rheum. 2004;50: 2615–21.
116. Marczinovits I, Kovacs L, Gyorgy A, et al. A peptide of human muscarinic acetylcholine receptor 3 is antigenic in primary Sjögren's syndrome. J Autoimmun. 2005;24:47–54.
117. Cavill D, Waterman SA, Gordon TP. Failure to detect antibodies to extracellular loop peptides of the muscarinic M3 receptor in primary Sjögren's syndrome. J Rheumatol. 2002;29:1342–4.
118. Dawson LJ, Allison HE, Stanbury J, Fitzgerald D, Smith PM. Putative anti-muscarinic antibodies cannot be detected in patients with primary Sjögren's syndrome using conventional immunological approaches. Rheumatology (Oxford) 2004;43:1488–95.
119. Budd DC, McDonald J, Emsley N, Cain K, Tobin AB. The C-terminal tail of the M3-muscarinic receptor possesses anti-apoptotic properties. J Biol Chem. 2003;278:19565–73.
120. Cha S, Singson E, Cornelius J, Yagna JP, Knot HJ, Peck AB. Muscarinic acetylcholine type-3 receptor desensitization due to chronic exposure to Sjögren's syndrome-associated autoantibodies. J Rheumatol. 2006;33:296–306.
121. Tayebati SK, El-Assouad D, Ricci A, Amenta F. Immunochemical and immunocytochemical characterization of cholinergic markers in human peripheral blood lymphocytes. J Neuroimmunol. 2002;132:147–55.
122. Main C, Blennerhassett P, Collins SM. Human recombinant interleukin 1 beta suppresses acetylcholine release from rat myenteric plexus. Gastroenterology 1993;104:1648–54.
123. Zoukhri D, Kublin CL. Impaired neurotransmitter release from lacrimal and salivary gland nerves of a murine model of Sjögren's syndrome. Invest Ophthalmol Vis Sci. 2001;42:925–32.
124. Dawson LJ, Christmas SE, Smith PM. An investigation of interactions between the immune system and stimulus-secretion coupling in mouse submandibular acinar cells. A possible mechanism to account for reduced salivary flow rates associated with the onset of Sjögren's syndrome. Rheumatology (Oxford) 2000;39:1226–33.
125. Konttinen YT, Halinen S, Hanemaaijer R, et al. Matrix metalloproteinase (MMP)-9 type IV collagenase/gelatinase implicated in the pathogenesis of Sjögren's syndrome. Matrix Biol. 1998;17:335–47.
126. Beroukas D, Goodfellow R, Hiscock J, Jonsson R, Gordon TP, Waterman SA. Up-regulation of M3-muscarinic receptors in labial salivary gland acini in primary Sjögren's syndrome. Lab Invest. 2002;82:203–10.
127. Agre P, King LS, Yasui M, et al. Aquaporin water channels—from atomic structure to clinical medicine. J Physiol. 2002;542:3–16.
128. Gresz V, Kwon TH, Hurley PT, et al. Identification and localization of aquaporin water channels in human salivary glands. Am J Physiol Gastrointest Liver Physiol. 2001;281:G247–54.
129. Nguyen KH, Brayer J, Cha S, et al. Evidence for antimuscarinic acetylcholine receptor antibody-mediated secretory dysfunction in nod mice. Arthritis Rheum. 2000;43:2297–306.
130. Krane CM, Melvin JE, Nguyen HV, et al. Salivary acinar cells from aquaporin 5-deficient mice have decreased membrane water permeability and altered cell volume regulation. J Biol Chem. 2001;276:23413–20.
131. Soyfoo MS, De Vriese C, Debaix H, et al. Modified aquaporin 5 expression and distribution in submandibular glands from NOD mice displaying autoimmune exocrinopathy. Arthritis Rheum. 2007;56:2566–74.
132. Steinfeld S, Cogan E, King LS, Agre P, Kiss R, Delporte C. Abnormal distribution of aquaporin-5 water channel protein in salivary glands from Sjögren's syndrome patients. Lab Invest. 2001;81:143–8.
133. Beroukas D, Hiscock J, Jonsson R, Waterman SA, Gordon TP. Subcellular distribution of aquaporin 5 in salivary glands in primary Sjögren's syndrome. Lancet 2001;358:1875–6.
134. Beroukas D, Hiscock J, Gannon BJ, Jonsson R, Gordon TP, Waterman SA. Selective down-regulation of aquaporin-1 in salivary glands in primary Sjögren's syndrome. Lab Invest. 2002;82:1547–52.
135. Kyewski B, Klein L. A central role for central tolerance. Annu Rev Immunol. 2006;24:571–606.
136. Burnet FM. The Nobel Lectures in Immunology. The Nobel Prize for Physiology or Medicine, 1960. Immunologic recognition of self. Scand J Immunol. 1991;33:3–13.
137. Nepom GT, Erlich H. MHC class-II molecules and autoimmunity. Annu Rev Immunol. 1991;9: 493–525.
138. Fernando MM, Stevens CR, Walsh EC, et al. Defining the role of the MHC in autoimmunity: a review and pooled analysis. PLoS Genet. 2008;4:e1000024.

139. Klareskog L, Ronnelid J, Lundberg K, Padyukov L, Alfredsson L. Immunity to citrullinated proteins in rheumatoid arthritis. Annu Rev Immunol. 2008;26:651–75.
140. Bolstad AI, Jonsson R. Genetic aspects of Sjögren's syndrome. Arthritis Res. 2002;4:353–9.
141. Harangi M, Kaminski WE, Fleck M, et al. Homozygosity for the 168His variant of the minor histocompatibility antigen HA-1 is associated with reduced risk of primary Sjögren's syndrome. Eur J Immunol. 2005;35:305–17.
142. Miceli-Richard C, Comets E, Loiseau P, Puechal X, Hachulla E, Mariette X. Association of an *IRF5* gene functional polymorphism with Sjögren's syndrome. Arthritis Rheum. 2007;56:3989–94.
143. Bolstad AI, Wargelius A, Nakken B, Haga HJ, Jonsson R. Fas and Fas ligand gene polymorphisms in primary Sjögren's syndrome. J Rheumatol. 2000;27:2397–405.
144. Magnusson V, Nakken B, Bolstad AI, Alarcon-Riquelme ME. Cytokine polymorphisms in systemic lupus erythematosus and Sjögren's syndrome. Scand J Immunol. 2001;54:55–61.
145. Gottenberg JE, Loiseau P, Azarian M, et al. CTLA-4 +49A/G and CT60 gene polymorphisms in primary Sjögren syndrome. Arthritis Res Ther. 2007;9:R24.
146. Miceli-Richard C, Dieude P, Hachulla E, Puechal X, Cornelis F, Mariette X. Tumour necrosis factor receptor 2 (TNFRSF1B) association study in Sjögren's syndrome. Ann Rheum Dis. 2007;66:1684–5.
147. Kahlmann D, Davalos-Misslitz AC, Ohl L, Stanke F, Witte T, Forster R. Genetic variants of chemokine receptor CCR7 in patients with systemic lupus erythematosus, Sjögren's syndrome and systemic sclerosis. BMC Genet. 2007;8:33.
148. Moutsopoulos HM, Papadopoulos GK. Possible viral implication in the pathogenesis of Sjögren's syndrome. Eur J Med. 1992;1:219–23.
149. Blank M, Barzilai O, Shoenfeld Y. Molecular mimicry and auto-immunity. Clin Rev Allergy Immunol. 2007;32:111–8.
150. Pflugfelder SC, Crouse CA, Monroy D, Yen M, Rowe M, Atherton SS. Epstein–Barr virus and the lacrimal gland pathology of Sjögren's syndrome. Am J Pathol. 1993;143:49–64.
151. Green JE, Hinrichs SH, Vogel J, Jay G. Exocrinopathy resembling Sjögren's syndrome in HTLV-1 tax transgenic mice. Nature 1989;341:72–4.
152. Haddad J, Deny P, Munz-Gotheil C, et al. Lymphocytic sialadenitis of Sjögren's syndrome associated with chronic hepatitis C virus liver disease. Lancet 1992;339:321–3.
153. Fleck M, Kern ER, Zhou T, Lang B, Mountz JD. Murine cytomegalovirus induces a Sjögren's syndrome-like disease in C57Bl/6-lpr/lpr mice. Arthritis Rheum. 1998;41:2175–84.
154. Fleck M, Zhang HG, Kern ER, Hsu HC, Muller-Ladner U, Mountz JD. Treatment of chronic sialadenitis in a murine model of Sjögren's syndrome by local fasL gene transfer. Arthritis Rheum. 2001;44:964–73.
155. Triantafyllopoulou A, Tapinos N, Moutsopoulos HM. Evidence for coxsackievirus infection in primary Sjögren's syndrome. Arthritis Rheum. 2004;50:2897–902.
156. Gottenberg JE, Pallier C, Ittah M, et al. Failure to confirm coxsackievirus infection in primary Sjögren's syndrome. Arthritis Rheum. 2006;54:2026–8.
157. Hjelmervik TO, Lindqvist AK, Petersen K, et al. The influence of the NOD Nss1/Idd5 loci on sialadenitis and gene expression in salivary glands of congenic mice. Arthritis Res Ther. 2007;9:R99.
158. Killedar SJ, Eckenrode SE, McIndoe RA, et al. Early pathogenic events associated with Sjögren's syndrome (SjS)-like disease of the NOD mouse using microarray analysis. Lab Invest. 2006;86:1243–60.
159. Theofilopoulos AN, Baccala R, Beutler B, Kono DH. Type I interferons (alpha/beta) in immunity and autoimmunity. Annu Rev Immunol. 2005;23:307–36.
160. Matzinger P. Friendly and dangerous signals: is the tissue in control? Nat Immunol. 2007;8:11–3.
161. Matzinger P. The danger model: a renewed sense of self. Science 2002;296:301–5.
162. Konttinen YT, Kasna-Ronkainen L. Sjögren's syndrome: viewpoint on pathogenesis. One of the reasons I was never asked to write a textbook chapter on it. Scand J Rheumatol. Suppl. 2002;116:15–22.
163. Ohlsson M, Jonsson R, Brokstad KA. Subcellular redistribution and surface exposure of the Ro52, Ro60 and La48 autoantigens during apoptosis in human ductal epithelial cells: a possible mechanism in the pathogenesis of Sjögren's syndrome. Scand J Immunol. 2002;56:456–69.
164. Rosen A, Casciola-Rosen L. Altered autoantigen structure in Sjögren's syndrome: implications for the pathogenesis of autoimmune tissue damage. Crit Rev Oral Biol Med. 2004;15:156–64.
165. Nagaraju K, Cox A, Casciola-Rosen L, Rosen A. Novel fragments of the Sjögren's syndrome autoantigens alpha-fodrin and type 3 muscarinic acetylcholine receptor generated during cytotoxic lymphocyte granule-induced cell death. Arthritis Rheum. 2001;44:2376–86.
166. Lovgren T, Eloranta ML, Kastner B, Wahren-Herlenius M, Alm GV, Ronnblom L. Induction of interferon-alpha by immune complexes or liposomes containing systemic lupus erythematosus autoantigen- and Sjögren's syndrome autoantigen-associated RNA. Arthritis Rheum. 2006;54:1917–27.
167. Nordmark G, Alm GV, Ronnblom L. Mechanisms of disease: primary Sjögren's syndrome and the

type I interferon system. Nat Clin Pract Rheumatol. 2006;2:262–9.

168. Scofield RH, Asfa S, Obeso D, Jonsson R, Kurien BT. Immunization with short peptides from the 60-kDa Ro antigen recapitulates the serological and pathological findings as well as the salivary gland dysfunction of Sjögren's syndrome. J Immunol. 2005;175:8409–14.
169. Kurien BT, Asfa S, Li C, Dorri Y, Jonsson R, Scofield RH. Induction of oral tolerance in experimental Sjögren's syndrome autoimmunity. Scand J Immunol. 2005;61:418–25.
170. Topfer F, Gordon T, McCluskey J. Intra- and intermolecular spreading of autoimmunity involving the nuclear self-antigens La (SS-B) and Ro (SS-A). Proc Natl Acad Sci USA. 1995;92:875–9.
171. Tseng CE, Chan EK, Miranda E, Gross M, Di Donato F, Buyon JP. The 52-kd protein as a target of intermolecular spreading of the immune response to components of the SS-A/Ro-SS-B/La complex. Arthritis Rheum. 1997;40:936–44.
172. Keech CL, Gordon TP, McCluskey J. The immune response to 52-kDa Ro and 60-kDa Ro is linked in experimental autoimmunity. J Immunol. 1996;157:3694–9.
173. Reynolds P, Gordon TP, Purcell AW, Jackson DC, McCluskey J. Hierarchical self-tolerance to T cell determinants within the ubiquitous nuclear self-antigen La (SS-B) permits induction of systemic autoimmunity in normal mice. J Exp Med. 1996;184:1857–70.
174. Masago R, Aiba-Masago S, Talal N, et al. Elevated proapoptotic Bax and caspase 3 activation in the NOD.scid model of Sjögren's syndrome. Arthritis Rheum. 2001;44:693–702.
175. Li H, Dai M, Zhuang Y. A T cell intrinsic role of Id3 in a mouse model for primary Sjögren's syndrome. Immunity. 2004;21:551–60.
176. Hayakawa I, Tedder TF, Zhuang Y. B-lymphocyte depletion ameliorates Sjögren's syndrome in Id3 knockout mice. Immunology 2007;122:73–9.
177. Sellam J, Miceli-Richard C, Gottenberg JE, et al. Is inhibitor of differentiation 3 involved in human primary Sjögren's syndrome? Rheumatology (Oxford) 2008;47:437–41.
178. Belkaid Y. Regulatory T cells and infection: a dangerous necessity. Nat Rev Immunol. 2007;7: 875–88.
179. Sakaguchi S. Naturally arising Foxp3-expressing $CD25^{+}CD4^{+}$ regulatory T cells in immunological tolerance to self and non-self. Nat Immunol. 2005;6:345–52.
180. Chatenoud L, Bluestone JA. CD3-specific antibodies: a portal to the treatment of autoimmunity. Nat Rev Immunol. 2007;7:622–32.
181. Zanin-Zhorov A, Cahalon L, Tal G, Margalit R, Lider O, Cohen IR. Heat shock protein 60 enhances $CD4^{+}$ $CD25^{+}$ regulatory T cell function via innate TLR2 signaling. J Clin Invest. 2006;116:2022–32.
182. Kulkarni AB, Huh CG, Becker D, et al. Transforming growth factor beta 1 null mutation in mice causes excessive inflammatory response and early death. Proc Natl Acad Sci USA. 1993;90:770–4.
183. Kok MR, Yamano S, Lodde BM, et al. Local adeno-associated virus-mediated interleukin 10 gene transfer has disease-modifying effects in a murine model of Sjögren's syndrome. Hum Gene Ther. 2003;14:1605–18.
184. Saito I, Haruta K, Shimuta M, et al. Fas ligand-mediated exocrinopathy resembling Sjögren's syndrome in mice transgenic for IL-10. J Immunol. 1999;162:2488–94.
185. Salam MA, Matin K, Matsumoto N, Tsuha Y, Hanada N, Senpuku H. E2f1 mutation induces early onset of diabetes and Sjögren's syndrome in nonobese diabetic mice. J Immunol. 2004;173:4908–18.
186. Setoguchi R, Hori S, Takahashi T, Sakaguchi S. Homeostatic maintenance of natural Foxp3(+) CD25(+) CD4(+) regulatory T cells by interleukin (IL)-2 and induction of autoimmune disease by IL-2 neutralization. J Exp Med. 2005;201:723–35.
187. Sharma R, Zheng L, Guo X, Fu SM, Ju ST, Jarjour WN. Novel animal models for Sjögren's syndrome: expression and transfer of salivary gland dysfunction from regulatory T cell-deficient mice. J Autoimmun. 2006;27:289–96.
188. Oak JS, Deane JA, Kharas MG, et al. Sjögren's syndrome-like disease in mice with T cells lacking class 1A phosphoinositide-3-kinase. Proc Natl Acad Sci USA. 2006;103:16882–7.
189. Merbl Y, Zucker-Toledano M, Quintana FJ, Cohen IR. Newborn humans manifest autoantibodies to defined self molecules detected by antigen microarray informatics. J Clin Invest. 2007;117:712–8.
190. Avrameas S, Ternynck T, Tsonis IA, Lymberi P. Naturally occurring B-cell autoreactivity: a critical overview. J Autoimmun. 2007;29:213–8.
191. Cohen IR. Autoimmunity to chaperonins in the pathogenesis of arthritis and diabetes. Annu Rev Immunol. 1991;9:567–89.
192. Cohen IR. The cognitive paradigm and the immunological homunculus. Immunol Today. 1992;13: 490–4.
193. Satpute SR, Durai M, Moudgil KD. Antigen-specific tolerogenic and immunomodulatory strategies for the treatment of autoimmune arthritis. Semin Arthritis Rheum. 2008;38(3):195–207.
194. van Eden W, van der Zee R, Prakken B. Heat-shock proteins induce T-cell regulation of chronic inflammation. Nat Rev Immunol. 2005;5:318–30.
195. Chatenoud L. Immune therapies of autoimmune diseases: are we approaching a real cure? Curr Opin Immunol. 2006;18:710–7.
196. Curtis JR, Xi J, Patkar N, Xie A, Saag KG, Martin C. Drug-specific and time-dependent risks of bacterial infection among patients with rheumatoid

arthritis who were exposed to tumor necrosis factor alpha antagonists. Arthritis Rheum. 2007;56: 4226–7.

197. Mackay F, Schneider P, Rennert P, Browning J. BAFF and APRIL: a tutorial on B cell survival. Annu Rev Immunol. 2003;21:231–64.
198. Groom J, Kalled SL, Cutler AH, et al. Association of BAFF/BLyS overexpression and altered B cell differentiation with Sjögren's syndrome. J Clin Invest. 2002;109:59–68.
199. Fletcher CA, Sutherland AP, Groom JR, et al. Development of nephritis but not sialadenitis in autoimmune-prone BAFF transgenic mice lacking marginal zone B cells. Eur J Immunol. 2006;36:2504–14.
200. Mariette X, Roux S, Zhang J, et al. The level of BLyS (BAFF) correlates with the titre of autoantibodies in human Sjögren's syndrome. Ann Rheum Dis. 2003;62:168–71.
201. Daridon C, Devauchelle V, Hutin P, et al. Aberrant expression of BAFF by B lymphocytes infiltrating the salivary glands of patients with primary Sjögren's syndrome. Arthritis Rheum. 2007;56:1134–44.
202. Ittah M, Miceli-Richard C, Eric Gottenberg J, et al. B cell-activating factor of the tumor necrosis factor family (BAFF) is expressed under stimulation by interferon in salivary gland epithelial cells in primary Sjögren's syndrome. Arthritis Res Ther. 2006;8:R51.
203. Szodoray P, Jellestad S, Teague MO, Jonsson R. Attenuated apoptosis of B cell activating factor-expressing cells in primary Sjögren's syndrome. Lab Invest. 2003;83:357–65.
204. Lavie F, Miceli-Richard C, Ittah M, Sellam J, Gottenberg JE, Mariette X. Increase of B cell-activating factor of the TNF family (BAFF) after rituximab treatment: insights into a new regulating system of BAFF production. Ann Rheum Dis. 2007;66:700–3.
205. Devauchelle-Pensec V, Pennec Y, Morvan J, et al. Improvement of Sjögren's syndrome after two infusions of rituximab (anti-CD20). Arthritis Rheum. 2007;57:310–7.
206. Laine M, Porola P, Udby L, et al. Low salivary dehydroepiandrosterone and androgen-regulated cysteine-rich secretory protein 3 levels in Sjögren's syndrome. Arthritis Rheum. 2007;56:2575–84.
207. Shim GJ, Warner M, Kim HJ, et al. Aromatase-deficient mice spontaneously develop a lymphoproliferative autoimmune disease resembling Sjögren's syndrome. Proc Natl Acad Sci USA. 2004;101:12628–33.
208. Grimaldi CM, Cleary J, Dagtas AS, Moussai D, Diamond B. Estrogen alters thresholds for B cell apoptosis and activation. J Clin Invest. 2002;109:1625–33.
209. Grimaldi CM, Michael DJ, Diamond B. Cutting edge: expansion and activation of a population of autoreactive marginal zone B cells in a model of estrogen-induced lupus. J Immunol. 2001;167: 1886–90.
210. Bynoe MS, Grimaldi CM, Diamond B. Estrogen up-regulates Bcl-2 and blocks tolerance induction of naive B cells. Proc Natl Acad Sci USA. 2000;97:2703–8.
211. Kuroki M, Okayama A, Nakamura S, et al. Detection of maternal–fetal microchimerism in the inflammatory lesions of patients with Sjögren's syndrome. Ann Rheum Dis. 2002;61:1041–6.
212. Endo Y, Negishi I, Ishikawa O. Possible contribution of microchimerism to the pathogenesis of Sjögren's syndrome. Rheumatology (Oxford) 2002;41:490–5.
213. Aractingi S, Sibilia J, Meignin V, et al. Presence of microchimerism in labial salivary glands in systemic sclerosis but not in Sjögren's syndrome. Arthritis Rheum. 2002;46:1039–43.
214. Devauchelle-Pensec V, Cagnard N, Pers JO, Youinou P, Saraux A, Chiocchia G. Gene expression profile in the salivary glands of primary Sjögren's syndrome patients before and after treatment with rituximab. Arthritis Rheum. 2010;62:2262–71.
215. Alevizos I, Alexander S, Turner RJ, Illei GG. MicroRNA expression profiles as biomarkers of minor salivary gland inflammation and dysfunction in Sjögren's syndrome. Arthritis Rheum. 2011;63:535–44.
216. Gonzalez S, Aguilera S, Alliende C, et al. Alterations in type I-hemidesmosome components suggest epigenetic control in salivary glands from Sjögren's syndrome patients. Arthritis Rheum. 2011.
217. Ewert P, Aguilera S, Alliende C, et al. Disruption of tight junction structure in salivary glands from Sjögren's syndrome patients is linked to proinflammatory cytokine exposure. Arthritis Rheum. 2010;62:1280–9.
218. Delaleu N, Nguyen CQ, Peck AB, Jonsson R. Sjögren's syndrome: studying the disease in mice. Arthritis Res Ther. 2011;13:217.
219. Garantziotis S, Hollingsworth JW, Zaas AK, Schwartz DA. The effect of toll-like receptors and toll-like receptor genetics in human disease. Annu Rev Med. 2008;59:343–59.
220. Mavragani CP, Crow MK. Activation of the type I interferon pathway in primary Sjögren's syndrome. J Autoimmun. 2010;35:225–31.
221. Higgs R, Lazzari E, Wynne C, et al. Self protection from anti-viral responses—Ro52 promotes degradation of the transcription factor IRF7 downstream of the viral Toll-like receptors. PLoS One 2010;5:e11776.
222. Ronnblom L, Alm GV, Eloranta ML. The type I interferon system in the development of lupus. Semin Immunol. 2011;23:113–21.
223. Miceli-Richard C, Gestermann N, Ittah M, et al. The CGGGG insertion/deletion polymorphism of

the IRF5 promoter is a strong risk factor for primary Sjögren's syndrome. Arthritis Rheum. 2009;60:1991–7.
224. Nordmark G, Kristjansdottir G, Theander E, et al. Association of EBF1, FAM167A(C8orf13)-BLK and TNFSF4 gene variants with primary Sjögren' syndrome. Genes Immun. 2011;12:100–9.
225. Vogelsang P, Brun JG, Oijordsbakken G, Skarstein K, Jonsson R, Appel S. Levels of plasmacytoid dendritic cells and type-2 myeloid dendritic cells are reduced in peripheral blood of patients with primary Sjögren's syndrome. Ann Rheum Dis. 2010;69:1235–8.
226. Katsifis GE, Rekka S, Moutsopoulos NM, Pillemer S, Wahl SM. Systemic and local interleukin-17 and linked cytokines associated with Sjögren's syndrome immunopathogenesis. Am J Pathol. 2009;175:1167–77.
227. Sakai A, Sugawara Y, Kuroishi T, Sasano T, Sugawara S. Identification of IL-18 and Th17 cells in salivary glands of patients with Sjögren's syndrome, and amplification of IL-17-mediated secretion of inflammatory cytokines from salivary gland cells by IL-18. J Immunol. 2008;181:2898–906.
228. Szyszko EA, Brokstad KA, Oijordsbakken G, Jonsson MV, Jonsson R, Skarstein K. Salivary glands of primary Sjögren's syndrome patients express factors vital for plasma cell survival. Arthritis Res Ther. 2011;13:R2.
229. Delaleu N, Jonsson MV, Jonsson R. Disease mechanisms of Sjögren's syndrome. Drug Discov Today: Dis Mech. 2004;1:329–36.

Otolaryngologic Manifestations of Sjögren's Syndrome

16

Jacqui E. Allen and Peter C. Belafsky

Abstract

Sjögren's syndrome (SS) is an insidious progressive autoimmune disease characterized by exocrinopathy and a predilection for women. It affects many organ systems; however, head and neck manifestations predominate and are frequently the initial presenting complaints. A high index of suspicion should be maintained to permit early diagnosis and minimize long-term complications of the disease. This chapter aims to review the otolaryngologic manifestations of Sjögren's syndrome, current diagnostic tools, and treatment.

Keywords

Sjögren's syndrome • Oral • Nasal • Laryngeal • Esophageal • Esophageal dysmotility • Laryngopharyngeal reflux • Xerostomia • Xerotrachea • Hyposalivation • Dental caries • Salivary gland lymphoma • Sialography • Salivary scintigraphy • Salivary MRI • Lip biopsy • Parotid biopsy • Autoimmune • Extra-glandular manifestations

16.1 Introduction

Sjögren's syndrome (SS) is an insidious progressive autoimmune disease. The disorder is characterized by exocrinopathy and is present in two forms, namely, primary Sjögren's syndrome (pSS) and secondary Sjögren's syndrome (sSS). Sjögren's syndrome is more common in women and affects up to 3% of the American population [1–3]. It is the second most common autoimmune disease after rheumatoid arthritis. The disorder has devastating effects and is responsible for dramatic reductions in quality of life.

Although symptoms may affect many organ systems, head and neck manifestations predominate and are frequently the initial presenting complaints [1, 4]. A high index of suspicion should be maintained to permit early diagnosis and minimize long-term complications of the disease. The purpose of this chapter is to review the otolaryngologic manifestations of Sjögren's syndrome.

P.C. Belafsky (✉)
The Center for Voice and Swallowing, University of California at Davis, Davis, CA, USA
e-mail: pbelafsky@sbcglobal.net

R.I. Fox, C.M. Fox (eds.), *Sjögren's Syndrome*, DOI 10.1007/978-1-60327-957-4_16,

16.2 Diagnosis

There is no single test for SS. There have been at least seven different sets of criteria proposed over the last quarter century [5]. The myriad of criteria has clouded the diagnostic waters and confused both patients and care givers alike. Delay between the onset of patient symptoms and the actual diagnosis may average greater than 6 years [1, 5]. The protracted time until diagnosis often exacerbates patient frustration. Clinicians should remain empathetic and work diligently to restore patient–physician confidence.

In recent years, trans-Atlantic discussion has resulted in the American–European Consensus Group criteria published in 2002 [5–9]. The criteria exhibit 95% sensitivity and specificity for diagnosis. These criteria include subjective and objective measures related to the sicca syndrome-type "glandular" manifestations—that is xerostomia and xerophthalmia caused by exocrine gland dysfunction (salivary and lacrimal glands, respectively) [1, 6]. Up to one-third of patients will also suffer extra-glandular manifestations that may affect diverse organ systems and be mistaken for other disease entities [2, 3]. Pulmonary, renal, cutaneous, and hematologic involvement have all been well documented [1–4, 9–11].

Workup in patients suspected of SS should include a comprehensive history and physical examination as listed in Table 16.1. Salivary gland enlargement is one of the most frequent physical examination findings encountered in the head and neck and is often one of the initial manifestations of the disease. Patients with diffuse parotid or submandibular gland enlargement and dry mucous membranes should be considered to have SS until proven otherwise. When examining the oral cavity and pharynx with a

Table 16.1 ORL workup and investigations

History
Xerostomia, xerophthalmia, salivary gland swelling and discomfort, sialadenitis, recurrent sinusitis, epistaxis, hyposmia, septal perforation, hearing loss, voice changes, symptoms of acid reflux, dysphagia, weight loss, regurgitations, odynophagia
Comorbidities, autoimmunity, family history, prior radiation
Medication list
Examination
Ophthalmic—corneal integrity, acuity, Schirmer's test, vital dye staining
Oral—angular cheilitis, fissured tongue, depapillation, dry mucosa, dental status, periodontal health, presence of fungal infection, salivary flow to massage, gland size, and texture. Positive Oral Allen's Test
Otologic—clinical tests of hearing, audiometry
Laryngeal—laryngoscopy, strobovideolaryngoscopy, tracheoscopy, subjective voice evaluation and objective acoustic analysis, laryngeal findings of reflux
Rhinologic—rhinoscopy, endoscopic examination, test of olfaction
Esophageal—esophagoscopy
Neck—thyroid gland, lymphadenopathy, submandibular, and parotid gland evaluation
Neurological—cranial nerve assessment
Laboratory testing
Autoantibody screening
Investigations
Ultrasound scanning of salivary and thyroid glands
Sialography, sialometry, sialochemistry
pH metry, manometry, impedance testing
Biopsies—labial glands, parotid glands, esophageal

wooden disposable tongue blade, the moisture in the mouth should not allow the blade to stick to the inner mucosa of the cheek. If the tongue blade does stick to the mucosa, oral moisture is poor and screening for SS is indicated. We refer to this as the Oral Allen Test.

Investigations in addition to normal serological markers include salivary gland ultrasound, computed tomography (CT), and sialography. Biopsies of affected minor or major salivary glands can be diagnostic and there is new evidence that suggests fine needle aspiration of the parotid gland can be diagnostic even when labial biopsies fail to demonstrate SS [12]. Pijpe and colleagues have compared parotid biopsy to labial biopsy and suggest it is equally specific and sensitive in the diagnosis of SS [13]. They site ease of harvest, low morbidity, and incidental diagnosis of lymphoma as advantages of parotid biopsy [13]. Distinct lesions palpable in glands must be biopsied promptly and may require ultrasound guidance. CT scanning allows assessment of both glands for lesions such as Warthin's tumors that may be seen bilaterally or for discreet lesions such as lymphoma. CT imaging also helps define the medial extent of a parotid mass into the parapharyngeal space (seen with deep lobe pleiomorphic adenomas) and helps identify cervical lymphadenopathy.

Recent publications have focused on new diagnostic techniques with the aim of early identification of Sjögren's development and knowledge that 15–26% of SS patients may not display typical xerostomia [1, 14]. Mignogna and colleagues suggest that sialochemistry, sialorrhea, early dental loss, and salivary gland swelling may occur well before development of hyposalivation and resultant xerostomia [14]. Hocevar et al. have suggested the use of an ultrasound scoring system (USS) to assist in the diagnosis given the non-invasive nature of the examination [15]. A recent publication further supports USS as a cheap, readily available, and non-invasive method of examining salivary glands in SS. Parenchymal inhomogeneity is said to be most specific for involvement of glands with SS [16, 17]. USS was suggested as a further diagnostic adjunct to the current American–European Consensus Group criteria [16]. Sialography involves filling the salivary gland ductal system with radio-opaque contrast media and obtaining plain X-ray films. A typical pattern of ductal ectasia with a "snowstorm" punctuate appearance of isolated acini can be seen in established Sjögren's syndrome. This is a technically demanding study requiring cannulation of Stenson's or Wharton's duct and is frequently painful [18, 19]. Salivary scintigraphy has been in use for more than 30 years and is non-invasive. It requires, however, the use of radioactive tracers and lacks quantitative parameters necessary to consistently establish a diagnosis [18]. The most reliable findings are a reduced parotid:submandibular gland uptake ratio (P:S ratio) and excretion fraction ratio less than 50% in the parotid (suggesting abnormal function). More than 25% of the gland mass must be lost to see a detectable difference. This is highly relevant in light of recent evidence that functional acini remain present in dysfunctional glands, suggesting neurohumoral mechanisms of reduced salivary flow [14]. It is used less commonly now, being replaced by CT scanning, USS, and magnetic resonance scans.

Magnetic resonance imaging and MR sialography (MRS) are fast becoming diagnostic modalities. They are highly sensitive (comparable to USS and better than scintigraphy), non-invasive, quickly performed, and not particularly operator-dependent. Performed with surface coils rather than head coils, the resolution is improved, particularly when the studies are combined. Excellent definition of the ductal system can be achieved and parenchymal changes noted [20, 21]. Furthermore Morimoto et al. have described dynamic MRS combining both morphological assessment and functional assessment (contrasting scans before and after citric acid stimulation) [22]. It is likely that MR studies will become more widespread in the diagnosis of salivary glandular abnormalities and SS [20–22].

The astute clinician employs a combination of serologic tests, imaging, and/or labial/parotid gland biopsy at an early stage to confirm diagnostic suspicion.

16.3 Head and Neck Manifestations

16.3.1 Ophthalmic

Dryness (xerophthalmia) is characteristic of SS and can lead to a variety of eye symptoms and signs. These will be described in detail in other chapters and will not be discussed here.

16.3.2 Oral

Xerostomia and oral pain are some of the most common presenting symptoms and key diagnostic features of SS [1, 2, 23]. However, there is a plethora of signs and symptoms that may be found in the oral cavity of Sjögren's syndrome patients (Table 16.2). Oral pain and dryness are debilitating and can markedly reduce quality of life by making speech and deglutition exceedingly difficult and uncomfortable [24]. Taste is reduced and atrophy of the lingual papillae may be seen. Hypersensitivity to spicy foods or strong tastes can occur, in some cases resulting in "burning mouth" or stomatopyrosis [24]. Hyposalivation caused by salivary dysfunction also threatens dentition, with early dental loss contributing to poor mastication and food intake. Periodontal disease is commonplace and requires meticulous dental hygiene to prevent complications (Fig. 16.1). Up to three quarters of SS patients may show signs of chronic erythematous candidiasis often affecting the palate or buccal region [1, 2, 23–25]. Extension of candida to the laryngopharynx and esophagus is also frequently encountered (Figs. 16.2 and 16.3). Distal chip, high definition video laryngoscopes, and ultrathin esophagoscopes have greatly increased our ability to diagnose subtle laryngeal and pharyngeal candidiasis often missed with traditional fiberoptic endoscopes. Regular dental examination is required and topical fluoride treatment may be used to delay caries formation [23]. Patients may be aware of poor oral health but often require education in correct oral care techniques [24].

Table 16.2 Oral manifestations of Sjögren's syndrome

Xerostomia
Dental caries
Periodontal disease
Early tooth loss
Mouth and throat pain
Denture problems
Difficulty swallowing and chewing
Chronic erythematous candidiasis
Stomatopyrosis
Halitosis
Dysgeusia
Salivary gland enlargement
Angular cheilitis
Oral ulceration
Lymphoma

Saliva has a critical immune role, protecting oral tissue from bacterial adherence, carrying immune proteins such as lysozyme, lactoferrin, and secretory IgA that control oral flora,

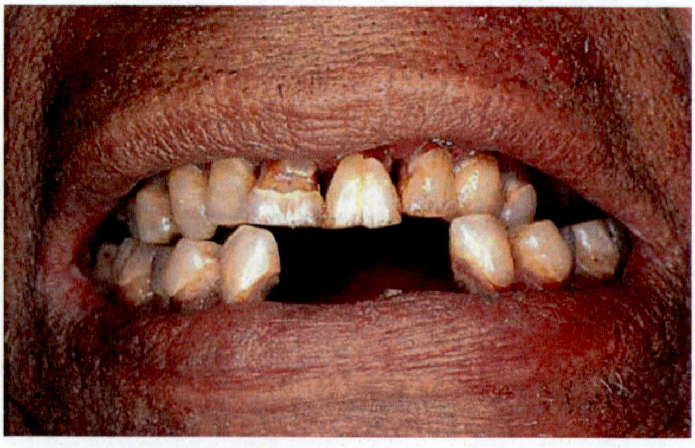

Fig. 16.1 Dental caries due to xerostomia

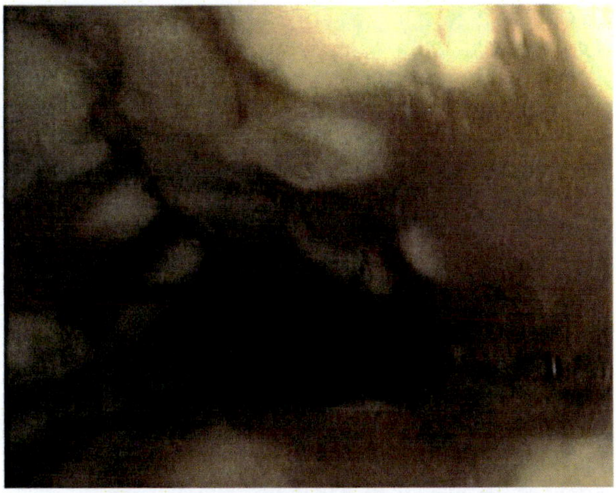

Fig. 16.2 Esophageal candidiasis in a patient with Sjögren's syndrome and dysphagia

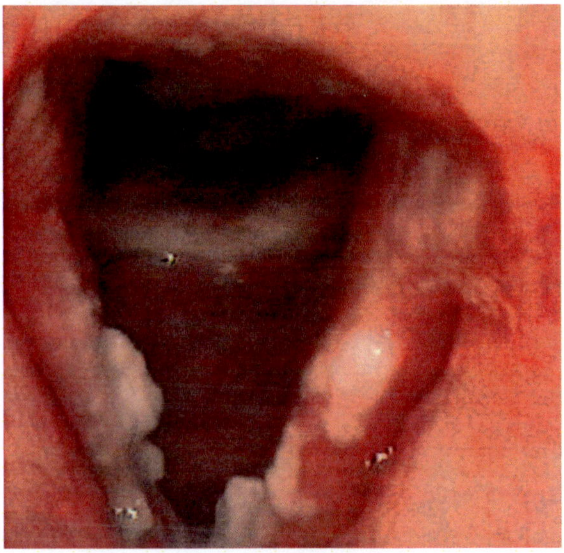

Fig. 16.3 Laryngeal candidiasis in a patient with Sjögren's syndrome

lubricate ingested material, and minimize traumatic damage [23–25]. Saliva flow also mechanically flushes the oral cavity and clears residue. It acts as a buffering solution stabilizing pH, is a solvent for ions critical to remineralization of teeth, and tastants that flavor food [1, 23–25]. The composition and flow rate of saliva are altered in SS [25]. The concentration of proteins is changed with a decrease in secretory IgA, which weakens the body's defense against plaque and caries [25]. Usually a total of 1.5 L of saliva is made per day. This can be reduced in SS to less than 30% of normal flow. This may be compounded by medications such as anticholinergics and diuretics [25]. Pijpe et al. also demonstrated a clear progressive loss of salivary function over time [26]. Patients frequently present with complaints of excessive throat clearing and the sensation of abundant throat mucus. The diminished viscosity of mucus often associated with SS can prolong hypopharyngeal transit of mucus through the pharynx and into the esophagus. Thus, although patients are making less saliva, what saliva they do produce adheres to the mucosa of the laryngopharynx and gives patients the sensation of excessive throat mucus. Patients often engage in habitual throat clearing in an ill-advised attempt to clear the thick mucus. This can exacerbate laryngeal and pharyngeal inflammation and produce laryngeal edema, which can aggravate the adherent mucus. Breaking people from this vicious cycle of habitual throat clearing is essential to optimize treatment outcomes.

Salivary gland enlargement is a frequent finding. Most often affecting the parotid gland, it may begin unilaterally but usually becomes bilateral. Gland size may fluctuate initially then become firm, rubbery, and consistently enlarged. Pain and tenderness of the glands are rare. Massage and heat application can be symptomatically helpful for patients and prevent stasis of saliva within ectatic ducts [1, 2, 23]. B-cell and T-cell infiltration of salivary tissue is found on histopathology, typically periductal in location. Although common thinking links acinar loss with T-cell and B-cell-mediated destruction (through cytokines and antibodies), neural loss or dysfunction may also be contributory, as antibodies against muscarinic receptors have been identified [7, 11, 23, 25]. Cholinergic muscarinic stimulation results in serous secretion from acini. If muscarinic M3 receptors are disabled by autoantibodies then gland secretion would be poor despite functional acini being present. This is supported by evidence of large numbers of morphologically intact acini in defunct glands of patients with severe xerostomia [11, 23, 25].

A variety of autoantibodies against different cellular components are identified in SS. Those against ribonucleoproteins known as anti-Ro (SSA) and anti-La (SSB) are seen commonly and are considered a diagnostic criteria [1, 6, 8, 9, 27, 28]. New studies have demonstrated the ability of anti-Ro and anti-La to penetrate cultured human salivary cells, induce DNA fragmentation and cleavage, and initiate caspase-driven apoptosis [28, 29]. This suggests a direct autoantibody-mediated targeted destruction of the glandular tissue resulting in dysfunctional glands and xerostomia.

Persistent glandular enlargement may be due to the development of lymphoproliferative disease within either the substance of the gland or intraparotid lymph nodes [30]. Studies previously suggested a 44-fold increased risk of development of lymphoma in patients with pSS [2, 30, 31]. More recently Theander and colleagues have reviewed over 500 patients with pSS and compared them to matched population controls. They found a 16-fold increased incidence of lymphoma and myeloma compared to the normal population [30]. The risk increased steadily with the longer duration of disease. Within the first 5 years after the initial diagnosis, the risk was elevated 6.4-fold. Greater than 10 years after the initial diagnosis, the risk of malignancy was 20.8 times the general population. A 5% lifetime risk for development of lymphoma is estimated [2, 30–32]. The strongest predictor of lymphoma was an altered $CD4^+/CD8^+$ ratio, with patients with $CD4^+$ lymphopenia showing significantly increased risk of death [30]. Other risk factors for malignancy development are hypergammaglobulinemia, purpura, and low C3 and C4 levels [1, 3, 8, 32–35]. Anti-B-cell therapy such as rituximab has shown some efficacy in treating SS patients including those with lymphomas [33].

16.3.3 Otologic

Approximately one-third of patients with primary or secondary SS have high frequency sensorineural hearing loss (SNHL) [2, 36–38]. Loss ranges from mild to severe and is not associated with an increased risk of retrocochlear pathology or correlated with the severity of disease or the level of autoantibodies [37–39]. Longer disease duration was associated with the level of hearing loss in one study [37]. A proposed mechanism is immune deposition within the stria vascularis, although no confirmatory evidence for this exists. In patients with other autoimmune disease, increased prevalence of high frequency SNHL has also been noted and, thus, may be a function of autoimmunity in general [11, 37, 38]. Possible autoantibodies to ciliar epitopes were identified in mice but not in humans as yet [11]. There is no evidence that otitis media is more prevalent in patients with SS compared to the general population. The high prevalence of hearing loss in patients with SS is underappreciated by most clinicians. The prevalence of hearing loss is elevated enough to warrant a baseline audiogram in all patients with an established diagnosis.

16.3.4 Rhinologic

There are no pathognomonic signs or symptoms of SS that are found in the nose or sinuses. However, the mucosal lining of the nasal cavity and sinus cavities are also subject to the xerosis that affects other sites. This can lead to epistaxis, crusting, and a poor sense of smell. Approximately 50% of patients may have nasal mucosal atrophy [40]. Research suggests that there is dissociation between the gel and sol layers within the mucociliary transport system of the nose. This leads to poor transport of mucus and particulate matter in the nose [41]. This presents clinically as nasal bleeding and crusting. There is no clear evidence to suggest an increased prevalence of sinusitis or septal perforation as seen in Wegener's granulomatosis. Smell may be decreased due to the lack of solvent for dissolving odorants.

Careful nasal hygiene with saline rinsing, misted saline sprays, and avoidance of drying medications such as decongestant sprays and anti-histamines are recommended. Petroleum-based ointments can also provide longer moisture protection by limiting drying of the mucosa and can be applied several times daily. These do not need to contain antibiotic—it is the viscosity and desiccation-retardant properties of the ointments that are beneficial. We have found over-the-counter steamers to be beneficial and frequently recommend applying three drops of eucalyptus oil to the water basin of the steamer as a form of "vapor therapy." Many herbal healers believe that eucalyptus oil can relieve the symptoms of colds and flu, sore throat, cough, and rhinitis. Empiric treatment of SS patients with eucalyptus vapor therapy has been beneficial in our practice. Clinical evidence is lacking.

16.3.5 Laryngeal

Dysphonia is relatively frequent and can be the presenting symptom in some patients with Sjögren's syndrome. We live in a communication age and voice problems can have devastating consequences on an individual's quality of life. Mucus is essential to normal mucosal vibration of the vocal folds. Mucus of high viscosity can adhere to the vocal folds and alter the normal frequency of a person's voice (Fig. 16.4). The voice can also become diplophonic, harsh, and raspy. Saliva, with its high concentration of bicarbonate, is essentially the body's endogenous antacid. All individuals reflux. Up to 50 reflux episodes from the stomach into the distal esophagus may be considered normal (physiologic reflux). Up to two reflux episodes (pH 4) into the laryngopharynx may also be considered normal. Patients with SS lack the innate buffering capacity of saliva. Even normal, physiologic amounts of reflux can cause extensive laryngeal damage and symptoms of laryngopharyngeal reflux (LPR) in patients

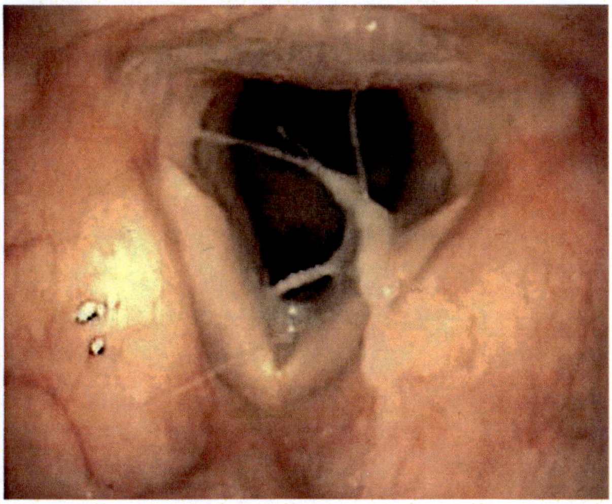

Fig. 16.4 Thick adherent endolaryngeal mucus in a person with Sjögren's syndrome

Table 16.3 Reflux symptom index

Within the last *month*, how did the following problems affect you?	0 = No problem 5 = Severe problem					
1. Hoarseness or a problem with your voice	0	1	2	3	4	5
2. Clearing your throat	0	1	2	3	4	5
3. Excess throat mucous or postnasal drip	0	1	2	3	4	5
4. Difficulty swallowing food, liquid, or pills	0	1	2	3	4	5
5. Coughing after you ate or after lying down	0	1	2	3	4	5
7. Troublesome or annoying cough	0	1	2	3	4	5
8. Sensations of something sticking in your throat or a lump in your throat	0	1	2	3	4	5
9. Heartburn, chest pain, indigestion, or stomach acid coming up	0	1	2	3	4	5
Total						

with SS. Symptoms of LPR include intermittent hoarseness, the sensation of a lump in the throat (globus), increased throat mucus, cough, the sensation of post nasal drip, and excessive throat clearing. General mucosal dryness can also result in xerotrachea and chronic cough [42]. The trachea, larynx, and pharynx are ill-equipped to handle even small amounts of acid and pepsin. This may exacerbate pre-existing edema, cough, and hoarseness [43]. We have validated a survey instrument for quantifying the symptoms of LPR (Table 16.3) [44]. The reflux symptom index (RSI) has been a valuable tool to establish the initial diagnosis and monitor treatment effectiveness in persons with LPR. The RSI has been adopted nationally and internationally [44–46]. Ogut et al. demonstrated significantly higher RSI scores and laryngeal reflux finding scores (endoscopic laryngeal inflammatory scale) in a controlled study of 77 patients with SS [46]. This suggests that persons with SS suffer from symptoms and laryngeal findings suggestive of LPR. The RSI has proven to be a very useful tool in monitoring treatment success in our patients with SS.

A specific rheumatologic laryngeal lesion termed the "bamboo node" has been described (Fig. 16.5). The bamboo node is a whitish yellow submucosal lesion in the mid-third of the fold and

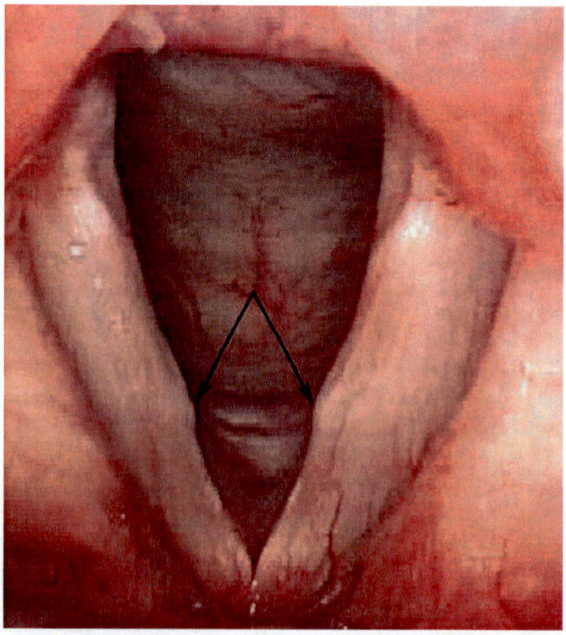

Fig. 16.5 Bamboo nodes on the vocal folds in a person with Sjögren's syndrome

has been identified in patients with autoimmune pathologies such as Sjögren's syndrome, rheumatoid arthritis, and systemic lupus erythematosus (SLE) [2, 47]. Murano describes two patients in whom this lesion was identified prior to the diagnosis of autoimmunity. Subsequent testing revealed one patient to have pSS and the other sSS associated with SLE. Microscopically the "node" seems to consist of eosinophilic material surrounded by a granulomatous reaction and fibrosis [47]. Murano suggests that identification of the bamboo node can be the first indication of the underlying systemic pathology in these cases and that voice quality is affected by the node due to stiffness and loss of the mucosal wave in the vocal fold at the site [47].

Vocal fold immobility in patients exhibiting SS findings may be due to either cricoarytenoid joint ankylosis or autoimmune neuropathy. In cases of secondary SSs that are associated with rheumatoid arthritis there may be cricoarytenoid joint ankylosis and rheumatoid bamboo nodes.

Treatment of laryngeal symptoms includes humidification, usually best achieved with personal steamers or nebulizer devices that aerosolize sterile water or saline, control of reflux (see below), and avoidance of other irritants to the larynx such as tobacco smoke and environmental pollutants. Drying medications including anti-cholinergic and anti-histamine preparations should be used with caution as they may aggravate the autoimmune xerotrachea and xerostomia already present. Anti-histamine medications may also thicken mucus, which can make it harder to clear. Dysphonia secondary to vocal fold immobility can be addressed by joint mobilization, vocal fold augmentation or, rarely, arytenoid adduction.

16.3.6 Esophageal

Dysphagia is a common symptom among SS patients. Reports suggest that anywhere from one-third to 80% of patients complain of difficulty swallowing [43, 48–52]. Multiple mechanisms contribute to swallowing difficulties in these patients (Table 16.4). Lack of saliva contributes to dysphagia both directly, by failing to adequately lubricate a bolus and indirectly by the inability to flush the esophagus and neutralize regurgitated acid content. Gastroesophageal and laryngopharyngeal refluxes occur, as in the normal population, but patients with SS lack the innate defenses to cope with acid and pepsin-containing refluxate.

Table 16.4 Mechanisms contributing to dysphagia in Sjögren's syndrome

Hyposalivation—poor lubrication, poor bolus transit, loss of salivary buffering, poor esophageal residue clearance Esophageal dysmotility—primary or secondary to prolonged acid clearance,
Gastroesophageal reflux (GER)
Esophageal seromucinous gland failure
Autonomic dysfunction
Webs and strictures
Esophagitis

Usually a three-tiered defense system protects the esophagus and larynx from gastric content. The combined valves of the upper and lower esophageal sphincters prevent gross volume reflux. Despite tonic closure in most situations the lower esophageal sphincter (LES) is known to experience transient relaxations (TLESR's) many times per day [53–56]. It is likely a venting mechanism to release gas and reduce pressure [43]. Investigators have demonstrated a hypotonic upper esophageal sphincter (UES) and LES (a risk factor for reflux) in up to 62% of patients with SS [46, 48]. Up to 50 acidification episodes ($pH < 4$) per 24 h is considered physiological reflux. Normal subjects respond to these episodes by secondary esophageal peristalsis to clear the majority of refluxate and by combined secretion from esophageal submucosal glands and saliva, which dilutes and neutralizes the acid component, flushing the remaining refluxate back into the stomach [43, 57]. The patient with SS lacks the buffering capacity and dilutional effects of saliva. This may result in esophagitis or other complications of reflux (stricture, esophageal spasm) in these patients (Fig. 16.6).

In addition, one-third of SS patients may experience esophageal dysmotility, exacerbating poor

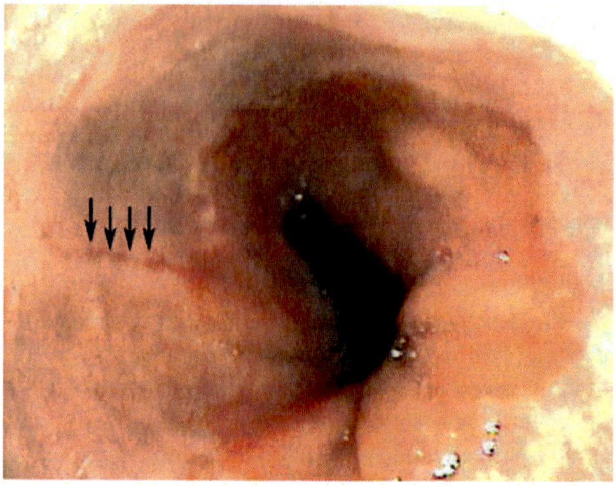

Fig. 16.6 Endoscopic view of grade B esophagitis in a patient with SS. *Arrows* show linear mucosal erosions

esophageal clearance [43, 48, 49, 52, 58, 59]. Increased esophageal intraluminal acid time may have deleterious effects on the esophagus, causing or worsening dysmotility and poor contractility, thus creating a vicious cycle [43, 48]. Motility disorders identified in the SS population cover a wide range of pathologies from achalasia to non-specific body dysmotility [48, 49, 58, 59]. Volter suggests that dysmotility is the result of GER and prolonged esophageal acid exposure rather than being a primary abnormality in these patients [48]. There is a general lack of consistency in findings surrounding dysmotility, however, with studies demonstrating contradictory results [48, 50–52, 59, 60]. Various investigators have reported increased and decreased LES pressures [49, 50, 59, 61]. The most consistent finding is of decreased esophageal body velocities [59, 61]. There may be difficulty comparing study findings as many older studies use different diagnostic criteria for defining SS (prior to the American–European Consensus Group criteria).

An esophageal web has been described in up to 10% of patients with SS [50]. This prevalence is higher than age-matched controls. Webs frequently cause solid food dysphagia and are very amenable to dilation. Autonomic neuropathy has also been detected in SS, particularly impaired parasympathetic function. This was significantly related to dysphagia symptoms [51]. Autonomic failure may impact submucosal gland secretory function, particularly if antibodies to muscarinic receptors are present [51]. Neuropathy, both central and peripheral, can be detected in some SS patients [1, 62]. It is possible that neural dysfunction contributes to myenteric plexus failure, secretory failure, and esophageal dysmotility. Myenteric plexus failure contributes to achalasia and this has been described in association with pSS [13, 62].

One of the most common medications prescribed for reflux—omeprazole—may decrease salivary flow and thus be less beneficial in SS patients [43].

Patients complaining of heartburn or dysphagia should undergo screening with esophagoscopy and videofluoroscopy. If the endoscopy and fluoroscopy do not identify the etiology of dysphagia, manometry is indicated. The advent of unsedated transnasal esophagoscopy (TNE) has greatly increased our ability to screen the esophagus in the office setting. The majority of complications of esophagoscopy are respiratory and cardiac events related to the intravenous sedation. Unsedated transnasal office esophagoscopy has greatly improved the safety and accessibility of endoscopic esophageal screening. Ambulatory pH testing may be useful if there are equivocal signs of reflux. Esophagitis, strictures, hiatal hernia, and Barrett's metaplasia (BM) can be identified and treated appropriately. All patients with BM must be biopsied and routinely followed to ensure there is no progression to adenocarcinoma.

The first-line treatment of reflux in persons with SS is behavioral modification. Exercise and weight loss in the overweight and out of shape is encouraged. Patients are instructed to limit the consumption of caffeine, alcohol, tobacco, peppermint, carbonated beverages, and other refluxogenic foods. The head of the bed should be elevated 30° and individuals should avoid lying down for 2–3 h after eating. If these modifications fail to control the reflux, pharmacologic treatment with H2-receptor antagonists or proton pump inhibitors (PPIs) is indicated. Aggressive acid suppression is often required and most clinicians recommend twice daily PPI as initial medical therapy. Patients are treated for 2–3 months and then tapered to a once-daily dosing regimen if possible. Proton pump inhibitors have a rebound effect that may last 2 months. It is important to counsel your patients not to go off of these medications abruptly. We recommend weaning off PPI over a 2-week period. Because of the absence of mucosal protection from saliva, a low threshold for esophageal screening should be maintained. Ambulatory pH testing is employed to ensure complete acid suppression and impedance monitoring may be considered to rule out non-acid reflux. There are no controlled trials evaluating the efficacy of prokinetic agents or secretogogues for esophageal dysfunction in SS and, therefore, it is unclear as to whether these might be helpful. Baclofen has been shown to decrease transient lower esophageal sphincter relaxation and may be of benefit in both acid and non-acid reflux [63–66]. Liquid alginate has been shown to form a physical barrier against reflux and may have some cytoprotective effects. We frequently recommend liquid alginate 30 cc after each meal and before bedtime. Anti-reflux surgery enhances LES tone and may cause dysphagia if there is preexisting esophageal dysmotility. Fundoplication surgery in patients with SS should be performed with caution.

16.3.7 Thyroid

Autoimmune thyroiditis and hypothyroidism have been associated with SS [67]. In patients diagnosed with autoimmune thyroiditis about 10% will also have SS [67]. This prevalence is high enough to recommend routine screening for SS in patients in whom autoimmune thyroiditis is indicated.

16.3.8 Neurological

Both central and peripheral neuropathies occur with increased prevalence in SS patients [2, 67]. Cranial nerves can be involved, particularly the trigeminal nerve. Autonomic function may also be affected. Dysfunction of parasympathetic nerves can exacerbate dryness of the upper respiratory mucosa by loss of cholinergic stimulation to the remaining functional glandular units.

16.4 Treatment

At this time treatment of SS is essentially symptomatic. Ensuring adequate hydration and avoidance of medications that exacerbate dryness are initial steps. Local attention to oral moisturization, dental hygiene, humidification, and eye care is essential [23]. Secretogogue medications such as pilocarpine (a muscarinic agonist) and the newer cevimeline (also a muscarinic agonist with increased M1 and M3 receptor specificity) have shown good efficacy in increasing saliva flow if functioning acini remain [8, 68–70]. They may also be effective in improving ocular dryness [69, 70]. Interferon-α in lozenge form was also trialed with some success, increasing salivary flow and decreasing lymphocytic infiltrate in tissue [71]. Monoclonal antibody therapy seemed to hold theoretical promise but trials with infliximab and etanercept have not delivered desired outcomes. The B-cell-depleting monoclonal antibody rituximab demonstrated subjective improvement in some patients but had a high rate of moderate-to-severe adverse effects [3, 8, 72]. In cases of widespread disease antirheumatic drugs and corticosteroids may be employed.

Targeted treatment for specific aspects of SS may also be required. Treatment of esophageal and extra-esophageal reflux requires combined lifestyle modifications, pharmacotherapy (proton pump inhibitors, alginates), and rarely surgery (fundoplication). Development of lymphoma requires directed treatment via a tertiary oncology service. Hearing loss may be assisted by appropriate hearing aids, and rhinologic and sinus symptoms may be minimized with saline nasal douching and humidification.

16.5 Conclusion

SS commonly presents with symptoms that involve the head and neck regions and may cause significant decrements in quality of life. The otolaryngologist is encouraged to have a high index of suspicion for Sjögren's syndrome and to investigate where appropriate in order to detect the disease at the earliest opportunity. Early treatment, although largely symptomatic, may reduce long-term sequelae and allow early intervention from the multiple disciplines that are involved in the care of the patient with Sjögren's syndrome.

Patient Handout

Recommendations for patients with *Sjögren's syndrome*

1. Eat an early dinner. Wait at least 2 h before lying down after a meal.
2. Elevate the head of your bed. This will get gravity on your side and help limit nighttime reflux. An inflatable wedge cushion is available for frequent travelers (www.sitincomfort.com).
3. Avoid eating large meals. Safer to eat small more frequent meals. Graze like a sheep.
4. Avoid caffeine and alcohol. Decaffeinated coffee is better, herbal tea is best. One glass of red wine in the evening is reasonable.
5. Avoid chocolate and peppermint.
6. Try chewing baking soda gum (Arm & Hammer Gum available at www.dentist.net). The gum chewing may promote saliva flow and the bicarbonate helps neutralize reflux. It is also good for your teeth.
7. Try products with liquid alginate; 30 cc of Gaviscon after meals and before bedtime can form a raft that floats on the stomach and physically inhibits gastroesophageal reflux.
8. Avoid carbonated beverages (even if without caffeine).
9. Avoid tight fitting clothing.
10. Try steam inhalations with a personal steamer two or three times daily (Vicks Personal Steam Inhaler available at www.amazon.com). You may add three drops of eucalyptus oil to the basin of the steamer.
11. Try nasal moisturizing gels (Ayr Saline Nasal Gel with Aloe available at www.drugstore.com).
12. Add low-fat sauces to help moisten dry foods and make them easier to swallow.
13. Take pills with a tall (10 oz) glass of water. If pills are difficult to swallow, consider having them made in liquid formulation with the assistance of a compounding pharmacy (www.ucprx.com).
14. Avoid spicy (acidic) foods.
15. Sleep with a cool mist humidifier next to the bed (available at www.drugstore.com).
16. If possible, avoid medications that dry you out (anti-histamines, some blood pressure medications, some anti-depressants, etc.).

References

1. Kassan SS, Moutsopoulos HM. Clinical manifestations and early diagnosis of Sjögren's syndrome. Arch Intern Med. 2004;164:1275–84.
2. Mahoney EJ, Speigel JH. Sjögren's disease. Otol Clin N Am. 2003;36:733–45.
3. Ng KP, Isenberg DA. Sjögren's syndrome. Diagnosis and therapeutic challenges in the elderly. Drugs Aging 2008;25(1):19–33.
4. Al-Hashimi I, Khuder S, Haghighat N, Zipp M. Frequency and predictive value of the clinical manifestations in Sjögren's syndrome. J Oral Pathol Med. 2001;30:1–6.
5. Manthorpe R. Sjögren's syndrome criteria. Ann Rheum Dis. 2002;61:482–4.
6. Vitali C, Bombardieri S, Jonsson R, et al. Classification criteria for Sjögren's syndrome: a revised version of the European criteria proposed by the American–European Consensus Group. Ann Rheum Dis. 2002; 61:554–8.

7. Fox RI. Clinical features, pathogenesis, and treatment of Sjögren's syndrome. Curr Op Rheum. 1996;8:438–45.
8. Jonsson R, Bolstad AI, Brokstad KA, Brun JG. Sjögren's syndrome—a plethora of clinical and immunological phenotypes with a complex genetic background. Ann NY Acad Sci. 2007;1108:433–47.
9. Srinivasan S, Slomovic AR. Sjögren syndrome. Comp Ophthamol Update. 2007;8:205–12.
10. Soy M, Piskin S. Cutaneous findings in patients with primary Sjögren's syndrome. Clin Rheum. 2007;26(8):1350–2.
11. Tucci M, Quatraro C, Silvestris F. Sjögren's syndrome: an autoimmune disorder with otolaryngological involvement. Acta Oto Ital. 2005;25:139–44.
12. McGuirt WF, Whang C, Moreland W. The role of parotid biopsy in the diagnosis of pediatric Sjögren's syndrome. Arch Oto Head Neck Surg. 2002;128:1279–81.
13. Pijpe J, Kalk WWI, Bootsma H, Spijkervet FKL, Kallenberg CGM, Vissink A. Progression of salivary gland dysfunction in patients with Sjögren's syndrome. Ann Rheum Dis. 2007;66:107–12.
14. Mignogna MD, Fedele S, Lo Russo L, Lo Muzio L, Wolff A. Sjögren's syndrome: the diagnostic potential of early oral manifestations preceding hyposalivation/xerostomia. J Oral Pathol Med. 2005;34:1–6.
15. Hocevar A, Rainer S, Rozman B, Zor P, Tomšic M. Ultrasonographic changes of major salivary glands in primary Sjögren's syndrome. Evaluation of a novel scoring system. Eur J Radiol. 2007;63:379–83.
16. Wernicke D, Hess H, Gromnica-Ihle E, Krause A, Schmidt WA. Ultrasonography of salivary glands—a highly specific imaging procedure for diagnosis of Sjögren's syndrome. J Rheum. 2008;35:285–93.
17. Salaffi F, Carotti M, Iagnocco A, et al. Ultrasonography of salivary glands in primary Sjögren's syndrome: a comparison with contrast sialography and scintigraphy. Rheumatology 2008;47:1244–9.
18. Booker J, Howarth D, Taylor L, Voutnis D, Sutherland D. Appropriate utilization of semi-quantitative analysis in salivary scintigraphy. Nuc Med. 2004;25:1203–10.
19. Decuzzi M, Tatulli F, Giampaolo M, et al. Sialocintigraphy versus ultrasonography of the salivary glands in patients first diagnosed with Sjögren's syndrome. Hell J Nucl Med. 2006;9(2):103–5.
20. Niemelä RK, Takalo R, Pääko E, et al. Ultrasonography of salivary glands in primary Sjögren's syndrome. A comparison with magnetic resonance imaging and magnetic resonance sialography of parotid glands. Rheumatology 2004;43:875–9.
21. Takagi Y, Sumi M, Van Cauteren M, Nakamura T. Fast and high-resolution MR sialography using a small surface coil. J Mag Res Imag. 2005;22:29–37.
22. Morimoto Y, Habu M, Tomoyose T, et al. Dynamic magnetic resonance sialography as a new diagnostic technique for patients with Sjögren's syndrome. Oral Dis. 1006;12:408–14.
23. Soto-Rojas AE, Kraus A. The oral side of Sjögren's syndrome. Diagnosis and treatment. Arch Med Res. 2002;33:95–106.
24. Soto-Rojas AE, Villa AR, Sifuentes-Osornio J, Alarcón-Segovia D, Kraus A. Oral manifestations in patients with Sjögren's syndrome. J Rheumatol. 1998;25:906–10.
25. Mathews SA, Kurien BT, Scofield RH. Oral manifestations of Sjögren's syndrome. J Dent Res. 2008;87(4):308–18.
26. Pijpe J, Kalk WWI, van der Wal JE, et al. Parotid gland biopsy compared with labial biopsy in the diagnosis of patients with primary Sjögren's syndrome. Rheumatology 2007;46:335–41.
27. Larché M. A short review of the pathogenesis of Sjögren's syndrome. Autoimmun Rev. 2006;5:132–5.
28. Lisi S, Sisto M, Scagliusi P, Mitolo V, D'Amore M. Sjögren's syndrome: anti-Ro and anti-La autoantibodies trigger apoptotic mechanism in the human salivary gland cell line, A-253. Panminerva Med. 2007;49:103–8.
29. Sisto M, Lisi S, Lofrumento D, D'Amore M, Scagliusi P, Mitolo V. Autoantibodies from Sjögren's syndrome trigger apoptosis in salivary gland cell line. Ann NY Acad Sci. 2007;1108:418–25.
30. Theander E, Henriksson G, Ljungberg O, Mandl T, Manthorpe R, Jacobsson LTH. Lymphoma and other malignancies in primary Sjögren's syndrome: a cohort study on cancer incidence and lymphoma predictors. Ann Rheum Dis. 2006;65:796–803.
31. Pariente D, Anaya JM, Combe B, et al. Non-Hodgkin's lymphoma associated with primary Sjögren's syndrome. Eur J Med. 1992;1:337–42.
32. Ioannidis JPA, Vassiliou V, Moutsopoulos HM. Long-term risk of mortality and lymphoproliferative disease and predictive classification of primary Sjögren's syndrome. Arth Rheum. 2002;46(3):741–7.
33. Mackay F, Groom JR, Tangye SG. An important role for B-cell activation factor and B cells in the pathogenesis of Sjögren's syndrome. Curr Opin Rheum. 2007;19(5):406–13.
34. Voulgarelis M, Dafni UG, Isenberg DA, Moutsopoulos HM. Malignant lymphoma in primary Sjögren's syndrome. Arth Rheum. 1999;42(8):1765–72.
35. Kauppi M, Pukkala E, Isomäki H. Elevated incidence of hematologic malignancies in patients with Sjögren's syndrome compared with patients with rheumatoid arthritis (Finland). Cancer Causes Control 1997;8:201–4.
36. Freeman SRM, Sheehan PZ, Thorpe MA, Rutka JA. Ear, nose and throat manifestations of Sjögren's syndrome: retrospective review of a multidisciplinary clinic. J Otol. 2005;34:20–4.
37. Ziavra N, Politi EN, Kastanioudakis I, Skevas A, Drosos AA. Hearing loss in Sjögren's syndrome

patients. A comparative study. Clin Exp Rheum. 2000;18:725–8.
38. Tumiati B, Casoli P, Parmeggiani A. Hearing loss in the Sjögren syndrome. Ann Int Med. 1997;126(6):450–3.
39. Boki KA, Ioannidis JPA, Segas JV, et al. How significant is sensorineural hearing loss in primary Sjögren's syndrome? An individually matched case–control study. J Rheumatol. 2001;28:798–801.
40. Alobid I, Guilemany JM, Mullol J. Nasal manifestations of systemic illnesses. Curr All Asth Rep. 2004;4:208–16.
41. Takeuchi K, Sakakura Y, Murai S, Majima Y. Nasal mucociliary clearance in Sjögren's syndrome. Dissociation in flow between sol and gel layers. Acta Otolaryngol. 1989;108:126–9.
42. Papiris SA, Maniati M, Constantopoulos SH, Roussos C, Moutsopoulos HM, Skopouli FN. Lung involvement in primary Sjögren's syndrome is mainly related to the small airway disease. Ann Rheum Dis. 1999;58:61–4.
43. Belafksy PC, Postma GN. The laryngeal and esophageal manifestations of Sjögren's syndrome. Curr Rheum Rep. 2003;5:297–303.
44. Belafsky PC, Postma GN, Koufman JA. Validity and reliability of the reflux symptom index (RSI). J Voice. 2002;16(2):274–7.
45. Ford CN. Evaluation and management of laryngopharyngeal reflux. JAMA 2005;294:1534–40.
46. Ogut F, Midilli R, Oder G, Engin EZ, Karci B, Kabasakal Y. Laryngeal findings and voice quality in Sjögren's syndrome. Auris Nas Larynx. 2005;32:375–80.
47. Murano E, Hosako-Naito Y, Oka T, Miyaji M, Kumada M, Niimi S. Bamboo node: primary vocal fold lesion as evidence of autoimmune disease. J Voice. 2001;15:441–50.
48. Volter F, Fain O, Mathieu E, Thomas M. Esophageal function and Sjögren's syndrome. Dig Dis Sci. 2004;49(2):248–53.
49. Palma R, Freire A, Freitas J, et al. Esophageal motility disorders in patients with Sjögren's syndrome. Dig Dis Sci. 1994;39(4):758–61.
50. Kjellén G, Fransson SG, Lindström F, Sökjer H, Tibbling L. Esophageal function, radiography, and dysphagia in Sjögren's syndrome. Dig Dis Sci. 1986;31(3):225–9.
51. Mandl T, Ekberg O, Wollmer P, Manthorpe R, Jacobsson LTH. Dysphagia and dysmotility of the pharynx and oesophagus in patients with primary Sjögren's syndrome. Scand J Rheumatol. 2007;36:394–401.
52. Türk T, Pirildar T, Tunç, Bor S, Doganavsargil E. Manometric assessment of esophageal motility in patients with primary Sjögren's syndrome. Rheumatol Int. 2005;25:246–9.
53. Dent J. Patterns of lower esophageal sphincter function associated with gastroesophageal reflux. Am J Med. 1997;103(5A):29S–32S.
54. Pope CE. The esophagus for the nonesophagologist. Am J Med. 1997;103(5A):19S–22S.
55. Biancani P, Sohn UD, Rich HG, Harnett KM, Behar J. Signal transduction pathways in esophageal and lower esophageal sphincter circular muscle. Am J Med. 1997;103(5A):23S–8S.
56. Pasricha PJ. Effect of sleep on gastroesophageal physiology and airway protective mechanisms. Am J Med. 2003;115(3A):114S–8S.
57. Shaker R, Hogan WJ. Reflex-mediated enhancement of airway protective mechanisms. Am J Med. 2000; 108(4A):8S–14S.
58. Tsianos EB, Chiras CD, Drosos AA, Moutsopoulos HM. Esophageal dysfunction in patients with primary Sjögren's syndrome. Ann Rheum Dis. 1985;44: 610–13.
59. Grande L, Lacima G, Ros E, Font J, Pera C. Esophageal motor function in primary Sjögren's syndrome. Am J Gastroenterol. 1993;88(3):378–81.
60. Sheikh SH, Shaw-Stiffel TA. The gastrointestinal manifestations of Sjögren's syndrome. Am J Gastroenterol. 1995;90(1):9–14.
61. Rosztóczy A, Kovács L, Wittmann T, Lonovics J, Pokorny G. Manometric assessment of impaired esophageal motor function in primary Sjögren's syndrome. Clin Exper Rheum. 2001;19:147–52.
62. Poglio F, Mongini T, Cocito D. Sensory ataxic neuropathy and esophageal achalasia in a patient with Sjögren's syndrome. Muscle Nerve 2007;35: 532–5.
63. Vela MF, Tutuian R, Katz PO, Castell DO. Baclofen decreases acid and non-acid post-prandial gastroesophageal reflux measured by combined multichannel intraluminal impedance and pH. Aliment Pharmacol Ther. 2003;17(2):243–51.
64. Richter JE. Novel medical therapies for gastroesophageal reflux disease beyond proton pump inhibitors. Gastroenterol Clin North Am. 2002; 31(4 Suppl):S111–6.
65. Holloway RH. Systemic pharmacomodulation of transient lower esophageal sphincter relaxations. Am J Med. 2001;(111 Suppl 8A):178S–85S.
66. Lehmann A, Antonsson M, Bremner-Danielson M, Flärd M, Hansson-Bränden L, Kärrberg L. Activation of the GABA(B) receptor inhibits transient lower esophageal sphincter relaxation in dogs. Gastroenterology 1999;117(5):1147–54.
67. Fox RI. Sjögren's syndrome. Lancet 2005;366: 321–31.
68. Fife RS, Chase WF, Dore RK, et al. Cevimeline for the treatment of xerostomia in patients with Sjögren's syndrome. Arch Int Med. 2002;162:1293–300.
69. Vivino FB, Al-Hashimi I, Khan Z, et al. Pilocarpine tablets for the treatment of dry mouth and dry eye symptoms in patients with Sjögren's syndrome. Arch Int Med. 1999;159:174–81.
70. Petrone D, Condemi JJ, Fife R, Gluck O, Cohen S, Dalgin P. A double-blind, randomized, placebo-controlled study of cevimeline in Sjögren's syndrome

patients with xerostomia and keratoconjunctivitis sicca. Arth Rheum. 2002;46(3):748–54.
71. Shiozawa S, Cummins JM, Fox PC. Opening the flood gates—interferon alpha treatment for Sjögren's syndrome. Biodrugs 2000;13(5):305–11.
72. Sankar V, Brennan MT, Kok MR, et al. Etanercept in Sjögren's syndrome. A twelve-week randomized, double-blind, placebo-controlled pilot clinical trial. Arth Rheum. 2004;50(7):2240–5.

Extraglandular Manifestations of Sjögren's Syndrome (SS): Dermatologic, Arthritic, Endocrine, Pulmonary, Cardiovascular, Gastroenterology, Renal, Urology, and Gynecologic Manifestations

17

Robert I. Fox

Abstract

Primary Sjögren's syndrome (1° SS) is an autoimmune disorder characterized by *dry eyes* (*keratoconjunctivitis sicca*) and *dry mouth* due to lymphocytic infiltrates of lacrimal and salivary glands. However, SS also affects many extraglandular systems. In SS patients, the pattern of extraglandular manifestations may have a close similarity with the vasculitic features seen in SLE patients that are mediated by immune complexes and complement. However, SS patients also have an increased frequency of lymphocytic infiltration into extraglandular tissues, as might be expected by their increased frequency of lymphoma in comparison to SLE patients. For example, SS patients need to be evaluated for interstitial nephritis (in contrast to the glomerulonephritis of SLE) or interstitial pneumonitis (in comparison to pleurisy of SLE). *This chapter will focus on the clinical extraglandular manifestations of primary SS* that are not specifically covered in other chapters. These extraglandular manifestations have led to a recently introduced "disease activity" and "organ damage index." The recognition of these extraglandular manifestations is important since they have prognostic and therapeutic implications. The differential diagnosis of these extraglandular manifestations includes overlapping features with other autoimmune diseases (particularly systemic lupus erythematosus (SLE), scleroderma, dermatomyositis, celiac sprue, and small- and medium-sized vessel vasculitis), infectious diseases that mimic autoimmune disease (particularly hepatitis C, HIV, syphilis, tuberculosis), and predisposition to drug toxicities that may involve extraglandular organs (particularly skin rashes, nephritis, pneumonitis, myositis, and hematopoietic abnormalities).

R.I. Fox (✉)
Rheumatology Clinic, Scripps Memorial Hospital
and Research Foundation, La Jolla, CA, USA
e-mail: robertfoxmd@mac.com

R.I. Fox, C.M. Fox (eds.), *Sjögren's Syndrome*, DOI 10.1007/978-1-60327-957-4_17,

Keywords
Sjögren's syndrome (SS)—[primary SS: 1°SS/secondary SS: 2° SS] • Systemic lupus erythematosus (SLE) • Vasculitis • Pneumonitis • Pericarditis • Pulmonary arterial hypertension • Hepatitis • Thromboembolic • Arthritis • Interstitial lung disease (ILD) • Non-specific interstitial pneumonitis (NSIP) • Interstitial nephritis (IN) • Interstitial cystitis (IC) • Lymphocytic interstitial pneumononitis (LIP) • Diffuse parenchymal lung disease (DPLD) • Autonomic neuropathy • Primary biliary cirrhosis (PBC) • Progressive multifocal leukoencephalopathy • Xerosis

17.1 Introduction

The care of the Sjögren's syndrome (SS) patient is often shared by multiple specialists beyond the rheumatologist, (see Table 17.1) including

- Dermatology
- Ophthalmology (see chapter)
- Oral medicine (see chapter)
- Otolaryngology (ENT) (see chapter)
- Hematology/oncology
- Neurology and psychology (see chapters)
- Orthopedic surgery
- Gastroenterology
- Urology
- Hematology
- Obstetrics and gynecology

Each of these specialist physicians reads different journals and rarely attends common educational meetings. Thus, the rheumatologist frequently becomes the central "quarterback" in the treatment of the SS patient, thus, must be familiar with a broad spectrum of diagnostic procedures and therapeutic approaches.

It is worth noting that in many parts of the world (as well as certain regions of the United States), the care of rheumatology patients is under the direction of family care physicians, orthopedic surgeons, and hematologists. Due in part to the current and increasing shortage of available rheumatologists and the time available per patient revisit, it is likely that that disorders such as Sjogren's syndrome will receive less attention in their clinical manifestations and therapy. On the other side of the coin, we have seen that the lack of familiarity with SS has led physicians to attribute other concurrent diseases (such as herpetic keratitis, heart attack, stroke, and septic or crystalline arthropathies) to their SS and thus not initiate appropriate care of the immediate problem.

In order to co-ordinate therapy between so many specialists and to avoid conflicting information/medications to the patient, we extensively use the *Internet and electronic transfer of files* to co-ordinating physicians. The patient also needs to be made an integral part of the educational and therapeutic treatment plan process.

17.2 Cutaneous/Dermatologic Manifestations

Cutaneous manifestations of SS include

- *dry skin*
- *immunologic inflammatory conditions such as vasculitis*
- *other associated skin conditions*

Complaints of dry skin occur in about 50% of SS patients [1–3]. It is unclear whether or not the xerosis is due to infiltrate of the eccrine or sebaceous glands or dysfunctional sweating [4]. In some cases, dryness of the skin has been associated with lymphocytic infiltrates in the eccrine glands [5].

The vascular findings of SS include benign hypergammaglobulinemic purpura of Waldenstrom, leukocytoclastic vasculitis, and urticarial vasculitis. The findings often occur on the legs.

Table 17.1 Extraglandular manifestations of Sjogren's syndrome included in this chapter

I. *Cutaneous*
• Skin dryness, hair loss (telo-effluvium), and scarring alopecia
• Maculopapular rashes
• Leukocytoclastic vasculitis
• Urticaria and urticarial vasculitis
• Raynaud's phenomena, digital ulceration, and acrocyanosis
• Infectious (including Herpes zoster)
• Embolic and thrombotic lesions
II. *Joints and muscles*
• Arthralgia/arthritis including overlap syndromes with rheumatoid arthritis, SLE, Jaccoud's arthritis, osteoarthritis, erosive osteoarthritis, and seronegative spondyloarthropathies
• Myalgias and myositis including overlap with SLE, polymyositis, inclusion body myositis, metabolic myopathies, and neuropathic myopathies; overlaps with myositis
• Fibromyalgia is covered in Chapter 21
III. *Endocrine*
• Thyroiditis, diabetes
• Adrenal insufficiency including autoimmune and catastrophic cardiolipin syndrome
• Androgen/estrogen replacement
• Autonomic neuropathy
IV. *Pulmonary*
• Interstitial pneumonitis
• Pleurisy and pleural effusions including lymphomatous
• Pulmonary hypertension and occult pulmonary emboli
• Lymphoproliferative manifestations [BALT (bronchial MALT lymphoma) will be covered in Chapter 20]
• Laryngotracheal reflux and motility disorders leading to aspiration are covered in Chapter 16
• Infections including tuberculosis that may mimic Sjögren's syndrome
• Infections including atypical mycobacterial pneumonitis
• Aspiration pneumonia in the SS patient with dysphagia
V. *Cardiovascular*
• Pericarditis and cardiomyopathy
• Anti-coagulant antibody
• Accelerated atherosclerosis including "precocious" carotid intimal thickening
• Autonomic neuropathy
VI. *Gastrointestinal*
• Gastroesophageal reflux and duodenal ulcer
• Motility disorders including laryngotracheal reflux will be covered in Chapter 16
• Celiac sprue, atrophic gastritis, and malabsorptive disorders
• Mesenteric vasculitis and ischemic colitis
• Irritable bowel syndrome and inflammatory bowel syndromes
VII. *Hepatic and pancreatic*
• Autoimmune hepatitis and biliary cirrhosis
• Pancreatitis

Table 17.1 (continued)

• Sclerosing cholangitis
• Occult presentation of hepatitis C virus
VIII. *Renal–urological*
• Interstitial nephritis
• Hypertensive crisis include "microvasculitis" with anti-cardiolipin antibody
• Hypertensive crisis due to pre-renal cause
• Glomerulonephritis due to mixed cryoglobulinemia and amyloid
IX. *Hematological*
• Leukopenia, agranulocytosis
• Thrombocytopenia and thrombocytosis
• Hemolytic anemia and pernicious anemia
• Cryoglobulinemia
• Lymphoma is covered in Chapter 20
X. *Obstetrical/gynecological*
• Neonatal heart block
• Issues of estrogen/androgen replacement
• Potential problems of pregnancy
• Vaginal dryness/dyspareunia
Finally, this chapter will address:
XI. *Differential diagnosis of extraglandular manifestations of SS*
• Most common area of diagnostic confusion between Sjögren's, scleroderma (progressive systemic sclerosis, PSS), polymyositis, and SLE
• Importance of ruling out other causes of morbidity including myocardial infarction, pulmonary emboli, and stroke
XII. *Manifestations and differential diagnosis in the pediatric population*
• Juvenile rheumatoid arthritis (JRA)
• Parotid gland swelling or lymphadenopathy
• Kawasaki disease
• Henoch–Schönlein purpura (HSP)

Hypergammaglobulemic purpura is relatively common in SS patients and may lead to sensory peripheral neuropathy [6–8].

In comparison, *among a large cohort of patients with hyperglobulinemic purpura—about 50%—have SS* [9]. The skin lesions are nonpalpable and often associated with rheumatoid factor (especially IgM-kappa monoclonal rheumatoid factor) containing VKIIIb subclass of light chains [10, 11].

Skin biopsies generally show ruptured blood vessels and deposition of complement. It has been assumed that immune complexes become trapped at the bifurcation of small blood vessels, leading to complement activation by the immune complex.

In one report, *cutaneous vasculitis was found in 52 out of 558 (9%) of patients with primary SS* [12] appearing as purpura, urticarial lesions, and maculopapules.

- Within the vasculitis group, 27% had *cryoglobulinemic vasculitis* and 21% had urticarial vasculitis.
- Most patients had small vessel vasculitis (leukocytoclastic), and only two had medium-sized vessel involvement.
- Compared to the patients without vasculitis, affected patients had a higher prevalence

of systemic involvement, positive anti-nuclear antibody (ANA), anti-Ro/SS-A antibodies, and rheumatoid factor.

Cryoglobulinemia was associated with worse outcome.

Features of cryoglobulinemia:

- o Cryoglobulins are immunoglobulins that precipitate from serum under laboratory conditions of cold.
- o The usual laboratory temperature used to precipitate cryoglobulins is 4°C.
- o *False-negative results in testing for cryoglobulins are common.*
- o Sensitive testing for cryoglobulins requires an experienced laboratory that is set up to perform the collection in proper condition.
- o While the patient is fasting (lipids can interfere with the assay), at least 20 mL of blood should be drawn into a tube that has not been treated with anti-coagulant.
- o The tube should be transported and centrifuged at 37°C, then kept for 72 h at 4°C.

Cryoglobulinemia is divided into *three clinical subsets*: types I, II, and III.

This classification is based on two features:

(1) The clonality of the IgM component
(2) The presence of rheumatoid factor activity

- In its clinical manifestations, *type I cryoglobulinemia* is usually quite distinct from types II and III.
- In contrast, substantial clinical overlap exists between types II and III.

Type I cryoglobulinemia is associated with a monoclonal component and is often associated with a hematopoietic malignancy.

The *symptoms of hyperviscosity are more common with type I* and increased chance that symptoms such as neuropathy may be related to amyloid.

Types II and III cryoglobulinemias are often termed "mixed" cryoglobulinemias, as they are composed of both IgG and IgM components. A low complement C4 (either as a C4 null patient or due to complement consumption) is common, so disproportionate decreases in C4 levels are commonly found.

In contrast to lupus glomerulonephritis, membranoproliferative glomerulonephritis due to cryoglobulinemia is usually a "later" presentation.

Vasculitis associated with mixed cryoglobulinemia involves both small-sized and medium-sized blood vessels. Small vessel disease is more common than medium vessel disease.

Vasculitis associated with mixed cryoglobulinemia may be caused by hepatitis C virus (HCV) infections and the diagnosis of SS does not rule out co-existent HCV.

It is also worth remembering that treatment with interferon-α (either standard form or pegylated), the cornerstone of HCV infection, may exacerbate type II mixed cryoglobulins in their cutaneous or other manifestations.

Additionally, ribavirin can exacerbate hemolytic anemia or renal manifestations during its first weeks of therapy. Plasmapheresis may be required in severe cases during the early phases of therapy.

Virtually, all patients with type II mixed cryoglobulinemia are rheumatoid factor positive. SS patients with monoclonal rheumatoid factor (RF) and type II mixed cryoglobulinemia have higher frequency of developing non-Hodgkin's lymphoma.

Peripheral nerve involvement is common in patients with cryoglobulinemic vasculitis, occurring in up to 80%. The most common type is a distal symmetric polyneuropathy with predilection for lower extremities. Mononeuritis multiplex may occur but is less common.

The *treatment of cryoglobulinemia* of any of the three types is directed whenever possible at the underlying cause. In some cases, the broad-spectrum immunosuppression and other measures must be employed with glucocorticoids, cytotoxic therapies, and plasma exchange.

Other authors have reported vasculitis in 30% of both primary and secondary SS patients [13]. *Palpable purpura* is also found in SS patients [14] with biopsies showing leukocytoclastic vasculitis [12] and may be associated with central nervous system involvement [15] or pulmonary involvement [16].

Mixed cryoglobulinemia also may be associated with leukocytoclastic vasculitis and should initiate a search for occult Hepatitis C infection [17].

Urticarial vasculitis has been reported in association with SS [18]. Urticarial vasculitis somewhat resembles urticaria, but lesions last typically for 3–4 days and can be painful. This type of vasculitis has also been reported in systemic lupus erythematosus (SLE) patients.

Histopathology of SS vasculitis lesions has demonstrated classic leukocytoclastic vasculitis with neutrophilic destruction of small vessel walls with fibrinoid necrosis and also a separate pattern of lymphocytic infiltrate of the vessel wall [15, 19].

Patients with anti-neutrophil cytoplasmic antibodies (ANCAs) are relatively uncommon in primary SS and when present are usually p-ANCAs (perinuclear antibodies). Caution must be used in interpreting the ANCA in SS patients since false-positive results may result from the presence of other anti-nuclear antibodies [20, 21].

Antibodies against endothelial cells have not only been found in a subset of SS patients, but are also detected in many other autoimmune disorders and are not closely associated with skin vasculitis [22]. Anti-cardiolipin antibodies are found in a subset of SS patients and are generally IgA isotype, with lower incidence of thrombosis than found in SLE patients [23].

Additional reported *non-vasculitic cutaneous manifestations* of SS include *vitiligo, anetoderma, alopecia, and cutaneous lymphomas* [24]. The presence of anetoderma has been associated with B-cell lymphomas [25].

Additional cutaneous features include subcutaneous amyloid [26, 27]. Erythema multiforme-like, erythema perstans-like, and erythema nodosum-like lesions [28] have been reported along with Sweet's syndrome [13, 24, 29, 30].

Raynaud's phenomenon has been reported in 30% of patients with primary SS, although the severe vasomotor instability should suggest the diagnosis of co-existent progressive systemic sclerosis (PSS) (usually characterized by telangiectasis and calcinosis) or cryoglobulinemia [29, 31–33].

Closely related digital skin lesions (which often exhibit T-cell infiltrates on biopsy of the nail beds) with vasospasm induced by cold exposure are termed "chilblains" or "perniosis," where there is a close association with anti-SS-A antibody, and the lesions may precede either SS or SLE by up to 10 years [34–36].

Attention to potential problems such as bland (atherosclerotic) or septic emboli, digital vasculopathy in smokers (Buerger's disease), and mononeuritis multiplex must be considered in the patient with cold cyanotic extremity. Severe ischemic or gangrenous changes, ulcerating dystrophic calcification with purulent or ulcerative changes, should suggest systemic sclerosis, deep tissue plane infection, and may constitute a medical/surgery emergency.

A subepidermal blistering *dermatosis* similar to bullous SLE, with antibodies to type VII collagen, has been reported in a patient with primary SS who did not fulfill the SLE criteria of the American Rheumatism Association at the time [37].

Among Asian SS patients, a specific cutaneous finding—annular erythema—of Sjögren's syndrome (AE–SS) has been reported in a relatively high proportion of patients [38–43], including those with childhood onset [44]. Although this eruption appears similar to subacute cutaneous lupus erythematosus (SCLE), histologically, it is distinguishable by coat sleeve-like infiltration of lymphocytes around the appendages, similar to gyrate erythema. A Caucasian female with SS was reported to have AE–SS [45]. Many of these patients have antibody to the 60-kDa epitope of SS-A.

Because many SS patients are often taking multiple medications, the differential diagnosis of cutaneous eruptions always includes drug eruption. Patients can also have infectious processes, especially if they are immunosuppressed due to treatment. A skin biopsy with direct immunofluorescence can be very helpful in distinguishing these latter two entities from vasculitis or other dermatoses associated with SS.

17.3 Joint and Muscle Manifestations—Arthralgia and Arthropathy

Approximately 50% of patients with primary SS have initial chief complaint of arthralgia (joint pain), with or without evidence of arthritis [1, 46]. Initially, the rheumatologist should consider whether these symptoms are due to underlying rheumatoid, psoriatic, spondyloarthritic, or infectious arthropathy.

Among SS patients lacking the above associated arthropathies, approximately 40% had synovitis and 10% had erosive changes on radiographs. The finding of high-titer anti-CCP peptide antibody was a strong predictor of erosive changes in SS patients [46].

The clinical features of *chronic arthritis* (over 6 weeks in duration) in the SS patient may present in a manner similar to *rheumatoid arthritis* with symmetric synovitis, positive rheumatoid factor, and positive anti-CCP antibody.

MRI has shown a higher frequency of erosions of the peripheral joints in "early" RA patients with sicca symptoms, although the significance and rate of progression in RA patients with sicca symptoms remain unknown.

The distinction between classic RA with secondary SS and primary SS with synovitis is difficult. Previous studies have suggested that RA patients with 2° SS often develop keratoconjunctivitis sicca (KCS) symptoms several years after the onset of RA, erosions detectable by standard radiographs; also, the finding of a dry, painful mouth in a RA patient (often on steroids and who has received concurrent antibiotic for some other reason) may indicate the development of oral candidiasis as the cause.

Also, in most *RA with secondary SS ocular symptoms are more prevalent than oral symptoms.*

Additionally, *HLA-DR4 is more common in RA patients* and this allele (or patients with the shared epitope) has an elevated frequency of RF. In comparison, most primary SS patients have the HLA-DR3 allele and this is associated with antibodies to SS-A/SS-B.

It is not uncommon for patients to have an "overlap" with both RA features and strong SS features. Although the haplotypes of a large cohort of these patients have not been presented, it is likely that they share both HLA-DR4 and HLA-DR3.

Monoarticular or pauciarticular arthropathy—with asymmetric joint involvement must always raise suspicion of septic joint or crystalline arthropathy.

Alternatively, overlap with seronegative arthropathies such as spondyloarthropathies including ankylosing spondylitis, reactive arthritis (Reiter's syndrome), inflammatory bowel disease, or psoriatic must be considered as having the potential for overlap with Sjögren's syndrome.

Lupus or Jaccoud's arthropathy—with primarily ligamentous laxity and joint subluxation [47, 48].

Osteoarthritis—that involves predominantly distal interphalangeal joints [47] may frequently occur in SS patients, who frequently give a history of similar onset of joint symptoms in the mother or other immediate family members.

Erosive osteoarthritis—that has a more aggressive course, radiological features, and treatment requirements than age-related osteoarthritis [49, 50].

It is estimated that about 20% of patients with severe RA have sicca symptoms (particularly eye involvement) and they are generally termed SS 2° RA. In SS patients with rheumatoid arthritis and secondary SS, the RA changes respond to etanercept but the sicca features remain unchanged [51].

In patients with RA and ocular complaints, concern for nodular scleritis (a vasculitis of the vessels of the globe) should be kept in the differential, as these constitute needs for immediate therapeutic intervention. The distribution of herpetic lesions in the ocular distribution of the trigeminal nerve (including a lesion on the tip of the nose) should raise suspicion. Pain may also be referred to the ear (Ramsey Hunt syndrome), indicating need for immediate evaluation and treatment.

The joint findings of RA generally precede the sicca findings by many years. However, the RA may have escaped earlier detection and a repeat of rheumatoid serology (including rheumatoid factor, anti-citrullinated peptide antibody) and X-rays may be required to look for occult RA [46].

In summary, the arthropathy associated most commonly with SS usually involves

- symmetric swelling
- intermittent flares
- generally affects hands and feet

Joint disease in SS is typically non-erosive and non-deforming. Due to the age distribution, *co-existent osteoarthritis of the distal interphalangeal joints is common*. However, SS patients may also develop severe *ulnar deviation of their hands* in the absence of erosions, reflecting inflammation of the tendonous sheaths. The use of a team approach with occupational therapy and orthopedic surgery with expertise in hand or feet is critical.

Rheumatoid factor is reported in approximately 40% of patients with SS and is associated with a significantly higher prevalence of articular symptoms (45 vs. 33% without articular complaints). Anti-cyclic citrullinated peptide antibodies are much less common in SS patients than in RA patients. However, their presence suggests a higher incidence of synovitis and subsequent erosive change [46].

The occurrence of *monoarticular arthritis*, especially of recent onset, should raise the possibility of a septic joint or crystalline arthropathy [47].

17.4 Endocrinopathic/Pancreatic Manifestations

17.4.1 Hypothyroidism

Hypothyroidism appears commonly in SS patients [52, 53].

Also, *among patients with autoimmune thyroid disease, SS may be present in about 10% of patients* [54].

Although SS patients may exhibit immune responses to pancreatic antigens, the incidence of clinically significant pancreatic disease is low [55]. SS patients have a blunted pituitary and adrenal response to test with corticotropin-releasing factor [56].

Patients with SS, being older and predominantly female, have a higher incidence of thyroid disease than the general population. Among 506 cases of primary SS reported in the medical literature from 1980 to 2000, the prevalence of *hypothyroidism, hyperthyroidism,* or any thyroid disease was 17, 6, and 29%, respectively [57]. This extends earlier reports of increased hypothyroidism in SS patients [58, 59]. However, in other well-designed studies of SS, there was no statistically significant difference in the overall prevalence of thyroid disease or any particular type of thyroid disease between cases and age-matched and sex-matched controls.

17.4.2 Adrenal

Adrenal insufficiency may occur in several autoimmune settings [60]. Most common is *iatrogenic adrenal suppression* in the patient who has been on steroids and may occur as frequently as 6 weeks of steroid therapy [61]. These patients are important to recognize due to their potential need for additional steroids at the time of surgery or sepsis. *Thrombois of the adrenals* may be due to cardiolipin syndrome and may lead to acute adrenal failure [21, 62].

A blunted response of the hypothalamic pituitary axis in SS patients has been reported [63]. This may in part be due to suppression of adrenal function by cytokines including interleukin-6 and may also involve a blunted response of the adrenergic sympathetic system [64].

Addison's disease due to presence of antibody against adrenal special antigen, particularly the 21-steroid hydroxylase, may occur [65]. There is a rare association termed "Tass" for thyroiditis, Addison's, Sjögren's syndrome, and sarcoidosis [66, 67].

Androgen deficiency in SS may be reflected in a low dehydroepiandrosterone (DHEA) and dehydroepiandrosterone-sulfate (DHEA-S) level patients [68]. This is postulated to occur at the level of adrenal androgen synthesis.

DHEA is a multifunctional steroid that has been implicated in a broad range of biological effects in humans and other mammals. Together with its sulfate ester (*DHEA-S*), it is the most abundant steroid in humans. DHEA is not only produced by adrenal glands, but also synthesized de novo in the brain. It acts on the androgen receptor both directly and through its metabolites, which include androstenediol and androstenedione, and can undergo further conversion to produce the androgen testosterone and the estrogens estrone and estradiol.

The low DHEA-S levels in SS may reflect a disease-mediated influence on adrenal steroid synthesis rather than a global effect on the entire hypopituitary adrenal axis. In the SS patients with low DHEA-S, the thyroid axis and gonadotropin secretion were similar in patients and controls [68].

Serum DHEA and DHEA-S are negatively correlated with serum interleukin-6 (IL-6) in SS and SLE patients. Also, IL-6 inhibits DHEA from the adrenals [69] in SLE and SS patients.

An additional finding of interest is the role that androgens play in both lacrimal and salivary glandular function. A recent study in SS patients demonstrated the diminished levels of an androgen-dependent saliva protein (crisp3) and suggested that DHEA or similar compounds may play an important role in salivary gland function by affecting aquaporin and other water channels [70].

Pillemer et al. [71] reported a pilot, double-blind trial of DHEA (200 mg/day) versus placebo for treatment of SS. In this study [71], randomization of SS patients resulted in 14 DHEA and 14 placebo group subjects. No significant differences were noted between the DHEA and placebo groups for dry eye symptoms, objective measures of ocular dryness, and stimulated salivary flow. Four DHEA and one placebo group patient dropped out because of adverse effects, generally increased acne. They concluded that DHEA treatment showed no evidence of efficacy in SS.

One positive finding in the Pillemer study [71] was statistically significant improvement in the dry mouth symptoms on visual analog scale (VAS) for the DHEA group compared with the placebo group. However, the improvement in the DHEA group represented only 9 mm on a 100-mm scale, i.e., 9% improvement, which, by the definition used in their study, is not clinically meaningful.

In 1988, a small, randomized, double-blind trial of another mild steroid androgen, *nandrolone decanoate*, showed some evidence of subjective, but not objective, improvement in primary SS [72]. Thus, an isolated effect of DHEA on symptoms of dry mouth cannot be ruled out.

DHEA levels are frequently decreased in SLE [73] and have been proposed to play a role in the fatigue and fibromyalgia symptoms that occur. These findings led to a study of DHEA in a controlled, double-blind treatment study. Although the study by a distinguished group of SLE researchers suggested a statistically significant beneficial effect of DHEA in "quality of life" in SLE [74], the same data were presented to the FDA for approval of DHEA and was turned down. Many patients will continue to purchase DHEA (or equivalents) which are available "over the counter" (OTC) as nutritional supplements, and physicians should caution their patients that *there may be significant variation in the actual DHEA content of these OTC preparations* [75].

17.4.3 Pancreas

Surprisingly, the incidence of insulin-dependent diabetes (type I diabetes) is not significantly increased, although diabetic patients with hyperglycemia frequently have complaints of dryness.

In the standard mouse model of diabetes (i.e., the NOD mouse), the genes predisposing to diabetes or to SS-like salivary infiltrates can be distinguished and selectively bred [76]. However, co-morbid conditions of steroid use including obesity are frequently present in the SS patient and lead to type II diabetes. However, as will be discussed in a subsequent chapter, the clinical features of SS neuropathy (peripheral, autonomic, and accelerated atherosclerotic) may closely overlap with diabetes and the latter condition may be made overt or exacerbated by steroids used to treat the SS.

17.5 Pulmonary Manifestations

17.5.1 Interstitial Pneumonitis

Interstitial lung disease (ILD), also known as *diffuse parenchymal lung disease (DPLD)*, refers to a group of lung diseases affecting the interstitium of the lung: alveolar epithelium, pulmonary capillary endothelium, basement membrane, perivascular, and perilymphatic tissues. The term ILD is used to distinguish these diseases from obstructive airway diseases.

Historically, the ILD associated with SS was termed LIP (lymphocytic interstitial pneumonitis) [77]. The *classification of interstitial pneumonitis* is undergoing change [78] with recognition of subsets including

- *Lymphocytic interstitial pneumonitis (LIP),* which is now recognized as a subset of non-specific interstitial pneumonitis (NSIP)
- *Usual Interstitial Pneumonitis (UIP)* that has a fibrotic feature on biopsy
- *Bronchiolitis obliterans* and *organizing pneumonia (BOOP)* and non-specific pneumonitis
- *Bronchial mucosal associated lymphoma (BALT)*

SS patients may have lymphomatous changes (both mucosal BALT and other forms of non-Hodgkin's lymphoma), and patients with LIP are at markedly increased risk of both types of lymphomas [79].

In patients with MALT lymphoma, *gastric lymphomas* may also be present and may regress when co-existent *Helicobacter pylori* infection is treated [80–82]. Also, *other causes of pulmonary changes that must be considered include hypersensitivity lung and drug toxicity* (including methotrexate, rituximab, or alkylating agents) as well as *opportunistic infections* in patients receiving immunosuppressive medications [83]. Of potential importance are reports of *pneumonitis* in patients receiving *infliximab* (including reactivated tuberclosis (TBC)) [84] and *rituximab* (perhaps a cytokine release syndrome) [85].

The differential diagnosis among connective tissue diseases includes the following

- o Systemic sclerosis even in the absence of skin changes
- o Dermatomyositis
- o Systemic lupus erythematosus including pulmonary hemorrhage
- o Rheumatoid arthritis
- o Sarcoidosis
- o Lymphoma
- o Tuberculosis and other opportunistic infections
- o Aspiration pneumonia
- o Post-operative pneumonias due to mucus plug inspissation of the airways
- o Pulmonary emboli and shock lung Acute Respiratory Distress Syndrome (ARDS)

Fischer et al. [86] recently reported a high frequency of NSIP patients who had a positive ANA (nucleolar pattern) with a novel antigen termed Th/Th0 and a forme fruste of calcinosis Raynaud's phenomena, esophageal dysfunction, limited scleroderma and telangiectasia (CREST) syndrome. Deterioration of ILD in patients should include consideration of pulmonary hypertension and recurrent pulmonary emboli (especially in the patient with anti-cardiolipin or other pro-coagulant states).

Other factors to be excluded in the differential diagnosis of ILD in SS patients include

- Inhaled substances
  - o Inorganic
    - ▪ Silicosis
    - ▪ Asbestosis
    - ▪ Berylliosis
  - o Organic
    - ▪ Hypersensitivity pneumonitis including molds
  - o Drug-induced
  - o Antibiotics
  - o Anti-arrhythmic agents
  - o Infection

- o Atypical pneumonia, including mycobacterial infections
- o Pneumocystis pneumonia (PCP)
- o Tuberculosis
- o Malignancy
- o Lymphangitic carcinomatosis

Investigation is tailored toward the symptoms and signs. Most patients have blood testing, chest X-ray, pulmonary function testing (including diffusing capacity, exercise oximetry and 6-min walk), and high-resolution CT of the thorax.

A lung biopsy is required if the clinical history and imaging are not clearly suggestive of a specific diagnosis or malignancy or if infection cannot otherwise be ruled out.

Initial treatment of ILDs includes corticosteroids (often starting at 60 mg/day), and occasionally cases of NSIP (non-specific interstitial pneumonia)—especially post-pneumonia—may revert to normal lung status [87].

However, most SS patients with a more chronic ILD require immunosuppressant treatment. The choice of immunosuppressant agent is always difficult, as ILD has also been associated with alkylators (i.e., cyclophosphamide), methotrexate, and mycophenolic acid.

Although double-blind studies have not been reported, the experience in SS follows the pattern of treatment often used in ILD involvement in PSS patients. Namely, patients may receive intravenous cyclophosphamide monthly for up to 6 months [88], followed by mycophenolic acid (mofetil) [89] in an effort to taper the corticosteroids. Patients with hypoxemia may be given supplemental oxygen and may be considered for lung transplant.

Magro et al. [90] suggested that antibodies with anti-endothelial properties may play a role in initiating and perpetuating the NSIP. Such a link between the humoral and fibroblast growth factor stimulating pathways would offer an approach to therapy.

Enlarged lymph nodes of the lung or other evidence of lymphoproliferative disease involving the upper airways is generally confined to patients with primary SS.

In addition, the importance of pulmonary lymphoid structures [91] has been recognized as part of the "extranodal" lymphoid infiltrates that were initially recognized as mucosa-associated lymphoid tumors ("MALT" lymphomas) in the stomach [92, 93]. These lesions need to be distinguished from sarcoidosis and tuberculosis.

17.6 Cardiac—Heart Disease Manifestations

17.6.1 Pericarditis

Pericarditis manifests as acute symptomatic disease with an exudative effusion and is a rare complication of primary SS [94, 95]. Echocardiographic evidence of prior pericarditis is more frequent, as illustrated by an echocardiographic study of 150 patients with definite or probable SS, among whom, one-third had increased pericardial echogenicity suggestive of prior pericarditis [96]. This finding has been confirmed in another study of 27 patients [96].

Among SS patients with a history of pericarditis, echocardiographic measurements indicated an unexpectedly high frequency of localized hypokinesia of the left ventricle, all with unspecific ECG changes, while only one without pericarditis showed this symptom. No patient had low voltage, ST–T elevation or conduction abnormalities.

17.6.2 Autonomic Manifestations

The autonomic neural system is a very complex interconnected organ system that comprises at least five components, whose functions are tightly interlinked:

- Parasympathetic cholinergic
- Sympathetic cholinergic
- Sympathetic noradrenergic
- Adrenomedullary hormonal
- Enteric motility

Suarez et al. [97] have developed a questionnaire containing 169 items concerning different aspects of autonomic symptoms

The *Composite Autonomic Symptom Scale (COMPASS)* with item-weighting was established; higher scores correlated with more or worse symptoms.

Cardiovascular tests suggestive of autonomic neuropathy such as

- response of blood pressure to sustained hand grip,
- valsalva maneuver,
- heart rate response to deep breathing, and
- heart rate and blood pressure response to standing—may be increased in SS patients [98].

Although there has been some difference in published reports regarding frequency and manifestations, the prevailing clinical experience supports the hypothesis that both SS and SLE patients are prone to autonomic neuropathy [99–103].

Beat-to-beat or heart rate variability (HRV) may reflect the dynamics of the interplay of the vagal nerve, sympathetic, parasympathetic, and intrinsic cardiac neuronal mechanisms. Time domain analysis of these variables has been used by athletes in training and recently were suggested as important markers that reflect the immune response on neural autonomic function [104–106].

Autonomic neuropathy involving gastric and bowel motility (also called *visceral neuropathy*) is usually thought to be associated with not only diabetes (types I and II), but also has increased frequency in SS patients [107]. Other internal organs such as the bladder muscles and the motility of the digestive tract may be affected. It has been suggested that circulating antibodies against muscarinic receptors, aquaporins, or other voltage-gated channels may play a role in these manifestations [108–111]. However, as demonstrated in the lacrimal and salivary gland, local cytokine release may interfere with the post-receptor signaling response.

17.6.3 Congenital Heart Block

Congenital heart block in infants may be associated with previously undiagnosed maternal primary Sjögren's syndrome [110, 112–117]. The autoantibody against SS-A 60-kDa or related p75 proteins may mediate the injury to the neonatal heart.

Heart block can also occur in adult SS patients and may be associated with antibodies against Purkinje fibers [118] or with antibodies to muscarinic M1 receptor [110, 119].

In summary, there is an increased incidence of congenital heart block in mothers bearing anti-SS antibody, although other autoantibodies have also been suggested as causative agents in this condition.

17.6.4 Accelerated Atherosclerosis

As has been demonstrated in SLE patients [120–122], *the late mortality is often due to accelerated atherosclerotic disease in SS patients* [123] and thus, *careful attention to lipid profiles is required.*

Similarly, other risk factors such as hypertension, diabetes, and perhaps elevations of homocysteine may also play a role. Leukopenia is associated with accelerated atherosclerosis, perhaps as a reflection of the ongoing intravascular coagulopathy that contributes to white blood cells "binding and rolling" along endothelial surfaces [124].

The recent emergence of CRP as a marker for cardiac and stroke is intriguing. Although most thoroughly studied as a predictor of erosions and disease activity of the joints in RA patients, the concept of CRP as a marker for intravascular inflammation and thus for accelerated atherosclerotic changes has received a great deal of recent attention. Indeed, the cardiologists have extended our familiar "normal" range of CRP to include lower levels of CRP (1–3 mg/L) as they measure "highly sensitive CRP (hsCRP)" as a measure of cardiovascular risk.

Indeed, an entirely new set of problems face the patient and rheumatologist, as the cardiologist pushes statins to higher levels in order to minimize the hsCRP with the instruction "better a little joint and muscle pain than a heart attack."

Thus, *the rheumatologist now must factor the statins into the differential diagnosis of myalgias (and mildly elevated CPK) in their evaluation of musculoskeletal symptoms.*

The interaction of fibrinogen, coagulation factors (such as factor XIII), CCP, CRP, and the antibody/complement system is gaining new importance as a system that may reflect both joint, muscle, and glandular inflammation as well perpetuate vasculopathy that predisposes to heart attack and stroke. The spectrum of coagulopathy that began with anti-cardiolipin antibodies, frequent miscarriages, and lupus anti-coagulants is growing broader [125].

17.7 Gastrointestinal Manifestations

Dysphagia is common in SS and is most often due to lack of saliva, but there have also been reports of esophageal dysmotility, similar to that seen in polymyositis or scleroderma [102, 126, 127].

Autonomic neuropathies may be present and patients exhibit bloating as a result of decreased motility. Since salivary flow is decreased, the flow of higher pH saliva is not available to neutralize the acidic secretions of the stomach. This predisposes patients to symptoms of gastroesophageal reflux and tracheal reflux, as described in Chapter 16. *This reflux may also present as hoarseness in talking or singing due to vocal cord irritation.*

Nausea, epigastric pain, and dyspepsia are other frequent complaints [79, 128]. Histological examination may show an atrophic gastritis, with an infiltrate of predominantly $CD4^{+}$ T cells. Achlorhydria and pernicious anemia can also occur. As noted above, autonomic neuropathy can affect bowel motility in SS patients [79, 111, 128].

17.8 Hepatic and Pancreatic Manifestations

There is an association between SS and hepatic abnormalities as evidenced by abnormal biochemical tests or biopsy features of primary biliary cirrhosis (PBC), portal tract fibrosis, or chronic active hepatitis [129–133].

Idiopathic portal hypertension has been associated with systemic sclerosis and Sjögren's syndrome [134]. The most common "mimic" of SS is *hepatitis C*, where patients may develop a positive ANA, RF, sicca symptoms, and extraarticular manifestations including mixed cryoglobulinemia. However, hepatitis C infection represents an "exclusion" to the current criteria of Sjögren's syndrome, so the hepatitis C-related manifestations will not be covered here, although the rheumatologist is urged to consider this infection in the diagnosis and screen for this virus.

Patients with PBC have an increased prevalence of sicca symptoms [132]. In one series, for example, all 14 subjects had either dry eyes or dry mouth; in another, the proportion was 47% [133].

The variation in frequency of PBC depends on several factors. The degree of elevation of liver function tests often determines whether either liver biopsy or anti-mitochondrial antibodies are determined [131]. Patients vary from asymptomatic to mild symptoms of pruritus all the way to end stages of cirrhosis.

It is important to recognize that *PBC has evolved into one of the leading causes for liver transplantation* and that this complication may be avoided by the use of bile salt-binding agents [129, 131, 132].

The molecular basis for sicca symptoms in PBC is not clear, but it is possible that hepatic and salivary gland damage share a similar pathology due to T lymphocytes that share a similar pattern of tissue "homing" receptors [135]. It is important to be aware of the association since there are other causes of abnormal liver function in SS—particularly autoimmune hepatitis, hepatitis C virus infection, and drug toxicity.

Autoimmune hepatitis may complicate SS [136]. Patients with elevated anti-smooth muscle antibody are most common, but others may have anti-liver/microsomal/kidney antibody.

In many patients, antibody profiles remain negative for these antibodies and diagnosis is confirmed by liver biopsy. The decision on what level of liver involvement deserves treatment is dependent in part on the findings in liver biopsy [136–138]. However, liver function abnormalities may not always be due to immune factors.

Consideration of liver toxicity due to methotrexate or leflunomide as well as herbal remedies must not be ignored. Rheumatologists must be aware that the majority of patients who use herbal (especially Chinese, Indian or African herbs) tend to not list these agents on the medication sheets, as they consider them "nutritional supplements"—not medicines [139, 140]. *Thus, the patient must be directly questioned about use of herbal or homeopathic remedies as well as other over-the-counter or "home" remedies.*

Celiac disease (gluten-sensitive enteropathy) may be more prevalent in patients with SS than in the general population. In a study of 111 patients with SS, histologically confirmed celiac disease was present in 5 patients, a rate that is approximately tenfold higher than that in the general European population [141–143].

Autoimmune pancreatitis has been reported in association with SS but is uncommon [144]. In SS patients with associated pancreatic and sclerosing cholangitis, there may be an elevation of IgG4 [145] and antibodies against carbonic anhydrase [146]. There may be subtle defects in the exocrine function of the pancreas of a higher proportion of SS patients lacking clinical features of pancreatitis, as indicated by decreased ability to digest particular substances such as decorin [147].

17.9 Renal/Urological Manifestations

Interstitial nephritis and glomerular disease can occur in SS.

The following is a brief summary:

- *Mild proteinuria and renal tubular dysfunction* can result in renal tubular acidosis and polyuria due to nephrogenic diabetes insipidus.
- *Glomerular involvement* is rare in SS.
- *Membranoproliferative glomerulonephritis* and *membranous nephropathy* may occur.
- *Co-existing systemic lupus erythematosus* or *mixed cryoglobulinemia* should be excluded in patients with clinical features or laboratory findings suggestive of glomerulonephritis.

Drugs can affect the kidneys in SS:

- *Interstitial nephritis (IN),* for example, can be due to *non-steroidal anti-inflammatory drugs* (see "NSAIDs: Acute renal failure and nephrotic syndrome").

  Interstitial nephritis is of particular interest in SS (IN is common in SS on provocative testing [148]). Some patients may present with hypokalemic paralysis [149], renal calculi, or osteomalacia [150].
- Deterioration in renal status should focus attention to medications including *non-steroidal anti-inflammatory agents.*
- Also, recently, a role for *Chinese herbs* in exacerbating renal disease has been recognized [151].

SS patients may develop *glomerulonephritis* (that is negative for anti-ds DNA antibodies), and this suggests the need to consider amyloidosis, immune complex disorder, or unappreciated SLE with error in lab testing [152].

1. Interstitial cystitis (IC) [153–156]—symptoms are more common in SS patients [156] and may be severe [154]. SS patients' bladder symptoms may be exacerbated by these patients' large fluid intake (due to dry mouth) and the antibodies to muscarinic cholinergic receptors found on bladder epithelial cells [157].

Women with SS may develop dysuria, urinary frequency, nocturia, and urgency—symptoms that are thought, in the absence of infection, to be due to interstitial cystitis. The frequency with which this symptom complex occurs was evaluated in a study of 870 Finnish women with SS and 1,304 population controls [158]. The presence of such urinary symptoms was 20-fold higher in those with SS (4.0 vs. 0.2% in controls).

17.10 Hematologic Manifestations

Autoimmune neutropenia, thrombocytopenia, and Coombs' positivity (hemolytic anemia) occur in patients with primary Sjögren's syndrome, similar to its occurrence in SLE [159].

Ramos-Casals et al. [160] have recently reported the incidence of these complications in a large SS cohort in Spain. Although uncommon, they responded well to rituximab therapy [161]. Older reports also note the beneficial response to splenectomy in refractory cases that did not respond to IV-gamma globulin [162].

Pure red blood cell aplasia has also been associated with SS [163].

Leukopenia is common in both SS and SLE.

Agranulocytosis is uncommon but is associated with SS.

Coppo et al. [164] reported seven patients with primary SS associated with a chronic (>6 months) agranulocytosis. They all had non-erosive arthritis and three had thrombocytopenia.

- o In vitro bone marrow culture was normal (four patients) or showed a decrease in colony-forming unit-granulocyte monocyte (CFU-GM) and colony-forming unit-erythroblast (CFU-E) (one patient).
- o Serum levels of granulocyte-colony-stimulating factor (G-CSF) concentrations were either normal or raised.
- o One patient was treated with steroids associated with intravenous immunoglobulins and achieved a lasting response.
- o Two other patients were treated with steroids and methotrexate, with poor efficacy.
- o Short courses of subcutaneous G-CSF produced a transient and mild response in all three patients.
- o Complete recovery of the neutrophils occurred temporarily during pregnancy in two patients.
- o After a mean follow up of 34.8 months (range 6–139) all patients were alive and none developed serious infections. Thus, a subset of patients with primary SS and non-destructive arthritis may develop a chronic but well-tolerated agranulocytosis that is usually poorly responsive to steroids and oral methotrexate.

17.11 Obstetrical/Gynecological Manifestations

Vaginal dryness often leads to painful intercourse (dyspareunia) and possible vaginal tearing leading to painful infection [165, 166]. It is important to be reassured that this does not occur in all Sjögren's patients, even those with severe mouth and eye dryness [167, 168].

Many women with Sjögren's syndrome are interested in the risks of pregnancy and risks to the baby. Obstetrical authorities report *slightly higher rates of recurrent fetal death and congenital heart block* in those pregnancies complicated by maternal autoimmune disease [169].

In rare patients, fetal loss has been associated with presence of the antibodies called "anti-phospholipid antibodies," "lupus anti-coagulant," and anti-cardiolipin antibodies [170–172].

Congenital heart block is an abnormality of the rate or rhythm of the fetal or infant heart. Certain autoantibodies, such as an antibody called "anti-SS-A," have been associated with congenital heart block in the newborn. These autoantibodies may be present in patients with systemic lupus erythematosus and with Sjögren's syndrome as well as in patients with no apparent disease. Antibodies other than anti-SS-A have also been associated with neonatal heart block [170, 172, 173].

However, it is important to reassure patients planning families that the vast majority of patients with Sjögren's syndrome have babies with no congenital abnormalities. Thus, we encourage family planning to be conducted without this being a major consideration.

Nevertheless, it is important for patients anticipating pregnancy (or those with multiple prior miscarriages) to have screening blood tests and that their pregnancies are supervised by obstetricians experienced in handling patients with autoimmune diseases. If a pregnant patient requires corticosteroids for their medical condition, we suggest dexamethasone (decadron, rather than prednisone) since it crosses the placenta and will provide protection to the fetus [174].

Abnormal PAP smears have been reported at higher frequency in women with SLE [175, 176], and it is likely that similar findings will occur in SS patients. The elevated frequency of abnormal PAP smears was more common among SLE patients than controls, even after adjusting for human papillomavirus (HPV) status. The use of immunosuppressant agents was not associated with abnormal PAP smears. Thus, it appears that SLE-associated immunosuppression increases susceptibility to HPV infection [176]. A potential link may be increased susceptibility to HPV infection in SLE (and SS) patients with a higher frequency of a particular allele in the TNF promoter.

17.12 Vasculitis

Vasculitis may affect virtually any organ in patients with SS (and these topics will be covered in other chapters), and this diagnosis is a "medical emergency" for both patient and rheumatologist. Thus, a brief overview is presented in this chapter. Vasculitis is generally classified by the size of the blood vessel affected and accompanied by increased erythrocyte sedimentation rate (ESR), elevated C-reactive protein (CRP), and anemia. The definite diagnosis of vasculitis is established after a biopsy of involved organ or tissue, such as skin, sinuses, lung, nerve, and kidney. An alternative to biopsy can be an angiogram or MRI angiography, which can demonstrate characteristic patterns of inflammation in affected blood vessels.

Overlaps of features of the major vasculitis have been reported in SS patients, including

- Kawasaki disease
- Behçet's disease
- Polyarteritis nodosa
- Wegener's granulomatosis
- Cryoglobulinemia including hepatitis C
- Takayasu's arteritis
- Churg–Strauss syndrome
- Giant cell arteritis (temporal arteritis)
- Henoch–Schönlein purpura

17.12.1 CNS Arteritis in the SS Patient

- *The clinical hallmarks*: headache, slowly evolving encephalopathy, and multifocal strokes.
- Fever, other constitutional symptoms, and extra-CNS manifestations are frequently absent.
- Acute-phase reactants tend to be normal in primary angiitis of the central nervous system (PACNS).
- Lumbar puncture typically reveals a lymphocytic pleocytosis.
- Magnetic resonance imaging (MRI) usually reveals multiple foci of strokes, some of which may be asymptomatic.
- *Caution should be exercised with use of medications :*
  - *Vasoconstrictive medications should be avoided in patients with presumed vasospasm and cranial vasculitis who present with headache and stroke-like symptoms.*
- *Caution in the ER:*
  - Vasoconstrictive drugs and medications such as sumatriptan and ergot derivatives may be given in the emergency room due to the presumptive diagnosis of "migraine."
  - Caution in interpreting vasospasm in MRI/MRA studies done in the emergency room, as these medications are generally given prior to the study.
- *Diet pills* (and use of herbal preparations principally used for weight reduction), nasal decongestants with pseudoephedrine, and serotonergic (SSRI) anti-depressants at high dose may trigger attacks of vasospasm.
- *Illicit drugs*: Anecdotal evidence also suggests that associations with cocaine, ecstasy (3,4-methylenedioxymethamphetamine), and marijuana have been identified as triggers of cranial vessel spasm and frank vasculitis and unfortunately, the use of these drugs is increasingly common in certain parts of this country and the world. The diagnosis of SS does not rule out the concurrent use of illicit drugs.

17.13 Differential Diagnosis of Extraglandular Manifestations of SS

There is a particularly close overlap between SS and a subset of SLE patients. This overlap is seen at several levels:

(a) SLE patients often have clinical symptoms of secondary SS.
(b) SLE and SS patients share an overlap of extraglandular manifestations, although this chapter will highlight the manifestations that are not shared.

(c) SLE patients often have anti-SS-A antibodies, making diagnosis often confusing.
(d) SS patients have similar genetic markers and respond to similar medications as SLE patients.

Often, there is a tendency for primary care physician to label every patient with a positive ANA as having SLE. There are specific criteria for primary SS (Table 17.2) that are distinct from SLE, scleroderma (PSS), and fibromyalgia. It is also recognized that some SS patients may lack anti-SS-A/SS-B antibody and may have other patterns such as anti-centromere, while still having features much more in common with SS than with scleroderma. Also, not every patient fits into a neat pigeon hole and a subset of patients have other autoimmune features that overlap, such as the RA patient with secondary SS.

Table 17.2 International consensus criteria for Sjögren's syndrome, systemic lupus erythematosus, and scleroderma

I. Primary SS
A. *Ocular symptoms (at least one present)*
1. Daily, persistent, troublesome dry eyes for more than 3 months
2. Recurrent sensation of sand or gravel in the eyes
3. Use of a tear substitute for more than three times a day
B. *Oral symptoms (at least one present)*
1. Daily feeling of dry mouth for at least 3 months
2. Recurrent feeling of swollen salivary glands as an adult
3. Need to drink liquids to aid in washing down dry foods
C. *Objective evidence of dry eyes (at least one present)*
1. Schirmer's-I test
2. Rose Bengal
3. Lacrimal gland biopsy with focus score $\geq$ 1
D. *Objective evidence of salivary gland involvement (at least one present)*
1. Salivary gland scintigraphy
2. Parotid sialography
3. Unstimulated whole sialometry ($\leq$ 1.5 mL/15 min)
E. *Laboratory abnormality (at least one present)*
1. Anti-SS-A or anti-SS-B antibody
2. Anti-nuclear antibody (ANA)
3. IgM rheumatoid factor (anti-IgG Fc)
• Diagnosis of primary Sjogren's syndrome requires four of six criteria, including a positive minor salivary gland biopsy or antibody to SS-A/SS-B.
• Exclusions include previous radiation to the head and neck lymphoma, sarcoidosis, hepatitis C infection, AIDS, graft-versus-host disease, and medications that can cause dryness.
• Diagnosis of secondary SS requires an established connective tissue disease and one sicca symptom plus two objective tests for dry mouth and dry eyes at the time of their clinical entry into study cohort.
• Diagnosis of SS can be made in patients who have no sicca symptoms if objective tests of ocular and oral dryness are fulfilled including either a minor salivary gland biopsy or anti-SS-A/SS-B antibody.
Diagnostic criteria of SLE
Criterion definition:
Malar rash
Rash over the cheeks

Table 17.2 (continued)

Discoid rash
Red raised patches
Photosensitivity
Reaction to sunlight, resulting in the development of or increase in skin rash
Oral ulcers
Ulcers in the nose or mouth, usually painless
Arthritis
Non-erosive arthritis involving two or more peripheral joints (arthritis in which the bones around the joints do not become destroyed)
Serositis
Pleuritis or pericarditis
Renal disorder
Excessive protein in the urine (greater than 0.5 g/day or 3+ on test sticks) and/or cellular casts (abnormal elements in the urine, derived from red and/or white cells and/or kidney tubule cells)
Neurologic
Seizures
(convulsions) and/or psychosis in the absence of drugs or metabolic disturbances which are known to cause such effects
Hematologic
Hemolytic anemia or leukopenia (white blood count below 4,000 cells per cubic millimeter) or lymphopenia (less than 1,500 lymphocytes per cubic millimeter) or thrombocytopenia (less than 100,000 platelets per cubic millimeter). The leukopenia and lymphopenia must be detected on two or more occasions. The thrombocytopenia must be detected in the absence of drugs known to induce it
Immunologic
Positive LE prep test, positive anti-DNA test, positive anti-Sm test, or false-positive syphilis test (VDRL)
Positive test for anti-nuclear antibodies in the absence of drugs known to induce it
Because many lupus symptoms mimic other illnesses, complaints are sometimes vague and may come and go, lupus can be difficult to diagnose. Diagnosis is usually made by a careful review of a person's entire medical history coupled with an analysis of the results obtained in routine laboratory tests and some specialized tests related to immune status. Currently, there is no single laboratory test that can determine whether a person has lupus or not. To assist the physician in the diagnosis of lupus, the American Rheumatism Association issued a list of 11 symptoms or signs that help distinguish lupus from other diseases. A person should have four or more of these symptoms to suspect lupus. The symptoms do not all have to occur at the same time.
Diagnostic criteria of progressive systemic sclerosis (scleroderma)
The American College of Rheumatology (ACR) criteria for the classification of scleroderma require *one major criterion* or *two minor criteria*, which are as follows:
Major criterion
Proximal scleroderma is characterized by symmetric thickening, tightening, and induration of the skin of the fingers and the skin that is proximal to the metacarpophalangeal or metatarsophalangeal joints. These changes may affect the entire extremity, face, neck, and trunk (thorax and abdomen).
Minor criteria
Sclerodactyly includes the above major criterion characteristics but is limited to only the fingers.
Digital pitting scars or a loss of substance from the finger pad: As a result of ischemia, depressed areas of the fingertips, or a loss of digital pad tissue occurs.
Bibasilar pulmonary fibrosis includes a bilateral reticular pattern of linear or lineonodular densities most pronounced in basilar portions of the lungs on standard chest roentgenograms. These densities may assume the appearance of diffuse mottling or a honeycomb lung and are not attributable to primary lung disease.

The diagnosis of SS (and distinction from an SLE patient) does alert the physician to particular glandular and extraglandular manifestations, particularly lymphocytic infiltrative and lymphoproliferative features. However, it is important that the physician does not become entangled with the semantics of "SLE vs. SS," especially when the therapeutic outcome will be the same medications.

Indeed in the majority of patients, SS is often considered "*incomplete*" *SLE* (possessing only four rather than five of the necessary diagnostic criteria for SLE), and many "older" patients who are diagnosed with SLE clinically actually have SS but have been labeled as lupus based on their positive ANA.

It is known that both SS and SLE share common genetic, autoantibody profiles, pathogenetic, and therapeutic response features (Fig. 17.1). However, the simplest distinction may be that many SLE clinical manifestations result due to immune complex formation and complement activation-mediated tissue damage (i.e., glomerulonephritis, pleural effusions, hemolytic anemia, thrombocytopenia, skin rashes), while *SS patients exhibit pathology that is characterized by tissue lymphocytic infiltrates* (interstitial pneumonitis, interstitial nephritis, lymphoma). A simplified comparison of extraglandular manifestations is shown in Fig. 17.2.

In this comparison of SS and SLE, the SS patients may have not only the immune complex manifestations of the SLE patient, but also exhibit additional disease manifestations that result from lymphocytic infiltration. The glandular and extraglandular tissue dysfunction result from the subsequent local cytokine and metalloproteinase production as well as direct tissue destruction accompanying the lymphocytic infiltrates.

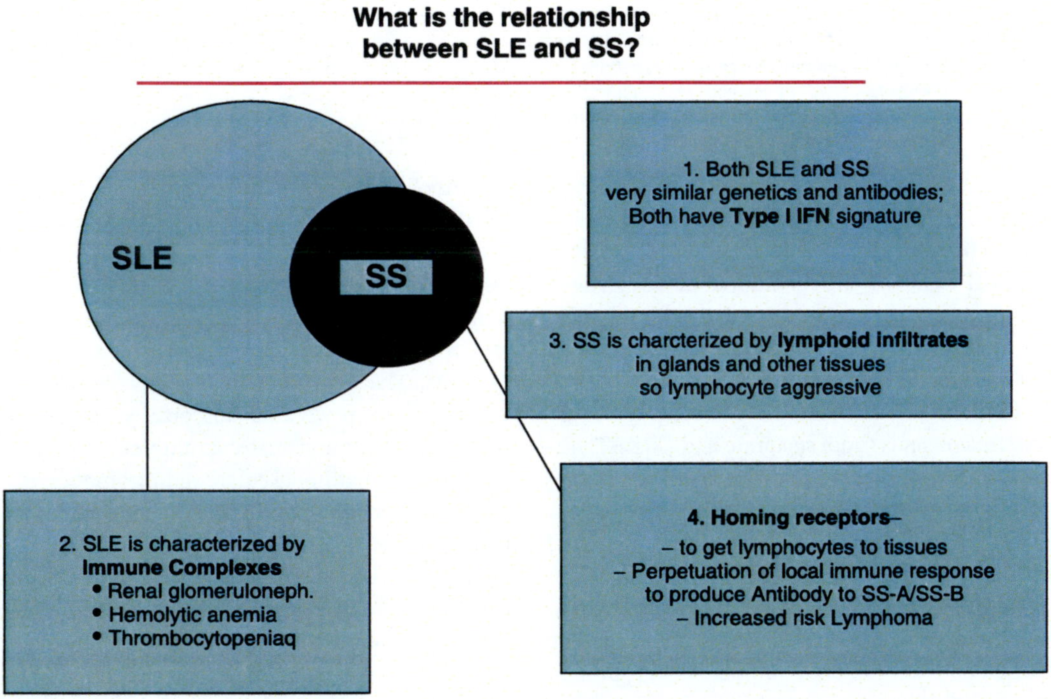

Fig. 17.1 What is the relationship between SLE and SS? One of the most difficult clinical distinctions is whether the patient has primary Sjögren's syndrome (SS) or systemic lupus erythematosus (SLE) with secondary SS. It is easiest to think of SLE to be composed of a series of clinical subsets that are characterized by their characteristic autoantibodies and associated HLA-DR associations. SS has close similarity to one of the subsets in SLE. Similarly, many older patients who are labeled "SLE" based on arthralgia, rashes, and a positive ANA probably have SS rather than SLE

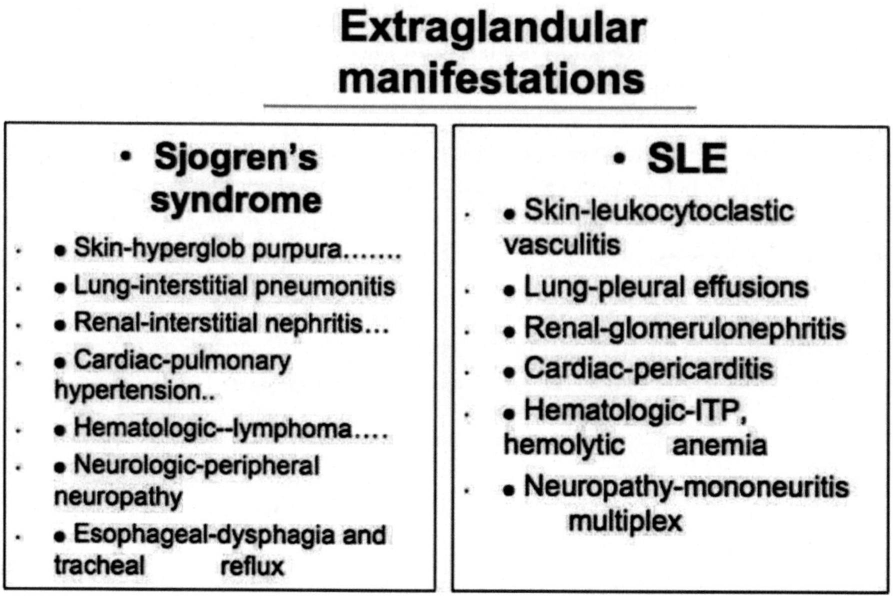

Fig. 17.2 Extraglandular manifestations in SS. Although the previous figure emphasizes the "overlap of symptoms" between SLE and SS, this figure demonstrates that the diagnosis of SS does lead to consideration of a slightly different pattern of extraglandular manifestations. Put most simply, many manifestations of SLE can be considered to develop as a result of antibody–antigen immune complexes and complement activation. In this simplified model, SS is considered a "lymphocyte" infiltrative disorder (as manifest by the salivary gland infiltrates on one hand and increased lymphoma at the extreme). This would lead to glomerulonephritis in SLE and interstitial nephritis in SS. Similarly, lung abnormalities would be pleural effusions in SLE and interstitial pneumonitis in SS. This figure proves several comparisons of extraglandular manifestations

As an overview of the contents of this chapter, Table 17.2 lists the current diagnostic criteria for SS (as well as SLE and scleroderma), a summary of reported extraglandular manifestations, and therapies. It will be seen that both the clinical manifestations and therapies have significant overlap among these disorders.

Similarly, SS patients show overlap with scleroderma patients (both systemic and CREST variants). The problems of diagnosis and therapy for Raynaud's phenomena, motility (esophageal) disorders, and interstitial tissue infiltrates such as lung represent challenges of diagnosis but again often come to the same diagnostic workup and therapeutic options. A subset of SS patients exhibit anti-centromere B antibodies but show far more clinical similarity to SS than the CREST. It needs to be remembered that the antibody profile is more closely tied to the genetic background (HLA-DR alleles) than to the clinical manifestations.

Although the normal diseases in the differential diagnosis of SS extraglandular manifestations are traditional autoimmune diseases such as RA, polymyositis, scleroderma, and SLE, it is important to recognize that SS also shows some overlap of features with disorders such as diabetes mellitus. The *neurological findings* in some SS patients (e.g., peripheral neuropathy, autonomic neuropathy, mononeuritis multiplex, increased frequency of cardiovascular, and thrombotic disease) often suggest parallels to diabetic pathogenesis with the latter disease's increased markers of vasculopathy and perivascular lymphocytic infiltrates on muscle/nerve biopsy as well as the findings of necrotizing vasculitis.

As the basis of a "uniform method of data collection" for determination of diagnostic and therapeutic tools, a set of "disease activity" and "organ damage" criteria have been proposed (Table 17.3).

Table 17.3 Sjögren's syndrome disease damage index

Item	Definition	Score
Oral/salivary damage		
Salivary flow impairment	Unstimulated whole saliva collection <1.5 ml/15 min, by standard method	1
Loss of teeth	Complete or almost complete	1
Ocular damage		
Tear flow impairment	Schirmer I test <5 mm in 5 min, by standard method†	1
Structural abnormalities	Corneal ulcers, cataracts, chronic blepharitis	1
Neurologic damage		
CNS involvemet	Long-lasting stable CNS involvement	2
Peripheral neuropathy	Long-lasting stable peripheral or autonomic system impairment	1
Pleropulmonary damage (any of the following)		2
Pleural fibrosis	Confirmed by imaging	
Interstitial fibrosis	Confirmed by imaging	
Significant irreversible functional damage	Confirmed by spirometry	
Renal impairment (any of the following)		2
Increased serum creatinine level or reduced GRF	Long-lasting stable abnormalities	
Tubular acidosis	Urinary pH >6 and serum bicarbonate <15 mmoles/L in 2 consecutive tests	
Nephrocalcinosis	Confirmed by imaging	
Lymphoproliferative disease (any of the following)		5
B cell lymphoma	Clinically and histologically confirmed	
Multiple myeloma	Clinically and histologically confirmed	
Waldenström's macroglobulinemia	Clinically and histologically confirmed	

17.13.1 Medications and Other Metabolic Disorders

Dry mouth can be caused by medications (anti-hypertensive, anti-histamine, parasympatholytic, psychotropic), amyloidosis, sarcoidosis, diabetes mellitus, infections, trauma, irradiation, or the cause could be psychogenic.

Endocrine disorders can affect the parotid gland, along with infections such as mumps, hepatitis C, or HIV. Pancreatitis, diabetes, cirrhosis, lymphoma, and lipid abnormalities can also lead to gland enlargement.

Neurological disorders associated with dryness can include multiple sclerosis.

In summary, the initial evaluation needs to determine if the patient presents with evidence suggestive of an objective autoimmune disease, not just a positive ANA, and this will involve specific autoantibody profiles, ophthalmologic studies, salivary flow studies, and/or minor lip biopsies. These studies are described in above chapters on ocular and oral manifestations of SS. It is important to remember that the ANA is more sensitive than specific and that symptoms of dryness may reflect medications (including over-the-counter or herbal drugs) or infections such as hepatitis B or C.

The patient may have SS, secondary to another autoimmune condition (RA, systemic sclerosis, etc.) or as part of an overlap syndrome with another autoimmune condition. Thus, other conditions that mimic SS need to be evaluated.

For the non-rheumatologist who wants to screen for SS, *the initial workup* should include *complete history and physical relevant to glandular and extraglandular manifestations and laboratory testing including ANA plus anti-SS-A antibody, CBC, ESR, comprehensive metabolic panel (including liver and renal evaluation), and rheumatoid factor. If indicated as workup for apparent lymphoproliferative manifestations or vasculitis, serum immunoglobulins and immunoelectrophoresis, thyroid and TSH, urinalysis, CXR, complement, ACE as well as serologies for Hep B, Hep C, and HIV may be helpful.*

17.14 Manifestations and Differential Diagnosis in the Pediatric Population

A. *SS can present as part of the spectrum of juvenile rheumatoid arthritis (JRA)*, also known as juvenile inflammatory arthritis (JIA).

B. *Parotid gland swelling or lymphadenopathy is a common presentation.*

The initial diagnosis is often includes mumps or infectious mononucleosis in which the swelling does not recede, which does not rapidly improve and the finding high-titer ANA.

C. *Differential diagnosis*

1. *Kawasaki disease*

In the initial differential of the child with prolonged fever, neck pain, and high ESR, a diagnosis of Kawasaki's disease should be considered.

Kawasaki's disease features can remain unrecognized for days after neck swelling develops.

- Neck swelling in Kawasaki's disease can represent superficial adenitis or more rarely, inflammation within the deeper tissue planes of the neck, including the retropharyngeal or parapharyngeal spaces.
- Despite the intensity of inflammation in these spaces and the decreased attenuation that can be observed on CT scan (suggesting an abscess), true abscesses do not develop in these areas.
- Most Kawasaki patients improve dramatically with intravenous gammaglobulin (IVIG) therapy.

Kawasaki's disease can occur in older children and adolescents, and these patients can be at risk for developing coronary artery disease. Older children are likely to experience a delay in diagnosis.

2. *Henoch–Schönlein purpura (HSP)* also must be considered in the diagnosis that presents with skin changes in the peripheral extremities or perineal region.
   - Polymorphous exanthema
   - Bilateral conjunctival injection
   - Changes of lips and oral cavity, with injection of oral and pharyngeal mucosa
   - Cervical lymphadenopathy

17.15 Summary

1. *Primary Sjögren's syndrome* (1° SS) is an autoimmune disorder characterized by

   dry eyes (keratoconjunctivitis sicca) and *dry mouth* due to lymphocytic infiltrates of lacrimal and salivary glands. However, SS is an autoimmune disorder that affects many extraglandular systems.
2. *Multiple extraglandular manifestations of primary SS* affect a myriad of organ systems and structures, including those covered in this chapter:
   - o *Dermatologic/integumentary/cutaneous*
     - skin dryness, vasculitis, urticaria, and Raynaud's phenomena
   - o *Joints and muscles*
     - arthralgia/arthritis and myalgia/myositis
   - o *Endocrinopathic*
     - increased incidence of thyroiditis and adrenal involvement (including Addisonian crisis)
   - o *Pulmonary*
     - interstitial pneumonitis and pulmonary hypertension
   - o *Cardiovascular*
     - pericarditis, cardiomyopathy, anti-coagulant antibodies, and accelerated atherosclerosis

- o *Gastrointestinal*
  - incidence of celiac sprue, atrophic gastritis and motility disorders
- o *Hepatic/pancreatic*
  - autoimmune hepatitis, pancreatic, and sclerosing cholangitis
- o *Renal/kidney*
  - interstitial nephritis and glomerulonephritis
- o *Urinary*
  - interstitial cystitis
- o *Obstetrical/gynecological*
  - neonatal heart block and problems of pregnancy as well as options for vaginal dryness/dyspareunia

3. *New international criteria have been developed for diagnosis, activity index and organ damage of SS.*
4. *The SS patient presents special needs at the time of surgery* due to dryness and risk of venoocclusive disease (Tables 17.4 and 17.5).

17.16 Late-Breaking Updates

In a recent study of SS patients with non-specific interstitial pneumonitis (NSIP) [177], SS patients generally developed characteristic clinical and respiratory features early in the course of their autoimmune disease. Thus, later onset of NSIP should suggest other etiologies including infection including tuberculosis, lymphoma, or drug toxicity [178–181]. Acute respiratory failure in SS patients may be the presenting manifestation of hypokalemic paralysis [182, 183].

Atopic dermatitis may be more common in SS patients, due to the added component of autoimmune anhidrosis [184]. An association of IgA anti-CCP antibodies (circular citrullinated peptide) was found with cutaneous vasculitis [185]. In patients with livedo reticularis, a relatively high incidence of anti-cardiolipin and anti-β2-glycoproteins was reported; surprisingly,

Table 17.4 Extraglandular manifestations of pSS

General manifestations	Main therapeutic modalities
Fatigue Sleep disorder Fibromyalgia	• Pentagabalin (Neurontin) • Pregabalin (Lyrica) • Duloxetine (Cymbalta) • Milnacipram (Savella) • Cognitive therapy and stress reduction • Avoid tricyclic anti-depressants due to dryness, exercise, and myofascial therapy
Cutaneous Dryness Vasculitis Cryoglobulinemia	• Moisturization • Recognition and treatment of yeast infection • Corticosteroids, agents to spare corticosteroids (methotrexate, leflunomide, mycophenolic acid (mofetil), rituximab)
Arthritis, arthralgia, and myalgia	• Acetaminophen • Non-steroidal agents and disalcid • Hydroxychloroquine (6–8 mg/kg/day) • Methotrexate (either oral or self-injected) • Leflunomide (20 mg/day) • Rituximab (dosing similar to RA)
Raynaud's phenomenon and acrocyanosis	• Avoidance of cold and stress exposure • Avoid sympathomimetic drugs (such as decongestants, amphetamines, diet pills, and herbs containing ephedra) • Calcium channel blockers • Ketanserin, a selective antagonist of the S2-serotonergic receptor • Sildenafil • Ilosprost
Circulating anti-coagulants	• Aspirin • Warfarin (if prior thrombotic episode) or lovenox

Table 17.4 (continued)

General manifestations	Main therapeutic modalities
Liver Primary biliary cirrhosis Autoimmune hepatitis Recognition of hepatitis C	• Ursodeoxycholic acid • Corticosteroids • Azathioprine • Aycophenolic acid
Pancreas (be aware that elevated amylase can be from glands) Sclerosing cholangitis (elevated serum levels of IgG4) Idiopathic (non-alcoholic) Pancreatitis Malabsorptive syndromes	• Corticosteroids • Ursodeoxycholic acid • Watch for strictures • Azathioprine • Mycophenolic acid • Rituximab
Kidney Interstitial nephritis Renal tubular acidosis Renal stones Glomerulonephritis Renal calculus	• Azathioprine • Mycophenolic acid • Oral potassium and sodium carbonate (3–12 g/day)
Gastrointestinal Atrophic gastritis Celiac sprue Gastroesophageal reflux Motility disorder	• Avoidance of gluten • Proton pump inhibitors • Promotility agents (Motillium, Reglan)
Accelerated atherosclerosis	Control hypertension, lipids with "tight" control
Vasculitis (cutaneous) Hyperglobulinemic purpura Mixed cryoglobulinemia Mononeuritis multiplex	Prednisolone (0.5–1.0 mg/kg body weight per day) Cyclophosphamide (0.5–1 g/m^2 of body surface/month) Rituximab Plasmapheresis
Endocrine Thyroid Adrenal Blunted hypothalamic axis Iatrogenic Addisonian "Androgen Deficiency"	 Thyroid replacement Corticosteroids and mineralocorticoids DHEA
Cardiac Pulmonary hypertension Pericarditis Autonomic neuropathy	 Endothelin receptor antagonists Iloprost Corticosteroids Midodrine, mineralocorticoids
Gynecology–obstetric Multiple miscarriage Congenital heart block Increased HPV	 Cardiolipin syndrome—lovenox Decadron Increased surveillance

there was relative overlap between subsets of patients with each autoantibody [186].

The sensation of nasal "congestion" in SS patients is common. This finding is frequently out of proportion to the observed patency of the airways and probably reflects the influence of neural sensory circuits that have dysfunction analogous to those innervating the eye and mouth [187].

Table 17.5 Precautions for the Sjögren's patient undergoing general anesthesia

I. Preoperative Period
A. Stop aspirin 1 week prior to surgery
B. Stop NSAIDs 3 days prior to surgery
C. Do not stop steroids
D. Notify anesthesiologist about specific problems with teeth, dentures, eyes, neck, sinuses, and lungs since this may affect the way intubation is performed
II. Day of surgery
A. Take all medications with you to hospital in their bottles
B. Be sure to ask anesthesiologist to use an ocular ointment (such as Refresh PM) during surgery and in post-operative recovery room
C. If receiving steroids, make sure these are taken on day of surgery either orally or through IV. In some cases, a higher dose is required
D. All right to use artificial salivas (such as Oasis Mouth Spray or MouthKote) to keep mouth moist on the day of surgery when "NPO" (nothing per mouth)
E. Ask anesthesiologist to use humidified oxygen in operating room and post-operative recovery room.
III. Post-operative days
A. Watch for yeast infections if receiving antibiotics
B. Use of artificial tears and salivas

Acknowledgments The authors are grateful for their collaboration in the care of our SS patients and their contributions to this chapter in the field of Dermatology (Dr. Alice Liu), Cardiology (Dr. Matthew Luck), Gynecology (Dr. John Willem), Dr. Abdul Khan (Nuclear Medicine), Dr. John Weston (Oral Medicine), Dr. Paul Michelson (Ophthalmology), and Drs. Edward Paradez, Donald Ritt, and Robert Goldklang (Gastroenterology) at Scripps Foundation for Medicine and Research. Also, we wish to thank Dr. Victor Test (Chest Medicine, University of California San Diego) and Dr. Julius Birnbaum (Department of Neurology, Johns Hopkins Medical Center). We also wish to remember the cardinal contributions of the late Professor Frank Howell, who started the combined Oral Medicine–Rheumatology–Ophthalmology Clinic at Scripps Clinic over 30 years ago, where many of the above contributors first learned the "myths and pearls" of Sjogren's syndrome reflected in this chapter.

References

1. Bloch KJ, Buchanan WW, Wohl MJ, Bunim JJ. Sjögren's syndrome: a clinical, pathological and serological study of 62 cases. Medicine (Baltimore) 1956;44:187–231.
2. Alexander EL, Provost TT. Cutaneous manifestations of primary Sjögren's syndrome: a reflection of vasculitis and association with anti-Ro (SSA) antibodies. J. Invest. Dermatol. 1983;80: 386–91.
3. Ito Y, Kanda N, Mitsui H, Watanabe T, Kobayashi S, Murayama S, et al. Cutaneous manifestations of Sjogren's syndrome associated with myasthenia gravis [letter]. Br J Dermatol. 1999;141(2):362–3.
4. Tapinos NI, Polihronis M, Tzioufas AG, Moutsopoulos HM. Sjogren's syndrome. Autoimmune epithelitis. Adv Exp Med Biol. 1999;455:127–34.
5. Sais G, Admella C, Fantova MJ, Montero JC. Lymphocytic autoimmune hidradenitis, cutaneous leucocytoclastic vasculitis and primary Sjogren's syndrome. Br J Dermatol. 1998;139(6):1073–6.
6. Gemignani F, Marbini A, Pavesi G, Di Vittorio S, Manganelli P, Cenacchi G, et al. Peripheral neuropathy associated with primary Sjogren's syndrome. J Neurol Neurosurg Psychiatry. 1994;57(8):983–6.
7. Hebbar M, Lassalle P, Janin A, Vanhee D, Bisiau S, Hatron PY, et al. E-selectin expression in salivary endothelial cells and sera from patients with systemic sclerosis. Role of resident mast cell-derived tumor necrosis factor alpha. Arthritis Rheum. 1995;38(3):406–12.
8. Cho CS, Park SH, Min JK, Lee SH, Kim HY. Clinical significances of antibodies to Ro/SS-A autoantigens and its subtypes in primary Sjogren's syndrome. Korean J Intern Med. 1997;12(2): 176–81.
9. Kyle R, Gleich G, Baynd E, et al. Benign hyperglobulinemic purpura of Waldenstrom. Medicine (Baltimore) 1971;50:113–23.
10. Fox RI, Carson DA, Chen P, Fong S. Characterization of a cross reactive idiotype in Sjögren's syndrome. Scand J Rheumatol. 1986;561:83–8.

11. Fox RI, Chen PP, Carson DA, Fong S. Expression of a cross reactive idiotype on rheumatoid factor in patients with Sjögren's syndrome. J Immunol. 1986;136:477–83.
12. Ramos-Casals M, Cervera R, Yague J, Garcia-Carrasco M, Trejo O, Jimenez S, et al. Cryoglobulinemia in primary Sjogren's syndrome: prevalence and clinical characteristics in a series of 115 patients. Semin Arthritis Rheum. 1998;28(3):200–5.
13. Bernacchi E, Amato L, Parodi A, Cottoni F, Rubegni P, De Pita O, et al. Sjogren's syndrome: a retrospective review of the cutaneous features of 93 patients by the Italian Group of Immunodermatology. Clin Exp Rheumatol. 2004;22(1):55–62.
14. Alexander E, Provost TT. Sjögren's syndrome. Association of cutaneous vasculitis with central nervous system disease. Arch. Dermatol. 1987;123:801–10.
15. Provost TT, Watson R, Simmons-O'Brien OBE. Anti-Ro(SS-A) antibody positive Sjogren's/lupus erythematosus overlap syndrome. Lupus. 1997;6(2):105–11.
16. Konishi M, Ohosone Y, Matsumura M, Oyamada Y, Yamaguchi K, Kawahara Y, et al. Mixed-cryoglobulinemia associated with cutaneous vasculitis and pulmonary symptoms. Intern Med. 1997;36(1):62–7.
17. Ferri C, La Civita L, Longombardo G, Zignego AL, Pasero G. Mixed cryoglobulinaemia: a crossroad between autoimmune and lymphoproliferative disorders. Lupus. 1998;7(4):275–9.
18. O'Donnell B, Black AK. Urticarial vasculitis. Int Angiol. 1995;14(2):166–74.
19. Provost TT, Watson R. Cutaneous manifestations of Sjogren's syndrome. Rheum Dis Clin North Am. 1992;18(3):609–16.
20. Merkel PA, Polisson RP, Chang Y, Skates SJ, Niles JL. Prevalence of antineutrophil cytoplasmic antibodies in a large inception cohort of patients with connective tissue disease. Ann Intern Med. 1997;126(11):866–73.
21. Merkel PA, Chang Y, Pierangeli SS, Convery K, Harris EN, Polisson RP. The prevalence and clinical associations of anticardiolipin antibodies in a large inception cohort of patients with connective tissue diseases. Am J Med. 1996;101(6): 576–83.
22. Navarro M, Cervera R, Font J, Reverter JC, Monteagudo J, Escolar G, et al. Anti-endothelial cell antibodies in systemic autoimmune diseases: prevalence and clinical significance. Lupus. 1997;6(6):521–6.
23. Asherson RA, Fei HM, Staub HL, Khamashta MA, Hughes GRV, Fox RI. Antiphospholipid antibodies and HLA associations in primary Sjögren's syndrome. Ann Rheum Dis. 1992;51:495–8.
24. Roguedas AM, Misery L, Sassolas B, Le Masson G, Pennec YL, Youinou P. Cutaneous manifestations of primary Sjogren's syndrome are underestimated. Clin Exp Rheumatol. 2004;22(5):632–6.
25. Jubert C, Cosnes A, Clerici T, Gaulard P, Andre P, Revuz J, et al. Sjogren's syndrome and cutaneous B cell lymphoma revealed by anetoderma. Arthritis Rheum. 1993;36(1):133–4.
26. Pablos JL, Cogolludo V, Pinedo F, Carreira PE. Subcutaneous nodular amyloidosis in Sjögren's syndrome. Scand J Rheumatol. 1993;22:250–1.
27. Yoneyama K, Tochigi N, Oikawa A, Shinkai H, Utani A. Primary localized cutaneous nodular amyloidosis in a patient with Sjogren's syndrome: a review of the literature. J Dermatol. 2005;32(2):120–3.
28. Yamamoto T, Katayama I, Nishioka K. Analysis of T cell receptor Vbeta repertoires of annular erythema associated with Sjogren's syndrome. Eur J Dermatol. 1998;8(4):248–51.
29. Ramos-Casals M, Anaya JM, Garcia-Carrasco M, Rosas J, Bove A, Claver G, et al. Cutaneous vasculitis in primary Sjogren syndrome: classification and clinical significance of 52 patients. Medicine (Baltimore) 2004;83(2):96–106.
30. Foster EN, Nguyen KK, Sheikh RA, Prindiville TP. Crohn's disease associated with Sweet's syndrome and Sjogren's syndrome treated with infliximab. Clin Dev Immunol. 2005;12(2):145–9.
31. Pirildar T, Tikiz C, Ozkaya S, Tarhan S, Utuk O, Tikiz H, et al. Endothelial dysfunction in patients with primary Sjogren's syndrome. Rheumatol Int. 2005;25(7):536–9.
32. Manoussakis MN, Georgopoulou C, Zintzaras E, Spyropoulou M, Stavropoulou A, Skopouli FN, et al. Sjogren's syndrome associated with systemic lupus erythematosus: clinical and laboratory profiles and comparison with primary Sjogren's syndrome. Arthritis Rheum. 2004;50(3): 882–91.
33. Tektonidou M, Kaskani E, Skopouli FN, Moutsopoulos HM. Microvascular abnormalities in Sjogren's syndrome: nailfold capillaroscopy. Rheumatology (Oxford) 1999;38(9):826–30.
34. Franceschini F, Calzavara-Pinton P, Quinzanini M, Cavazzana I, Bettoni L, Zane C, et al. Chilblain lupus erythematosus is associated with antibodies to SSA/Ro. Lupus 1999;8(3):215.
35. Millard LG, Rowell NR. Chilblain lupus erythematosus (Hutchinson): a clinical and laboratory study of 17 patients. Br J Dermatol. 1978;98(5):497–506.
36. Rustin MHA, Newton JA, Smith NP, Dowd PM. The treatment of chilblains with nifedipine: the results of a pilot study, a double-blind placebo-controlled randomized study and a long-term open trial. Br J Dermatol. 1989;120(2):267–275.
37. Gyulai R, Kiss M, Mehravaran M, Kovacs L, Pokorny G, Husz S, et al. Atypical autoimmune blistering dermatosis associated with Sjogren's syndrome. Acta Derm Venereol. 2002;82(6): 462–4.

38. Ruzicka T, Faes J, Bergner T, Peter RU, Braun-Falco O. Annular erythema associated with Sjogren's syndrome: a variant of systemic lupus erythematosus. J Am Acad Dermatol. 1991;25(3):557–60.
39. Mori K, Iijima M, Koike H, Hattori N, Tanaka F, Watanabe H, et al. The wide spectrum of clinical manifestations in Sjogren's syndrome-associated neuropathy. Brain 2005;128(Pt 11):2518–34.
40. Watanabe T, Tsuchida T, Furue M, Yoshinoya S. Annular erythema, dermatomyositis, and Sjogren's syndrome. Int J Dermatol. 1996;35(4):285–7.
41. Watanabe T, Tsuchida T, Ito Y, Kanda N, Ueda Y, Tamaki K. Annular erythema associated with lupus erythematosus/Sjogren's syndrome. J Am Acad Dermatol. 1997;36(2 Pt 1):214–8.
42. Katayama Y, Kohriyama K. Telomerase activity in peripheral blood mononuclear cells of systemic connective tissue diseases. J Rheumatol. 2001;28(2):288–91.
43. Katayama I, Yamamoto T, Otoyama K, Matsunaga T, Nishioka K. Clinical and immunological analysis of annular erythema associated with Sjogren syndrome. Dermatology. 1994;189 (Suppl 1): 14–7.
44. Miyagawa S, Iida T, Fukumoto T, Matsunaga T, Yoshioka A, Shirai T. Anti-Ro/SSA-associated annular erythema in childhood. Br J Dermatol. 1995;133(5):779–82.
45. Haimowitz JE, McCauliffe DP, Seykora J, Werth VP. Annular erythema of Sjogren's syndrome in a white woman. J Am Acad Dermatol. 2000;42(6):1069–72.
46. Atzeni F, Sarzi-Puttini P, Lama N, Bonacci E, Bobbio-Pallavicini F, Montecucco C, et al. Anti-cyclic citrullinated peptide antibodies in primary Sjogren syndrome may be associated with non-erosive synovitis. Arthritis Res Ther. 2008;10(3):R51.
47. Buchanan WW. Systemic disorders with rheumatic manifestations. Current Opin Rheumatol. 1992;4(1):57.
48. M'Rad S, Ben Miled K, Makni S, Kchir M, Ennafaa M, Harmel A, et al. Jaccoud's arthropathy in primary Sjögren's syndrome with benign hypergammaglobulinaemic purpura. Eur J Med. 1993;2(6):373–375.
49. Punzi L, Ramonda R, Sfriso P. Erosive osteoarthritis. Best Pract Res Clin Rheumatol. 2004;18(5):739–758.
50. Shuckett R, Russell ML, Gladman DD. Atypical erosive osteoarthritis and Sjogren's syndrome. Br Med J. 1986;45(4):281–288.
51. Sankar V, Brennan MT, Kok MR, Leakan RA, Smith JA, Manny J, et al. Etanercept in Sjogren's syndrome: a twelve-week randomized, double-blind, placebo-controlled pilot clinical trial. Arthritis Rheum. 2004;50(7):2240–5.
52. D'Arbonneau F, Ansart S, Le Berre R, Dueymes M, Youinou P, Pennec YL. Thyroid dysfunction in primary Sjogren's syndrome: a long-term follow up study. Arthritis Rheum. 2003;49(6):804–9.
53. Perez B, Kraus A, Lopez G, Cifuentes M, Alarcon-Segovia D. Autoimmune thyroid disease in primary Sjogren's syndrome. Am J Med. 1995;99(5):480–4.
54. Tektonidou MG, Anapliotou M, Vlachoyiannopoulos P, Moutsopoulos HM. Presence of systemic autoimmune disorders in patients with autoimmune thyroid diseases. Ann Rheum Dis. 2004;63(9):1159–61.
55. Nishimori I, Okazaki K, Yamamoto Y, Morita M, Tamura S, Yamamoto Y. Specific cellular immune responses to pancreatic antigen in chronic pancreatitis and Sjögren's syndrome. J Clin Immunol. 1993;13(4):265–271.
56. Johnson EO, Vlachoyiannopoulos PG, Skopouli FN, Tzioufas AG, Moutsopoulos HM. Hypofunction of the stress axis in Sjogren's syndrome. J Rheumatol. 1998;25(8):1508–14.
57. Jara LJ, Navarro C, Brito-Zeron Mdel P, Garcia-Carrasco M, Escarcega RO, Ramos-Casals M. Thyroid disease in Sjogren's syndrome. Clin Rheumatol. 2007;26(10):1601–6.
58. Lazarus MN, Isenberg DA. Development of additional autoimmune diseases in a population of patients with primary Sjogren's syndrome. Ann Rheum Dis. 2005;64(7):1062–4.
59. Caron P, Lassoued S, Dromer C, Oksman F, Fournie A. Prevalence of thyroid abnormalities in patients with rheumatoid arthritis. Thyroidol Clin Exp. 1992;4(3):99–102.
60. Johnson EO, Skopouli FN, Moutsopoulos HM. Neuroendocrine manifestations in Sjogren's syndrome [in process citation]. Rheum Dis Clin North Am. 2000;26(4):927–49.
61. Yocum DE. Glucocorticosteroids in rheumatoid arthritis: lessons for the future. Br J Rheumatol. 1998;37(11):1145–7.
62. Arroyo RA, Ridley DJ, Brey RL, et al. Anticardiolipin antibodies in patients with primary Sjögren's syndrome. Arthritis Rheum. 1989;32:S73 (Abstr).
63. Ali SR, Johnson FB, Luke JL, Kalasinsky VF. Characterization of silicone breast implant biopsies by Fourier transform infrared mapping. Cell Mol Biol (Noisy-le-grand). 1998;44(1):75–80.
64. Torpy DJ, Papanicolaou DA, Lotsikas AJ, Wilder RL, Chrousos GP, Pillemer SR. Responses of the sympathetic nervous system and the hypothalamic–pituitary–adrenal axis to interleukin-6: a pilot study in fibromyalgia. Arthritis Rheum. 2000;43(4):872–80.
65. Winqvist O, Karlsson FA, Kampe O. 21-Hydroxylase, a major autoantigen in idiopathic Addison's disease. Lancet 1992;339(8809): 1559–62.
66. Deheinzelin D, de Carvalho CR, Tomazini ME, Barbas FJV, Saldiva PH. Association of Sjogren's syndrome and sarcoidosis. Report of a case. Sarcoidosis 1988;5(1):68–70.

67. Seinfeld ED, Sharma OP. TASS syndrome: unusual association of thyroiditis, Addison's disease, Sjögren's syndrome and sarcoidosis. J R Soc Med. 1983;76(10):883.
68. Valtysdottir ST, Wide L, Hallgren R. Low serum dehydroepiandrosterone sulfate in women with primary Sjogren's syndrome as an isolated sign of impaired HPA axis function. J Rheumatol. 2001;28(6):1259–65.
69. Schadlich PK, Zeidler H, Zink A, Gromnica-Ihle E, Schneider M, Straub C, et al. Modelling cost effectiveness and cost utility of sequential DMARD therapy including leflunomide for rheumatoid arthritis in Germany: II. The contribution of leflunomide to efficiency. Pharmacoeconomics 2005;23(4):395–420.
70. Laine M, Porola P, Udby L, Kjeldsen L, Cowland JB, Borregaard N, et al. Low salivary dehydroepiandrosterone and androgen-regulated cysteine-rich secretory protein 3 levels in Sjogren's syndrome. Arthritis Rheum. 2007;56(8):2575–84.
71. Pillemer SR, Brennan MT, Sankar V, Leakan RA, Smith JA, Grisius M, et al. Pilot clinical trial of dehydroepiandrosterone (DHEA) versus placebo for Sjogren's syndrome. Arthritis Rheum. 2004;51(4):601–4.
72. Drosos A, Andonopoulos A, Costopoulos J, Papadimitriou C, Moutsopoulos HM. Prevalence of primary Sjögren's syndrome in an elderly population. Br. J. Rheumatol. 1988;27:123–127.
73. Petri MA, Lahita RG, van Vollenhoven RF, Merrill J, Schiff M, Ginzler EM, et al. Effects of prasterone on corticosteroid requirements of women with systemic lupus erythematosus. Arthritis Rheum. 2002;46(7):1820–1829.
74. Van Vollenhoven RF. Dehydroepiandrosterone in systemic lupus erythematosus. Rheum Dis Clin North Am. 2000;26(2):349–362.
75. Nippoldt TB, Nair KS. Is there a case for DHEA replacement? Baillière's Clin Endocrinol Metabol. 1998;12(3):507–520.
76. Johansson AC, Nakken B, Sundler M, Lindqvist AK, Johannesson M, Alarcon-Riquelme M, et al. The genetic control of sialadenitis versus arthritis in a NOD.Q×B10.Q F2 cross. Eur J Immunol. 2002;32(1):243–50.
77. Quismorio FP, Jr. Pulmonary involvement in primary Sjogren's syndrome. Curr Opin Pulm Med. 1996;2(5):424–8.
78. Battista G, Zompatori M, Poletti V, Canini R. Thoracic manifestations of the less common collagen diseases. A pictorial essay. Radiol Med (Torino). 2003;106(5–6):445–51; quiz 452–3.
79. Constantopoulos SH, Tsianos EV, Moutsopoulos HM. Pulmonary and gastrointestinal manifestations of Sjogren's syndrome. Rheum Dis Clin North Am. 1992;18(3):617–35.
80. Isaacson PG. Extranodal lymphomas: the MALT concept. Verh Dtsch Ges Pathol. 1992;76:14–23.
81. Spencer J, Wotherspoon AC. Gastric MALT lymphoma and *Helicobacter pylori*. Cancer Surv. 1997;30:213–31.
82. Nishimura M, Miyajima S, Okada N. Salivary gland MALT lymphoma associated with *Helicobacter pylori* infection in a patient with Sjogren's syndrome [in process citation]. J Dermatol. 2000;27(7):450–2.
83. Kim EA, Lee KS, Johkoh T, Kim TS, Suh GY, Kwon OJ, et al. Interstitial lung diseases associated with collagen vascular diseases: radiologic and histopathologic findings. Radiographics 2002;22 Spec No:S151–65.
84. Chatterjee S. Severe interstitial pneumonitis associated with infliximab therapy. Scand J Rheumatol. 2004;33(4):276–7.
85. Swords R, Power D, Fay M, O'Donnell R, Murphy PT. Interstitial pneumonitis following rituximab therapy for immune thrombocytopenic purpura (ITP). Am J Hematol. 2004;77(1):103–4.
86. Fischer A, Pfalzgraf FJ, Feghali-Bostwick CA, Wright TM, Curran-Everett D, West SG, et al. Anti-Th/To-positivity in a cohort of patients with idiopathic pulmonary fibrosis. J Rheumatol. 2006;33(8):1600–5.
87. Kim DS, Collard HR, King Jr TE. Classification and natural history of the idiopathic interstitial pneumonias. Am Thoracic Soc 2006;285.
88. Tashkin DP, Elashoff R, Clements PJ, Goldin J, Roth MD, Furst DE, et al. Cyclophosphamide versus placebo in scleroderma lung disease. N Engl J Med. 2006;354(25):2655.
89. Liossis SN, Solomou EE, Sikakis PP. Lyn deficiency in B cells from patients with systemic lupus erythematosus: comment on the article by Flores-Borja et al. Arthritis Rheum. 2006;54(6):2036–2037.
90. Magro CM, Ross P, Marsh CB, Allen JN, Liff D, Knight DA, et al. The role of anti-endothelial cell antibody-mediated microvascular injury in the evolution of pulmonary fibrosis in the setting of collagen vascular disease. Am J Clin Pathol. 2007;127(2):237–47.
91. Lee JC, Kumar S, Griswold DE, Underwood DC, Votta BJ, Adams JL. Inhibition of p38 MAP kinase as a therapeutic strategy. Immunopharmacology 2000;47(2–3):185–201.
92. Papiris SA, Kalomenidis I, Malagari K, Kapotsis GE, Harhalakis N, Manali ED, et al. Extranodal marginal zone B-cell lymphoma of the lung in Sjogren's syndrome patients: reappraisal of clinical, radiological, and pathology findings. Respir Med. 2007;101(1):84–92.
93. Cho CS, Cho ML, Chen PP, Min SY, Hwang SY, Park KS, et al. Antiphospholipid antibodies induce monocyte chemoattractant protein-1 in endothelial cells. J Immunol. 2002;168(8):4209–15.
94. Gyongyosi M, Pokorny G, Jambrik Z, Kovacs L, Kovacs A, Makula E, et al. Cardiac manifestations

in primary Sjogren's syndrome. Ann Rheum Dis. 1996;55(7):450–4.
95. Kelly CA, Foster H, Pal B, Gardiner P, Malcolm AJ, Charles P, et al. Primary Sjogren's syndrome in north east England—a longitudinal study. Rheumatology 1991;30(6):437–442.
96. {Akpek E-B, 1979 #9; French, 2003 #8; Graves, 2003 #10; Jacobs, 1988 #11; Khurrum Baig, 2004 #2; Kiang, 1998 #5; Perry, 1997 #6; Pucci, 2002 #4; Smith, 1981 #12; Tang-Liu, 2005 #1; Temprano, 2005 #7}. The American College of Rheumatology response criteria for proliferative and membranous renal disease in systemic lupus erythematosus clinical trials. Arthritis Rheum. 2006;54(2):421–32.
97. Suarez GA, Opfer-Gehrking TL, Offord KP, Atkinson EJ, O'Brien PC, Low PA. The autonomic symptom profile: a new instrument to assess autonomic symptoms. Neurology 1999;52(3):523.
98. Andonopoulos AP, Christodoulou J, Ballas C, Bounas A, Alexopoulos D. Autonomic cardiovascular neuropathy in Sjogren's syndrome. A controlled study. J Rheumatol. 1998;25(12):2385–8.
99. Mandl T, Granberg V, Apelqvist J, Wollmer P, Manthorpe R, Jacobsson LTH. Autonomic nervous symptoms in primary Sjogren's syndrome. Rheumatology 2008;47(6):914.
100. Stojanovich L, Milovanovich B, de Luka SR, Popovich-Kuzmanovich D, Bisenich V, Djukanovich B, et al. Cardiovascular autonomic dysfunction in systemic lupus, rheumatoid arthritis, primary Sjogren syndrome and other autoimmune diseases. Lupus 2007;16(3):181–5.
101. Mellgren SI, Goransson LG, Omdal R. Primary Sjogren's syndrome associated neuropathy. Can J Neurol Sci. 2007;34(3):280–7.
102. Mandl T, Ekberg O, Wollmer P, Manthorpe R, Jacobsson LT. Dysphagia and dysmotility of the pharynx and oesophagus in patients with primary Sjogren's syndrome. Scand J Rheumatol. 2007;36(5):394–401.
103. Shalimar, Handa R, Deepak KK, Bhatia M, Aggarwal P, Pandey RM. Autonomic dysfunction in systemic lupus erythematosus. Rheumatol Int. 2006;26(9):837–40.
104. Akinci A, Çeliker A, Baykal E, Teziç T. Heart rate variability in diabetic children: sensitivity of the time-and frequency-domain methods. Pediatr Cardiol. 1993;14(3):140–146.
105. Evrengül H, Dursunoglu D, Cobankara V, Polat B, Seleci D, Kabukcu S, et al. Heart rate variability in patients with rheumatoid arthritis. Rheumatol Int. 2004;24(4):198–202.
106. Tumiati B, Perazzoli F, Negro A, Pantaleoni M, Regolisti G. Heart rate variability in patients with Sjogren's syndrome. Clin Rheumatol. 2000;19(6):477–80.
107. Wright RA, Grant IA, Low PA. Autonomic neuropathy associated with sicca complex. J Auton Nerv Syst. 1999;75(1):70–76.
108. Kovacs L, Marczinovits I, Gyorgy A, Toth GK, Dorgai L, Pal J, et al. Clinical associations of autoantibodies to human muscarinic acetylcholine receptor 3213-228 in primary Sjogren's syndrome. Rheumatology (Oxford) 2005;44(8):1021–5.
109. Gordon TP, Bolstad AI, Rischmueller M, Jonsson R, Waterman SA. Autoantibodies in primary Sjogren's syndrome: new insights into mechanisms of autoantibody diversification and disease pathogenesis. Autoimmunity 2001;34(2):123–32.
110. Borda E, Sterin-Borda L. Autoantibodies against neonatal heart M1 muscarinic acetylcholine receptor in children with congenital heart block. J Autoimmun. 2001;16(2):143–50.
111. Waterman SA, Gordon TP, Rischmueller M. Inhibitory effects of muscarinic receptor autoantibodies on parasympathetic neurotransmission in Sjogren's syndrome. Arthritis Rheum. 2000;43(7):1647–54.
112. Escobar MC, Gomez-Puerta JA, Albert D, Ferrer Q, Girona J. Recurrent congenital heart block in neonatal lupus. Clin Rheumatol. 2007;26:1161–3.
113. Ruffatti A, Favaro M, Cozzi F, Tonello M, Grava C, Lazzarin P, et al. Anti-SSA/Ro-related congenital heart block in two family members of different generations: comment on the article by Clancy et al. Arthritis Rheum. 2005;52(5):1623–5; author reply 1625–6.
114. Haga HJ, Gjesdal CG, Koksvik HS, Skomsvoll JF, Irgens LM, Ostensen M. Pregnancy outcome in patients with primary Sjogren's syndrome. A case–control study. J Rheumatol. 2005;32(9):1734–1736.
115. Eronen M, Heikkila P, Teramo K. Congenital complete heart block in the fetus: hemodynamic features, antenatal treatment, and outcome in six cases. Pediatr Cardiol. 2001;22(5):385–92.
116. Yamada H, Kato EH, Ebina Y, Moriwaki M, Yamamoto R, Furuta I, et al. Fetal treatment of congenital heart block ascribed to anti-SSA antibody: case reports with observation of cardiohemodynamics and review of the literature. Am J Reprod Immunol. 1999;42(4):226–32.
117. Borda E, Leiros CP, Bacman S, Berra A, Sterin-Borda L. Sjogren autoantibodies modify neonatal cardiac function via M1 muscarinic acetylcholine receptor activation. Int J Cardiol. 1999;70(1): 23–32.
118. Obbiassi M, Brucato A, Meroni PL, Vismara A, Lettino M, Poloni F, et al. Antibodies to cardiac Purkinje cells: further characterization in autoimmune diseases and atrioventricular heart block. Clin Immunol Immunopathol. 1987;42(2): 141–50.
119. Ryberg AT, Warfvinge G, Axelsson L, Soukup O, Gotrick B, Tobin G. Expression of muscarinic receptor subtypes in salivary glands of rats, sheep and man. Arch Oral Biol. 2008;53(1):66–74.
120. Asanuma Y, Chung CP, Oeser A, Shintani A, Stanley E, Raggi P, et al. Increased concentration of proatherogenic inflammatory cytokines in systemic

lupus erythematosus: relationship to cardiovascular risk factors. J Rheumatol. 2006;33(3):539–45.
121. Sander GE, Giles TD. Cardiovascular complications of collagen vascular disease. Curr Treat Options Cardiovasc Med. 2002;4(2):151–159.
122. Petri M. Long-term outcomes in lupus. Am J Manag Care. 2001;7(16 Suppl):S480–5.
123. Shoenfeld Y, Gerli R, Doria A, Matsuura E, Cerinic MM, Ronda N, Jara LJ, Abu-Shakra M, Meroni PL, Sherer Y. 2005. Accelerated atherosclerosis in autoimmune rheumatic diseases. *Circulation* 112:3337.
124. Kurien BT, Newland J, Paczkowski C, Moore KL, Scofield RH. Association of neutropenia in systemic lupus erythematosus (SLE) with anti-Ro and binding of an immunologically cross-reactive neutrophil membrane antigen. Clin Exp Immunol. 2000;120(1):209–17.
125. D'Cruz DP, Khamashta MA, Hughes GR. Systemic lupus erythematosus. Lancet 2007;369(9561):587–96.
126. Belafsky PC, Postma GN. The laryngeal and esophageal manifestations of Sjogren's syndrome. Curr Rheumatol Rep. 2003;5(4):297–303.
127. Rosztoczy A, Kovacs L, Wittmann T, Lonovics J, Pokorny G. Manometric assessment of impaired esophageal motor function in primary Sjogren's syndrome. Clin Exp Rheumatol. 2001;19(2):147–52.
128. Sheikh SH, Shaw-Stiffel TA. The gastrointestinal manifestations of Sjogren's syndrome. Am J Gastroenterol. 1995;90(1):9–14.
129. Fox RA, Scheuer PJ, Sherlock S. Asymptomatic primary biliary cirrhosis. Br Med J. 1973;14(6):444–7.
130. Fujikura S, Davis PA, Prindiville T, Leung P, Fox RI, Gershwin ME. Autoantibodies to purified mitochondrial 2 OXO acid dehydrogenases in patients with Sjögren's syndrome. J. Rheum. 1990;17:1453–7.
131. Inoue K, Hirohara J, Nakano T, Seki T, Sasaki H, Higuchi K, et al. Prediction of prognosis of primary biliary cirrhosis in Japan. Liver 1995;15(2):70–7.
132. Kaplan MM. Primary biliary cirrhosis. N Engl J Med. 1996;335(21):1570–80.
133. Tsianos EV, Hoofnagle JH, Fox PC, Alspaugh M, et al. Sjögren's syndrome in patients with primary biliary cirrhosis. Hepatology 1990;11:730–4.
134. Kogawa H, Migita K, Ito M, Takii Y, Daikoku M, Nakao M, Miyashita T, Kimura H, Ezaki H, Nakamura M. Idiopathic portal hypertension associated with systemic sclerosis and Sjogren's syndrome. Clin Rheumatol. 2005;24:544–7.
135. Fujikura S, Davis PA, Prindiville T, Leung P, Fox RI, Gershwin ME. Sjogren's syndrome and primary biliary cirrhosis: presence of autoantibodies to purified mitochondrial 2-oxo acid dehydrogenases. J Rheumatol. 1990;17(11):1453–7.
136. Katayama Y, Kohriyama K, Kirizuka K, Nishizaki H, Fujii H, Tanji Y. Sjogren's syndrome complicated with autoimmune hepatitis and antiphospholipid antibody syndrome [see comments]. Intern Med. 2000;39(1):73–6.
137. Al-Khalidi JA, Czaja AJ. Current concepts in the diagnosis, pathogenesis, and treatment of autoimmune hepatitis. Mayo Clin Proc. 2001;76(12):1237–52.
138. Ben-Ari Z, Czaja AJ. Autoimmune hepatitis and its variant syndromes. Gut. 2001;49(4):589–94.
139. Chan K. Some aspects of toxic contaminants in herbal medicines. Chemosphere. 2003;52(9):1361–71.
140. Ernst E. Toxic heavy metals and undeclared drugs in Asian herbal medicines. Trends Pharmacol Sci. 2002;23(3):136–9.
141. Iltanen S, Collin P, Korpela M, Holm K, Partanen J, Polvi A, et al. Celiac disease and markers of celiac disease latency in patients with primary Sjögren's syndrome. Am J Gastroenterol. 1999;94(4):1042–6.
142. Lee SK, Green PHR. Celiac sprue (the great modern-day imposter). Curr Opin Rheumatol. 2006;18(1):101.
143. Liden M, Kristjansson G, Valtysdottir S, Hallgren R. Gluten sensitivity in patients with primary Sjogren's syndrome. Scand J Gastroenterol. 2007;42(8):962–7.
144. Pearson RK, Longnecker DS, Chari ST, Smyrk TC, Okazaki K, Frulloni L, et al. Controversies in clinical pancreatology: autoimmune pancreatitis: does it exist? Pancreas 2003;27(1):1.
145. Hamano H, Kawa S, Horiuchi A, Unno H, Furuya N, Akamatsu T, Fukushima M, Nikaido T, Nakayama K, Usuda N. High serum IgG4 concentrations in patients with sclerosing pancreatitis. N Engl J Med In: 2001;344:732–8.
146. Nishimori I, Yamamoto Y, Okazaki K, Morita M, Onodera M, Kino J, et al. Identification of autoantibodies to a pancreatic antigen in patients with idiopathic chronic pancreatitis and Sjogren's syndrome. Pancreas 1994;9(3):374.
147. Coll J, Navarro S, Tomas R, Elena M, Martinez E. Exocrine pancreatic function in Sjogren's syndrome. Arch Intern Med. 1989;149(4):848.
148. Gamron S, Barberis G, Onetti CM, Strusberg I, Hliba E, Martellotto G, et al. Mesangial nephropathy in Sjogren's syndrome. Scand J Rheumatol. 2000;29(1):65–7.
149. Siamopoulos KC, Elisaf M, Moutsopoulos HM. Hypokalaemic paralysis as the presenting manifestation of primary Sjogren's syndrome. Nephrol Dial Transplant. 1994;9(8):1176–8.
150. Fulop M, Mackay M. Renal tubular acidosis, Sjogren syndrome, and bone disease. Arch Intern Med. 2004;164(8):905–9.
151. Nishimagi E, Kawaguchi Y, Terai C, Kajiyama H, Hara M, Kamatani N. Progressive interstitial renal fibrosis due to Chinese herbs in a patient with calcinosis Raynaud esophageal sclerodactyly telangiectasia (CREST) syndrome. Intern Med. 2001;40(10):1059–63.

152. Dabadghao S, Aggarwal A, Arora P, Pandey R, Misra R. Glomerulonephritis leading to end stage renal disease in a patient with primary Sjogren syndrome. Clin Exp Rheumatol. 1995;13(4): 509–11.
153. Sugai S. Interstitial cystitis and Sjogren's syndrome. Intern Med. 2004;43(3):174–6.
154. Shibata S, Ubara Y, Sawa N, Tagami T, Hosino J, Yokota M, et al. Severe interstitial cystitis associated with Sjogren's syndrome. Intern Med. 2004;43(3):248–52.
155. van de Merwe JP, Yamada T, Sakamoto Y. Systemic aspects of interstitial cystitis, immunology and linkage with autoimmune disorders. Int J Urol. 2003;10 Suppl:S35–8.
156. Leppilahti M, Tammela TL, Huhtala H, Kiilholma P, Leppilahti K, Auvinen A. Interstitial cystitis-like urinary symptoms among patients with Sjogren's syndrome: a population-based study in Finland. Am J Med. 2003;115(1):62–5.
157. Beroukas D, Hiscock J, Jonsson R, Waterman SA, Gordon TP. Subcellular distribution of aquaporin 5 in salivary glands in primary Sjogren's syndrome. Lancet 2001;358(9296):1875–6.
158. van de Merwe JP. Interstitial cystitis and systemic autoimmune diseases. Nat Clin Pract Urol. 2007;4(9):484–91.
159. Klepfish A, Friedman J, Schechter Y, Schattner A. Autoimmune neutropenia, thrombocytopenia and Coombs positivity in a patient with primary Sjogren's syndrome. Rheumatology (Oxford) 2001;40(8):948–9.
160. Ramos-Casals M, Solans R, Rosas J, Camps MT, Gil A, Del Pino-Montes J, et al. Primary Sjogren syndrome in Spain: clinical and immunologic expression in 1010 patients. Medicine (Baltimore) 2008;87(4):210–9.
161. Seror R, Sordet C, Guillevin L, Hachulla E, Masson C, Ittah M, Candon S, Le Guern V, Aouba A, Sibilia J. Tolerance and efficacy of rituximab and changes in serum B cell biomarkers in patients with systemic complications of primary Sjogren's syndrome. Ann Rheum Dis. 2007;66:351–7.
162. Bourgeois E, Caulier MT, Rose C, Dupriez B, Bauters F, Fenaux P. Role of splenectomy in the treatment of myelodysplastic syndromes with peripheral thrombocytopenia: a report on six cases. Leukemia 2001;15(6):950–3.
163. Assimakopoulos SF, Michalopoulou S, Melachrinou M, Giannakoulas N, Papakonstantinou C, Lekkou A, et al. Primary Sjogren syndrome complicated by autoimmune hemolytic anemia and pure red cell aplasia. Am J Med Sci. 2007;334(6): 493–6.
164. Coppo P, Sibilia J, Maloisel F, Schlageter MH, Voyer AL, Gouilleux-Gruart V, et al. Primary Sjogren's syndrome associated agranulocytosis: a benign disorder? Ann Rheum Dis. 2003;62(5): 476–8.
165. Mulherin DM, Sheeran TP, Kumararatne DS, Speculand B, Luesley D, Situnayake RD. Sjogren's syndrome in women presenting with chronic dyspareunia. Br J Obstet Gynaecol. 1997;104(9): 1019–23.
166. Tayal SC, Watson PG. Dyspareunia in undiagnosed Sjogren's syndrome. Br J Clin Pract. 1996;50(1):57–8.
167. Graziottin A. Clinical approach to dyspareunia. J Sex Marital Ther. 2001;27(5):489–501.
168. Skopouli FN, Papanikolaou S, Malamou-Mitsi V, Papanikolaou N, Moutsopoulos HM. Obstetric and gynaecological profile in patients with primary Sjogren's syndrome. Ann Rheum Dis. 1994;53(9):569–73.
169. Infante-Rivard C, David M, Gauthier R, Rivard GE. Lupus anticoagulants, anticardiolipin antibodies, and fetal loss. A case–control study. N Engl J Med 1991;325:1063–1066.
170. Buyon JP, Clancy RM. Neonatal lupus syndromes. Curr Opin Rheumatol. 2003;15(5):535.
171. Chan EK, Di Donato F, Hamel JC, Tseng CE, Buyon JP. 52-kD SS-A/Ro: genomic structure and identification of an alternatively spliced transcript encoding a novel leucine zipper-minus autoantigen expressed in fetal and adult heart. J Exp Med. 1995;182(4):983–92.
172. Buyon JP, Petri MA, Kim MY, Kalunian KC, Grossman J, Hahn BH, et al. The effect of combined estrogen and progesterone hormone replacement therapy on disease activity in systemic lupus erythematosus: a randomized trial. Ann Intern Med. 2005;142(12 Part 1):953–962.
173. Buyon JP, Kalunian KC, Skovron ML, Petri M, Lahita R, Merrill J, et al. Can women with systemic lupus erythematosus safely use exogenous estrogens? JCR 1995;1(4):205.
174. McGee DC, Rnc MSN, Pnnp R. Steroid use during pregnancy. J Perinat Neonatal Nurs. 2002;16(2): 26.
175. Tam LS, Li EK, Wong CK, Lam CW, Szeto CC. Double-blind, randomized, placebo-controlled pilot study of leflunomide in systemic lupus erythematosus. Lupus 2004;13(8):601–4.
176. Petry KU, Köchel H, Bode U, Schedel I, Niesert S, Glaubitz M, et al. Human papillomavirus is associated with the frequent detection of warty and basaloid high-grade neoplasia of the vulva and cervical neoplasia among immunocompromised women. Gynecol Oncol. 1996;60(1):30–4.
177. Romagnoli M, Nannini C, Piciucchi S, Girelli F, Gurioli C, Casoni G, Ravaglia C, Tomassetti S, Gavelli G, Carloni A. Idiopathic NSIP: an interstitial lung disease associated with autoimmune disorders? Eur Respir J. 2011;325.
178. Kim JY, Park SH, Kim SK, Hyun DS, Kum YS, Jung KJ, Choe JY. Lymphocytic interstitial pneumonia in primary sjögren's syndrome: a case report. J Intern Med. 2011;26:108–11.

179. Henriet A, Diot E, Marchand-Adam S, de Muret A, Favelle O, Crestani B, Diot P. Organising pneumonia can be the inaugural manifestation in connective tissue diseases, including Sjögren's syndrome. Eur Respir Rev. 2010;19:161.
180. Leung CC, Feller-Kopman D, Niederman MS, Spiro SG. Year in review 2010: tuberculosis, pleural diseases, respiratory infections. Respirology 2011;16:564–73.
181. Dokwal C. Pulmonary manifestations of collagen vascular disease. Pulse 2011;4:16–21.
182. Pandey S. Acute neuromuscular respiratory failure. Arch Neurol. 2011;68:398.
183. Julian M, Chakravorty T, Dyer P. Primary Sjögren's disease and its complications presenting with progressive paralysis. BMJ Case Rep. 2011;10: 1136–1138.
184. Kitaba S, Matsui S, Iimuro E, Nishioka M, Kijima A, Umegaki N, Murota H, Katayama I. Four cases of atopic dermatitis complicated by Sjögren's syndrome: link between dry skin and autoimmune anhidrosis. Allergol Int Official J Jpn Soc Allergol. 2011.
185. Haga HJ, Terp Andersen D, Peen E. Prevalence of IgA class antibodies to cyclic citrullinated peptide (anti-CCP) in patients with primary Sjögren's syndrome, and its association to clinical manifestations. Clin Rheumatol. 30(3):369–72.
186. Feng S, Jin P, Shao C. The significance of anticardiolipin antibody and immunologic abnormality in livedoid vasculitis. Int J Dermatol. 2011;50:21–3.
187. Baraniuk JN. Subjective nasal fullness and objective congestion Proc Am Thorac Soc. 2011;8(1): 62–9.

18 Therapy of Dermatologic, Renal, Cardiovascular, Pulmonary, Gynecologic, Gastro-enterologic, Urologic and Fibromyalgia Manifestations Including Special Considerations at the Time of Surgery

Robert I. Fox and Carla M. Fox

Abstract

Therapy of Sjögren's syndrome (SS) patients requires attention to different clinical manifestations. These include treatment of

1. *Dry eyes and mouth* (glandular manifestations);
2. *Dermatologic manifestations* including dryness of other mucous membranes, including vaginal dryness;
3. *Non-visceral manifestation* of arthralgia/arthritis and myalgia/myositis;
4. *Visceral manifestations* that include immune complex-like deposition tissue injuries and "lupus-like" signs/symptoms that may affect lung, heart, abdomen, urologic, kidney, and neurologic systems;
5. *Visceral manifestations that reflect the lymphocytic infiltrative processes* in SS that reflect the "aggressive" lymphocyte, such as interstitial pneumonitis, autoimmune hepatitis, interstitial nephritis, lymphadenopathy, and lymphoma;
6. *Vague symptoms of fatigue*, which have been termed fibromyalgia or chronic fatigue syndrome and which greatly influence the patient's quality of life;
7. *Increased risk of atherosclerosis and thrombotic disease*, where late cardiovascular complications exceed the risk expected for elevations of standard risk factors such as lipid profiles and hypertension;
8. This chapter will also review the particular *needs of the SS patient at the time of surgery* (with attention to avoiding complications due to dry eyes/mouth and poor dentition) *and the current recommendations regarding vaccinations*.

R.I. Fox (✉)
Rheumatology Clinic, Scripps Memorial Hospital
and Research Foundation, La Jolla, CA, USA
e-mail: robertfoxmd@mac.com

R.I. Fox, C.M. Fox (eds.), *Sjögren's Syndrome*, DOI 10.1007/978-1-60327-957-4_18,

Keywords
Sjögren's syndrome (SS) (primary SS [1°SS], Secondary SS [2° SS]) • Arthralgia • Myalgia • Raynaud's phenomenon • Oral candidiasis • Dysphagia • Gastroesophageal reflux disease (GERD) • Lymphadenopathy • BK/JC virus/multifocal leukoencephalopathy • Vasculitis skin lesions • Pneumonitis • Neuropathy • Nephritis • Monoclonal antibody • Human anti-chimeric antibodies (HACAs) • Estrogen replacement therapy • Non-specific Interstitial pneumonitis (NSIP) • Erythrocyte sedimentation rate (ESR) • Herpes "shingles" vaccine • Sicca symptoms • Lymphoma • Tumor necrosis factor inhibitor

18.1 Introduction

Primary Sjögren's syndrome (SS) usually has a benign course centered on sicca features and general musculoskeletal features that are managed symptomatically [1]. However, a subset of SS patients develops more severe extraglandular disease that warrants close monitoring and aggressive treatment [2, 3]. Although the extraglandular manifestations often show a similarity to systemic lupus erythematosus (SLE), there are important differences between the types of clinical presentations that may be present in the SS and SLE patient [4]. Both SS and SLE patients exhibit constitutional symptoms (fatigue, arthralgia, myalgia, low-grade temperatures, lymphadenopathy) that are treated in a similar manner using NSAIDs and hydroxychloroquine [5]. SS patients develop skin rashes including leukocytoclastic vasculitis, Raynaud's phenomenon, and hematologic complications, which also receive treatment regimens similar to SLE.

However, it is important to distinguish between the SS and SLE because there are important differences in the treatment of each set of patients [2, 5]. In particular, the issue of lymphoproliferation (including increased risk of lymphoma) and a higher prevalence of lymphocytic infiltrative disease (interstitial nephritis, autoimmune hepatitis, and interstitial pneumonitis) occur in the SS patient as well as a different type of particular skin rashes (hyperglobulinemic purpura and anetoderma) and the risk of lymphoma. Also, the types and incidence and type of neuropathies (peripheral and central), including demyelinating disorders, may differ in the SS and SLE patient. Further, the SS patient may exhibit overlap with other autoimmune disorders including rheumatoid arthritis (RA), scleroderma, polymyositis, polyarteritis nodosa-like vasculitis, and primary biliary cirrhosis, which will require particular therapies.

This chapter will emphasize the "day-to-day" approach that we pursue at our clinic for treatment of common questions in SS patients. A summary of extraglandular manifestations discussed in this chapter is presented in Table 18.1. This chapter will supplement the other contributions in this book on "Traditional Oral Therapies of SS," "Biologic Therapies Including CD20, CD20 and BAFF," and novel "Emerging Therapies: Tyrosine Kinase and Jak Kinases, Gene Therapy and microRNA targets." Also, the specific treatment of neuropathies, fibromyalgia, and ENT manifestations is covered in more detail in additional chapters of this book.

Due to increasing specialization and subspecialization of medicine, SS patients are increasingly turning to the rheumatologist to co-ordinate and manage a vast array of intricate medical issues. Indeed, rheumatologists are finding themselves not only playing the central "quarterback" in the treatment of the SS patient, but also increasingly becoming some patients' *primary care provider*, treating an array of problems associated with very complicated patients.

Further, other specialists (including emergency room physicians or orthopedic surgeons) are unclear what extraglandular manifestations may be the result of SS, as they try to sort through the patient's complaint of chest pain or

Table 18.1 Therapy for systemic features of pSS—general manifestations and main therapeutic modalities

Extraglandular manifestations	Main therapeutic modalities
Cutaneous Dryness Vasculitis SLE and discoid LE-like rashes Overlap with scleroderma Cryoglobulinemia Raynaud's phenomenon Arterial emboli Manifestations of drug use Thrombotic—arterial and venous Acrocyanosis (exacerbated in smokers—Buerger's disease) Arthritis Overlap with RA Osteoarthritis SLE-like subluxations without erosion Erosive osteoarthritis Jaccoud's arthritis	Moisturizers Hydroxychloroquine Steroids (topical and oral) Methotrexate, leflunomide Rituximab Cyclophosphamide Avoidance of cold and stress exposure Avoid sympathomimetic drugs (such as decongestants, amphetamines, diet pills, herbs containing ephedra) Calcium channel blockers Ketanserin, a selective antagonist of the S2-serotonergic receptor, Sildenafil citrate, ilosprost Acetaminophen Non-steroidal agents and disalcid Hydroxychloroquine (6–8 mg/kg/day) Methotrexate (either oral or self-injected) Leflunomide (20 mg/day) Rituximab (dosing similar to RA)
Circulating anti-coagulants and coagulopathies Anti-cardiolipin antibody Lupus anti-coagulant *Factor deficiency* Exacerbating anti-coagulant (Factor VL, protein S, protein C, prothrombin mutation, homocysteine, MTHR mutation)	Aspirin, warfarin (if prior thrombotic episode), or lovenox
Liver Mild non-progressive elevation of liver function tests associated with lymphocytic infiltrates Primary biliary cirrhosis Autoimmune hepatitis Recognition of viral hepatitis including A, B, and C Steatosis Liver toxins including herbal and nutritional supplement	Ursodeoxycholic acid Corticosteroids Azathioprine Mycophenolic acid
Pancreas Sclerosing cholangitis (elevated serum levels of IgG4) Idiopathic (non-alcoholic) pancreatitis Malabsorptive syndromes Macroamylasemia (from salivary glands)	Corticosteroids Ursodeoxycholic acid Watch for strictures Azathioprine Mycophenolic acid Rituximab
Kidney glomerulonephritis including Amyloid, cryoglobulinemia, immune complex (including unrecognized SLE) Interstitial nephritis, renal tubular acidosis with periodic paralysis (low K), metabolic acidosis, renal stones (nephrocalcinosis), glomerulonephritis, renal calculus Obstructive nephropathy	Cyclophosphamide Azathioprine Mycophenolic acid Oral potassium and sodium carbonate (3–12 g/day) Rituximab
Bladder Interstitial cystitis Cystitis due to prior therapy (i.e., cyclophosphamide) Polyuria due to polydipsia	Pentosan polysulfate sodium Recognition of anti-cholinergics exacerbating sicca symptoms

Table 18.1 (continued)

Extraglandular manifestations	Main therapeutic modalities
Upper airway and lung chronic cough Vasomotor rhinitis and postnasal drip Laryngotracheal reflux Hoarseness Voice disorder and larynx irritation	Mucolytics including Guaifenesin (glyceryl guaiacolate) Humidification, room air purifiers Neurontin (low dose) Avoidance of caffeine and alcohol Elevation of head of bed Nasal lavage
Bronchial lymphocytic infiltrative leading to Decrease aqueous and abnormal mucus production	Bactroban nasal ointment
Lung parenchymal infiltrates NSIP, UIP, DIP Bronchial and/or bronchiolar involvement (common, indolent course)	Cyclophosphamide Prednisolone Mycophenolic acid Azathioprine Rituximab
Gastrointestinal atrophic gastritis Celiac sprue Gastroesophageal reflux Motility disorder	Avoidance of gluten Proton pump inhibitors Promotility agents (Motilium, Reglan) Vitamin B_{12}
Accelerated atherosclerosis Similar to early mortality of SLE patients with stroke and heart attack	Control hypertension, lipid levels with "tight" control of blood pressure, diet, weight, smoking, and statins
Vasculitis (cutaneous) Hyperglobulinemic purpura Mixed cryoglobulinemia Mononeuritis multiplex	Prednisolone (0.5–1.0 mg/kg body weight per day) Cyclophosphamide (0.5–1 g/m^2 of body surface/month) Rituximab Plasmapheresis
Endocrine Thyroid—hypo and hyper including recognition of exophthalmia causing failure of lid closure (exposure keratitis)	Thyroid replacement Treatment of Grave's myxedema Corticosteroids Mineralocorticoids or proamitine DHEA
Adrenal including Blunted hypothalamic axis Iatrogenic Addisonian due to chronic steroids Addisonian secondary to catastrophic phospholipid syndrome "Androgen Deficiency" Unrecognized diabetes	
Cardiac Pulmonary hypertension Pericarditis Autonomic neuropathy Accelerated atherosclerosis	Corticosteroids DMARDs to spare corticosteroids Endothelin receptor antagonists Iloprost Midodrine Mineralocorticoids
Central nervous system disease Stroke (thrombotic, embolic) Ganglionic neuropathy Demyelinating (multiple sclerosis) brain or cord Devic's syndrome (IgG4) Depression, seizures, and other manifestations similar to CNS lupus Cranial neuropathy including trigeminal neuralgia	Pulse steroids (1 g methylprednisolone for 3 consecutive days) Prednisolone (0.5–1.0 mg/kg body weight per day) Cyclophosphamide (0.5–1 g/m^2 of body surface/month) Azathioprine (2 mg/kg body weight per day) Rituximab
Peripheral neuropathy Sensory neuropathy including	SSRI, SNSRI Pentagabalin and pregabalin Duloxetine Aware that tricyclics agents will exacerbate dryness

Table 18.1 (continued)

Extraglandular manifestations	Main therapeutic modalities
"Burning mouth syndrome" Axonal neuropathy (anti-Mag) Ganglionic neuropathy Paraneoplastic (ANNA-1 and ANNA-2) Hearing loss (anti-cochlear) Taste loss Vitamin deficiency or toxicity Toxicity of herbal or nutritional supplements	
Infectious and postinfectious neuropathy Transverse myelitis Paravertebral abscess Guillain–Barre	If not infectious Plasmapheresis Intravenous gammaglobulin If recurrent Steroids (1 g methylprednisolone for 3 consecutive days) Cyclophosphamide (0.5–1 g/m^2 of body surface/month) Azathioprine (2 mg/kg body weight per day)
Gynecology–Obstetric Multiple miscarriage Congenital heart block Increased HPV	Cardiolipin syndrome-lovenox Decadron Increased surveillance
Lymphoproliferative Swelling of parotid including Mickulicz syndrome (elevated serum levels of IgG4), submandibular Lymphadenopathy	If biopsy does not indicate lymphoma Hydroxychloroquine Corticosteroids Methotrexate and leflunomide Rituximab
Fatigue Sleep disorder Fibromyalgia	• Pregabalin (Neurontin) • Pregabalin (Lyrica) • Duloxetine (Cymbalta) • Milnacipran (Ixel, Savella, Dalcipran, Toledomin) • Cognitive therapy and stress reduction • Avoid tricyclic anti-depressants due to dryness, exercise, myofascial therapy

Note: It is noted that most of these therapies have not been established by "evidence-based" medicine using double-blind trials. However, the case reports and response in patients with related disorders such as systemic lupus erythematosus have led to their use

fever. Thus, it is more critical than ever that rheumatologists educate their patients and other specialists about the therapy of SS and its wide spectrum of extraglandular manifestations, diagnostic procedures, and therapeutic approaches. Further, rheumatologists need to further educate themselves about the procedures used by other specialists.

Although we are advocates of evidence-based medicine, it should be recognized that most of the studies in therapy of extraglandular manifestations of SS are largely based on small series of patients from single institutions or small multicenter open-label trials. Thus, this chapter represents the current approach we use for treatment of patients at our Sjögren's clinic. Fortunately, an international consortium of rheumatologists and other SS specialists are developing a standardized disease activity/damage index that will greatly facilitate the uniform standards of diagnosis, therapy, and prognosis.

18.2 Treatment and Management of Cutaneous Manifestations

18.2.1 Treatment of Dry Skin

Treatment of dry skin in Sjögren's syndrome is similar to managing *xerosis* in other conditions.

1. The patient should *moisturize* with a fragrance-free cream moisturizer once or twice a day. Moisturizing is performed immediately after bathing or showering, while the skin is still damp, to prevent further evaporation from the skin.
   Sometimes in cases of extreme dryness, an *ointment* is suggested for its barrier and protective properties (such as petrolatum jelly or Aquaphor).
   If ointment is used, then application should be to damp skin because the ointment itself does not contain water.
   Excess greasiness can be blotted with a towel.
   Sometimes a moisturizing cream with β-hydroxy acid or α-hydroxy acid or urea can add extra moisture, but in cases of cracks in the skin, these will sting and irritate.
2. Excessive, long, hot showers or baths should be avoided in addition to heavily fragranced cleansers.
3. Cleansing of the skin—The usual recommendation is to cleanse with a moisturizing soap such as Dove® fragrance-free bar or a soap-free cleanser such as Cetaphil® gentle cleanser or Aquanil® cleanser.
   If the xerosis leads to *pruritis*, then safe anti-pruritus topical treatments are recommended. The therapeutic approach is similar to contact dermatitis or eczema. Topical steroids and immodulary creams or sprays are initially preferred. Mirtazapine also has some anti-pruritic effect to its strong antagonism of the H1 receptor.
4. *Over-the-counter lotions* containing menthol, camphor (Sarna Anti-Itch Lotion®), 2% lidocaine (Neutrogena Norwegian Formula Soothing Relief Anti-Itch Moisturizer®), and pramoxine (Aveeno Anti-Itch Concentrated Lotion®) are readily available.
5. *Oral anti-histamines* should be used with caution because of their anti-cholinergic effects. Fexofenadine (Allegra) does not cross the blood–brain barrier and may have slightly less dryness as a side effect. Over-the-counter sleeping medications that contain hydroxyzine (Atarax) or diphenhydramine (Benadryl) are very drying and may contribute to sleep disturbance.
6. *Topical corticosteroids*—We generally do not like to use topical corticosteroids (especially on the face) for more than a couple of weeks at a time, especially the ultra-potent ones, but even the mid-potent ones. In the case of inflammatory skin findings, local treatment with potent topical steroids can augment systemic treatments.
   Sometimes topical corticosteroids are used for pruritis, but their use should be limited due to long-term side effects such as skin atrophy, tachyphylaxis, and absorption.
7. We always suggest *constant daily sun protection* for patients with autoimmune conditions. Because the wavelength of light causing sun sensitivity in autoimmune conditions may not be in the UVB spectrum (290–320 nm), *patients should use a broad-spectrum sunscreen.*
   - SPF factors refer to UVB protection only, so patients cannot count on simply the SPF factor.
   - Most sunscreens available now have added UVA protection (290–320 nm), commonly from chemical UVA-absorbing compounds such as Parsol 1789 (avobenzone).
8. We prefer *physical sun blocks* because wavelengths outside of both UVB and UVA may affect the patient with autoimmune disease.
   Physical sun blocks contain titanium dioxide or zinc oxide, which reflects rays.
   One commonly available sun block is Neutrogena Sensitive Skin Sun Block SPF-30®, which uses purely titanium dioxide as its active ingredient.
9. The most effective protection is *sun protective clothing* because it will not wear off as sunscreens do.
   Obviously, avoiding excess sun contact altogether is prudent, such as trying to stay indoors during the intense sunlight hours of 10:00 a.m.–4 p.m.
10. *Routine skin checks for skin cancers*—In addition to the hunt for actinic keratosis

and squamous cell carcinomas that may be increased in frequency in SS patients [6] and melanomas, the physician needs to look for cutaneous B-lymphoma and anetoderma, a condition that is frequently associated with increased risk of occult lymphoma or plasmacytoma.

18.2.2 Raynaud's Phenomena

18.2.2.1 Raynaud's Phenomena Reported in 30% of Patients with Primary SS

The clinical course of Raynaud's phenomena in most SS patients is often milder than in patients with scleroderma [6]. Raynaud's phenomenon is often an early sign and may be apparent before symptoms of clinical sicca are apparent. However, some SS patients do develop severe Raynaud's phenomenon and digital ulcers even though they lack other clinical features suggestive of scleroderma [6]. The use of protection including gloves, especially when spending excess time in the freezer section of the supermarket, and moisturizers to prevent skin cracking must be emphasized. The use of moisturizers to the fingertips is increasingly important because SS patients spend increasing amounts of time using either their computer keyboard or "text messaging" on their cell phones (explaining in part the sudden increase in trauma pain in the thumbs used for "keying text" to other friends). Avoidance of caffeine, smoking, and herbal medications also may play a role in improvement of symptoms. The use of 3-omega fatty acids and other anti-oxidants may prove helpful [7].

18.2.2.2 Pharmacologic Treatment of Raynaud's Phenomena

Of SS patients with Raynaud's phenomena, about half will require pharmacologic treatment [6]. Initial therapy uses calcium channel blockers. In patients with low baseline blood pressure or symptoms of autonomic orthostatic hypotension, it is important to start dosing at low levels and increase gradually. For more severe cases, treatment is similar to that used in PSS, including ganglionic blocks, iloprost, and use of endothelin antagonists and sildenafil [8–11].

18.3 Arthralgia/Arthritis

The joint symptoms of SS frequently can be considered along the points of a square that encompasses

1. Osteoarthritis (including "erosive osteoarthritis," which may have earlier age of onset and more rapid progression);
2. Rheumatoid arthritis with its joint distribution and tendency to erosive, deforming disease;
3. Systemic lupus and Jaccoud's-type arthritis where erosive changes on radiography are less likely even though the patient presents with typical swollen joints and also with tendon subluxation or rheumatoid-like nodules;
4. Patients may also have peripheral neuropathy and distal myopathy that contribute to their joint symptoms and require additional therapeutic modalities.

The approach to arthralgias and arthritis is similar to the SLE patients with each of the above conditions.

Symptoms are initially treated with salicylates (including disalcid or trilisate) or non-steroidal agents (NSAIDs) of cox1 and cox2 types [2]. Many SS patients have decreased tolerance of NSAIDs, probably due to *dysphagia* secondary to decreased salivary flow and esophageal motility [12]. They also have increased frequency of GERD and tracheal reflux, discussed in Chapter 16 which is exacerbated by the NSAIDs.

Among the "slow-acting" drugs (previously termed disease-modifying anti-rheumatic drugs (DMARDs)), *anti-malarials* (hydroxychloroquine) have proven useful in decreasing the arthralgia, myalgia, and lymphadenopathy in SS patients and in tapering the steroids [13, 14]. Hydroxychloroquine's action is similar to its benefit in some SLE patients, and flare in arthralgia is noted when patients are withdrawn from their hydroxychloroquine [15]. However, many patients are unable to take hydroxychloroquine due to difficulty in swallowing the medication because of its bitter taste. This is particularly true with the generic form of the drug, which is often a "milled" tablet (manufactured with a fine dust coating of the drug still on the pills' surface) with a taste quite bitter to the patient who has less saliva. The "branded" Plaquenil is a polished tablet and may be tolerated in patients who cannot take the generic version.

We have used *hydroxychloroquine* (6–8 mg/kg/day) in SS patients when there is elevation of erythrocyte sedimentation rate (ESR) and arthralgias or myalgia. Indeed, hydroxychloroquine is used in SS much as it is used in SLE as a "platform" for therapy and immune modulation of non-visceral manifestations.

In a European study, Kruize et al. [16] also found that hydroxychloroquine improved ESR and arthralgias but did not increase tear flow volumes. When taken at the proper dose (6–8 mg/kg/day), hydroxychloroquine has a very good safety record, although there remains a remote possibility (probably less than 1:1,000) [17] of significant build-up in the eye. For this reason, periodic eye checks (generally every 6–12 months) are recommended so that the medicine can be discontinued if there is any significant build-up.

In patients in whom arthralgia/arthritis persists, we will next use methotrexate (MTX) given as a weekly dose. We generally start at methotrexate 7.5 mg/week as an oral dose, taken with daily folic acid 1 mg. In patients where doses of methotrexate exceed 15 mg/week, we generally advise the patient to use self-injection of MTX to ensure absorption and because this minimizes gastric toxicity. Again, folic acid 1 mg/day is taken. However, the possible CNS side effects of MTX at higher dose (described by the patient as "just not feeling right") on the day of MTX should be checked. It is also common to use a combination of hydroxychloroquine plus methotrexate when either drug alone is insufficient.

In patients unable to tolerate methotrexate, our next choice is often leflunomide [2, 18]. Leflunomide is started at dose 20 mg/day. We do not use the initial loading dose of 100 mg/day for 5 days because it leads to a greater incidence of drug discontinuation due to diarrhea or other gastrointestinal side effects. The combination of methotrexate plus leflunomide also has been used, similar to their combined benefits in RA patients. We check liver function tests monthly for at least the first 3 months and then go to every 3-month safety checks. We advise patients about risks of alcohol and overweight patients about risks of hepatic fatty infiltrates as co-factors in toxicity.

Previous studies in SS have utilized sulfasalazine [19] and azathioprine [20], but these agents seem less well-tolerated and less effective in SS patients than in RA or spondyloarthropathy patients [2]. In some SS patients with joint symptoms, *cyclosporine* has been reported [21], but the tendency toward interstitial nephritis at doses above 3 mg/kg/day in many Sjögren's patients limits the usefulness of the drug.

As in SLE patients, treatment with corticosteroids is effective but limited by their usual side effects including osteoporosis, diabetes, cardiovascular, and mood disruption. However, it is worth noting that increased tear flow, salivary flow, and neuropathic symptoms have been reported in patients receiving relatively high-dose steroids [22]. This is important since it indicates the partial reversibility of the processes as a therapeutic goal. In patients with prednisone dose more than 5 mg/day, we add a bisphosphonate (such as risedronate) to prevent osteoporosis.

In addition to the expected problems associated with steroids, SS patients have increased problems with corticosteroids including acceleration of their periodontal disease and oral candidiasis as a result of their dry mouth. Also, it is unclear if steroids may promote accelerated atherosclerosis [23].

18.4 Therapeutic Management of Pulmonary Manifestations

18.4.1 Chronic Cough

The most common respiratory manifestation is a dry cough and hoarseness. This may be partly due to "bronchial sicca" with decreased bronchial secretions. Other factors may include laryngo-tracheal reflux. These changes can be observed on bronchoscopy tracheolaryngeal examinations. Symptomatic treatment with room humidifiers, air purifiers, and nasal lavage may prove helpful. Belafsky discusses these problems more fully in Chapter 16.

18.4.2 Non-specific Interstitial Pneumonitis (NSIP)

SS patients may have interstitial infiltrates on their chest radiograph that are found incidentally or upon evaluation of dyspnea [24, 25]. Pulmonary function tests have shown abnormalities including a restrictive pattern in small airways and cellular abnormalities in bronchoalveolar lavage fluid even in patients without respiratory complaints [26, 27]. Long-term prospective controlled studies are needed to determine the clinical course and significance of these findings. However, many of the patients at 5-year follow up will show little progression [28, 29]. Other reports indicate a progressive fibrotic lung process similar to scleroderma pneumonitis [30]. Thus, we follow SS patients for progression of their infiltrates on high-resolution CAT scan. In general, our SS population is representative of tertiary referral center and thus a higher percentage of patients have progressive disease. We have treated these SS patients as having NSIP, an entity that now encompasses the previous lymphocytic interstitial pneumonitis (LIP).

Initial therapy with corticosteroids in NSIP and SS has been effective, but the tapering of steroids may lead to relapse.

- Cyclophosphamide therapy has been reported as useful in SS patients with rapidly progressive NSIP or patients who relapse rapidly when steroids are tapered [31]. However, several of our SS patients have required cyclophosphamide, but it is not possible to determine if we have made any difference in these "open" trials. Mycophenolic acid (1 g bid) has also been used in hopes of slowing progression.
- We need to remember that both alkylator and methotrexate therapy may cause pneumonitis.
- Sudden deterioration should raise the possibility of intercurrent infection, including atypical mycobacterial infection.

Our approach to therapy has been based on uncontrolled case reports of NSIP in SS that include *cyclophosphamide*, *mycophenolic acid*, and *cyclosporine* [31]. It should be noted that *interstitial pneumonitis has been reported after rituximab therapy* [32]. Thus, therapies used to treat other manifestations of SS may contribute to the NSIP.

18.5 Renal Manifestations

18.5.1 Interstitial Nephritis

The clinical manifestations of the interstitial nephritis include a variable, but generally mild elevation in the plasma creatinine concentration, a relatively benign urinalysis, and abnormalities in tubular function, including the Fanconi syndrome, type 1 (distal) renal tubular acidosis (RTA), nephrogenic diabetes insipidus (tubular resistance to anti-diuretic hormone), and hypokalemia [33, 34]. Anemia may be prominent due to decreased erythropoietin production.

A course of corticosteroids is frequently beneficial unless irreversible tubulointerstitial injury has occurred. An improvement in the plasma creatinine concentration should be observed within a few weeks of the initiation of corticosteroids if the damage is reversible. Progression to end-stage renal disease is a rare event [35].

If the symptoms relapse after steroids are tapered, then azathioprine [36] or mycophenolic acid [37] has been suggested. Also, rituximab has been reported to improve nephritis with decrease in severity of renal biopsy [38].

Type 1 renal tubular acidosis [39]—A defect in distal acidification occurs in up to 25% of patients with Sjögren's syndrome. The associated metabolic acidosis is usually mild, but some patients present with a plasma bicarbonate concentration below 10 meq/L and a plasma potassium concentration below 1.5–2.0 meq/L due to concurrent urinary potassium wasting.

Muscle paralysis and respiratory arrest have been reported as consequences of the severe hypokalemia [40]; in some cases, hypokalemic paralysis has been the presenting symptom of Sjögren's syndrome [41].

The mechanism by which Sjögren's syndrome leads to type 1 RTA is incompletely understood. A possible mechanism is the presence of high titers of an autoantibody directed against carbonic anhydrase II; inhibition of this enzyme would result in the generation within the cell of fewer hydrogen ions available for secretion.

Nephrogenic diabetes insipidus [42, 43]—Polyuria and polydipsia due to nephrogenic diabetes insipidus are other manifestations of impaired tubular function in Sjögren's syndrome. Once again, patients may present with these complaints rather than a sicca syndrome. It is, therefore, important to exclude Sjögren's syndrome in any adult with symptomatic nephrogenic diabetes insipidus who does not have the two most common causes of this disorder—chronic lithium ingestion or hypercalcemia.

Hypokalemia without renal tubular acidosis [44]—The tubular injury induced by the interstitial nephritis indirectly leads to potassium wasting and potentially severe hypokalemia. The primary defect is thought to be sodium wasting, which has two effects that augment potassium secretion: it increases sodium delivery to the potassium secretory site in the collecting tubules and, via volume depletion, enhances the release of aldosterone. The use of spironolactone may be helpful in these patients.

18.5.1.1 Glomerular Disease

Glomerular involvement is much less common than interstitial nephritis in Sjögren's syndrome [45, 46]. Membranoproliferative glomerulonephritis and membranous nephropathy are the most common. The pathogenesis of the glomerular disease, including the possible etiologic relationship to Sjögren's syndrome, is unclear, but may be related to the deposition of circulating immune complexes. Other etiologies are mixed cryoglobulinemia and amyloid. Optimal therapy is uncertain. Some patients with membranoproliferative glomerulonephritis, for example, have been treated with prednisone without or with cytotoxic therapy (such as cyclophosphamide) with varying success; in one case, spontaneous remission occurred. As in SLE patients, mycophenolic acid is being used to treat SS glomerulonephritis as an alternative to cyclophosphamide. Azathioprine has also been used as a steroid-sparing drug in patients with glomerulonephritis.

In patients with glomerulonephritis due to mixed cryoglobulinemia, plasmapheresis, and cytotoxic therapy may be required [47].

18.6 Gastrointestinal Manifestations

18.6.1 Mesenteric Vasculitis

Mesenteric vasculitis may occur in SS patients, similar to patients with SLE in the setting of a generalized vasculitis [48]. The vasculitis associated with SS or systemic lupus erythematosus (SLE) involves small-sized and medium-sized vessels and involves the gastrointestinal tract. Lower abdominal pain secondary to mesenteric vasculitis is generally an insidious symptom that may be intermittent for months prior to the development of an acute abdomen with nausea, vomiting, diarrhea, GI bleeding, and fever [49]. Risk factors for the development of mesenteric vasculitis include peripheral vasculitis and central nervous system vasculitis. Patients with an acute presentation may also have mesenteric thrombosis and infarction often in association with anti-phospholipid antibodies.

Mesenteric vasculitis is a potentially life-threatening disorder. In addition to the possible development of necrotic segments of bowel, patients may suffer septic complications and bowel perforation. Current therapy of severe SS vasculitis is more aggressive and typically consists of intravenous pulse methylprednisolone and pulse cyclophosphamide [50].

These patients can also present acutely with small bowel obstruction secondary to strictures, resembling Crohn's disease or intussusception, or with massive gastrointestinal bleeding secondary to aneurysm formation. Bowel infarction, perforation, and peritonitis are rare complications of chronic intestinal ischemia due to vasculitis [50].

In addition to mesenteric ischemia, systemic vasculitis can also cause ischemic hepatitis, pancreatitis, cholecystitis, and less commonly gastritis or esophagitis. Treatment of mesenteric vasculitis in SS is similar to that used in polyarteritis nodosa with corticosteroids and cyclophosphamide, which has led to a dramatic improvement in patient survival and relief of symptoms [49].

The differential diagnosis should include Henoch–Schönlein purpura (HSP), which is a small vessel vasculitis that typically occurs in children, although all ages can be affected. Patients classically exhibit lower extremity purpura, arthritis, and hematuria, which can all be mistaken for vasculitis in the setting of SS.

18.6.2 Primary Biliary Cirrhosis

Primary biliary cirrhosis patients have a high frequency of sicca complaints and, due to their frequently positive anti-nuclear antibody (ANA), may be labeled as SS patients [51, 52]. In some studies there is an increased frequency of overlap PBC-associated autoantibodies (anti-mitochondrial antibody) and those antibodies found in SS patients. Primary biliary cirrhosis (PBC) is characterized by an ongoing immunologic attack on the intralobular bile ducts that eventually leads to cirrhosis and liver failure.

There are a number of complications that occur in PBC that require therapy. These include the following:

- Pruritis associated with bile salts
- Metabolic bone disease
- Hypercholesterolemia and xanthomas
- Malabsorption vitamin deficiencies
- Hypothyroidism anemia

The role of immunosuppressive drugs remains unproven, although ursodeoxycholic acid has been shown to halt disease progression [53]. Colchicine has also been reported as helpful [54].

Symptomatic steatorrhea due to bile acid insufficiency can be partially corrected by restricting dietary fat. Medium-chain triglycerides (MCTs) can be added if caloric supplementation is required to maintain body weight. The digestion and absorption of MCTs are not nearly as dependent upon bile acids as are the long-chain fatty acids, which are the major constituent of dietary triglycerides. Each milliliter of MCT oil contains 7.5 calories. Most patients can tolerate 60 mL/day without difficulty. MCT oil can be taken directly by the teaspoon or can be used as salad oil or as a substitute for shortening in cooking.

If pancreatic insufficiency is suspected, it is easier to treat with pancreatic enzyme replacement than it is to diagnose. Preparations such as Pancrease and pancrelipase (Creon) taken with meals are usually effective.

Deficiencies of fat-soluble vitamins—Patients with PBC may have malabsorption of the fat-soluble vitamins A, D, E, and K. Deficiencies of vitamin E are uncommon except in patients with advanced disease awaiting liver transplantation. In comparison, vitamin A deficiency occurs in approximately 30% of patients but is rarely symptomatic. It correlates directly with serum retinol-binding protein and albumin levels and inversely with serum bilirubin levels. Vitamin A deficiency usually responds to dietary supplements of vitamin A, 15,000 units/day (three times the recommended daily allowance). In exceptional cases, as in the patient with night blindness, parenteral vitamin A may be required.

Vitamin D deficiency, if untreated, can lead to osteomalacia. It is best detected by measuring the serum concentration of calcitriol (25-hydroxyvitamin D), the metabolite of vitamin D produced in the liver. Serum levels of vitamin D and calcitriol (the most active form of vitamin D) are usually normal in PBC except for patients who are deeply jaundiced and who are candidates for liver transplantation.

Annual measurement of serum vitamin A and calcidiol levels is sufficient in patients whose serum bilirubin concentration is elevated. Less frequent measurements, e.g., every 2–3 years, is sufficient in patients with normal serum bilirubin levels. Measurements should be obtained more frequently in patients whose values are just above the lower limit of normal.

Clinically important vitamin K deficiency rarely occurs in PBC unless the patient regularly takes cholestyramine and is deeply jaundiced. The prothrombin time is normal in most patients until late in the course of the disease when there are signs of liver failure. Only these patients require vitamin K supplementation.

Celiac Sprue [55]—Serologic studies are now used to further confirm the diagnosis of celiac disease. These include the ELISA for IgA antibodies to gliadin and the immunofluorescence test for IgA antibodies to endomysium, a structure of the smooth muscle connective tissue, the presence of which is virtually pathognomonic for celiac disease. Using these methods, the incidence of celiac sprue is elevated in SS patients [56]. Treatment includes avoidance of gluten as well as attention to the consequences of malabsorption that are similar to the nutrient and vitamin deficiencies described above.

Gastroparesis [57] is defined as delayed gastric emptying, and patients often complain of bloating. Its true prevalence in SS is unknown; however, it is estimated that up to 20% of SS patients may have some slowing of gastric motility. Concurrent lactose intolerance also may play a role. SS patients should be cautious in prolonged use of this drug since a recent analysis suggested that metoclopramide is the most common cause of drug-induced movement disorders. Another analysis of study data by the FDA showed that about 20% of patients in that study that used metoclopramide took it for longer than 3 months. The FDA only approves metoclopramide for 4- to 12-week short-term treatment. *Domperidone* (trade names *Motilium, Motillium, Motinorm*, and *Costi*) is an antidopaminergic drug used as a prokinetic agent used in Canada and Europe [58]. Higher acetylcholine levels increase gastrointestinal peristalsis and further increase pressure on the lower esophageal sphincter, thereby stimulating gastrointestinal motility, accelerating gastric emptying, and improving gastro-duodenal coordination. It should be noted that the FDA turned down an application for domperidone in the USA, even though the FDA's division of gastrointestinal drugs had approved domperidone. Individual incidents of problems with the drug include cardiac arrhythmia and potential interaction with other medications has been reported.

The association between delayed gastric emptying and SS is not straightforward. Delayed gastric emptying is present in 25–40% of patients with functional dyspepsia, a condition affecting approximately 20% of Western population with increased frequency in patients with fibromyalgia.

In addition, the magnitude of the delay in gastric emptying is often modest and not well correlated with symptoms, except possibly bloating. One possible explanation for the poor correlation between delayed gastric emptying and symptoms in SS may be involvement of the afferent sensory nerve fibers by autonomic neuropathy thereby decreasing perception of symptoms.

Also, bloating is a common symptom in SS patients and may be due to the increased amount of air swallowed with food due to their dysphagia as a result of decreased saliva. Concurrent lactose intolerance also may play a role in non-specific gastrointestinal symptoms. It is estimated that 75% of adults worldwide show some decrease in lactase activity during adulthood, although there is no clear evidence for an increased frequency in SS patients. Due to difficulty in swallowing other solid foods, the diet in SS patients may be skewed toward "softer foods" including milk and derived products such as yogurt. The frequency of decreased lactase activity ranges from as little as 5% in northern Europe, up to 71% for Sicily, to more than 90% in some African and Asian countries. Disaccharides cannot be absorbed through the wall of the small intestine into the bloodstream, so in the absence of lactase, lactose present in ingested dairy products remains uncleaved and passes intact into the colon. The operons of enteric bacteria quickly switch over to lactose metabolism, and the resulting in vivo fermentation produces copious amounts of gas (a mixture of hydrogen, carbon dioxide, and methane). It results in symptoms including abdominal pain, bloating, flatulence, diarrhea, nausea, and acid reflux. As milk products are a common source of calcium and vitamin D (which is supplemented in milk), osteoporosis may be accelerated in these individuals.

Pancreatitis and sclerosing cholangitis (PSC) [59–62]—Primary sclerosing cholangitis is a chronic progressive disorder of unknown etiology that is characterized by inflammation, fibrosis, and stricturing of medium-sized and large-sized ducts in the intrahepatic and extrahepatic biliary tree. The great majority of cases have underlying ulcerative colitis, but the syndrome has also been reported in increased frequency in SS patients. A variety of immunosuppressive and anti-inflammatory agents have been studied in patients with PSC, including ursodeoxycholic acid, steroids, cyclosporine, methotrexate, azathioprine and 6-mercaptopurine, tacrolimus, D-penicillamine, and more recently etanercept (that failed to show benefit). Unfortunately, none has been shown conclusively proven to alter the natural history of this disorder. Initial small studies with each of these agents looked promising but subsequent larger studies failed to confirm the initial enthusiasm. Among the agents listed above, a result from recent randomized trials of high-dose ursodeoxycholic acid has suggested promise.

18.7 Urologic

Painful bladder syndrome (PBS)/interstitial cystitis (IC) has been reported in SS and the patients have increased urinary frequency and urgency [63–65]. Large volumes of fluid consumed due to dry mouth compound the problems of interstitial cystitis.

Amitriptyline is commonly prescribed for relief of PBS/IC symptoms. However, its anticholinergic side effects increase dryness and thus it is poorly tolerated in SS patients. However, only a minority of patients in the amitriptyline group experienced greater than 30% decrease in symptom score, suggesting that benefits are modest.

Pentosan polysulfate sodium—Pentosan polysulfate sodium (PPS) is the only oral medication approved by the United States Food and Drug Administration (FDA) for treatment of IC. The approved dose is 100 mg three times daily, although off-label treatment using 200 mg twice daily is clinically common. The medication is a protein that is supposed to be filtered by the kidneys and appear in the urine so that it can reconstitute the deficient glycosaminoglycan (GAG) layer over the urothelium. In fact, only a tiny proportion of the drug is absorbed by the gastrointestinal tract and excreted in the urine. If the patient is scheduled for surgery, it is worth noting that this medication can lead to altered platelet function [66] and may contribute to thrombocytopenia [67].

Other therapies of interstitial cystitis that have been reported include

- Intravesical heparin and lidocaine
- Intravesical dimethyl sulfoxide (DMSO)
- Hydrodistension, however, there are risks of hydrodistension that includes bleeding (from ruptured vessels) and, rarely, rupture of the bladder wall

18.8 Therapeutic Management of Obstetrical/Gynecological Manifestations

18.8.1 Vaginal Dryness [68–72]

A gynecologic exam is useful to rule out other causes of painful intercourse and other causes of vaginal dryness.

When it does occur as part of Sjögren's syndrome, the spouse or partner needs to be reassured that this is a "physiological" problem and not related to a failure of sexual arousal. The Sjögren's patient currently has many more options regarding safe and effective vaginal lubrication than ever before.

Lubricants such as Maxilube® and Astroglide® have slightly different characteristics when compared with KY Brand® jelly or Surgilube® and yet share the common characteristics of being water soluble and non-irritating.

This also holds true for the new non-hormonal vaginal moisturizer Replens®, which may be used unassociated with intercourse. For those patients who do not like the gel-type lubricants, there is now available Lubrin® vaginal inserts. Sterile lubricants such as Astroglide®, KY Brand® jelly, or Surgilube® are helpful (should be liberally applied to *both* partners for maximal comfort) [73, 74]. Unscented vaginal lubricants are preferred.

Finding the right preparation for a specific individual is often a matter of trial and error inasmuch as satisfaction with each lubricant is a matter of personal preference. The patient needs to be frank with her physician regarding her satisfaction or dissatisfaction with a particular preparation. The external use of preparations containing petrolatum or oils that "seal in" moisture, such as Vaseline® or cocoa butter, may lead to maceration of the vaginal lining and are to be avoided.

Vaginal dryness in perimenopausal or *postmenopausal women* is often related to vaginal atrophy because of declining estrogen levels and therefore responds to vaginal estrogen creams such as Estrace®. Cortisone creams are not beneficial in this situation.

If *vaginal yeast infection* occurs, prompt treatment with clotrimazole topical cream, vaginal suppositories (Gynelotrimin®), or oral gluconazole 150 mg is safe and effective.

On the external vulvar surface, dryness may be treated with lubricating creams as would other skin surface. Several patients have reported considerable satisfaction with the use of a thin film of vitamin E oil [75], used on the vulva once or twice a day.

An issue of concern to female Sjögren's patients has been whether or not estrogen replacement therapy at the time of menopause is harmful to their condition [76]. With regards to estrogen replacement in general, the clinical evidence is controversial whether the risks of blocking osteoporosis and reducing cardiovascular mortality adequately offset the small increase in risk in breast cancer.

It is also worth noting that the *subset of women who had previous hysterectomy/ovariectomy were not found to have increased risk of breast cancer on receiving estrogen replacement* [77].

Of importance, some women feel that estrogen replacement improves their quality of life in terms of mood elevation by reducing hot flashes and hormone-related vaginal dryness [78–80]. Part of this improvement may relate to the interconversion of hormones to include dehydroepiandrosterone (DHEA), which appears to have beneficial effects on local mucosal surfaces [81] as well as affect [82].

Earlier investigators were concerned that estrogen might have a negative influence on Sjögren's or SLE based on animal studies. At our clinic, we have not seen any deterioration of Sjögren's syndrome related to either estrogen replacement therapy or low estrogen forms of oral contraceptives.

Because of this, we encourage adequate estrogen replacement for the properly screened postmenopausal Sjögren's patient who feels that it improves their quality of life. Although the data have not been formally collected in SS, there have been extensive trials on the use of oral contraceptives and estrogen replacement in SLE patients [78, 79, 83]. These studies have indicated safety in terms of breast cancer and disease activity. However, *caution with regard to blood clot risk remains, particularly in the patient with circulating anti-coagulants or a past history of thromboembolic disease.*

Nonetheless, estrogens would not be the agent of choice to deal with either postmenopausal osteoporosis or elevated lipid profiles. Other therapeutic alternatives for osteoporosis (alendronate, Fosamax®, and risedronate, Actonel®) and other agents for lowering cholesterol (such as statins) are now available, and estrogens are now not the agents of choice for these medical issues.

18.9 Special Precautions at the Time of Surgery

SS patients have particularly unique needs at the time of surgery. These precautions are summarized in Table 17.5. *Patients with ocular dryness are at increased risk for corneal abrasions in operating rooms* (that generally have low humidity) and particularly in the postoperative recovery room, where non-humidified oxygen is blown across their face at a time when they are still too groggy to have adequate blink reflex.

Therefore, we have recommended application of an ocular ointment or gel prior to surgery.

Patients are subject to severe dryness of the mouth as a consequence of their disease but are told to be "NPO" for at least 12 h before surgery (and often longer if they are a later operative case in the day). We have found that patients can safely use their oral mouth sprays for comfort, while not having the risk of gastric contents and aspiration during anesthesia. If possible, patients should request from their surgeons that they be placed in an early slot in the OR schedule.

The anesthesiologist will need to take special precautions with oral intubations, as these patients have fragile teeth and often have expensive dental reconstructions including implants.

Therefore, it is important for the patient to make certain that a "heads-up" note is recorded in, or better yet, on the front of the chart.

Patients with SS often have very dry upper airways and minimal use of anti-cholinergic agents to control tracheal secretions. The tenacious mucus secretions may predispose to "mucus" plus inspissations and postoperative obstructions.

The use of *humidified oxygen* and mucolytics may help minimize this process.

Although anesthesiologists and surgeons are familiar with precautions regarding NSAIDs and bleeding risk, they are often less familiar with the relatively long duration of agents such as the new biologic agents. Although most of the literature about increased rate of infection after joint replacements deals with TNF inhibitors, it is likely that similar caveats will apply to additional biologic agents as they become available.

Finally, *steroid coverage for "stress" levels* may be required in patients on chronic steroids. Also, *oral candida* is quite common in the post-operative patient who has been on steroids and recent antibiotic therapy.

Patients should also be permitted to have their eye and mouth moisturizers and other appropriate remedies at bedside if inpatient.

18.10 Vaccinations in the SS Patient

Vaccine preventable infectious diseases remain a significant source of morbidity and mortality in immunocompromised hosts including SLE and SS patients, but special considerations may limit the benefit that this group derives from vaccination [84]. Pneumococcal, hepatitis A/B and non-live influenza vaccines are recommended, particularly prior to the initiation of biologic agents. Although the antibody titers may be diminished after vaccination, the level of protection is generally considered adequate to justify the expense and risk of vaccination even after the biologic agent has been given. In the particular case of hepatitis B vaccine, experience in SLE patients has suggested the need for testing the patient's antibody response after two vaccinations and to determine if a third vaccination is necessary. Patients with past history of allergy (including urticarial reactions) to prior vaccines or to egg protein, it is important for the rheumatologist counsel the patient about risks. Although there are anecdotal reports of serious flares of disease in SLE patients after vaccination, these incidents appear to be uncommon. One particular problem for the rheumatologist is the identification of the SS patient with history of neurologic manifestations including myelitis that may have had onset after a previous vaccine where chemoprophylaxis may be chosen over vaccination.

Live vaccines are generally contraindicated in immunocompromised patients including those receiving immunosuppressive medications. One of the most frequent questions for the rheumatologist is the risk/benefit in the use of the herpes zoster vaccine. The zoster vaccine is not licensed for use in immunocompromised people, even though this population is at especially high risk for the development of herpes zoster. This is because the group people who are mildly immunosuppressed (including patients with diabetes or who are receiving low-dose corticosteroids, tumor-necrosis-factor blockers, and other immunomodulatory drugs) were excluded from the initial zoster vaccine trials. Thus, the safety and efficacy of the vaccine has not been firmly established patients who are at higher risk for herpes zoster. Further, the efficacy of the vaccine in people who have had a previous episode of herpes zoster is unknown, since this population was also excluded from the large zoster vaccine trial. Thus, there remains a debate about whether zoster vaccine is "cost-effective" in these patients as well as potential medical-legal concerns if complications do develop.

The Center for Communicable Disease emphasizes that the level of protection is "partial" even in non-immune compromised people. Thus, the physician needs to educate the SS patient to pursue prompt anti-viral treatment if symptoms of herpetic viral reactivation should occur even though a zoster vaccination has been given. This may be particularly important in the SS patient where the patient may mistake symptoms of a unilateral flare of ocular pain as a result of their keratoconjunctivitis sicca or corneal abrasion. The finding of paresthesia (and particular a vesicular lesion) in the opthalmic dermatome should be treated promptly and requires an immediate slit lamp evaluation to determine if characteristic lesions of herpetic keratitis are present.

Among SS patients taking immunosuppressant medications (including biologic agents), no clear guidelines have been provided although experience in rheumatoid arthritis (RA) patients on biologic agents suggests benefit of vaccination, especially prior to initiating the immunosuppressive therapy. Another question is the SS patient's risk from the exposure to live attenuated flu vaccine (LAV) or polio vaccine given to children or other family members. In clinical practice, this has not proven to be a substantial risk.

In world travelers or military personnel, the risk from yellow fever and cholera infections may be substantial. The yellow fever vaccine (usually 17D) has been well tolerated in both SLE and SS patients. Although a live cholera vaccine is available, a recombinant cholera toxin B subunit vaccine has been recommended as safe and equally effective. Unfortunately, no vaccine is yet available for dengue or Chikungunya, which remain endemic in certain parts of the world.

According to the Center for Disease Control Guidelines (http://www.cdc.gov/vaccines/), individuals with a history of allergy to prior vaccines and a history of Guillain–Barre require careful monitoring if a vaccine is required. Also, patients with history of allergy to prior vaccines, including components grown in chicken eggs, should be given the vaccines with caution.

Patients with defects in host defense and those receiving exogenous immunosuppression agents may have suboptimal responses to certain vaccinations.

This has been demonstrated as found impaired immune responses to vaccines among patients receiving long-term immunosuppressive therapy, but postvaccination antibody titers are usually sufficient to provide protection for the majority of immunized individuals [85].

Vaccines against influenza and pneumococcus appear to be safe and immunogenic in SLE patients and their routine administration should be encouraged [86].

This is important in SLE and SS patients because many are functionally "asplenic" [87].

Patients should receive pneumococcal vaccine prior to rituximab.

Clinicians' concerns about adverse effects, including the possibility of exacerbating rheumatologic disease, may also limit the number of patients to whom potentially effective vaccines are offered.

The evidence for and against exacerbation of underlying rheumatologic disease and the use of postexposure prophylaxis with anti-microbials or immune globulins for selected infections have been an area of debate [88]. Although there appears to be a temporal association with some disease flares, the causal association has not been established [89, 90].

18.11 Summary

SS presents an immense time investment to manage the unique extraglandular manifestations of SS, and these manifestations will be unique to each patient.

With rheumatologists increasingly taking the lead in being both the diagnostician and clinician managing the broad spectrum of extraglandular manifestations of SS, it is paramount that rheumatologists broaden their knowledge base of SS and its wide spectrum of extraglandular manifestations, diagnostic procedures, and therapeutic approaches.

Among the many manifestations rheumatologists can expect to see and treat include *sicca symptoms* (including eyes, mouth, vagina), *arthralgias, myalgias, dysphagia, elevation of erythrocyte sedimentation rate (ESR),* and *polyclonal hyperglobulinemia, vasculitic skin lesions, pneumonitis, neuropathy, nephritis, lymphoma, interstitial pneumonitis, multifocal leukoencephalopathy, Raynaud's phenomenon, and fibromyalgia.*

18.12 Late-Breaking Updates

Botulism toxin injection may provide a novel therapy for non-suppurative parotitis due to cystic changes of the gland [91].

The unusual respiratory manifestation of pulmonary veno-occlusive disease in SS patients may respond to immunosuppressive therapy with azathioprine [92]. Another usual respiratory manifestation termed "shrinking lung syndrome" associated with SS may respond to steroids and azathioprine [93]. Shrinking lung syndrome is characterized by small lung volumes, elevation of the diaphragm, and restrictive physiology without parenchymal involvement. Pleural adhesions and pain probably play a significant role in the pathogenesis.

A comprehensive review of the evaluation and treatment of pregnant patients with SS or SLE outlines the pre-natal workup and the results with therapy for those with anti-cardiolipin antibodies [94]. A high frequency of patients continuing to take medications with teratogenic potential were noted, due to inadequate counseling by physicians. Heparin plus aspirin was found beneficial in patients with risk for anti-phospholipid syndrome and decadron for neonatal heart block.

A retrospective study found that interstitial nephritis is more frequent than clinically diagnosed and that early recognition/treatment may slow or prevent progression [95]. In patients with suspicion of interstitial nephritis, renal biopsy was reported to be underutilized.

References

1. Mavragani CP, Moutsopoulos HM. Conventional therapy of Sjogren's syndrome. Clin Rev Allergy Immunol. 2007;32(3):284–91.
2. Thanou-Stavraki A, James JA. Primary Sjogren's syndrome: current and prospective therapies. Semin Arthritis Rheum. 2008;37(5):273–92.
3. Sugai S, Masaki Y. Current and prospective treatment options for Sjogren's syndrome. Expert Rev Clin Immunol. 2008;4(4):469–79.
4. Moutsopoulos HM. Sjogren's syndrome or autoimmune epithelitis? Clin Rev Allergy Immunol. 2007;32(3):199–200.
5. Isenberg DA. Systemic lupus erythematosus and Sjogren's syndrome: historical perspective and ongoing concerns. Arthritis Rheum. 2004;50(3): 681–3.
6. Fox RI, Liu AY. Sjogren's syndrome in dermatology. Clin Dermatol. 2006;24(5):393–413.
7. Ho M, Maple C, Bancroft A, McLaren M, Belch JJF. The beneficial effects of omega-3 and omega-6 essential fatty acid supplementation on red blood cell rheology. Prostaglandins, Leukot Essent Fatty Acids. 1999;61(1):13–7.
8. Launay D, Hachulla E, Hatron PY, Jais X, Simonneau G, Humbert M. Pulmonary arterial hypertension: a rare complication of primary Sjogren syndrome: report of 9 new cases and review of the literature. Medicine 2007;86(5):299–315.
9. Hachulla E, Coghlan JG. A new era in the management of pulmonary arterial hypertension related to scleroderma: endothelin receptor antagonism. Ann Rheum Dis. 2004;63(9):1009–14.
10. Badesch DB, McLaughlin VV, Delcroix M, et al. Prostanoid therapy for pulmonary arterial hypertension. J Am Coll Cardiol. 2004;43(12 Suppl S):56S–61S.
11. Leighton C. Drug treatment of scleroderma. Drugs 2001;61(3):419–27.
12. Belafsky PC, Postma GN. The laryngeal and esophageal manifestations of Sjogren's syndrome. Curr Rheumatol Rep. 2003;5(4):297–303.
13. Fox RI, Chan E, Benton L, Fong S, Friedlaender M, Howell FV. Treatment of primary Sjögren's syndrome with hydroxychloroquine. Am J Med. 1988;85:62–7.
14. Fox RI, Dixon R, Guarrasi V, Krubel S. Treatment of primary Sjogren's syndrome with

hydroxychloroquine: a retrospective, open-label study. Lupus 1996;5 Suppl 1:S31–6.
15. Wallace D. Antimalarial agents and lupus. Rheum Dis Clinics NA. 1994;20:243–63.
16. Kruize A, Hene R, Kallenberg C, et al. Hydroxychloroquine treatment for primary Sjögren's syndrome: a two year double blind crossover trial. Ann Rheum Dis. 1993;52:360–4.
17. Bernstein HN. Ocular safety of hydroxychloroquine. Ann Ophthalmol. 1991;23:292–6.
18. van Woerkom JM, Kruize AA, Geenen R, et al. Safety and efficacy of leflunomide in primary Sjogren's syndrome: a phase II pilot study. BMJ 2007;66(8):1026.
19. Imai F, Suzuki T, Ishibashi T, Ohno S, Tanaka M, Dohi Y. Sulfasalazine therapy for hypergammaglobulinemia in patients with Sjögren's syndrome. Arerug [Allergy] 1994;43(1):68.
20. Price EJ, Rigby SP, Clancy U, Venables PJW. A double blind placebo controlled trial of azathioprine in the treatment of primary Sjögren's syndrome. J Rheumatol. 1998;25(5):896–9.
21. Dalavanga YA, Detrick B, Hooks JJ, Drosos AA, Moutsopoulos HM. Effect of cyclosporin A (CyA) on the immunopathological lesion of the minor salivary glands from patients with Sjögren's syndrome. Ann Rheum Dis. 1990;46:89–92.
22. Zandbelt MM, van den Hoogen FHJ, De Wilde PC, van den Berg PJS, Schneider HGF, van de Putte LBA. Reversibility of histological and immunohistological abnormalities in sublabial salivary gland biopsy specimens following treatment with corticosteroids in Sjogren's syndrome. Ann Rheum Dis. 2001;60(5):511–3.
23. Wallberg-Jonsson S, Ohman ML, Dahlqvist SR. Cardiovascular morbidity and mortality in patients with seropositive rheumatoid arthritis in Northern Sweden. J Rheumatol. 1997;24(3):445.
24. Cottin V, Donsbeck AV, Revel D, Loire R, Cordier JF. Nonspecific interstitial pneumonia individualization of a clinicopathologic entity in a series of 12 patients. Am J Resp Crit Care Med. 1998;158(4):1286–93.
25. Vourlekis JS, Brown KK, Schwarz MI. Acute interstitial pneumonitis: current understanding regarding diagnosis, pathogenesis, and natural history. Semin Resp Crit Care Med. 2001;22(4):399–408.
26. Quismorio FP, Jr. Pulmonary involvement in primary Sjogren's syndrome. Curr Opin Pulm Med. 1996;2(5):424–8.
27. Vourlekis JS, Schwarz MI, Cool CD, Tuder RM, King TE, Brown KK. Nonspecific interstitial pneumonitis as the sole histologic expression of hypersensitivity pneumonitis. Am J Med. 2002;112(6): 490–3.
28. Strimlan CV, Rosenow EC, Divertie MB, Harrison EG. Pulmonary manifestations of Sjogren's syndrome. Chest 1976;70(3):354–61.
29. Ito I, Nagai S, Kitaichi M, Nicholson AG, Johkoh T, Noma S, et al. Pulmonary manifestations of primary Sjogren's syndrome: a clinical, radiologic, and pathologic study. Am J Resp Crit Care Med. 2005;171(6):632–8.
30. Sauty A, Rochat T, Schoch OD, Hamacher J, Kurt AM, Dayer JM, et al. Pulmonary fibrosis with predominant CD8 lymphocytic alveolitis and anti-Jo-1 antibodies. Eur Resp J. 1997;10(12):2907–12.
31. Yamanaka H, Matsuda Y, Tanaka M, et al. Serum matrix metalloproteinase 3 as a predictor of the degree of joint destruction during the six months after measurement, in patients with early rheumatoid arthritis. Arthritis Rheum. 2000;43(4):852–8.
32. Burton C, Kaczmarski R, Jan-Mohamed R, Benyunes MC, Multani PS, Saunders A. Interstitial pneumonitis related to rituximab therapy. N Engl J Med. 2003;348(26):2690–1.
33. Kaufman I, Schwartz D, Caspi D, Paran D. Sjogren's syndrome—not just sicca: renal involvement in Sjogren's syndrome. Scand J Rheumatol. 2008;37(3):213–8.
34. Goules A, Masouridi S, Tzioufas AG, Ioannidis JP, Skopouli FN, Moutsopoulos HM. Clinically significant and biopsy-documented renal involvement in primary Sjogren syndrome. Medicine 2000;79(4):241–9.
35. Adam FU, Torun D, Bolat F, Zumrutdal A, Sezer S, Ozdemir FN. Acute renal failure due to mesangial proliferative glomerulonephritis in a pregnant woman with primary Sjogren's syndrome. Clin Rheumatol. 2006;25(1):75–9.
36. Goules A, Masouridi S, Tzioufas AG, Ioannidis J, Skopouli FN, Moutsopoulos HM. Clinically significant and biopsy-documented renal involvement in primary Sjogren syndrome. Medicine 2000;79(4):241.
37. Willeke P, Schlüter B, Becker H, Schotte H, Domschke W, Gaubitz M. Mycophenolate sodium treatment in patients with primary Sjögren syndrome: a pilot trial. Arthritis Res Ther. 2007;9(6):R115.
38. Devauchelle-Pensec V, Pennec Y, Morvan J, et al. Improvement of Sjogren's syndrome after two infusions of rituximab (anti-CD20). Arthritis Rheum. 2007;57(2).
39. Fox RI, Wilson C. Sjögren's syndrome: The association of interstitial nephritis and keratoconjunctivitis. New York, NY: Karger; 1993.
40. Dowd JE, Lipsky PE. Sjogren's syndrome presenting as hypokalemic periodic paralysis. Arthritis Rheum. 1993;36(12).
41. Pessler F, Emery H, Dai L, et al. The spectrum of renal tubular acidosis in paediatric Sjogren syndrome. Rheumatology 2006;45(1):85–91.
42. Nagayama Y, Shigeno M, Nakagawa Y, et al. Acquired nephrogenic diabetes insipidus secondary to distal renal tubular acidosis and nephrocalcinosis associated with Sjögren's syndrome. J Endocrinol Invest. 1994;17(8):659–63.
43. Bossini N, Savoldi S, Franceschini F, Mombelloni S, Baronio M, Cavazzana I, Viola BF, Valzorio B,

Mazzucchelli C, Cattaneo R. Clinical and morphological features of kidney involvement in primary Sjögren's syndrome. Nephrol Dial Transplant. 2001;16:2328.
44. Mason A, Golding PL. Hyperglobulinaemic renal tubular acidosis: a report of nine cases. BMJ 1970;3(5715):143.
45. Johnson RJ, Gretch DR, Yamabe H, et al. Membranoproliferative glomerulonephritis associated with hepatitis C virus infection. N Engl J Med. 1993;328(7):465–70.
46. Cortez MS, Sturgill BC, Bolton WK. Membranoproliferative glomerulonephritis with primary Sjögren's syndrome. Am J Kidney Dis. 1995;25(4):632.
47. Suzuki H, Hickling P, Lyons CBA. A case of primary Sjogren's syndrome, complicated by cryoglobulinaemic glomerulonephritis, pericardial and pleural effusions. Br Soc Rheumatol. 1996; 35(1):72–5.
48. Turner HE, Myszor MF, Bradlow A, David J. Lupus or lupoid hepatitis with mesenteric vasculitis. Br Soc Rheumatol. 1996;35(12):1309–11.
49. Bailey M, Chapin W, Licht H, Reynolds JC. The effects of vasculitis on the gastrointestinal tract and liver. Gastroenterol Clin N Am. 1998;27(4): 747–82.
50. Scott DGI. Classification and treatment of systemic vasculitis. Br Soc Rheumatol. 1988; 27(4):251–3.
51. Alarcon-Segovia D, Diaz-Jouanen E, Fishbein E. Features of Sjogren's syndrome in primary biliary cirrhosis. Ann Internal Med. 1973;79(1):31.
52. Tsianos EV, Hoofnagle JH, Fox PC, et al. Sjogren's syndrome in patients with primary biliary cirrhosis. Hepatology 1990;11(5):730–4.
53. Goulis J, Leandro G, Burroughs AK. Randomised controlled trials of ursodeoxycholic-acid therapy for primary biliary cirrhosis: a meta-analysis. Lancet 1999;354(9184):1053–60.
54. Bodenheimer H, Schaffner F, Pezzullo J. Evaluation of colchicine therapy in primary biliary cirrhosis. Gastroenterology 1988;95(1):124–9.
55. Lee SK, Green PHR. Celiac sprue (the great modern-day imposter). Curr Opin Rheumatol. 2006;18(1):101.
56. Farrell RJ, Kelly CP. Diagnosis of celiac sprue. Am J Gastroenterol. 2001;96(12):3237–46.
57. Mandl T, Granberg V, Apelqvist J, Wollmer P, Manthorpe R, Jacobsson LTH. Autonomic nervous symptoms in primary Sjogren's syndrome. Rheumatology 2008;47(6):914.
58. Koch KL, Stern RM, Stewart WR, Vasey MW. Gastric emptying and gastric myoelectrical activity in patients with diabetic gastroparesis: effect of long-term domperidone treatment. Am J Gastroenterol. 1989;84(9):1069.
59. Beuers U, Spengler U, Kruis W, et al. Ursodeoxycholic acid for treatment of primary sclerosing cholangitis: a placebo-controlled trial. Hepatology 1992;16(3):707–14.
60. Angulo P, Batts KP, Jorgensen RA, LaRusso NA, Lindor KD. Oral budesonide in the treatment of primary sclerosing cholangitis. Am J Gastroenterol. 2000;95(9):2333–37.
61. Knox TA, Kaplan MM. A double-blind controlled trial of oral-pulse methotrexate therapy in the treatment of primary sclerosing cholangitis. Gastroenterology 1994;106(2):494–9.
62. Thiel DH, Carroll P, Abu-Elmagd K, et al. Tacrolimus (FK 506), a treatment for primary sclerosing cholangitis: results of an open-label preliminary trial. Am J Gastroenterol. 1995;90(3):455–9.
63. Waterman SA, Gordon TP, Rischmueller M. Inhibitory effects of muscarinic receptor autoantibodies on parasympathetic neurotransmission in Sjogren's syndrome. Arthritis Rheum. 2000;43(7):1647–54.
64. Leppilahti M, Tammela TLJ, Huhtala H, Kiilholma P, Leppilahti K, Auvinen A. Interstitial cystitis-like urinary symptoms among patients with Sjögren's syndrome: a population-based study in Finland. Am J Med. 2003;115(1):62–5.
65. Van De Merwe JP, Yamada T, Sakamoto Y. Systemic aspects of interstitial cystitis, immunology and linkage with autoimmune disorders. Int J Urol. 2003;10:S35.
66. Esquivel CO, Bergqvist D, Björck CG, Nilsson B. Comparison between commercial heparin, low molecular weight heparin and pentosan polysulfate on hemostasis and platelets in vivo. Thromb Res. 1982;28(3):389.
67. Goad KE, Horne MDK, Gralnick HR. Pentosan-induced thrombocytopenia: support for an immune complex mechanism. Br J Haematol. 1994;88(4):803–8.
68. Skopouli FN, Papanikolaou S, Malamou-Mitsi V, Papanikolaou N, Moutsopoulos HM. Obstetric and gynaecological profile in patients with primary Sjogren's syndrome. Br Med J. 1994;53(9): 569–73.
69. Valtysdottir ST, Wide L, Hallgren R. Mental well-being and quality of sexual life in women with primary Sjogren's syndrome are related to circulating dehydroepiandrosterone sulphate. Ann Rheum Dis. 2003;62(9):875–9.
70. Mulherin DM, Sheeran TP, Kumararatne DS, Speculand B, Luesley D, Situnayake RD. Sjogren's syndrome in women presenting with chronic dyspareunia. BJOG 1997;104(9):1019–23.
71. Saad SC, Pietrzykowski JE, Lewis SS, et al. Vaginal lubrication in women with scleroderma and Sjogren's syndrome. Sex Disabil. 1999;17(2):103–13.
72. Lehrer S, Bogursky E, Yemini M, Kase NG, Birkenfeld A. Gynecologic manifestations of Sjögren's syndrome. Am J Obstet Gyn. 1994;170: 835–9.
73. Carsons S. A review and update of Sjogren's syndrome: manifestations, diagnosis, and treatment. Am J Manag Care. 2001;7(14 Supp):433–43.

74. Graziottin A. Clinical approach to dyspareunia. J Sex Marital Ther. 2001;27(5):489–501.
75. Fleming Cole N, Toy EC, Baker B. Sjogren's syndrome. Primary Care Update Ob/Gyns. 2001;8(1):48–51.
76. Johnson EO, Skopouli FN, Moutsopoulos HM. Neuroendocrine manifestations in Sjogren's syndrome. Rheum Dis Clin N Am. 2000;26(4):927–49.
77. Colditz GA, Hankinson SE, Hunter DJ, et al. The use of estrogens and progestins and the risk of breast cancer in postmenopausal women. N Engl J Med. 1995;332(24):1589–93.
78. Buyon JP, Kalunian KC, Skovron ML, et al. Can women with systemic lupus erythematosus safely use exogenous estrogens? J Clin Rheumatol. 1995;1(4):205.
79. Buyon JP, Petri MA, Kim MY, et al. The effect of combined estrogen and progesterone hormone replacement therapy on disease activity in systemic lupus erythematosus: a randomized trial. Ann Internal Med. 2005;142(12 Part 1):953–62.
80. Petri M. Long-term outcomes in lupus. Am J Manag Care. 2001;7(16 Suppl):S480–5.
81. Sullivan DA, Belanger A, Cermak JM, et al. Are women with Sjögren's syndrome androgen-deficient? J Rheumatol. 2003;30(11):2413–9.
82. Petri MA, Lahita RG, van Vollenhoven RF, et al. Effects of prasterone on corticosteroid requirements of women with systemic lupus erythematosus. Arthritis Rheum. 2002;46(7):1820–9.
83. Petri M. Exogenous estrogen in systemic lupus erythematosus: oral contraceptives and hormone replacement therapy. Lupus 2001;10(3):222–6.
84. Avery RK. Vaccination of the immunosuppressed adult patient with rheumatologic disease. Rheum Dis Clin N Am. 1999;25(3):567–84.
85. Gluck T, Muller-Ladner U, Plotkin S. Vaccination in patients with chronic rheumatic or autoimmune diseases. Clin Infect Dis. 2008;46(9):1459–65.
86. Elkayam O, Paran D, Caspi D, et al. Immunogenicity and safety of pneumococcal vaccination in patients with rheumatoid arthritis or systemic lupus erythematosus. Clin Infect Dis. 2001;34(2):147–53.
87. Pines A, Kaplinsky N, Olchovsky D, Holtzman E, Frankl O. Hyposplenism in systemic lupus erythematosus. Br Soc Rheumatol. 1983;22(3):176–8.
88. Iyngkaran P, Limaye V, Hill C, Henderson D, Pile KD, Rischmueller M. Rheumatoid vasculitis following influenza vaccination. Br Soc Rheumatol. 2003;42(7):907–9.
89. Aron-Maor A, Shoenfeld Y. Vaccination and systemic lupus erythematosus: the bidirectional dilemmas. Lupus 2001;10(3):237.
90. Maillefert JF, Sibilia J, Toussirot E, Vignon E, Eschard JP, Lorcerie B, et al. Rheumatic disorders developed after hepatitis B vaccination. Br Soc Rheumatol. 1999;38(10):978–83.
91. Daniel SJ, Diamond M. Botulinum toxin injection. Otolaryngol Head Neck Surg. 2011;145:180–1.
92. Naniwa T, Takeda Y. Long-term remission of pulmonary veno-occlusive disease associated with primary Sjögren's syndrome following immunosuppressive therapy. Modern Rheumatol 2011;1–4.
93. Carmier D, Diot E, Diot P. 2011. Shrinking lung syndrome: recognition, pathophysiology and therapeutic strategy. Expert Rev Respirat Med 5: 33–9.
94. Gillis JAZ, Panopalis P, Schmajuk G, Ramsey Goldman R, Yazdany J. 2011. Systematic review of the literature informing the systemic lupus erythematosus indicators project: Reproductive health care quality indicators. Arthritis Care Res 63: 17–30.
95. Maripuri S, Grande JP, Osborn TG, Fervenza FC, Matteson EL, Donadio JV, Hogan MC. 2009. Renal involvement in primary Sjögren's syndrome: a clinicopathologic study. Clin J Am Soc Nephrol 4:1423.

Current Treatment of Extraglandular Manifestations with Disease-Modifying and Immunosuppressive Agents

19

Athanasios G. Tzioufas and
Haralampos M. Moutsopoulos

Abstract

Sjögren's syndrome is a chronic autoimmune disorder, characterized by lymphocytic infiltration and impaired function of the exocrine glands, mainly the salivary and lacrimal glands, resulting in dry mouth and eyes. The syndrome is seen alone (primary Sjögren's syndrome) or in association with another connective tissue disease (secondary Sjögren's syndrome). Systemic features, resulting from cutaneous, respiratory, renal, hepatic, neurologic, and vascular involvement, often occur. Two types of primary Sjögren's syndrome are currently recognized: a benign disease that affects quality of life and a systemic syndrome associated with increased morbidity and mortality as well as a high risk of malignant transformation (non-Hodgkin's B-cell lymphomas). For these patients a close follow-up is required. Traditional treatments of the extraglandular manifestations include a variety of drugs, originated mainly from the treatment armamentarium of other systemic autoimmune rheumatic disease, including rheumatoid arthritis and systemic lupus erythematosus. Traditional disease-modifying antirheumatic drugs are used empirically, but their efficacy in primary Sjögren's syndrome is limited. Systemic immunosuppressives are reserved for treatment of severe extraepithelial manifestations of the disease.

Keywords

Sjögren's syndrome • Systemic disease • Extraglandular • Vasculitis • Treatment

19.1 Introduction

Sjögren's syndrome (SS) is a chronic, slowly progressing autoimmune disease, affecting 0.5–1.0% of the population, predominantly middle-aged women [1]. SS is characterized by lymphocytic infiltration of the exocrine glands, mainly the lacrimal and salivary glands resulting in impaired secretory function. Systemic features of cutaneous, respiratory, renal, hepatic, neurologic, and vascular nature are seen in more than 50% of patients. The syndrome can present either alone (connoted primary Sjögren's syndrome

A.G. Tzioufas (✉)
Department of Pathophysiology, School of Medicine, University of Athens, Athens, Greece
e-mail: agtzi@med.uoa.gr

R.I. Fox, C.M. Fox (eds.), *Sjögren's Syndrome*, DOI 10.1007/978-1-60327-957-4_19,

[pSS]) or in association with another systemic autoimmune disease, for example, rheumatoid arthritis, systemic lupus erythematosus, and systemic sclerosis (secondary Sjögren's syndrome [sSS]) [2].

Prognosis and appropriate treatment planning are important issues because of the complexity and varying nature of the disease [3]. During the past few years, two types of Sjögren's syndrome have been identified: a localized disease that affects quality of life and a systemic syndrome that is associated with increased morbidity and mortality due to the high risk of malignant transformation. Systemic Sjögren's syndrome is defined by the presence of palpable purpura, mixed monoclonal cryoglobulinemia, and low complement C4 levels at presentation [4]. So far, treatment for both types of Sjögren's syndrome is empiric. Nevertheless, a more frequent and thorough follow-up plan is needed for patients who are at increased risk of severe disease.

In Chapter 19, we discuss the current treatments for the systemic manifestations of the disease, excluding the treatment with the newer biologic agents that will be discussed in Chapter.

19.2 Extraglandular Manifestations and Outcome of Patients

Systemic manifestations are seen frequently in primary Sjögren's syndrome patients and may include general symptoms such as easy fatigue, low-grade fever, myalgias, and arthralgias and other organ involvement. Easy fatigue is often a severe problem affecting the quality of life of patients with Sjögren's syndrome [5].

The extraglandular manifestations in primary Sjögren's syndrome can be divided into two major categories.

1. The periepithelial organ involvement, such as interstitial nephritis, liver involvement, and obstructive bronchiolitis, is the result of lymphocytic invasion in the epithelia of organs beyond the affected exocrine glands. These clinical features appear early in the disease and usually have a stable and benign course.
2. The extraepithelial manifestations are produced from an immune complex deposition as a result of the ongoing B-cell hyperreactivity. Clinical findings associated with this process include palpable purpura, glomerulonephritis, and peripheral neuropathy, and they are associated with increased morbidity and risk for lymphoma development.

Based on this classification, the prognostic factors of outcome and survival have been determined. Skopouli et al. [4] studied the evolution of the clinical picture and laboratory profile, the incidence, and predictors for systemic disease, as well as the impact of clinical and laboratory findings on overall survival of the disease in a prospective cohort study of 261 Greek patients with primary Sjögren's syndrome followed for 10 years. The results were compared with the general Greek population, adjusting for age and sex. The glandular manifestations of the syndrome were typically present at the time of diagnosis, and the serological profile of patients did not significantly change during the follow-up. The extraglandular manifestations were grouped into two different populations with regard to disease outcome. Arthritis, Raynaud's phenomenon, interstitial nephritis, and lung and liver involvement appear early in the disease process. Purpura, glomerulonephritis, decreased C4 complement levels, and mixed monoclonal cryoglobulinemia were identified as adverse prognostic factors (Table 19.1). The overall mortality of patients with primary Sjögren's syndrome compared with that of the general population was

Table 19.1 Extraglandular manifestations of pSS. Cumulative prevalence of extraglandular manifestations in primary Sjögren's syndrome [4]

	Percent
Arthralgias/arthritis	75
Raynaud's phenomenon	48
Pulmonary involvement	29
Kidney involvement	
Interstitial nephritis	9
Glomerulonephritis	2
Liver involvement	4
Peripheral neuropathy	2
Myositis	1
Central nervous system disease	0
Lymphoma	4

Table 19.2 Therapy for systemic features of pSS with DMARDs and immunosuppressive agents

General manifestations	Main therapeutic modalities
Fatigue	Tricyclic antidepressants, exercise, myofascial therapy
Arthritis	Hydroxychloroquine, methotrexate
Raynaud's phenomenon	Avoidance of cold and stress exposure, calcium channel blockers
Periepithelial organ involvement	
Liver Primary biliary cirrhosis	Ursodeoxycholic acid
Autoimmune hepatitis	Corticosteroids, prednisolone (0.5–1.0 mg/kg body weight per day) Azathioprine (2 mg/kg body weight per day)
Kidney Interstitial nephritis, tubular dysfunction of renal tubular acidosis	Oral potassium and sodium carbonate (3–12 g per day)
Lung Bronchial and/or bronchiolar involvement (common, indolent course)	*Mucolytics* Small effect of steroids and β(beta)-agonists
Extraepithelial organ involvement	
Kidney Immune complex-mediated glomerulonephritis	Prednisolone (0.5–1.0 mg/kg body weight per day) Intravenous cyclophosphamide (0.5–1 g/m^2 of body surface/month)
Vasculitis	Prednisolone (0.5–1.0 mg/kg body weight per day) Cyclophosphamide (0.5–1 g/m^2 of body surface/month) Plasmapheresis
Lung Interstitial lung disease	Azathioprine (2 mg/kg body weight per day)
Central nervous system disease	Pulse steroids (1 g methylprednisolone for 3 consecutive days) Prednisolone (0.5–1.0 mg/kg body weight per day) Cyclophosphamide (0.5–1 g/m^2 of body surface/month) Azathioprine (2 mg/kg body weight per day)
Peripheral neuropathy	Steroids (1 g methylprednisolone for 3 consecutive days) Cyclophosphamide (0.5–1 g/m^2 of body surface/month) Azathioprine (2 mg/kg body weight per day) Plasmapheresis Intravenous gammaglobulin

increased only in patients with adverse predictors. Similar results were reported by two other important studies that identified hypocomplementemia and palpable purpura as significant predictors of death, largely due to lymphoproliferative malignancy [6, 7].

19.3 Management of Extraglandular Manifestations

The treatment of the systemic manifestations of Sjögren's syndrome is not evidence-based because of the lack of large, controlled, randomized studies. Instead, most of the regimens given are largely empiric and case dependent (Table 19.2) [8]. Most of the traditional disease-modifying antirheumatic drugs (DMARDs) used in rheumatoid arthritis and systemic lupus erythematosus have been tried also in pSS with limited results, both in sicca syndrome and as disease-modifying agents. These regimens, however, may be beneficial for the management of more severe, systemic manifestations often observed in pSS [9].

19.3.1 Fatigue

Fatigue is observed in approximately 50% of patients with Sjögren's syndrome and manifests as an increased need for resting hours [10, 11]. In these patients, concomitant hypothyroidism, fibromyalgia, lymphoma, or underlying depression should be considered. In cases of fibromyalgia, tricyclic antidepressants should be carefully used because they can exacerbate the dryness of patients; regular exercise and myofascial therapy could be of benefit [8].

19.3.2 Musculoskeletal

A half of patients with pSS experience intermittent episodes of arthritis during the course of their disease. In some instances, arthritis may precede sicca manifestations. Articular signs and symptoms include arthralgias, morning stiffness, intermittent synovitis, and chronic polyarthritis, which may sometimes lead to Jaccoud's arthropathy [12]. In contrast to rheumatoid arthritis, radiographs of the hands usually do not reveal bone erosions.

Hydroxychloroquine has been successfully used for the treatment of constitutional and musculoskeletal symptoms as well as non-vasculitic cutaneous lesions in pSS. Its mechanism of action is not yet clarified, but experimental data have shown that hydroxychloroquine interferes with antigen presentation [13] and the production of pro-inflammatory cytokines (IL-1α and IL-6) [14]. Hydroxychloroquine may also inhibit glandular cholinesterase that may contribute to glandular hypofunction in SS [15]. In terms of laboratory findings, hydroxychloroquine has been shown to improve the levels of IgG, erythrocyte sedimentation rate, antinuclear antibody, rheumatoid factor, and IL-6 [16–20].

pSS patients should not be treated with steroids for long-time periods because, in addition to their well-known side effects, steroids may also accelerate the periodontal disease and oral candidiasis [21].

Methotrexate, the most widely used DMARD in rheumatoid arthritis, has also been used for the treatment of polyarticular inflammatory arthritis of pSS. An open-label, non-controlled trial by Skopouli et al. in 17 patients with pSS showed improvement in sicca symptoms, frequency of parotid gland enlargement, and purpura but no benefit in objective parameters of dry eyes and mouth [22]. Immunoglobulin levels, autoantibody positivity, cryoglobulins, or complement levels remained unaffected. Persistent asymptomatic elevations of liver enzymes that occurred in methotrexate-treated individuals in higher frequency in pSS, compared with rheumatoid arthritis, led to dose reduction or discontinuation of treatment in 41% of patients. Other DMARDs including azathioprine, sulfasalazine, leflunomide, and cyclosporine have not shown any significant effect [9].

19.3.3 Raynaud's Phenomenon

Raynaud's phenomenon is the most common manifestation of the skin, seen in one-third of patients with pSS. It usually precedes sicca manifestations by many years, and, therefore, patients with Raynaud's phenomenon should be regularly followed-up for subjective sicca manifestations. Patients with Raynaud's phenomenon present with swollen hands, but, in contrast to those with scleroderma, they do not develop telangiectasias or digital ulcers. Hand radiographs of these patients may show small tissue calcifications. Furthermore, these patients present more frequently with non-erosive arthritis, compared to those without Raynaud's phenomenon [23]. For the treatment of Raynaud's phenomenon, avoidance of physical and emotional stress, along with administration of calcium channel blockers or angiotensin-converting enzyme inhibitors, seems to be sufficient measures [23, 24].

19.3.4 Gastrointestinal Manifestations

Patients with Sjögren's syndrome may frequently present with varying degrees of esophageal dysmotility, mainly manifesting as gastroesophageal reflux [25]. They may also develop laryngopharyngeal reflux, a newly recognized disease that produces local symptoms and laryngeal changes caused by the reflux of gastric contents into the upper aerodigestive tract [26]. Unlike classic gastroesophageal reflux, esophagitis, heartburn, or complaints of regurgitation are rare symptoms. Treatment options include gastric acid suppression and lifestyle modifications.

19.3.5 Liver Involvement

The liver is affected in a small number (5%) of patients with pSS. These patients present with elevated liver enzymes and antimitochondrial antibodies [27, 28]. The liver biopsy discloses histopathologic lesions of stage I primary biliary cirrhosis. In these patients, ursodeoxycholic acid can be of some benefit. Autoimmune hepatitis can also occur, requiring treatment with prednisolone and azathioprine [29].

19.3.6 Lung Involvement

Manifestations from the tracheobronchial tree are frequent but rarely clinically important. They can present either with dry cough secondary to dryness of the tracheobronchial mucosa (xerotrachea) or dyspnea due to airway obstruction or interstitial lung disease. The major finding of lung involvement is small airways obstruction, which is frequently associated with mild hypoxemia. Chest radiography shows mild interstitial-like changes, and high-resolution computed tomography (CT) of the lung in patients with abnormal chest radiography reveals wall thickening at the segmental bronchi. Transbronchial and/or endobronchial biopsy specimens discloses peribronchial and/or peribronchiolar mononuclear inflammation [30]. Non-specific interstitial pneumonia (NSIP) is also a common pathologic finding [31]. However, severe interstitial disease in Sjögren's syndrome is rare and is appreciated only after a complete functional and radiological evaluation of the patient. In most patients, the use of β(beta)-agonists and corticosteroids demonstrated little benefit. In rare cases of interstitial lung disease, prednisolone administration, with or without an immunosuppressive agent (azathioprine), might be a viable option.

19.3.7 Kidney Involvement

Clinically significant and biopsy-documented renal disease is observed in approximately 5% of patients with pSS [32]. Two forms of renal involvement have been described, interstitial nephritis or glomerulonephritis. Subclinical involvement of the renal tubules can be seen in one-third of patients, as attested by an abnormal urine acidification test. Renal biopsy typically reveals interstitial lymphocytic infiltration. Most patients present with hyposthenuria and hypokalemic, hyperchloremic distal renal tubular acidosis, reflecting interstitial infiltration and destruction by lymphocytes. Distal tubular acidosis may be clinically silent, but if left untreated, significant renal tubular acidosis may lead to renal stones, nephrocalcinosis, and compromised renal function. Such patients may present with recurrent renal colic and/or hypokalemic muscular weakness. Less commonly, Sjögren's syndrome patients have proximal tubular acidosis with Fanconi's syndrome. Hypokalemic hyperchloremic acidosis, the most serious manifestation of tubular dysfunction, can be treated with oral potassium and sodium bicarbonate [33, 34].

Membranous or membranoproliferative glomerulonephritis in Sjögren's syndrome has been described in few patients. Cryoglobulinemia, associated with hypocomplementemia, is a consistent serological finding in these cases [35]. Interstitial nephritis is usually an early feature of the syndrome, whereas glomerulonephritis is a late sequel [32]. Glomerulonephritis is mainly treated with prednisolone and/or pulse intravenous cyclophosphamide. In cases of treatment of refractory disease, caution is required, however, because the use of cytotoxic agents is associated with a 100-fold increase in the incidence of lymphoma in patients with Sjögren's syndrome [36].

19.3.8 Neurologic Involvement

Peripheral neurologic involvement is found in 5–10% of patients with pSS. In contrast, the presence of central nervous system involvement is a matter of debate with descriptions ranging from "undetectable" to "quite common" and a variety of reported clinical manifestations, including multiple sclerosis-like disease, stroke, transverse myelitis, or psychiatric manifestations [37, 38]. Because of the rarity of cases, controlled therapeutic trials are lacking. However, immunosuppressive treatments with pulse intravenous cyclophosphamide, in combination with steroids, are currently considered the treatment strategy of choice [39]. The early institution of treatment during the course of the disease is crucial and mostly beneficial [40]. Azathioprine, methotrexate, mycophenolate mofetil, or cyclosporine may be used in the failure or intolerance of cyclophosphamide. In the case of progressing neurologic symptoms, IVIg and plasmapheresis may be considered [39].

The peripheral, primary sensory neuropathies usually respond poorly to treatment (reviewed in Ref. [9]); however, stabilization of symptoms, spontaneous or after treatment, is often seen [41]. In multiple mononeuropathies, nerve biopsy frequently reveals vasculitis, which may explain the efficacy of steroids and immunosuppressive drugs. In contrast, steroids appear to have a poor effect in axonal polyneuropathies [38]. IVIg has recently demonstrated benefit [42–44], even in cases resistant to treatment or long-standing sensory neuropathy [45, 46]. A recent work has shown that IVIg improves SS-related dysautonomia, by anti-idiotypic antibodies neutralizing serum IgG against the muscarinic M3 receptors [47]. Case presentations of patients with sensory neuropathy treated with plasmapheresis [48] have been reported.

19.3.9 Hematologic Involvement

Patients with pSS present with hypergammaglobulinemia and mild asymptomatic autoimmune cytopenias. Serious manifestations, such as severe cytopenias, may occur infrequently and warrant more aggressive treatment [49]. Steroids are the first-line treatment for autoimmune cytopenias with the additional steroid-sparing agent azathioprine or danazol [49, 50]. Cyclophosphamide, or methotrexate, has been reported in cases of autoimmune hemolytic anemia, thrombocytopenia, and agranulocytosis, respectively [50, 51]. IVIg in combination with cyclosporine has been tried in agranulocytosis complicating pSS [51, 52].

19.4 Conclusions

The systemic manifestations of pSS are observed in more than 50% of patients comprising the main factors for increased morbidity of the disease. Extraglandular manifestations are divided into periepithelial (liver, lung, and interstitial nephritis) and extraepithelial (palpable purpura, nervous system involvement, and glomerulonephritis) with the latter being the main prognostic factors for poor outcome. Their treatment remains mostly empiric and symptom-based. Current immunosuppressive therapies appear to be unable to modify the course of the disease. The association of traditional treatments with newer promising biologic agents is still an unaddressed question. To this end, well-constructed epidemiologic and basic science data are needed to move treatment of this disorder from the empiric to a more scientific, etiologic approach.

References

1. Dafni UG, Tzioufas AG, Staikos P, Skopouli FN, Moutsopoulos HM. Prevalence of Sjögren's syndrome in a closed rural community. Ann Rheum Dis. 1997;56:521–5.
2. Tzioufas AG, Voulgarelis M. Update on Sjögren's syndrome autoimmune epithelitis: from classification to increased neoplasias. Best Pract Res Clin Rheumatol. 2007;21:989–1010.
3. Kassan SS, Moutsopoulos HM. Clinical manifestations and early diagnosis of Sjögren's syndrome. Arch Intern Med. 2004;164:1275–84.
4. Skopouli FN, Dafni U, Ioannidis JP, Moutsopoulos HM. Clinical evolution, and morbidity and mortality

of primary Sjögren's syndrome. Semin Arthritis Rheum. 2000;29: 296–304.
5. Strombeck B, Ekdahl C, Manthorpe R, Jacobsson LT. Physical capacity in women with primary Sjogren's syndrome: a controlled study. Arthritis Rheum. 2003;49:681–8.
6. Ioannidis JP, Vassiliou VA, Moutsopoulos HM. Long-term risk of mortality and lymphoproliferative disease and predictive classification of primary Sjogren's syndrome. Arthritis Rheum. 2002; 46:741–7.
7. Theander E, Manthorpe R, Jacobsson LT. Mortality and causes of death in primary Sjogren's syndrome: a prospective cohort study. Arthritis Rheum. 2004;50:1262–9.
8. Mavragani CP, Moutsopoulos NM, Moutsopoulos HM. The management of Sjögren's syndrome. Nat Clin Pract Rheumatol. 2006;2:252–61.
9. Thanou-Stavraki A, James JA. Primary Sjogren's syndrome: current and prospective therapies. Semin Arthritis Rheum. 2008;37:273–92.
10. Barendregt PJ, Visser MR, Smets EM, et al. Fatigue in primary Sjögren's syndrome. Ann Rheum Dis. 1998;57:291–5.
11. d'Elia HF, Rehnberg E, Kvist G, Ericsson A, Konttinen Y, Mannerkorpi K. Fatigue and blood pressure in primary Sjogren's syndrome. Scand J Rheumatol. 2008;37:284–92.
12. M'Rad S, Ben Miled K, Makni S, et al. Jaccoud's arthropathy in primary Sjögren's syndrome with benign hypergammaglobulinaemic purpura. Eur J Med. 1993;2:373–5.
13. Fox RI, Kang HI. Mechanism of action of antimalarial drugs: inhibition of antigen processing and presentation. Lupus 1993;2:S9–12.
14. Sperber K, Quraishi H, Kalb TH, Panja A, Stecher V, Mayer L. Selective regulation of cytokine secretion by hydroxychloroquine: inhibition of interleukin 1 alpha (IL-1-alpha) and IL-6 in human monocytes and T cells. J Rheumatol. 1993;20: 803–8.
15. Dawson LJ, Caulfield VL, Stanbury JB, Field AE, Christmas SE, Smith PM. Hydroxychloroquine therapy in patients with primary Sjogren's syndrome may improve salivary gland hypofunction by inhibition of glandular cholinesterase. Rheumatology 2005;44:449–55.
16. Lakhanpal S, Duffy J, Griffing WL, Conn DL, Luthra HS. Sjogren's syndrome: treatment with D-penicillamine and hydroxychloroquine. J Rheumatol. 1985;12:1028–9.
17. Fox RI, Chan E, Benton L, Fong S, Friedlaender M, Howell FV. Treatment of primary Sjogren's syndrome with hydroxychloroquine. Am J Med. 1988;85:62–7.
18. Kruize AA, Hene RJ, Kallenberg CG, et al. Hydroxychloroquine treatment for primary Sjogren's syndrome: a two year double blind crossover trial. Ann Rheum Dis. 1993;52:360–4.
19. Fox RI, Dixon R, Guarrasi V, Krubel S. Treatment of primary Sjogren's syndrome with hydroxychloroquine: a retrospective, open-label study. Lupus 1996;5:S31–6.
20. Tishler M, Yaron I, Shirazi I, Yaron M. Hydroxychloroquine treatment for primary Sjogren's syndrome: its effect on salivary and serum inflammatory markers. Ann Rheum Dis. 1999;58:253–6.
21. Fox RI. Sjogren's syndrome. Lancet. 2005;366: 321–31.
22. Skopouli FN, Jagiello P, Tsifetaki N, Moutsopoulos HM. Methotrexate in primary Sjogren's syndrome. Clin Exp Rheumatol. 1996;14:555–8.
23. Skopouli FN, Talal A, Galanopoulou V, et al. Raynaud's phenomenon in primary Sjögren's syndrome. J Rheumatol. 1990;17:618–20.
24. Garcia-Carrasco M, Sisó A, Ramos-Casals M, et al. Raynaud's phenomenon in primary Sjögren's syndrome. Prevalence and clinical characteristics in a series of 320 patients. J Rheumatol. 2002;29:726–30.
25. Volter F, Fain O, Mathieu E, Thomas M. Esophageal function and Sjögren's syndrome. Dig Dis Sci. 2004;49:248–53.
26. Ford CN. Evaluation and management of laryngopharyngeal reflux. JAMA 2005;294:1534–40.
27. Skopouli FN, Barbatis C, Moutsopoulos HM. Liver involvement in primary Sjögren's syndrome. Br J Rheumatol. 1994;33:745–8.
28. Hatzis GS, Fragoulis GE, Karatzaferis A, Delladetsima I, Barbatis C, Moutsopoulos HM. Prevalence and long term course of primary biliary cirrhosis in primary Sjögren's syndrome. J Rheumatol. 2008;35:2012–6.
29. Matsumoto T, Morizane T, Aoki Y, et al. Autoimmune hepatitis in primary Sjogren's syndrome: pathological study of the livers and labial salivary glands in 17 patients with primary Sjogren's syndrome. Pathol Int. 2005;55:70–6.
30. Papiris SA, Maniati M, Constantopoulos SH, Roussos C, Moutsopoulos HM, Skopouli FN. Lung involvement in primary Sjögren's syndrome is mainly related to the small airway disease. Ann Rheum Dis. 1999;58:61–4
31. Ito I, Nagai S, Kitaichi M, et al. Pulmonary manifestations of primary Sjogren's syndrome: a clinical, radiologic, and pathologic study. Am J Respir Crit Care Med. 2005;171:632–8.
32. Goules A, Masouridi S, Tzioufas AG, Ioannidis JP, Skopouli FN, Moutsopoulos HM. Clinically significant and biopsy-documented renal involvement in primary Sjögren syndrome. Medicine 2000;79: 241–9
33. Pessler F, Emery H, Dai L, et al. The spectrum of renal tubular acidosis in paediatric Sjögren syndrome. Rheumatology 2006;45:85–91
34. Siamopoulos KC, Mavridis AK, Elisaf M, Drosos AA, Moutsopoulos HM. Kidney involvement in primary Sjögren's syndrome. Scand J Rheumatol Suppl. 1986;61:156–60

35. Moutsopoulos HM, Balow JE, Lawley TJ, Stahl NI, Antonovych TT, Chused TM. Immune complex glomerulonephritis in sicca syndrome. Am J Med. 1978;64:955–60.
36. Linardaki G, Moutsopoulos HM. The uncertain role of immuno-suppressive agents in Sjögren's syndrome. Cleve Clin J Med. 1997;64: 523–6.
37. Soliotis FC, Mavragani CP, Moutsopoulos HM. Central nervous system involvement in Sjogren's syndrome. Ann Rheum Dis. 2004;63:616–20.
38. Delalande S, de Seze J, Fauchais AL, et al. Neurologic manifestations in primary Sjögren syndrome: a study of 82 patients. Medicine 2004;83:280–91.
39. Rogers SJ, Williams CS, Roman GC. Myelopathy in Sjogren's syndrome: role of nonsteroidal immunosuppressants. Drugs 2004;64:123–32.
40. de Seze J, Delalande S, Fauchais AL, et al. Myelopathies secondary to Sjogren's syndrome: treatment with monthly intravenous cyclophosphamide associated with corticosteroids. J Rheumatol. 2006;33:709–11.
41. Font J, Ramos-Casals M, de la Red G, et al. Pure sensory neuropathy in primary Sjogren's syndrome. Long-term prospective follow-up and review of the literature. J Rheumatol. 2003;30:1552–7.
42. Molina JA, Benito-Leon J, Bermejo F, Jimenez-Jimenez FJ, Olivan J. Intravenous immunoglobulin therapy in sensory neuropathy associated with Sjogren's syndrome. J Neurol Neurosurg Psychiatry. 1996;60:699.
43. Pascual J, Cid C, Berciano J. High-dose i.v. immunoglobulin for peripheral neuropathy associated with Sjogren's syndrome. Neurology 1998;51:650–1.
44. Kizawa M, Mori K, Iijima M, Koike H, Hattori N, Sobue G. Intravenous immunoglobulin treatment in painful sensory neuropathy without sensory ataxia associated with Sjogren's syndrome. J Neurol Neurosurg Psychiatry. 2006;77:967–9.
45. Takahashi Y, Takata T, Hoshino M, Sakurai M, Kanazawa I. Benefit of IVIG for long-standing ataxic sensory neuronopathy with Sjogren's syndrome. Neurology 2003;60:503–5.
46. Wolfe GI, Nations SP, Burns DK, Herbelin LL, Barohn RJ. Benefit of IVIg for long-standing ataxic sensory neuronopathy with Sjogren's syndrome. Neurology 2003;61:873.
47. Cavill D, Waterman SA, Gordon TP. Antiidiotypic antibodies neutralize auto-antibodies that inhibit cholinergic neurotransmission. Arthritis Rheum. 2003;48:3597–602.
48. Chen WH, Yeh JH, Chiu HC. Plasmapheresis in the treatment of ataxic sensory neuropathy associated with Sjogren's syndrome. Eur Neurol. 2001;45: 270–4.
49. Ramos-Casals M, Font J, Garcia-Carrasco M, et al. Primary Sjogren syndrome: hematologic patterns of disease expression. Medicine 2002;81:281–92.
50. Schattner A, Friedman J, Klepfish A, Berrebi A. Immune cytopenias as the presenting finding in primary Sjogren's syndrome. QJM 2000;93: 825–9.
51. Friedman J, Klepfish A, Miller EB, Ognenovski V, Ike RW, Schattner A. Agranulocytosis in Sjogren's syndrome: two case reports and analysis of 11 additional reported cases. Semin Arthritis Rheum. 2002;31:338–45.
52. Coppo P, Sibilia J, Maloisel F, et al. Primary Sjogren's syndrome associated agranulocytosis: a benign disorder? Ann Rheum Dis. 2003;62: 476–8.

20 Lymphoproliferation and Lymphoma in Sjögren's Syndrome

Justin Pijpe, Hendrika Bootsma, and Gustaaf W. van Imhoff

Abstract

A multidisciplinary approach is necessary for evaluation and treatment of patients with mucosa-associated lymphoid tissue (MALT)-type lymphoma and associated Sjögren's syndrome (MALT–SS). If asymptomatic MALT lymphoma is detected in a parotid biopsy by chance during a routine diagnostic procedure for SS, and there are no severe extraglandular manifestations of SS present, staging and treatment of MALT lymphoma may probably be deferred. In other patients with MALT–SS both SS activity and symptoms of MALT lymphoma (e.g., large swelling, pain) should be taken into account to guide treatment. Future clinical studies in MALT–SS patients should determine the clinical significance of asymptomatic clonal B-cell infiltrate in patients with SS and the place of maintenance treatment with monoclonal antibodies in long-term disease control.

Keywords

Sjögren's syndrome • MALT lymphoma • Treatment

20.1 Introduction

Sjögren's syndrome (SS) is a systemic autoimmune disease characterized by chronic inflammation of salivary and lacrimal glands, frequently accompanied by systemic symptoms. Five percent of patients with SS develop malignant B-cell lymphoma, 48–75% of which are of mucosa-associated lymphoid tissue (MALT)-type. These B-cell lymphomas are most frequently located in the parotid gland [1–3]. A recent analysis showed that SS was associated with a 6.6-fold increased risk of non-Hodgkin lymphoma, and secondary SS yielded a higher risk than the primary form [4]. Moreover, this study showed a 1,000-fold increase in relative risk of MALT lymphoma localized in the parotid glands in patients with SS. This finding is consistent with biological evidence of antigen-driven clonal B-cell expansions in the affected salivary glands. An immune reaction to specific antigenic stimulation is also believed to play an important

J. Pijpe (✉)
Department of Oral and Maxillofacial Surgery, Catharina Hospital Eindhoven, Eindhoven, The Netherlands;
University Medical Center, Groningen, The Netherlands
e-mail: j.pijpe@gmail.com

R.I. Fox, C.M. Fox (eds.), *Sjögren's Syndrome*, DOI 10.1007/978-1-60327-957-4_20,

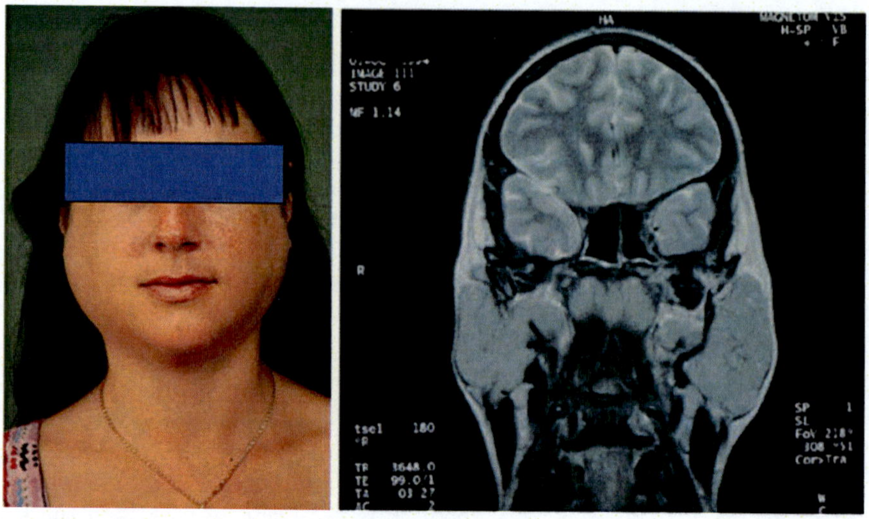

Fig. 20.1 **a** Enlarged parotid gland in a patient with SS and MALT lymphoma. **b** Coronal MRI of same patient showing cystic enlarged parotid glands and bilateral lymphadenopathy

role in other MALT lymphomas, such as *Helicobacter pylori* in gastric MALT lymphoma, *Borrelia burgdorferi* in skin, and *Chlamydia trachomatis* in ocular MALT lymphoma [5]. Apart from persistently enlarged parotid glands (Fig. 20.1a), the emergence of lymphoma in SS (MALT–SS) is frequently heralded by extraglandular manifestations of SS (e.g., palpable purpura, vasculitis, renal involvement, and peripheral neuropathy). None of these features are specific, but any of them should raise suspicion, particularly if accompanied by features such as monoclonal gammopathy, reduced levels of complement C4, $CD4^+$ T lymphocytopenia, or cryoglobulinemia (Table 20.1) [6–10]. Ioannidis et al. demonstrated that lymphoproliferative disease was independently predicted by parotid gland enlargement, palpable purpura, and low C4 levels [7].

In general, MALT lymphoma is an indolent disease, with a reported 5-year overall survival between 86 and 95%, without significant difference in clinical course between localized and disseminated disease [12, 13]. Recurrences may involve extranodal or nodal sites and transformation into aggressive diffuse large B-cell lymphoma is rare, occurring in less than 10% of the cases [14].

The traditional Ann Arbor staging system, mainly designed for nodal lymphoma, is not very informative for patients with MALT lymphoma. For instance, involvement of multiple extranodal sites, i.e., multiple salivary glands in case of MALT–SS, may neither reflect truly disseminated disease as in nodal lymphoma types nor confer inferior prognosis associated with stage IV disease in nodal lymphoma [5]. MALT–SS is often localized at one or more salivary sites (usually the parotid gland[s]), but can occur also in other extranodal sites, such as the orbital adnexa and stomach [15, 16]. Dissemination of MALT–SS is usually detected in local draining lymph nodes. Distant lymph nodes, other mucosal sites, or bone marrow is seldomly involved [17].

Table 20.1 Risk factors for lymphoma development in SS [11]

• Persistent parotid gland enlargement
• Palpable purpura
• Low C3, C4
• Cryoglobulinemia
• Monoclonal paraproteinemia
• Increased β(beta)-2 microglobulin
• Lymphocytopenia
• Hypoglobulinemia

In our experience with the follow-up of 35 patients with MALT–SS, 25 patients (71%) showed only localization of lymphoma in the salivary glands, 6 patients (17%) showed local regional nodal dissemination, and bone marrow involvement was observed in only 1 patient (3%). Of the remaining three patients, there was lacrimal gland involvement in two and involvement of the stomach in one. No transformation into diffuse large B-cell lymphoma was observed.

Overall survival does not seem to be influenced by its spreading to other MALT organs, although involvement of lymph nodes might be an adverse prognostic factor for transformation into high-grade lymphoma [13, 17].

The relative infrequency and heterogeneity of MALT lymphomas in general, with their clinical presentation varying according to the site of involvement, make it difficult to define optimal treatment of these lymphomas. There is increasing evidence that antibiotics can be used as initial treatment of MALT lymphoma associated with microbial pathogens, such as gastric MALT lymphoma associated with *H. pylori* [18–21]. In other MALT lymphomas, local treatment (surgery or radiotherapy) results in excellent disease control in symptomatic local disease [5]. In the head and neck region, however, conventional radiotherapy (25–39 Gy) may lead to significant residual xerostomia, especially when the salivary glands are irradiated [22, 23]. An alternative might be low-dose 2 × 2 Gy involved field radiotherapy, which is very effective in follicular lymphoma [24], and experience with this therapy in the treatment of MALT seems promising [15, 25]. For symptomatic disseminated disease chemotherapy is commonly used, with 75% complete remission rate and 5-year event-free survival and overall survival rates at 50 and 75%, respectively [12, 13, 26–28]. Rituximab, a chimeric murine/human anti-CD20 monoclonal antibody, has proven to be highly efficacious in patients with indolent and aggressive B-cell lymphoma, alone or in combination with chemotherapy [15, 29–32].

At present, no clear guidelines exist for the management of patients with MALT–SS. These patients usually show an uncomplicated clinical course with a median overall survival of 6.4 years, both treated and untreated patients showed the same overall survival [3]. A retrospective analysis reported no significant differences in outcomes among MALT–SS patients undergoing surgery, radiotherapy, and chemotherapy [17]. Rituximab has also been used effectively in patients with MALT lymphoma, with or without associated SS [33–37].

In our view, morbidity in patients with MALT–SS is not only determined by lymphoma, but also, maybe even more, by extraglandular activity of SS. Therefore, in patients with MALT–SS, both lymphoma and SS disease activity need to be addressed—not only clinical characteristics of the lymphoma, but also the severity of SS manifestations might determine the choice of treatment.

20.2 Diagnosis

MALT lymphoma in patients with SS is part of a spectrum from indolent asymptomatic lymphoma without disease activity of SS, up to locally disseminated lymphoma with severe extraglandular SS manifestations. Patients suspected of SS should undergo complete SS diagnostics according to the latest consensus criteria [38]. In the European–American consensus criteria for diagnosing SS, pre-existent lymphoma is considered to be an exclusion criterion, because lymphoma of the parotid gland can cause mouth dryness and parotid gland swelling [38]. This criterion should be reconsidered with respect to the exclusion of MALT lymphoma, as this type of lymphoma could be considered as a continuum of SS. The majority of these lymphomas are associated with SS or other autoimmune diseases [17, 39]. Therefore, patients with MALT lymphoma of the salivary glands should also be further evaluated for SS, especially since patients with MALT lymphoma and associated SS usually have a more severe form of SS. Vasculitis, peripheral nerve involvement, nephritis, fever, anemia, and lymphopenia are observed significantly more often in MALT–SS patients than in the general SS population [3].

Patients must be evaluated by a multidisciplinary team, consisting of a rheumatologist/

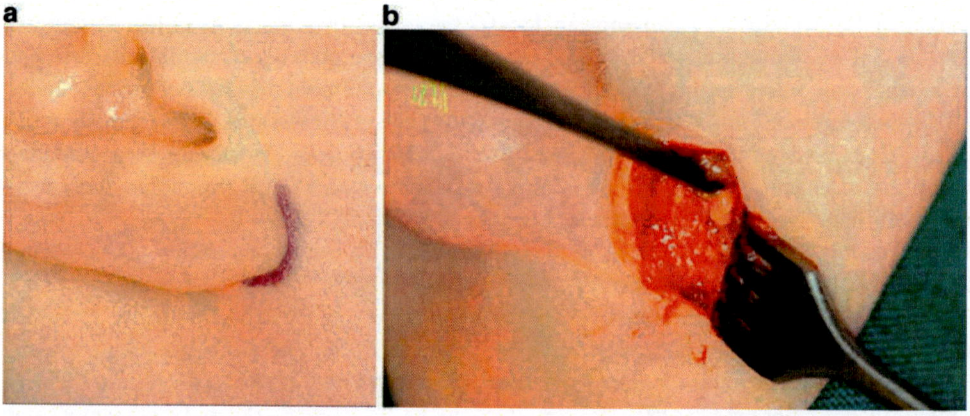

Fig. 20.2 Biopsy technique of parotid gland according to the technique described by Kraaijenhagen [47]. In short, a 1-cm skin incision is performed around the lower earlobe under local anesthesia. After blunt dissection to the parotid gland, an incisional biopsy is taken. The wound is closed in layers, no post-operative drape is applied

internist, ophthalmologist, oral and maxillofacial surgeon or ENT specialist, and a pathologist. Serological analysis should not only focus on anti-SSA/SSB autoantibodies, but also on IgM-Rf, immunoglobulins, complements C3 and C4, cryoglobulins, and monoclonal protein. Detection of early MALT lymphoma in the major salivary glands of patients with SS is often difficult because histopathological features are subtle, and monoclonal expansion does not necessarily indicate presence of malignant lymphoma. Whether monoclonal B-cell populations in lymphoepithelial lesions represent lymphoma or more benign types of expansion remains controversial [40].

We recently showed that for the diagnosis of SS, an incision of the parotid gland has the same diagnostic potential comparable with that of the labial salivary gland (for the technique, see Fig. 20.2) [41]. An incision biopsy of the parotid gland for the diagnosis of SS might lead to early detection of MALT lymphoma, but the clinical relevance of asymptomatic early MALT detection is not known. We studied 11 patients who underwent a parotid biopsy for the diagnostic work-up of SS, in whom MALT lymphoma was detected by chance [42]. There was no clinical suspicion of lymphoma (e.g., no parotid gland swelling). These patients generally had localized disease and showed no progression during follow-up when left untreated. Although localization of lymphoma in the labial glands has been described incidentally [43], the parotid gland is the location of preference, and this must be kept in mind when performing an incision biopsy of the parotid gland in the routine diagnosis of SS. In patients with a persistent swelling of the parotid gland with or without SS, fine-needle aspiration (FNA) is the evaluation of choice to differ between benign or malignant disease. FNA and immunophenotyping by flow cytometry are complementary and might be useful in the differential diagnosis of non-Hodgkin lymphoma [44, 45], however, final diagnosis and subtyping of non-Hodgkin lymphoma requires an incision biopsy or a superficial parotidectomy [46]. Imaging of MALT lymphoma is described in Fig. 20.1.

20.3 Staging and Evaluation of Treatment Response

It is debatable whether it is necessary to perform full staging in patients with MALT–SS, including CT scans of thorax and abdomen and bone marrow biopsy. Bone marrow involvement is rare in the patients described and probably does neither influence prognosis nor treatment [12]. Although in MALT–SS the lymphoma usually arises in the main target of the autoimmune disease, i.e., the parotid gland, localization in other mucosal sites can occur [16]. Furthermore, these extranodal localizations are often difficult to detect by CT scan. It might be advisable to evaluate salivary glands by imaging or biopsy in patients with SS and MALT lymphoma localized at other extranodal sites. Imaging of MALT lymphoma of the parotid gland by MRI often reveals a localized or a diffuse lesion in the gland accompanied by multiple cysts, which probably represent focal dilatations of salivary ducts resulting from compression of terminal ducts by the lymphoma (Fig. 20.1b) [48].

Criteria for response to treatment in patients with MALT–SS are not standardized. The International Working Group response criteria for non-Hodgkin lymphoma [49] are not sufficient, as both MALT and SS activity must be evaluated in order to monitor clinically relevant response to treatment. Response criteria for lymphoma of the salivary gland should be based on clinical, radiological, and pathological criteria. Physical examination of head and neck, in combination with CT scan or MRI, is recommended to determine salivary gland involvement and locoregional lymphadenopathy. Post-treatment parotid biopsies may offer an additional method for evaluating treatment and have low morbidity [50]. However, criteria for the diagnosis of residual disease and complete remission of MALT in biopsies are not clearly defined. As in gastric MALT lymphoma after *H. pylori* eradication, residual lymphoid infiltrate may still be present in parotid gland tissue in patients with SS, making evaluation of histological response difficult [51]. Moreover, these infiltrates will most likely never completely disappear in SS as they are an integral part of the ongoing autoimmune disease. Moreover, the clinical significance of these infiltrates, as in case of finding MALT lymphoma by chance in parotid biopsies during work-up for SS, is not well defined.

20.4 Treatment

There is no evidence-based treatment for SS. Corticosteroids and disease-modifying antirheumatic drugs (DMARDs) have no major effect on disease course of SS [52], although in selected patients prednisone seems to improve salivary flow and clinical and histological features [53–55]. Cyclophosphamide, with or without prednisone, has been shown to be effective in patients with renal involvement and in different other severe extraglandular complications of SS, such as systemic vasculitis and polyneuropathy [6, 56, 57]. Currently, B-cell-directed therapies (B-cell depletion) seem very promising [58]. Rituximab, alone or in combination with cyclophosphamide and prednisone (R–CP), has also been reported to be of benefit in patients with secondary SS [36, 59, 60]. A recent review showed rituximab to be efficient regarding its effects on systemic complications and fatigue in patients with SS [61]. Currently, rituximab is standard of care for treatment of symptomatic disseminated B-cell lymphoma. It is usually combined with chemotherapy, although it is effective as single agent as well in selected cases of indolent lymphoma including MALT lymphoma [62].

No clear guidelines are available for the treatment of patients with MALT–SS. In our view the choice of treatment should be based on the philosophy that MALT–SS and SS are manifestations of the same disease and therefore should be treated (if at all) keeping both SS activity and MALT symptomatology in mind. Current guidelines for management and treatment of patients with MALT–SS in our center are depicted in Fig. 20.3 and are based on our own experience [42]. In patients with asymptomatic MALT lymphoma without high SS disease activity (e.g., only arthralgia, fatigue, and/or Raynaud's phenomenon), "watchful waiting" seems a suitable option. Especially in these patients, surgery or radiotherapy might even be more harmful than close monitoring without treatment. In patients with symptomatic MALT lymphoma, e.g., a persistent disabling parotid gland swelling, but with low SS disease activity, local treatment with low-dose involved field radiotherapy (2×2 or 1×4 Gy) might be sufficient, but experience with this approach in MALT lymphoma is rare. We treated a patient with disabling MALT lymphoma of the parotid gland with 2×2 Gy radiotherapy of the head and neck, which led to decrease

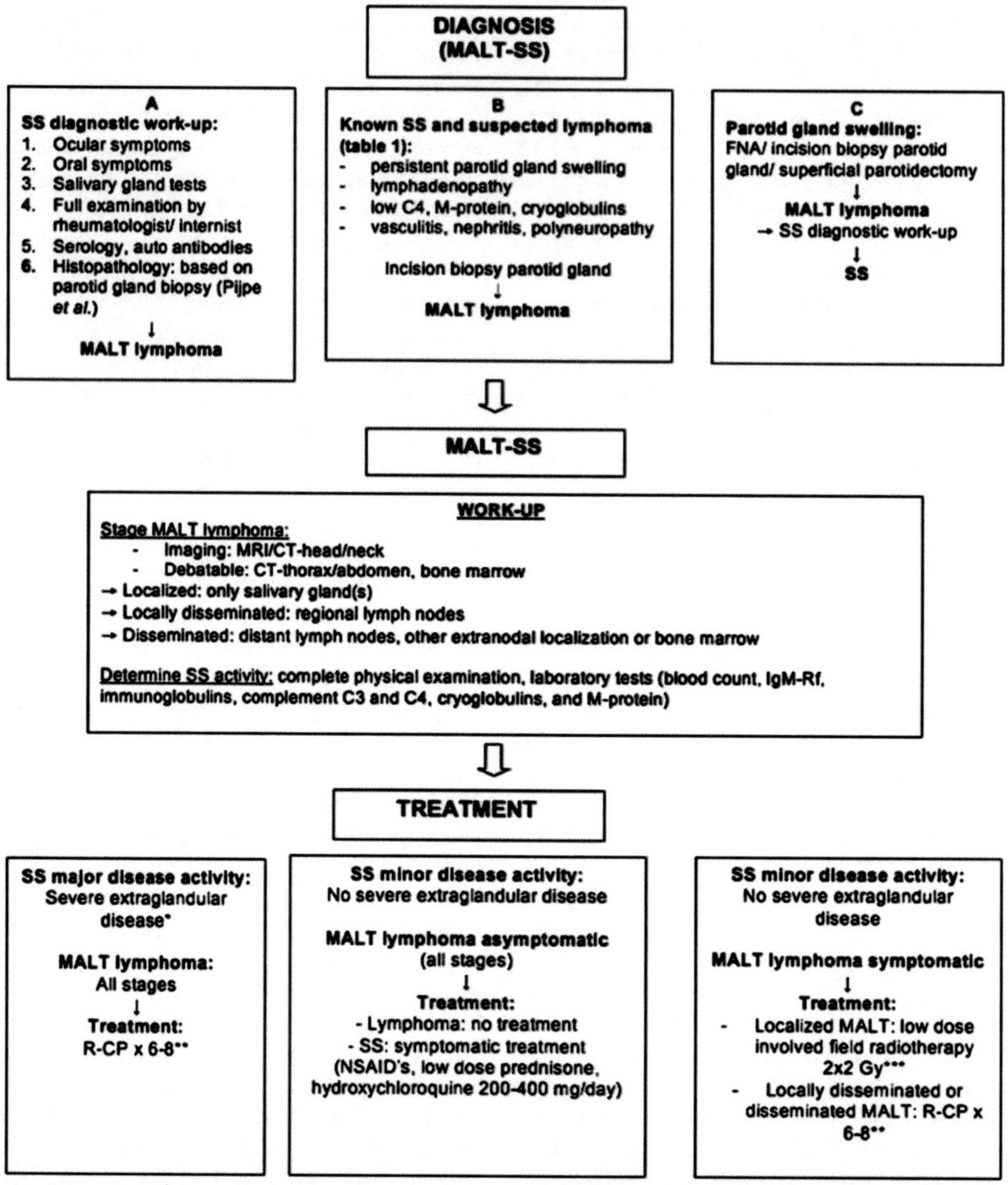

Fig. 20.3 Diagnosis of MALT–SS: clinical algorithm leading to MALT–SS diagnosis. **a** Patients in whom MALT–SS is diagnosed by chance at routine diagnostic biopsy for SS diagnosis. **b** Patients with known SS and strong clinical suspicion of lymphoma. **c** Patients with unknown parotid gland swelling; MALT–SS: patient with MALT lymphoma and associated Sjögren's syndrome (SS); FNA: fine-needle aspiration; *extraglandular disease: polyarthritis/myositis, glomerulonephritis, nervous system involvement, cryoglobulinemic vasculitis, other severe organ involvement, and serological abnormalities: cryoglobulinemia, C4 < 0.10 g/L; **R–CP: six intravenous infusions of 375 mg/m^2 of rituximab and 6–8 cycles of CP, given every 3 weeks. For schedule see Czuczman et al. [60]. ***Patients receive a dose of 4 Gy, either as 2×2 Gy, after an interval of 48 h, or as an single fraction of 4 Gy [24]

of swelling and an improvement of salivary gland function (Fig. 20.4). It is hypothesized that low-dose radiotherapy diminishes the obstruction of salivary secretion created by the lymphoma, but does not damage the salivary parenchyma. Further studies investigating this are necessary.

High initial SS disease activity seems to constitute an adverse prognostic factor for

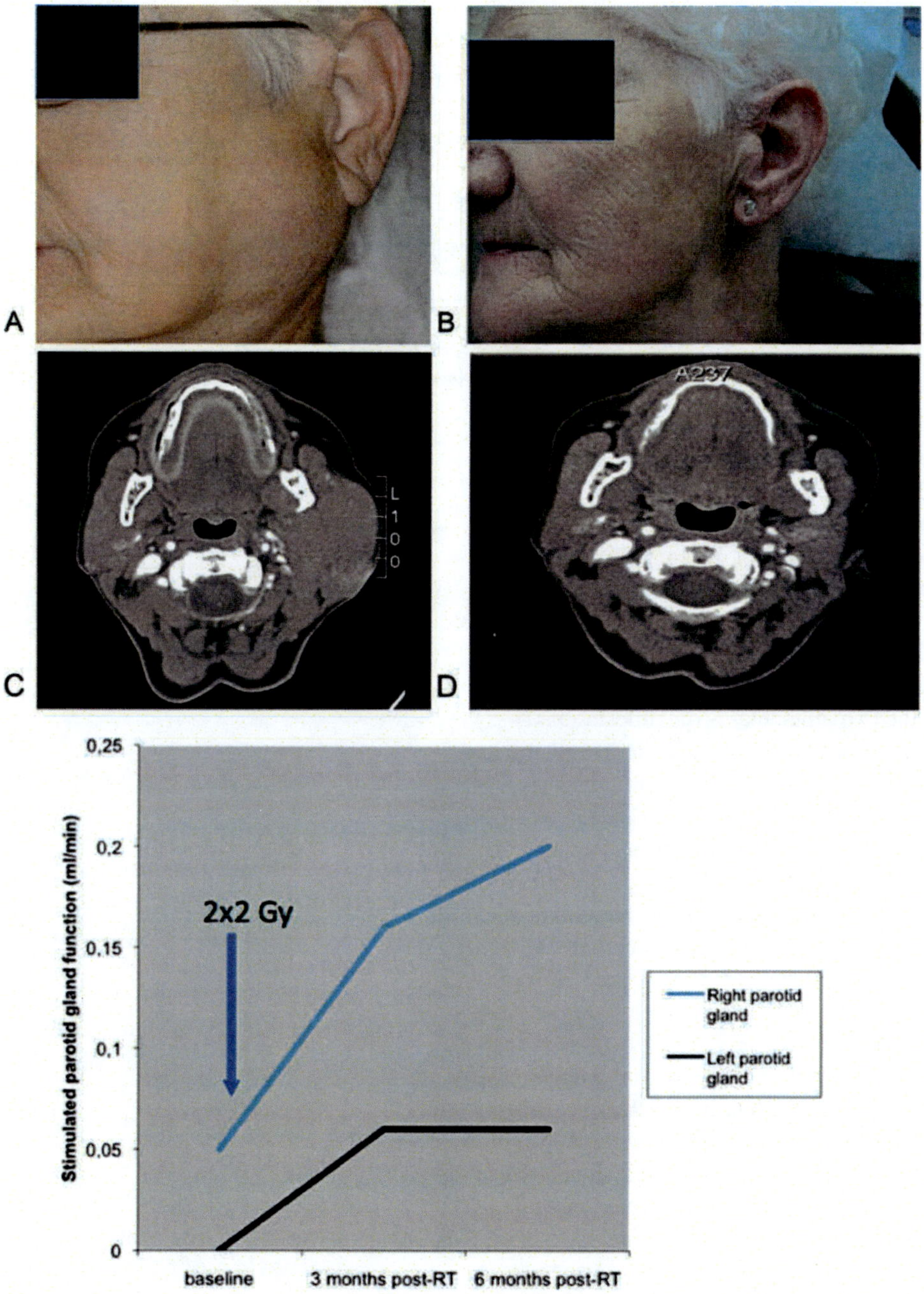

Fig. 20.4 **a** Patient with MALT lymphoma of the left parotid gland. **b** Same patient 3 months after 2×2 Gy low-dose involved field radiotherapy. **c**, **d** Axial MRI before and after radiotherapy showing regression of MALT lymphoma. **e** Parotid salivary gland function (mL/min) of the left and right parotid gland at baseline, 3 and 6 months after radiotherapy

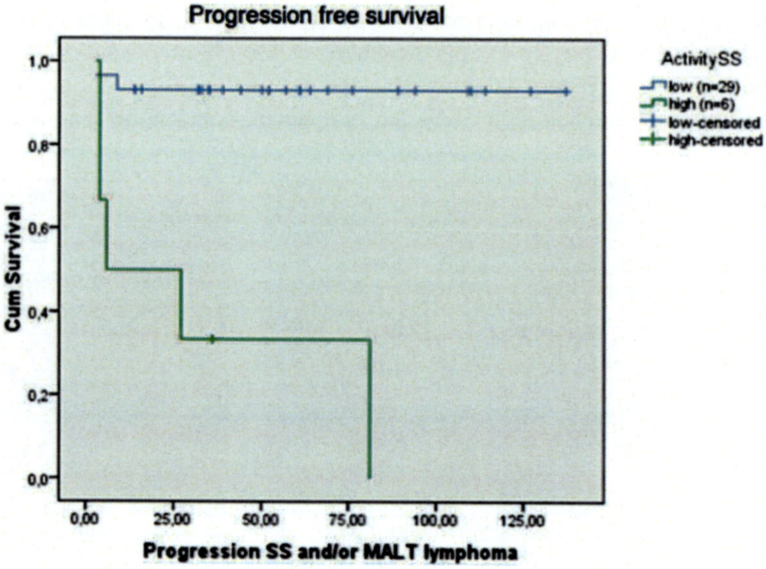

Fig. 20.5 Progression-free survival in patients with MALT–SS and low SS disease activity ($n = 29$) and in patients with MALT–SS and high disease activity ($n = 6$), $p < 0.05$. Events are defined as progression of MALT lymphoma and/or increased SS activity with extraglandular disease

development of lymphoma or progression of extraglandular SS activity (Fig. 20.5) [42]. Our experience suggests that rituximab monotherapy may not be sufficient in the long-term treatment of patients with MALT lymphoma and SS with severe extraglandular manifestations, such as vasculitis, nephritis, or polyneuropathy. Specifically, rituximab alone may be insufficient for the control of the extraglandular SS manifestations.

In our experience treatment in these patients should include more intensive immunosuppressive therapy, for instance, a combination of rituximab with cyclophosphamide and prednisone (R–CP). This combination therapy is effective in the treatment of both indolent lymphoma and autoimmune disease and usually consists of 6–8 intravenous infusions of 375 mg/m^2 of rituximab and 750 mg/m^2 of cyclophosphamide, one infusion given every 3–4 weeks, in combination with 100 mg prednisone for 5 days [59, 60]. We chose to exclude vincristine because of polyneuropathy as side effect. In patients with indolent non-Hodgkin's lymphoma, maintenance therapy with antibodies after induction therapy with rituximab or cyclophosphamide, vincristine, and prednisone prolongs the time to progression but does not prolong survival [62]. Furthermore, the optimal maintenance regimen remains to be determined [63].

20.5 Summary/Pearls

20.5.1 Risk Factors for MALT–SS Development

- Persistent parotid gland swelling, palpable purpura, low levels of C4, and severe extraglandular manifestations (Table 20.1).

20.5.2 Diagnostic Work-up of MALT–SS

- Diagnosis of MALT lymphoma requires histology (parotid gland biopsy).
- Imaging (MRI) in patients with MALT lymphoma shows a diffuse or localized lesion in the gland with multiple cysts.
- Patients with MALT lymphoma of salivary glands must also be evaluated for SS activity.
- Relevance of full systemic staging and bone marrow biopsy is questionable.
- Cervical lymph node involvement is associated with worse prognosis.

20.5.3 Treatment and response evaluation of MALT–SS

- Treatment strategy is dependent on both SS disease activity and MALT symptomatology (see Fig. 20.3).

- In patients with asymptomatic MALT lymphoma and low SS disease activity treatment can be deferred. In these patients watchful waiting is indicated.
- Response evaluation of treatment should include both lymphoma and SS parameters.

References

1. Kassan SS, Thomas TL, Moutsopoulos HM, et al. Increased risk of lymphoma in sicca syndrome. Ann Intern Med. 1978;89:888–92.
2. Tzioufas AG, Boumba DS, Skopouli FN, Moutsopoulos HM. Mixed monoclonal cryoglobulinemia and monoclonal rheumatoid factor cross-reactive idiotypes as predictive factors for the development of lymphoma in primary Sjögren's syndrome. Arthritis Rheum. 1996;39:767–72.
3. Voulgarelis M, Dafni UG, Isenberg DA, Moutsopoulos HM. Malignant lymphoma in primary Sjögren's syndrome: a multicenter, retrospective, clinical study by the European Concerted Action on Sjögren's Syndrome. Arthritis Rheum. 1999;42:1765–72.
4. Ekstrom Smedby K, Vajdic CM, Falster M, et al. Autoimmune disorders and risk of non-Hodgkin lymphoma subtypes: a pooled analysis within the InterLymph Consortium. Blood 2008;111: 4029–38.
5. Thieblemont C. Clinical presentation and management of marginal zone lymphomas. Hematology (Am Soc Hematol Educ Program) 2005;307–13.
6. Fox RI. Sjögren's syndrome. Lancet 2005;366: 321–31.
7. Ioannidis JP, Vassiliou VA, Moutsopoulos HM. Long-term risk of mortality and lymphoproliferative disease and predictive classification of primary Sjögren's syndrome. Arthritis Rheum. 2002;46: 741–7.
8. Ramos-Casals M, Brito-Zeron P, Yague J, et al. Hypocomplementaemia as an immunological marker of morbidity and mortality in patients with primary Sjögren's syndrome. Rheumatology 2005;44:89–94.
9. Theander E, Manthorpe R, Jacobsson LT. Mortality and causes of death in primary Sjögren's syndrome: a prospective cohort study. Arthritis Rheum. 2004;50:1262–9.
10. Theander E, Henriksson G, Ljungberg O, Mandl T, Manthorpe R, Jacobsson LT. Lymphoma and other malignancies in primary Sjögren's syndrome: a cohort study on cancer incidence and lymphoma predictors. Ann Rheum Dis. 2006;65:796–803.
11. Voulgarelis M, Tzioufas AG, Moutsopoulos HM. Mortality in Sjögren's syndrome. Clin Exp Rheumatol. 2008;26(5 Suppl 51):S66–S71.
12. Thieblemont C, Berger F, Dumontet C, et al. Mucosa-associated lymphoid tissue lymphoma is a disseminated disease in one third of 158 patients analyzed. Blood 2000;95:802–6.
13. Zucca E, Conconi A, Pedrinis E, et al. Nongastric marginal zone B-cell lymphoma of mucosa-associated lymphoid tissue. Blood 2003;101:2489–95.
14. Thieblemont C, Bastion Y, Berger F, et al. Mucosa-associated lymphoid tissue gastrointestinal and non-gastrointestinal lymphoma behavior: analysis of 108 patients. J Clin Oncol. 1997;15:1624–30.
15. Coupland SE, Krause L, Delecluse HJ, et al. Lymphoproliferative lesions of the ocular adnexa. Analysis of 112 cases. Ophthalmology 1998;105:1430–41.
16. Royer B, Cazals-Hatem D, Sibilia J, et al. Lymphomas in patients with Sjögren's syndrome are marginal zone B-cell neoplasms, arise in diverse extranodal and nodal sites, and are not associated with viruses. Blood 1997; 90:766–75.
17. Ambrosetti A, Zanotti R, Pattaro C, et al. Most cases of primary salivary mucosa-associated lymphoid tissue lymphoma are associated either with Sjögren syndrome or hepatitis C virus infection. Br J Haematol. 2004;126:43–9.
18. Du MQ, Isaccson PG. Gastric MALT lymphoma: from aetiology to treatment. Lancet Oncol. 2002; 3:97–104.
19. Ferreri AJ, Guidoboni M, Ponzoni M, et al. Evidence for an association between *Chlamydia psittaci* and ocular adnexal lymphomas. J Natl Cancer Inst. 2004;96:586–94.
20. Lecuit M, Abachin E, Martin A, et al. Immunoproliferative small intestinal disease associated with *Campylobacter jejuni*. N Engl J Med. 2004;350:239–48.
21. Roggero E, Zucca E, Mainetti C, et al. Eradication of *Borrelia burgdorferi* infection in primary marginal zone B-cell lymphoma of the skin. Hum Pathol. 2000;31:263–8.
22. Tsang RW, Gospodarowicz MK, Pintilie M, et al. Localized mucosa-associated lymphoid tissue lymphoma treated with radiation therapy has excellent clinical outcome. J Clin Oncol. 2003;21: 4157–64.
23. Vissink A, Jansma J, Spijkervet FKL, Burlage FR, Coppes RP. Oral sequelae of head and neck radiotherapy. Crit Rev Oral Biol Med. 2003;14:199–212.
24. Haas RL, Poortmans P, de Jong D, et al. High response rates and lasting remissions after low-dose involved field radiotherapy in indolent lymphomas. J Clin Oncol. 2003;21:2474–80.
25. Luthy SK, Ng AK, Silver B, et al. Response to low-dose involved-field radiotherapy in patients with non-Hodgkin's lymphoma. Ann Oncol. 2008;19:2043–47.
26. Hammel P, Haioun C, Chaumette MT, et al. Efficacy of single-agent chemotherapy in low-grade B-cell mucosa-associated lymphoid tissue lymphoma

with prominent gastric expression. J Clin Oncol. 1995;13:2524–9.
27. Thieblemont C, de la Fouchardiere A, Coiffier B. Nongastric mucosa-associated lymphoid tissue lymphomas. Clin Lymphoma. 2003;3:212–24.
28. Zinzani PL, Magagnoli M, Galieni P, et al. Nongastrointestinal low-grade mucosa-associated lymphoid tissue lymphoma: analysis of 75 patients. J Clin Oncol. 1999;17:1254.
29. Coiffier B, Lepage E, Briere J, et al. CHOP chemotherapy plus rituximab compared with CHOP alone in elderly patients with diffuse large-B-cell lymphoma. N Engl J Med. 2002;346: 235–42.
30. Maloney DG, Grillo-Lopez AJ, White CA, et al. IDEC-C2B8 (Rituximab) anti-CD20 monoclonal antibody therapy in patients with relapsed low-grade non-Hodgkin's lymphoma. Blood 1997;90: 2188–95.
31. Marcus R, Imrie K, Belch A, et al. CVP chemotherapy plus rituximab compared with CVP as first-line treatment for advanced follicular lymphoma. Blood 2005;105:1417–23.
32. Valencak J, Weihsengruber F, Rappersberger K, et al. Rituximab monotherapy for primary cutaneous B-cell lymphoma: response and follow-up in 16 patients. Ann Oncol. 2009; 20:326–30.
33. Conconi A, Martinelli G, Thieblemont C, et al. Clinical activity of rituximab in extranodal marginal zone B-cell lymphoma of MALT type. Blood 2003;102:2741–5.
34. Martinelli G, Laszlo D, Ferreri AJ, et al. Clinical activity of rituximab in gastric marginal zone non-Hodgkin's lymphoma resistant to or not eligible for anti-*Helicobacter pylori* therapy. J Clin Oncol. 2005;23:1979–83.
35. Nuckel H, Meller D, Steuhl KP, Duhrsen U. Anti-CD20 monoclonal antibody therapy in relapsed MALT lymphoma of the conjunctiva. Eur J Haematol. 2004;73:258–62.
36. Pijpe J, Van Imhoff GW, Spijkervet FKL, et al. Rituximab treatment in patients with primary Sjögren's syndrome: an open-label phase II study. Arthritis Rheum. 2005;52:2740–50.
37. Raderer M, Jager G, Brugger S, et al. Rituximab for treatment of advanced extranodal marginal zone B cell lymphoma of the mucosa-associated lymphoid tissue lymphoma. Oncology 2003;65:306–10.
38. Vitali C, Bombardieri S, Jonsson R, et al. Classification criteria for Sjögren's syndrome: a revised version of the European criteria proposed by the American–European Consensus Group. Ann Rheum Dis. 2002;61:554–8.
39. Cavalli F, Isaacson PG, Gascoyne RD, Zucca E. MALT lymphomas. Hematology (Am Soc Hematol Educ Program) 2001;241–58.
40. Voulgarelis M, Moutsopoulos HM. Malignant lymphoma in primary Sjögren's syndrome. Isr Med Assoc J. 2001;3:761–6.
41. Pijpe J, Kalk WWI, Van der Wal JE, et al. Parotid gland biopsy compared with labial biopsy in the diagnosis of patients with primary Sjögren's syndrome. Rheumatology 2007;46:335–41.
42. Pijpe J, Bootsma H, Vissink A, et al. Treatment of MALT lymphoma in Sjögren's syndrome: a retrospective clinical study and a proposal for treatment guidelines. Oral Oncol. 2007;2:P270.
43. Van Mello NM, Pillemer SR, Tak PP, Sankar V. B cell MALT lymphoma diagnosed by labial minor salivary gland biopsy in patients screened for Sjögren's syndrome. Ann Rheum Dis. 2005;64: 471–3.
44. Meda BA, Buss DH, Woodruff RD, et al. Diagnosis and subclassification of primary and recurrent lymphoma. The usefulness and limitations of combined fine-needle aspiration cytomorphology and flow cytometry. Am J Clin Pathol. 2000;113: 688–99.
45. Sergi B, Contucci AM, Corina L, Paludetti G. Value of fine-needle aspiration cytology of parotid gland masses. Laryngoscope 2004;114:789.
46. Gross M, Ben Yaacov A, Rund D, Elidan J. Role of open incisional biopsy in parotid tumors. Acta Otolaryngol. 2004;124:758–60.
47. Kraaijenhagen HA. Letter: technique for parotid biopsy. J Oral Surg. 1975;33:328.
48. Ando M, Matsuzaki M, Murofushi T. Mucosa-associated lymphoid tissue lymphoma presented as diffuse swelling of the parotid gland. Am J Otolaryngol. 2005;26:285–88.
49. Cheson BD, Pfistner B, Juweid ME, et al. Revised response criteria for malignant lymphoma. J Clin Oncol. 2007;25:579–86.
50. Pijpe J, Van Imhoff GW, Vissink A, et al. Changes in salivary gland immunohistology and function after rituximab mono-therapy in a patient with Sjögren's syndrome and associated MALT-lymphoma. Ann Rheum Dis. 2005;64:958–60.
51. Fischbach W, Goebeler-Kolve M, Starostik P, Greiner A, Muller-Hermelink HK. Minimal residual low-grade gastric MALT-type lymphoma after eradication of *Helicobacter pylori*. Lancet 2002;360:547–8.
52. Jonsson R, Haga HJ, Gordon TP. Current concepts on diagnosis, autoantibodies and therapy in Sjögren's syndrome. Scand J Rheumatol. 2000;29:341–8.
53. Fox PC, Datiles M, Atkinson JC, et al. Prednisone and piroxicam for treatment of primary Sjögren's syndrome. Clin Exp Rheumatol. 1993;11:149–56.
54. Miyawaki S, Nishiyama S, Matoba K. Efficacy of low-dose prednisolone maintenance for saliva production and serological abnormalities in patients with primary Sjögren's syndrome. Intern Med. 1999;38:938–43.
55. Zandbelt MM, van den Hoogen FH, de Wilde PC, van den Berg PJ, Schneider HG, van de Putte LB. Reversibility of histological and immunohistological abnormalities in sublabial salivary gland biopsy specimens following treatment with corticosteroids

in Sjögren's syndrome. Ann Rheum Dis. 2001;60: 511–3.
56. Kastrup O, Maschke M, Diener HC. Pulse-cyclophosphamide in the treatment of ataxic sensory and cranial nerve neuropathy associated with Sjögren's syndrome. Clin Neurol Neurosurg. 2005;107:440–1.
57. Williams CS, Butler E, Roman GC. Treatment of myelopathy in Sjogren syndrome with a combination of prednisone and cyclophosphamide. Arch Neurol. 2001;58:815–9.
58. Meijer JM, Pijpe J, Bootsma H, Vissink A, Kallenberg CGM. The future of biologic agents in the treatment of Sjögren's syndrome. Clin Rev Allergy Immunol. 2007;32:292–7.
59. Chambers SA, Isenberg D. Anti-B cell therapy (rituximab) in the treatment of autoimmune diseases. Lupus 2005;14:210–4.
60. Czuczman MS, Grillo-Lopez AJ, White CA, et al. Treatment of patients with low-grade B-cell lymphoma with the combination of chimeric anti-CD20 monoclonal antibody and CHOP chemotherapy. J Clin Oncol. 1999;17:268–76.
61. Isaksen K, Jonsson R, Omdal R. Anti-CD20 treatment in primary Sjögren's syndrome. Scand J Immunol. 2008;68:554–64.
62. Cheson BD, Leonard JP. Monoclonal antibody therapy for B-cell non-Hodgkin's lymphoma. N Engl J Med. 2008;359:613–26.
63. Hainsworth JD, Litchy S, Shaffer DW, Lackey VL, Grimaldi M, Greco FA. Maximizing therapeutic benefit of rituximab: maintenance therapy versus re-treatment at progression in patients with indolent non-Hodgkin's lymphoma—a randomized phase II trial of the Minnie Pearl Cancer Research Network. J Clin Oncol. 2005;23(6):1088–95.

Fatigue, Dryness, and Quality of Life as Clinical Trial Outcomes in Primary Sjögren's Syndrome

21

Simon J. Bowman

Abstract

Although dryness symptoms are regarded as the defining features of Sjögren's syndrome (SS), fatigue is also a common and often disabling symptom for many patients. The biologic mechanisms of fatigue in SS or in other rheumatic diseases are poorly understood. Low mood associated with having a chronic disease plays a part. Attempts to show correlations between fatigue levels and the levels of cytokines or other biologic parameters or with clinical measures of "disease activity" have not generated a clear answer. Much fatigue research has focused on the measurement and classification of fatigue features and a number of fatigue questionnaires have been developed. Although we can now, therefore, "measure" fatigue levels, there is no proven therapy for fatigue in SS, and considerable debate as to whether a biological or a psychosocial approach is more appropriate. Our understanding of dryness symptoms has been complicated by the lack of correlation between the level of symptoms and the degree of objective dryness measured by standard tests in groups of patients. This has generated a lack of certainty as to what is the goal of therapy in SS—improvement in symptoms or in physical measures of tear and/or salivary flow or histological features in the exocrine glands, or some combination of all of these. What is clear from a number of studies is that patients with SS have reduced levels of health-related quality of life comparable to that of rheumatoid arthritis or systemic lupus erythematosus. Despite these limitations, however, there has been considerable progress in symptom assessment, and this should lay the groundwork for clinical trials of therapeutic agents over the next few years.

Keywords

Sjögren's syndrome • Fatigue • Patient symptoms • Clinical trials

S.J. Bowman (✉)
Department of Rheumatology, University Hospitals
Birmingham, Birmingham, England
e-mail: simon.bowman@uhb.nhs.uk

R.I. Fox, C.M. Fox (eds.), *Sjögren's Syndrome*, DOI 10.1007/978-1-60327-957-4_21,

21.1 Introduction

Sicca (dryness) symptoms, reflecting reduced saliva and/or tear production, are the key features of primary Sjögren's syndrome (pSS) and are reported by most patients [1]. Fatigue, however, is also a major problem and is often the symptom that patients complain about most bitterly. It is found in approximately 70% of patients and, as we will discuss below, is associated with a reduced sense of well-being (health-related quality of life/health status) [2–4]. Other common patient-reported extraglandular symptoms identified in our and other studies include arthralgia, myalgia, and Raynaud's phenomenon [5–8].

In this chapter we will review the features of patient-reported symptoms in pSS, particularly fatigue and dryness, the extent to which they are associated with objective assessment of the disease, potential therapies for these symptoms, and the challenges of outcome assessment in clinical therapeutic trials in pSS.

Although patients with rheumatoid arthritis (RA), systemic lupus erythematosus (SLE), or systemic sclerosis/scleroderma (SSc) who also have secondary Sjögren's syndrome can have some or many of these symptoms, this chapter will focus only on primary Sjögren's syndrome (pSS).

21.2 What Is Fatigue?

The concept of fatigue can be approached in several different ways. In physiological terms isolated muscles demonstrate progressive biochemical (and measurable) fatigability with continued use, or if an individual person exercises, they are fatigued afterward, at least in part, from chemical changes in their muscles. In sports science, for example, this can be formally assessed in a standardized manner in a sports science laboratory.

In patients with a myopathic or neuropathic process, muscles can be weak, and some patients may feel fatigued as a consequence. Another patient, however, can have weakness but without having a perception of fatigue. One important point, therefore, is to recognize that the concept of fatigue is a global one experienced by the patient as a whole, not simply the symptom component of biological muscle weakness.

There are also mental components of fatigue with difficulty in thinking or concentrating. The term "brain-fog" is sometimes used. As we will discuss below, this is typically assessed using patient-completed questionnaires, although formal psychometric testing could be considered in parallel with this.

Furthermore, it is important to recognize that fatigue is common in the general population [9] and, in population terms, "disease-related" fatigue is the component of fatigue that is in excess of that already present in the background population. This, however, only deals with "quantity," and it is also important to consider whether there are qualitative features of the fatigue that differ between conditions or from the background fatigue described in the general population. This is where questionnaires that attempt to probe into different features of what is meant by fatigue can be helpful over and above a single question asking about the amount or "severity" of the fatigue and will be discussed in detail below.

Fatigue can be a presentation of medical conditions such as hypothyroidism, anemia, or of sleep deprivation or a whole range of other disorders or medications (biological fatigue), or a manifestation of psychosocial factors such as psychiatric morbidity (e.g., depression) or social factors (life events, family circumstances). It can also be a feature of a personality disorder or be medically unexplained (chronic fatigue syndrome) [9, 10]. Fatigue is also commonly reported by patients with other rheumatic diseases such as RA and SLE [2–4].

21.3 Potential Causes of Fatigue in pSS

21.3.1 Biological

21.3.1.1 Cytokines

In terms of how disease activity or biological factors might contribute to fatigue in pSS, one approach is to look for associations between levels of fatigue and biological measures. A small number of studies have looked at this in pSS by examining correlations in cross-sectional studies between levels of fatigue and levels of inflammatory markers (ESR, CRP), antibodies (immunoglobulin levels, anti-Ro/La antibody titres), or cytokines such as IL-1β(beta), IL-2, IL-6, IL-10, and TNF-α(alpha), [3, 11, 12]. These studies have not, however, identified definitive associations between fatigue and serological parameters in pSS. One study of 16 patients with pSS suggested that patients with pSS and myalgia had diminished cytokine release from peripheral blood mononuclear cells in vitro and increased serum levels of IL-18 [13]. There is, however, an important distinction between pSS and RA and SLE. In rheumatoid arthritis, for example, cytokines such as TNF-α(alpha), IL-1β(beta), and IL-6 (and the ESR and CRP) have clear relationships with disease activity and disease-modifying anti-rheumatic drugs and anti-TNF therapies reduce fatigue levels as part of their beneficial effects on disease activity [14]. In pSS "flares" are less well described, and, if they occur, are less common and less severe [15]. The raised ESR in pSS is mainly associated with antibody levels rather than clinical markers of disease activity [5] and there is no obvious link between the CRP level and systemic disease activity [5]. To this extent, therefore, existing serological markers in pSS such as immunoglobulin or anti-Ro/La antibody levels are more akin to the rheumatoid factor in RA, which is not a marker of disease activity per se.

Even in RA, however, the associations between disease activity and fatigue are relatively modest with the best predictors of fatigue being pain, depressive symptoms, and female sex [16]. In our study to develop and validate a systemic disease activity score, the Sjögren's systemic clinical activity index (SCAI) [5], we demonstrated correlations between fatigue, arthritis, and Raynaud's phenomenon domains of the SCAI and comparable domains of the Profile of Fatigue and Discomfort (PROFAD) measure. There was not, however, a clear relationship between total fatigue and a total disease activity score, although at this point our assessment of systemic disease activity is still advancing and this may become clearer as our tools develop.

Nevertheless, in comparing fatigue in pSS to that in RA and SLE the appropriate comparison is with the background levels of chronic fatigue in these conditions, rather than with the intermittently increased fatigue associated with increased disease activity. Since we do not know which cytokines might be involved in pSS, we are in the semi-darkness at present in terms of which cytokines to study. Currently, most of the focus in pSS at present is in the role of B cells and hence cytokines such as BlyS/BAFF would be logical to evaluate [17]. Our previous studies developing the PROFAD [2] have also shown that there is a very similar character or Profile of Fatigue among patients with pSS to that seen in patients with SLE [2]. While this does not directly address the core issue of biological versus psychosocial contributors to fatigue in pSS, it does suggest that fatigue in pSS has similar characteristics to that in SLE and may share a similar etiopathogenesis. Given our lack of understanding of many aspects of etiopathogenesis, the redundancy of many cytokines and the inherent difficulties of disentangling psychosocial components, this may not be an area of research to expect quick answers, although the development of large-scale patient registries combining data on clinical, serological, genetic, and symptom may lead to some progress over the next few years.

21.3.1.2 Neuroendocrine

Another approach has been to examine the relationship between fatigue and neuroendocrine factors—particularly the hypothalamic–pituitary axis (HPA). There is a large and conflicting body of literature, particularly in the idiopathic chronic fatigue syndrome, arguing whether or not an underactive HPA, e.g., resulting in low cortisol levels, is related to chronic fatigue in some patients. There is some limited evidence of an underactive HPA in pSS with low cortisol and/or low dehydroepiandrosterone levels, suggested as a cause of reduced well-being [18, 19]. Another related consideration is that of autonomic dysfunction found in some patients with pSS. In a recent study of 48 women with pSS, there was an inverse relationship between diastolic blood pressure and fatigue levels [20]. The hypothesis is that autonomic dysfunction predisposes to lower blood pressure and this in turn may predispose to increased fatigue levels. Again this needs to be investigated in larger groups of patients and with more detailed studies before this can be regarded as definitive.

21.3.1.3 Sleep

Lack of sleep is a potential biological cause of fatigue. It would be logical, therefore, to hypothesize that oral dryness in particular might lead to increased waking at night and therefore disturbed sleep and hence fatigue. Another possibility is that drinking water before bed to reduce dryness symptoms might lead to waking up at night to pass urine. There are studies in pSS investigating sleep disturbance. These include a study of 65 patients (predating the American–European consensus criteria) demonstrating severe sleep disturbance in 75% using a 10-item Mini Sleep Questionnaire, but no relationship with clinical or laboratory parameters [21]. In this study, 55% of these patients were regarded as also having fibromyalgia (see below), which may suggest the involvement of psychosocial factors rather than pure biological ones. In another questionnaire-based study of 40 patients, sleep disturbance was more common than in comparator groups of controls or RA patients, as was fatigue [22]. At least in terms of difficulty in falling asleep the reported issues were muscular tension and restless legs, however, rather than dryness symptoms. In another study of 76 patients sleep disturbance assessed by the Epworth Sleepiness Scale was commoner in pSS than in patients with osteoarthritis even though there was no difference in fatigue measured by the Functional Assessment of Chronic Illness Therapy-Fatigue (FACIT-F) scale [23]. This study was focused on urinary symptoms as a potential marker of anti-muscarinic antibody-related autonomic dysfunction and found a correlation between urological symptoms and daytime sleepiness.

These studies did not focus on the possible relationships between sleepiness and sicca symptoms and this is an area still to be studied in detail. In addition, these studies assessed sleep using questionnaires and it would be of particular interest to compare these data with objective measures of sleep such as polysomnography.

21.3.2 Psychosocial

21.3.2.1 Depression

Valtysdottir et al. identified higher levels of depression in 62 pSS patients than in 38 RA patients or 63 healthy controls using the Hospital Anxiety And Depression Scale (HADS) [24], although the finding of similar depression scores for RA patients and healthy controls in this study differs from other studies in which RA is associated with an increased prevalence of low mood [25]. Nevertheless, another study of 40 patients with pSS using the HADS also showed a higher prevalence of clinical depression risk compared with controls [26]. In a study of 49 pSS patients, correlations were found between depression measured by the Zung depression scale and dimensions of reduced motivation and mental fatigue measured by the Multidimensional Fatigue Inventory (MFI) [3]. In our patients with pSS there was a similar prevalence of low mood to that in patients with RA and SLE, which was greater than in matched controls [2]. Furthermore, when anxiety and depression (measured by the HADS) were controlled, the differences between patient groups and controls were largely maintained. We did not identify any significant correlations between fatigue or pain and the HADS, i.e., the fatigue levels identified could not be accounted for by levels of depression. In another study of 111 patients with pSS, fatigue and pain correlated with quality of life and psychological distress [27]. One issue to be aware of is that some of the questions in depression or anxiety scales can reflect features of the disease (e.g., dry mouth as a feature of anxiety). The scores from such a questionnaire may overestimate the prevalence of anxiety or depression—so-called criterion contamination [25].

What these studies show, overall, is an increased prevalence of depressive/low mood symptoms in pSS, as might be expected in a chronic rheumatic disease, but that there is still some uncertainty as to the extent to which symptoms of fatigue and pain in pSS correlate with symptoms of low mood and psychological distress.

21.3.2.2 Fibromyalgia

Fibromyalgia (FMA) is another area of potential controversy due to the wildly different reported prevalence of FMA in pSS. Vitali et al. identified FMA in 14 out of 30 patients (47%) [28]. In another Italian study, the prevalence was 22% [29]. In a single-center UK study, however, the prevalence was reported as 7–12% dependent on the criteria used and 5% in a comparator group of SLE patients [30]. In our UK cohort, the prevalence was 4.4% in pSS, 4.5% in SLE, 1.4% in RA, and 0% in the controls [2]. One potential explanation for these differences is the extent to which narrower criteria, such as the American College of Rheumatology (ACR) criteria, were used for the diagnosis of FMA. Similar controversies apply to SLE where many studies suggest a comparable prevalence of FMA of approximately 5% [2, 30], while other studies suggest a higher figure (e.g., 22% in Ref. [31]). Another possibility is that these are "real" differences in FMA prevalence but reflect cultural factors in different countries. Nevertheless, the two UK studies are consistent in methodology and results in demonstrating a prevalence of 5–12% of patients fulfilling ACR criteria for fibromyalgia and demonstrating that fibromyalgia does not, of itself, account for the symptoms of fatigue in pSS [2, 15].

21.4 Measurement of Fatigue and Other Extraglandular Symptoms

The simplest way of measuring fatigue (or indeed other symptoms such as joint/muscle pain or Raynaud's phenomenon) is to use a 10-cm visual analog scale (VAS) or Likert rating scale (0, 1, 2, 3, etc.) asking the patient to rate their fatigue (e.g., from "none" at minimum to "worst fatigue imaginable" at most). Another approach is to use a questionnaire comprising a series of questions, each of which addresses some different component of the symptom under evaluation. Some of these fatigue questionnaires, e.g., FACIT-F scale [32] and the Fatigue Severity Scale (FSS) [33] are described as "uni-dimensional," i.e., they give a total score for fatigue much as the fatigue VAS does. In the context of clinical trials in rheumatoid arthritis, there is evidence that a VAS may be just as effective as using a longer questionnaire [34], particularly in relation to sensitivity to change. This may well be the case in therapeutic studies in pSS as well [35]. One might conclude, therefore, that a simple VAS is all that is needed as a primary outcome measure for the symptom of interest. Using even a simple, uni-dimensional, fatigue questionnaire in parallel with the VAS, however, offers reassurance that the VAS findings are valid and can, therefore, be a useful confirmatory secondary outcome tool.

Other questionnaires are "multidimensional," i.e., they have a series of domains or subscales that try and assess different aspects of fatigue [2, 36–40]. In some of these questionnaires a total score can also be calculated. The individual questions that make-up these questionnaires and the resulting domains offer a useful insight into what is meant by the term fatigue. One common theme is the differentiation of physical fatigue (e.g., lack of energy, difficulty in getting started, easily worn out, feeling weak) and mental fatigue (e.g., difficulty in concentrating or thinking) and, although the exact phraseology differs between questionnaires, these two basic concepts are reflected in all five of the above multidimensional fatigue questionnaires. In addition some questionnaires such as the Fatigue Assessment Instrument (FAI) [37], Piper Fatigue Scale (PFS) [38], and Fatigue Impact Scale [40] explore other concepts such as fatigue severity, the consequences of fatigue on daily activities, or the emotional consequences of fatigue.

In practical terms, however, such as the consideration of fatigue as a potential outcome in clinical trials [35], as will be discussed below, the predominant concepts are that of "total" or "global" fatigue measured either by the

VAS, or by questionnaires and the domains of "physical fatigue" and "mental fatigue" typically measured by multidimensional questionnaires. Another widely used questionnaire in rheumatology research is the Medical Outcomes Study Short-Form 36-item questionnaire (SF-36) [41] (see below). This eight domain questionnaire includes a "vitality" domain, which generally correlates reasonably well with fatigue questionnaires [2]. Fatigue, however, is just one component of health-related quality of life and should not be equated as an identical concept.

In terms of the decision as to which questionnaire to use to measure fatigue (and other symptoms) the reality is that in comparing "like-to-like," e.g., the physical fatigue or mental fatigue domains of two different questionnaires, they are likely to generate very similar results, e.g., MFI versus PROFAD [42]. One important note is that fatigue in pSS/RA measured by VAS appears to correlate better with "somatic fatigue" domain scores of multidimensional fatigue questionnaires than with "mental fatigue" domain scores [43–45]. It looks, therefore, as though patients with pSS or RA generally associate the term "fatigue" (e.g., measured by the VAS) primarily with physical rather than mental fatigue.

In order to examine how best to measure fatigue as well as other symptoms in pSS we started in 2000 by reviewing the literature and interviewing patients to get an idea of key disease symptoms. We then constructed and refined a symptom questionnaire, which was then completed by patients with pSS, RA, SLE, and community controls without rheumatic disease. This included a wide range of symptoms including constitutional, pulmonary, neurological, urological, and other general and organ-specific symptoms of potential relevance to pSS. By eliminating symptoms that were either infrequent, or common to the community control group (i.e., not disease specific), we were able to produce a Profile of Fatigue and Discomfort (PROFAD) that captured the symptomatic component of pSS [2]. This demonstrated a very similar background Profile of Fatigue among pSS and SLE patients with the RA group showing higher levels of physical fatigue (likely related to the physical component of arthritis) and clearly different to controls (Fig. 21.1).

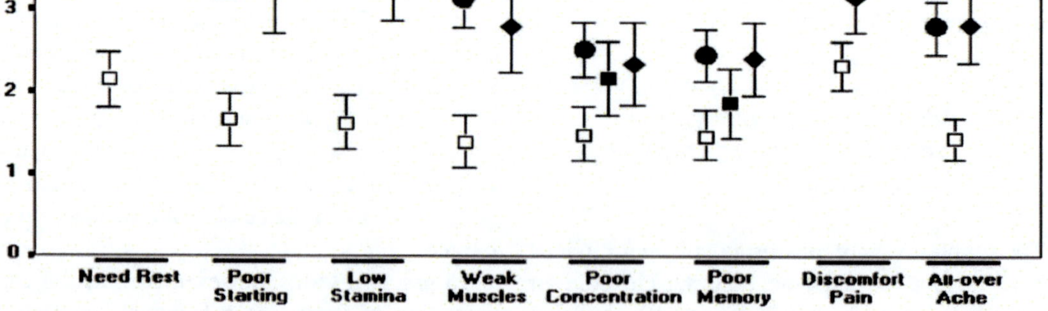

Fig. 21.1 Mean and 95% confidence intervals for fatigue and general discomfort ratings at worst in the Sjögren's-based questionnaire tool (7 = worst imaginable) for healthy controls and three disease groups. Reproduced with permission from Ref. [2]

Clearly our bias is to recommend the use of a questionnaire developed specifically to capture the symptoms of pSS in preference to a questionnaire developed for other diseases, but the practical reality is that in capturing similar data many of these questionnaires generate similar results and therefore the choice depends on the personal preferences of the researcher rather than there being one gold standard option.

21.5 Health Status/Health-Related Quality of Life

Quality of life (QOL) is a difficult to define concept but in general terms it describes an overall concept of "well-being." This might include concepts of basic need such as access to clean water, food and shelter, psychological state, state of health, and relationships. It is not straightforward to measure in absolute terms—how does one compare the quality of life of a Kalahari bushman with that of a New York banker? Nevertheless attempts have been made to devise questionnaires that measure QOL such as the World Health Organization Quality of Life Questionnaire (WHOQOL) [46]. This has four principal domains: physical (PHY), psychological (PSY), social relationships (SOC), and environment (ENV). Another more limited concept is that of "health-related QOL" or "health-status" where the focus is on assessing how a disease affects an individual or group in a general way. The SF-36 [41] is probably the most widely used questionnaire designed to evaluate health-related quality of life in individuals with medical disorders. The 36-question items have been split among eight domains, namely, general health (GH), physical functioning (PF), role-functioning physical (RP), bodily pain (BP), social functioning (SF), role-functioning emotional (RE), mental health (MH), and vitality (VT). There are now a series of papers in pSS showing fairly globally reduced SF-36 scores (i.e., lower health-related quality of life) compared to the general population and comparable to that of patients with SLE and rheumatoid arthritis [2, 4, 27, 47–49]. In our study [2], as well as reduced health-related quality of life/health status, we also demonstrated similar reductions in general quality of life measured by the WHOQOL-BREF [46] (Fig. 21.2).

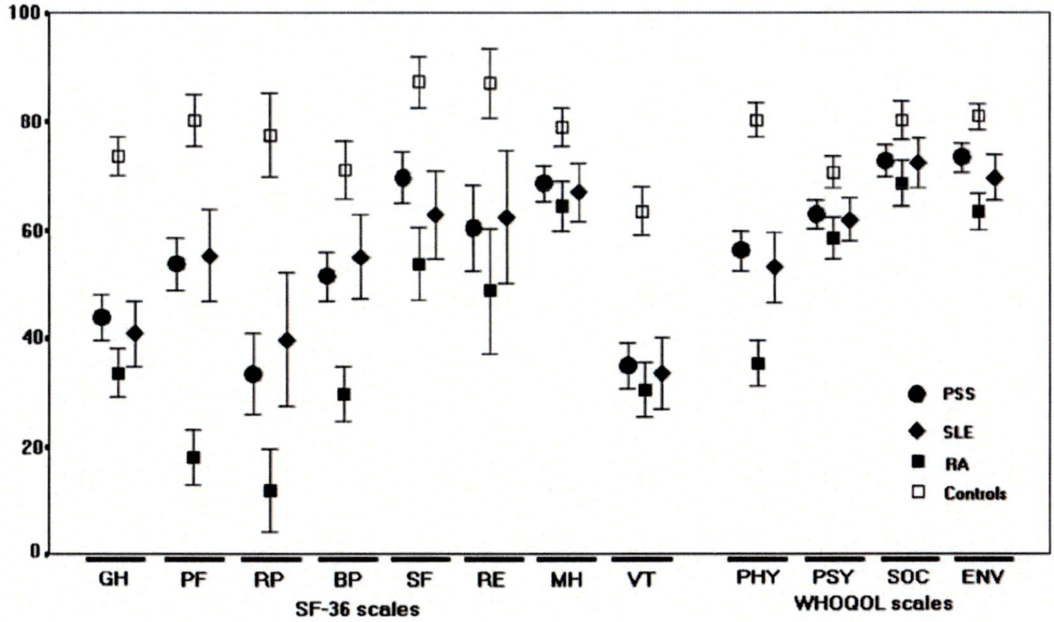

Fig. 21.2 Mean and 95% confidence intervals for SF-36 subscales and WHOQOL-BREF domains for healthy controls and three disease groups. Reproduced with permission from Ref. [2]

21.6 Potential Approaches to Treatment of Fatigue and Other Extraglandular Symptoms

Although hydroxychloroquine is frequently prescribed to treat fatigue in pSS, formal studies have been small in scale [50, 51] and there has never been a fully powered, double-blind, randomized, controlled clinical trial (RCT) of hydroxychloroquine in pSS. This omission, however, should be rectified following a French trial currently in progress (www.clinicaltrials.gov, Identifier: NCT00632866).

Infliximab has been studied in an RCT of 103 patients with pSS [52]. The outcome chosen was an ad hoc composite of VAS of fatigue, pain, and dryness in which patients had to score >50 mm on at least two of these at baseline and demonstrate a 30% improvement at 10 weeks compared with baseline for at least two of the three components. The study outcome was negative, both in terms of this composite outcome and in terms of each of the individual components suggesting that TNF-α(alpha) is not a key driver of inflammation as it is in RA.

Results from another double-blind RCT, this time of dehydroepiandrosterone (DHEA) (see also the above section on the hypothalamic–pituitary axis), were reported by Hartkamp et al. [53]. Patients in both active therapy and placebo groups showed improvement in primary outcomes of fatigue, mental well-being, and depressive mood but without any difference between active treatment and placebo.

Taking a non-biological therapeutic approach, Strombeck et al. [54] examined the effect of exercise on fatigue and aerobic exercise capacity in nine patients with pSS over a 12-week period compared with ten patients who did not pursue an exercise regime over this period. Both of these components as well as depression improved although there was no relationship between the improvement in fatigue and in aerobic capacity in individual patients. This study suggests that non-medical approaches to treating fatigue may be successful.

Pilot clinical data for anti-CD20 (a B-cell marker) therapy, rituximab [35, 55–59], as well as from an open-label study of anti-CD22 antibody (epratuzumab) [60] paint an intriguing picture. In our study [35], 17 patients with pSS and a score on fatigue visual analog scale (VAS) > 50 mm were randomized to receive either two infusions of rituximab or placebo; patients also received oral and intravenous steroids. The results demonstrated significant improvement from baseline in fatigue VAS in the rituximab-treated group ($p < 0.001$) in contrast to the placebo group ($p = 0.147$), which became more apparent over time (see Figs. 21.3 and 21.4). There was also a significant difference between the groups at 6 months in the social functioning score of SF-36 ($p = 0.01$) and a trend to significant difference in the mental health domain score of SF-36 ($p = 0.06$). These data and studies by other groups suggest potential benefit in treating fatigue [35, 55, 58–60], dryness symptoms [55, 56], and systemic features [57]. If, therefore, fatigue improves following biologic therapy, one could argue that, in contradistinction to the above studies, this might suggest a biological mechanism for at least part of the fatigue symptoms in pSS.

21.7 Measurement of Dryness (Sicca) Symptoms

Dryness is the key symptom of Sjögren's syndrome with oral and ocular dryness as the most common and most troublesome components [1]. As with fatigue, pain, or other extraglandular symptoms, the simplest way to measure dryness is with a VAS, but questionnaires can add detail and reliability. A number of dryness questionnaires have been developed, although many are screening questionnaires to identify the presence or absence of dryness symptoms in the community or as part of classification criteria for Sjögren's syndrome [61, 62]. There are, however, a number of questionnaires that have been developed to quantify oral [63–70] and ocular

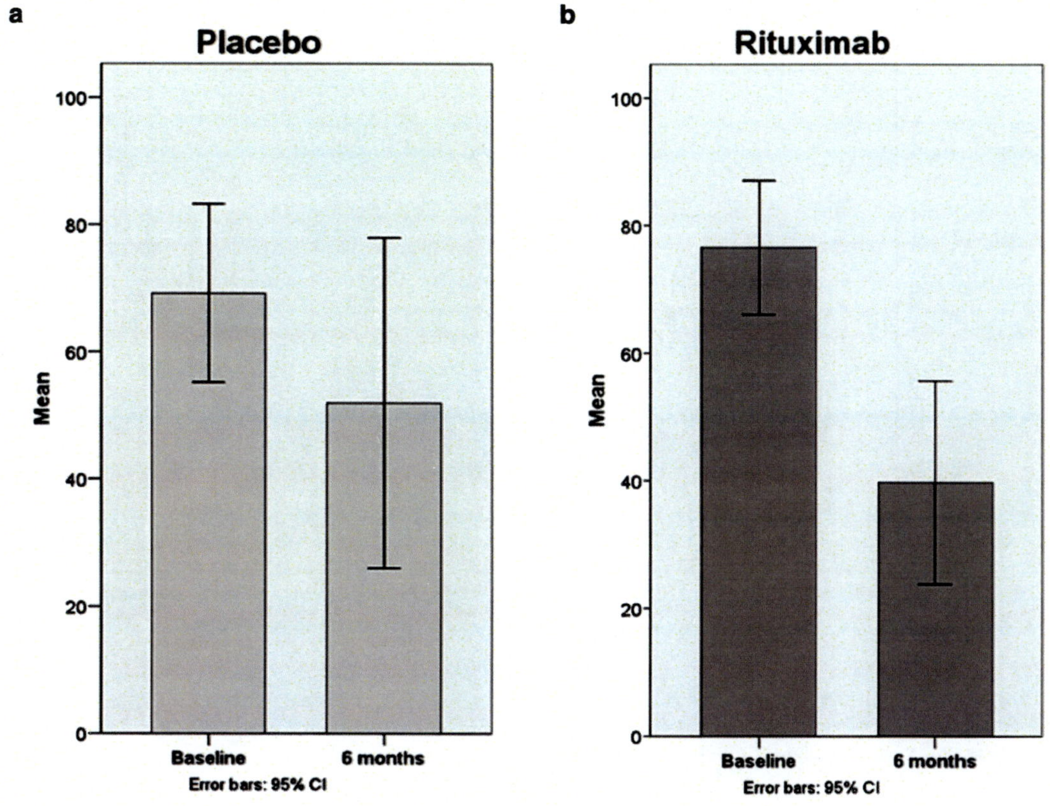

Fig. 21.3 Mean fatigue VAS at baseline and 6 months. Reproduced with permission from Ref. [35]

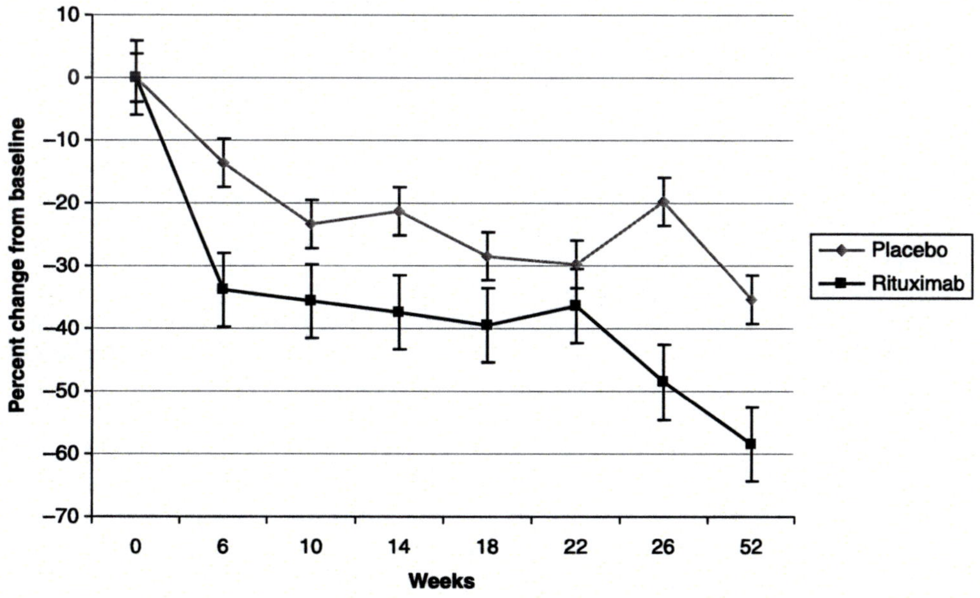

Fig. 21.4 Change in fatigue VAS from baseline. Reproduced with permission from Ref. [35]

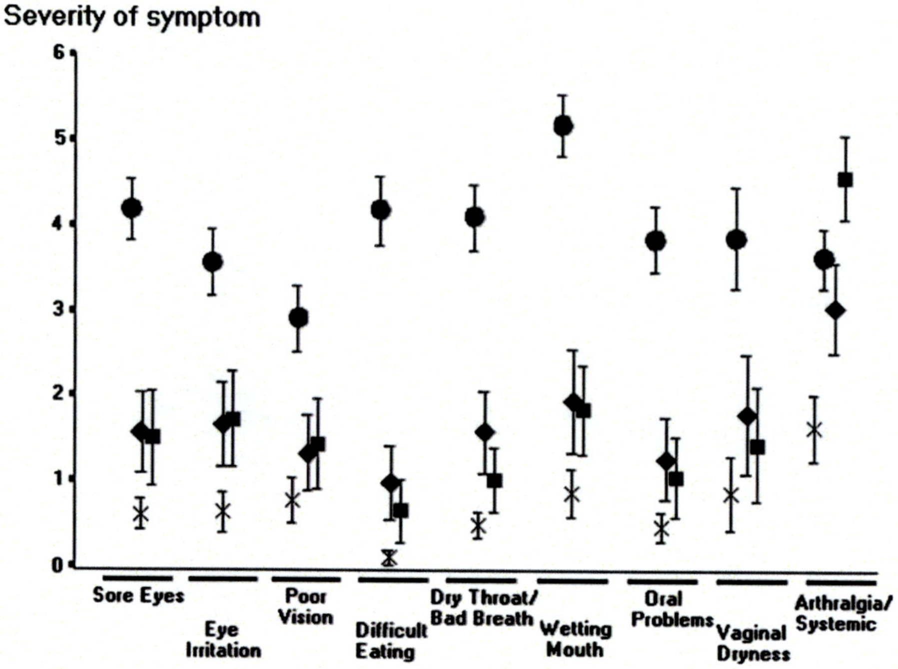

Fig. 21.5 Mean and 95% confidence intervals for ratings of discomfort at their worst over the last 2 weeks (7 = worst discomfort imaginable) for groups diagnosed with PSS, SLE, RA, and healthy controls. • PSS ($n = 78$–112); ♦ SLE ($n = 48$–53); ■ RA ($n = 39$–50); □ controls ($n =$ 58–77)

[69–72] dryness, although this list is not exclusive. Data from the Sicca Symptoms Inventory (SSI) is presented in Fig. 21.5 demonstrating higher levels of oral, ocular, vaginal, and cutaneous dryness than controls. As with fatigue questionnaires, some of these sicca questionnaires are uni-dimensional [63, 64, 67] whereas others are multidimensional [65, 66, 68, 69, 71, 72] and some also include questions on vaginal, cutaneous, bronchial, and/or nasal dryness.

There have been relatively few studies directly comparing different sicca questionnaires. In our study developing the Sicca Symptoms Inventory (SSI) [69] we identified similarities between the SSI and Xerostomia Inventory. The National Eye Institute Visual Function 25-item (NEI-VFQ-25) Questionnaire has also been shown to correlate with results using the ocular surface disease index (OSDI) [72]. It is likely, however, that as with the measurement of fatigue and pain, using a VAS of dryness as the primary outcome measure along with a dryness questionnaire as a confirmatory secondary outcome measure is the most logical approach. This still leaves the question as to which component of dryness to choose? To some extent this will depend on the study medication and the research question. In a recent study, our patients demonstrated a close correlation between oral and global dryness VASs [45], and our preference at this time is to use oral rather than global dryness as the principal measure of sicca in a clinical trial, but this is by no means fixed in stone.

21.8 Data from Existing Clinical Studies Addressing Dryness in pSS

The largest trial of systemic therapy of oral and ocular dryness in SS was performed by Vivino et al. in 1999 [70]. They studied 373 patients with primary or secondary SS randomized to placebo or pilocarpine. Pilocarpine is a muscarinic agonist that stimulates exocrine glands. Pilocarpine was effective in stimulating salivary flow at the start and throughout the study, although with no increase in basal or stimulated flow rates at the end of the study. Nevertheless, from a symptomatic perspective, patients on the 5 mg qds dose had a significantly higher likelihood of responding as assessed by symptomatic measures of global dryness of eyes and mouth and multiple individual dryness symptom items. Similar data are available from studies of cevimeline, another muscarinic agonist licensed in the USA and Japan for the treatment of dryness in pSS [73, 74].

Interferon-α lozenges have also been studied for improvement in salivary function in an open-label study [75]. Salivary flow and histological features improved but patient-related outcomes were not reported. In a combined report from two phase III double-blind randomized controlled studies by Cummins et al. [76] of 497 patients with pSS, improvement in unstimulated whole salivary flow and 7 of 8 symptoms of oral dryness were observed although the chosen primary endpoints of an improvement in both stimulated whole salivary flow and a VAS of oral dryness did not show statistically significant improvement.

Topical cyclosporine emulsion has also been studied in two large studies of ocular dryness [77, 78]. In the smaller study [77], the 0.1% dose was most consistent in improving some objective and some subjective endpoints and the 0.05% dose in improving patient symptoms including the OSDI. In the larger study of 877 patients by Sall et al. [78], Schirmer's tear test with anesthetic and corneal staining at 6 months improved significantly more in the active treatment groups compared with placebo, whereas Schirmer's test without anesthetic and the OSDI improved with both active drug and the placebo (vehicle alone) although other subjective measures (blurred vision, artificial tear usage, and physician global assessment) did show greater benefit from the active drug. These studies suggest that both the vehicle and active drug have beneficial effects with some added benefit from the cyclosporine component.

Two open-label studies of rituximab have suggested potential benefit for sicca features [5, 55]. More recently a double-blind study of 30 patients showed improvement in both stimulated flow rate and oral dryness VAS in the active but not placebo group. This is potentially very positive support for larger studies of anti-B-cell agents in pSS.

21.9 Conclusion: Clinical Trial Outcomes

The development of questionnaire tools for dryness and fatigue symptoms as well as the availability of new biological therapies has opened the possibility of conducting clinical trials of these therapies in pSS. At the present time, anti-B-cell therapies such as rituximab are the logical agent of choice and a number of studies are in progress or planned. There are, however, some remaining challenges with regard to assessment, particularly in relation to the choice of primary outcome, which is regarded as absolutely critical in an early clinical trial of a therapeutic product.

1. One question is whether to choose dryness or fatigue symptoms or a composite of both (or to include health-related quality of life and pain as well). In two expert workshops, fatigue was felt to be a particularly important outcome domain [79, 80]. We have also shown that fatigue can improve following systemic therapy [35] and there is increasing interest in its use as a secondary outcome measure in RA [14, 81]. Nevertheless, there is some reluctance to rely on it exclusively. Other approaches, therefore, are to use it as part of a composite symptomatic outcome measure [52] or to incorporate it into, or alongside, a systemic activity measure [5, 82].
2. The second issue is what constitutes meaningful clinical improvement? In rheumatoid arthritis the American College of Rheumatology response criteria require a minimum 20% improvement (ACR-20) in the number of tender and swollen joints and other parameters [83]. The ACR-50 and ACR-70 are similar but require 50% and 70% improvement in the above parameters, respectively. These criteria were developed through an analysis of the results of pre-existing trials that used different outcome measures and a

process of developing a broad consensus of experts. They have stood the test of time over the past decade and are now used in every RA trial. We now need to develop equivalent response criteria in pSS.

3. There is a relatively weak correlation between dryness symptoms and objective measures of lacrimal and salivary flow [84]. This poses a dilemma in a clinical trial context—should the primary outcome be improvement in salivary/lacrimal flow or improvement in symptoms or both? Other uncertainties include with a placebo group response rate for improvement in symptoms of approximately 30% [35, 70] what is the minimum clinically meaningful response in the active group that should be reflected in the definition of the primary outcome? Another issue to be aware of is that salivary flow can be measured either as basal (unstimulated) flow or as stimulated flow (e.g., in response to a sharp stimulus such as lemon drops or a pastille). Mechanistically, reduced unstimulated basal flow has been regarded as the main deficit in pSS but several successful clinical trials have used stimulated salivary flow in preference to this [59, 70].

Some of these issues will be addressed by a collaborative European League against Rheumatism (EULAR) sponsored project (Vitali C, Mariette X, Bowman SJ, et al.) to develop and validate consensus disease activity and patient-reported outcome measures based on our previous work [2, 5, 45, 69, 82, 85]. Part of this project will evaluate the relative importance to patients of fatigue and the common dryness symptoms as well as assessing what is minimally significant change. Information from this study as well as data from recent and current trials will inform the design of future phase II/III trials and the development of effective therapy for this debilitating condition.

Acknowledgments A variation of this article has also been published in *Rheumatic Disease Clinics of North America 2008*. Figures in this article have been reprinted with permission from *Annals of the Rheumatic Diseases and the Journal of Rheumatology and Rheumatology* (Oxford).

References

1. Jonsson R, Bowman SJ, Gordon TP. Sjögren's syndrome. In: Arthritis and allied conditions, Koopman WJ, Moreland LW, editors, 15th ed. Philadelphia, PA: Lippincott Williams & Wilkins; 2005, pp. 1681–705.
2. Bowman SJ, Booth DA, Platts RG, UK Sjögren's Interest Group. Measurement of fatigue and discomfort in primary Sjögren's syndrome using a new questionnaire tool. Rheumatology 2004;43:758–64.
3. Barendregt PJ, Visser MR, Smets EM, et al. Fatigue in primary Sjögren's syndrome. Ann Rheum Dis. 1998;57:291–5.
4. Strömbeck B, Ekdahl C, Manthorpe R, Wikström I, Jacobsson L. Health-related quality of life in primary Sjögren's syndrome, rheumatoid arthritis and fibromyalgia compared to normal population data using SF-36. Scand J Rheumatol. 2000;29:20–8.
5. Bowman SJ, Sutcliffe N, Isenberg DA, et al. Sjögren's systemic clinical activity index (SCAI): a systemic disease activity measure for use in clinical trials in primary Sjögren's syndrome. Rheumatology 2007;46:1845–51.
6. Skopouli FN, Dafni U, Ioannidis JPA. Clinical evolution and morbidity and mortality of primary Sjögren's syndrome. Semin Arthritis Rheum. 2000;29:296–304.
7. Pertovaara M, Pukkala E, Laippala P, Miettinen A, Pasternack A. A longitudinal cohort study of Finnish patients with primary Sjögren's syndrome: clinical, immunological, and epidemiological aspects. Ann Rheum Dis. 2001;60:467–72.
8. Davidson BKS, Kelly CA, Griffiths ID. Primary Sjögren's syndrome in the North East of England: a long-term follow-up study. Rheumatology 1999;38:245–53.
9. Bates DW, Schmitt W, Buchwald D, et al. Prevalence of fatigue and chronic fatigue syndrome in a primary care practice. Arch Int Med. 1993;153:2759–65.
10. Wessely S, Hotopf M, Sharpe M. Chronic fatigue and its syndromes. Oxford: Oxford University Press; 1998.
11. Hartkamp A, Geenen R, Bijl M, Kruize AA, Godaert GL, Derksen RH. Serum cytokine levels related to multiple dimensions of fatigue in patients with primary Sjogren's syndrome. Ann Rheum Dis. 2004;63:1335–7.
12. Bax HI, Vriesendorp TM, Kallenberg CGM, Kalk WWI. Fatigue and immune activity in Sjogren's syndrome. Ann Rheum Dis. 2002;61:284.
13. Eriksson P, Andersson C, Ekerfelt C, Ernerudh J, Skogh T. Sjogren's syndrome with myalgia is associated with subnormal secretion of cytokines by peripheral blood mononuclear cells. J Rheumatol. 2004;31:729–35.
14. Wolfe F, Michaud K, Pincus T. Fatigue, rheumatoid arthritis, anti-tumour necrosis factor therapy:

an investigation in 24,831 patients. J Rheumatol. 2004;31:2115–20.
15. Stevens RJ, Hamburger J, Ainsworth JR, Holmes G, Bowman SJ. Flares of systemic disease in primary Sjögren's syndrome. Rheumatology 2005;44:402–3.
16. Huyser BA, Parker JC, Thoreson R, et al. Predictors of subjective fatigue among individuals with rheumatoid arthritis. Arthritis Rheum. 1998;41:2230–7.
17. Gottenberg JE, Busson M, Cohen-Solal J, et al. Correlation of serum B lymphocyte stimulator and beta2 microglobulin with autoantibody secretion and systemic involvement in primary Sjogren's syndrome. Ann Rheum Dis. 2005;64:1050–5.
18. Johnson EO, Kostandi M, Moutsopoulos HM. Hypothalamic–pituitary–adrenal axis function in Sjogren's syndrome: mechanisms of neuroendocrine and immune system homeostasis. Ann NY Acad Sci. 2006;1088:41–51.
19. Valtysdottir ST, Wilde L, Hallgren R. Low serum dehydroepiandrosterone sulfate in women with primary Sjögren's syndrome as an isolated sign of impaired HPA axis function. J Rheumatol. 2001:28;1259–65.
20. D'Elia HF, Rehnberg E, Kvist G, Ericsson A, Konttinen YT, Mannerkorpi K. Fatigue and blood pressure in primary Sjogren's syndrome. Scand J Rheumatol. 2008:37;284–92.
21. Tischler M, Barak Y, Paran D, Yaron M. Sleep disturbance, fibromyalgia and primary Sjogren's syndrome. Clin Exp Rheumatol. 1997;15:71–4.
22. Gudbjornsson B, Broman JE, Hetta J, Hallgren R, Sleep disturbances in patients with primary Sjögren's syndrome. Br J Rheumatol. 1993;32:1072–6.
23. Walker J, Gordon T, Lester S, et al. Increased severity of lower urinary tract symptoms and daytime somnolence in primary Sjögren's syndrome. J Rheumatol. 2003;30:2406–12.
24. Valtysdottir ST, Gudbjornsson B, Lindqvist U, Hallgren R, Hetta J. Anxiety and depression in patients with primary Sjogren's syndrome. J Rheumatol. 2000;27:165–9.
25. Pincus T, Griffith J, Pearce S, Isenberg D. Prevalence of self-reported depression in patients with rheumatoid arthritis. Br J Rheumatol. 1996;35:879–83.
26. Stevenson HA, Jones ME, Rostron JL, Longman LP, Field EA. UK patients with primary Sjögren's syndrome are at increased risk from clinical depression. Gerodontology 2004;21:141–5.
27. Champey J, Corruble E, Gottenberg JE, et al. Quality of life and psychological status in patients with primary Sjögren's syndrome and sicca symptoms without autoimmune features. Arthritis Rheum. 2006;55:451–7.
28. Vitali C, Tavoni A, Neri R, Castrogiovanni P, Pasero G, Bombardieri S. Fibromyalgia features in patients with primary Sjogren's syndrome. Evidence of a relationship with psychological depression. Scand J Rheumatol. 1989;18:21–7.
29. Ostuni P, Botsios C, Sfriso P, et al. Prevalence and clinical features of fibromyalgia in systemic lupus erythematosus, systemic sclerosis and Sjogren's syndrome. Minerva Med. 2002;93:203–9.
30. Giles I, Isenberg D. Fatigue in primary Sjögren's syndrome: is there a link with the fibromyalgia syndrome? Ann Rheum Dis. 2000;59:875–8.
31. Middleton GD, McFarlin JE, Lipsky PE. The prevalence and clinical impact of fibromyalgia in systemic lupus erythematosus. Arthritis Rheum. 1994;37:1181–8.
32. Yellen SB, Cella DF, Webster K, Blendowski C, Kaplan E. Measuring fatigue and other anemia-related symptoms with the Functional Assessment of Cancer Therapy (FACT) measurement system. J Pain Symptom Manage. 1997;13:63–74.
33. Krupp LB, LaRocca NG, Muir-Nash J, Steinberg AD. The fatigue severity scale. Arch Neurol. 1989;46:1121–3.
34. Wolfe F. Fatigue assessments in rheumatoid arthritis: comparative performance of visual analogue scales and longer fatigue questionnaires in 7760 patients. J Rheumatol. 2004;31:1896–902.
35. Dass S, Bowman SJ, Vital, et al. Reduction of fatigue in Sjögren's syndrome with rituximab: results of a randomised, double-blind, placebo controlled pilot study. Ann Rheum Dis. 2008;67:1541–4.
36. Smets EMA, Garssen B, Bonke B, De Haes JCJM. The Multidimensional Fatigue Inventory (MFI) psychometric qualities of an instrument to assess fatigue. J Psychosomatic Res. 1995;39:315–25.
37. Schwartz JE, Jandorf L, Krupp LB. The measurement of fatigue: a new instrument. J Psychosomatic Res. 1993;37:753–62.
38. Piper BF, Dibble SL, Dodd MJ, et al. The revised Piper Fatigue Scale: psychometric evaluation in women with breast cancer. Oncol Nurs Forum. 1998;25:677–84.
39. Chalder T, Berelowitz G, Pawlikowska T, et al. Development of a fatigue scale. J Psychosomatic Res. 1993;37:147–53.
40. Fisk JD, Ritvo PG, Ross L, Haase DA, Marrie TJ, Schlech WF. Measuring the functional impact of fatigue: initial validation of the Fatigue Impact Scale. Clin Infect Dis. 1994;18(Suppl 1):S79–83.
41. Ware JE, Snow KK, Kosinski M, Gandek B. SF-36 health survey. Manual and interpretation guide. Boston, MA: The Health Institute, New England Medical Centre; 1993.
42. Goodchild CE, Treharne GJ, Booth DA, Kitas GD, Bowman SJ. Measuring fatigue among women with Sjögren's syndrome or rheumatoid arthritis: a comparison of the Profile of Fatigue (ProF) and the Multidimensional Fatigue Inventory (MFI). Musculoskelet Care. 2008;6:41–8.
43. Lwin C T-T, Bishay M, Platts RG, Booth DA, Bowman SJ. The assessment of fatigue in primary Sjögren's syndrome. Scand J Rheumatol. 2003;32: 1–5.
44. Strombeck B, Theander E, Jacobsson LT. Assessment of fatigue in primary Sjogren's syndrome: the

Swedish version of the Profile of Fatigue. Scand J Rheumatol. 2005;34:455–9.
45. Bowman SJ, Hamburger J, Richards A, Barry RJ, Rauz S. Patient reported outcomes in primary Sjögren's syndrome (PSS): comparison of the long & short versions of the Profile of Fatigue & Discomfort–Sicca Symptoms Inventory (PROFAD–SSI). Rheumatology 2009;48(2):140–143.
46. The WHOQOL Group. Development of the World Health Organization WHOQOL-BREF quality of life assessment. Psychol Med. 1998;28:551–8.
47. Thomas E, Hay EM, Hajeer A, Silman AJ. Sjögren's syndrome: a community-based study of prevalence and impact. Br J Rheumatol. 1998;37:1069–76.
48. Stewart CM, Berg KM, Cha S, Reeves WH. Salivary dysfunction and quality of life in Sjogren's syndrome: a critical oral:systemic connection. J Am Dent Assoc. 2008;139:291–9.
49. Tensing EK, Solovieva SA, Tervahartiala T, et al. Fatigue and health profile in sicca syndrome of Sjögren's and non-Sjögren's syndrome origin. Clin Exp Rheumatol. 2001;19:313–6.
50. Fox RI, Dixon R, Guarrasi V, Krubel S. Treatment of primary Sjogren's syndrome with hydroxychloroquine: a retrospective, open-label study. Lupus. 1996;5(Suppl 1):S31–6.
51. Kruize AA, Hene RJ, Kallenberg CGM, et al. Hydroxychloroquine treatment for primary Sjögren's syndrome: a two year double blind crossover trial. Ann Rheum Dis. 1993;52:360–4.
52. Mariette X, Ravaud P, Steinfeld S, et al. Inefficacy of infliximab in primary Sjögren's syndrome. Arthritis Rheum. 2004;50:1270–6.
53. Hartkamp A, Geenen R, Godaert GL, et al. Effect of dehydroepiandrosterone administration on fatigue, well-being, and functioning in women with primary Sjögren's syndrome: a randomised controlled trial. Ann Rheum Dis. 2008;67:91–7.
54. Strombeck BE, Theander E, Jacobsson LTH. Effects of exercise on aerobic capacity and fatigue in women with primary Sjögren's syndrome. Rheumatology 2007;46:868–71.
55. Devauchelle-Pensec V, Pennec Y, Morvan J, et al. Improvement of Sjogren's syndrome after two infusions of rituximab (anti-CD20). Arthritis Care Res. 2007;57:310–7.
56. Pijpe J, van Imhoff GW, Spijkervet FK, et al. Rituximab treatment in patients with primary Sjogren's syndrome: an open-label phase II study. Arthritis Rheum. 2005;52:2740–50.
57. Seror R, Sordet C, Guillevin L, et al. Tolerance and efficacy of rituximab and changes in serum B cell biomarkers in patients with systemic complications of primary Sjögren's syndrome. Ann Rheum Dis. 2007;66:351–7.
58. Levesque MC, Luning Prak N, St. Clair EW, et al. Longitudinal analysis of lymphocyte subsets in patients with primary Sjogren's syndrome (pSS) treated with rituximab: results from an open-label clinical trial. Arthritis Rheum. 2007;56(Suppl):S445.
59. Meijer JM, Vissink A, Meiners PM, Spijkervet FKL, Kallenberg CGM, Bootsma H. Rituximab treatment in primary Sjogren's syndrome: a double-blind placebo controlled trial. ACR 2008. Abstract 713.
60. Steinfeld SD, Tant L, Burmester G, et al. Epratuzimab (humanised anti-CD22 antibody) in primary Sjogren's syndrome: a cohort study on cancer incidence and lymphoma predictors. Ann Rheum Dis. 2006;65:796–803.
61. McMonnies CW. Key questions in a dry eye history. J Am Optometric Assoc. 1986;57:512–7.
62. Vitali C, Bombardieri S, Jonsson R, et al. Classification criteria for Sjögren's syndrome: a revised version of the European criteria proposed by the American–European Consensus Group. Ann Rheum Dis. 2002;61:554–8.
63. Fox PC, Busch KA, Baum BJ. Subjective reports of xerostomia and objective measures of salivary gland performance. J Am Dent Assoc. 1987;115:581–4.
64. Pai S, Ghezzi EM, Ship JA. Development of a visual analogue scale questionnaire for subjective assessment of salivary dysfunction. Oral Surg Oral Med Oral Pathol Oral Radiol Endod. 2001;91:311–6.
65. Henson BS, Inglehart MR, Eisbruch A, Ship JA. Preserved salivary output and xerostomia-related quality of life in head and neck cancer patients receiving parotid-sparing radiotherapy. Oral Oncol. 2001;37:84–93.
66. Slade GD, Spencer AJ. Development and evaluation of the Oral Health Impact Profile. Comm Dent Health. 1994;11:3–11.
67. Thomson WM, Chalmers JM, Spencer AJ, Williams SM. The Xerostomia Inventory: a multi-item approach to measuring dry mouth. Comm Dent Health. 1999;16:12–7.
68. Field EA, Rostron JL, Longman LP, Bowman SJ, Lowe D, Rogers SN. The development and initial validation of the Liverpool Sicca Index to assess symptoms and dysfunction in patients with primary Sjogren's syndrome. J Oral Pathol Med. 2003;32:154–62.
69. Bowman SJ, Booth DA, Platts RG, Field A, Rostron J, UK Sjögren's Interest Group. Validation of the Sicca Symptoms Inventory (SSI) for clinical studies of Sjögren's syndrome. J Rheumatol. 2003;30: 1259–66.
70. Vivino FB, Al-Hashimi I, Khan Z, et al. Pilocarpine tablets for the treatment of dry mouth and dry eye symptoms in patients with Sjögren's syndrome. Arch Int Med. 1999;159:174–81.
71. Schiffman RM, Christianson MD, Jacobsen G, Hirsch JD, Reis BL. Reliability and validity of the ocular surface disease index. Arch Ophthalmol. 2000;118:615–21.
72. Vitale S, Goodman LA, Reed GF, Smith JA. Comparison of the NEI–VFQ and OSDI questionnaires in patients with Sjögren's syndrome-related dry eye. Health Qual Life Outcomes. 2004;2:44.
73. Fife RS, Chase WF, Dore RK, et al. Cevimeline for the treatment of xerostomia in patients with Sjögren's

syndrome. A randomized trial. Arch Intern Med. 2002;162:1293–300.

74. Petrone D, Condemi JJ, Fife R, et al. A double-blind, randomized, placebo-controlled study of cevimeline in Sjögren's syndrome patients with xerostomia and keratoconjunctivitis sicca. Arthritis Rheum. 2002;46:748–54.
75. Shiozawa S, Tanaka Y, Shiozawa K. Single-blinded controlled trial of low-dose oral IFN-a for the treatment of xerostomia in patients with Sjogren's syndrome. J Interferon Cytokine Res. 1998;18:255–62.
76. Cummins MJ, Papas A, Kammer GM, Fox PC. Treatment of primary Sjogren's syndrome with low-dose human interferon α administered by the oromucosal route: combined phase III results. Arthritis Rheum. 2003;49:585–93.
77. Stevenson D, Tauber J, Reis BL. Efficacy and safety of cyclosporin A ophthalmic emulsion in the treatment of moderate-to-severe dry eye disease: a dose-ranging, randomised trial. The Cyclosporin A Phase 2 Study Group. Ophthalmology 2000;107:967–74.
78. Sall K, Stevenson OD, Mundorf TK, Reis BL, CsA Phase 3 Study Group. Two multicenter, randomised studies of the efficacy and safety of cyclosporine ophthalmic emulsion in moderate to severe dry eye disease. Ophthalmology 2000;107:631–9.
79. Bowman S, Pillemer S, Jonsson, et al. Revisiting Sjögren's syndrome in the new millennium: perspectives on assessment and outcome measures. Report of a workshop held on 23 March 2000 at Oxford, UK. Rheumatology 2001;40:1180–8.
80. Pillemer SR, Smith J, Fox PC, Bowman SJ. Outcome measures for Sjögren's syndrome, April 10–11, 2003, Bethesda, Maryland, USA. J Rheumatol. 2005;32:143–9.
81. Wells G, Li T, Maxwell L, Maclean R, Tugwell P. Responsiveness of patient reported outcomes including fatigue, sleep quality, activity limitation, and quality of life following treatment with abatacept for rheumatoid arthritis. Ann Rheum Dis. 2008;67: 260–5.
82. Vitali C, Palombi G, Baldini C, et al. Sjögren's syndrome disease damage index and disease activity index: scoring systems for the assessment of disease damage and disease activity in Sjögren's syndrome, derived from an analysis of a cohort of Italian patients. Arthritis Rheum. 2007;56:2223–31.
83. Felson DT, Anderson JJ, Boers M, et al. American College of Rheumatology. Preliminary definition of improvement in rheumatoid arthritis. Arthritis Rheum. 1995;38:727–35.
84. Hay EM, Thomas E, Pal B, Hajeer A, Chambers H, Silman AJ. Weak association between subjective symptoms of and objective testing for dry eyes and dry mouth: results from a population based study. Ann Rheum Dis. 1998;57:20–4.
85. Barry RJ, Sutcliffe N, Isenberg DA, et al. The Sjögren's syndrome damage index—a damage index for use in clinical trials and observational studies in primary Sjögren's syndrome. Rheumatology 2008;47:1193–8.

The Neurological Manifestations of Sjögren's Syndrome: Diagnosis and Treatment

22

Robert I. Fox and Julius Birnbaum

Abstract

This chapter addresses the following:

(a) clinical neurological presentation,
(b) laboratory investigation, and
(c) treatment of peripheral and central nervous system diseases associated with Sjögren's syndrome.

Keywords

Peripheral neuropathy • Cognitive dysfunction • Polyneuropathy • Myopathy • Cerebrovascular disease • Mononeuritis multiplex • Anti-cardiolipin syndrome • Vasculitis • Vasculopathy • Cryoglobulinemia • IgM paraproteinemic neuropathy • Demyelinating polyneuropathy • Dysesthesia • Ataxia • and sensory ataxic neuropathy • Athetosis • Areflexia • Dysarthria • Vasculitic neuropathy • Diabetic and non-diabetic radiculoplexus neuropathies • Autoimmune autonomic neuropathy • Paraneoplastic autonomic neuropathy • Amyloid neuropathy • Sporadic amyloid and genetically determined amyloidosis • Hypocomplementemia • Albumin-cytological dissociation • Aseptic meningoencephalitis • Acute cerebellar ataxia • Cerebral venous thrombosis • Hypertrophic cranial pachymeningitis • Lymphocytic hypophysitis • Acute transverse myelitis

Abbreviations

SS	Sjögren's syndrome
PNS	Peripheral nervous system
CNS	Central nervous system
ACL	Anti-cardiolipin
APLS	Anti-phospholipid antibodies syndrome
FMS	Fibromyalgia syndrome
MGUS	Monoclonal gammopathy of unknown significance
CIDP	Chronic inflammatory demyelinating polyneuropathy
PML	Progressive multifocal leukoencephalopathy
NMO	Neuromyelitis optica (Devic's syndrome)

R.I. Fox (✉)
Rheumatology Clinic, Scripps Memorial Hospital and Research Foundation, La Jolla, CA, USA
e-mail: robertfoxmd@mac.com

R.I. Fox, C.M. Fox (eds.), *Sjögren's Syndrome*, DOI 10.1007/978-1-60327-957-4_22,

22.1 Introduction

Neurologists occupy an invaluable role in partnering with rheumatologists, to facilitate the diagnosis of Sjögren's patients, to prioritize and interpret diagnostic studies, and help with the management of an eclectic array of central nervous system (CNS) and peripheral nervous system (PNS) manifestations. There is considerable evidence for the involvement of the nervous system in Sjögren's syndrome (SS) [1]. The pathogenic processes include the acquired immune system (T-cell and B-cell-mediated factors) and the innate immune system (including complement and coagulation systems as well as release of cytokines/chemokines).

Clinically, there is a very wide range in the reported prevalence of *central and peripheral neurological manifestations* associated with Sjögren's syndrome. *Complaints of peripheral neuropathy, fatigue, and impaired cognitive function* may occur in up to 70% of patients and *are often listed as the most important clinical extraglandular features in their impaired quality of life assessment (see* Chapter 21).

A wide range of peripheral neuropathies may be found in SS (described further in sections below). These include (Table 22.1)

- Small fiber neuropathies, an exquisitely painful neuropathy which affects unmyelinated nerves
- Axonal polyneuropathies, which can exclusively affect sensory nerves (i.e., axonal sensory neuropathy), which can exclusively affect motor nerves (i.e., axonal motor neuropathy), or which can affect sensory as well as motor nerves (i.e., sensorimotor polyneuropathies)
- Ganglionopathies (i.e., also called sensory neuronopathy or ataxic neuropathies)—loss of proprioception, resulting in "deafferentation," due to dysfunction of the dorsal root ganglia. Such severe deafferentation can cause pseudoathetoid movements, which can be misdiagnosed as a movement disorder
- Vasculitic neuropathies
- Cranial neuropathies (as described below)
- Autonomic neuropathies

Symptoms of muscle or nerve pain [2] may not correlate well with objective testing on standard electromyography (EMG) studies which are most sensitive for large fibers or myelinated A-fibers, in comparison to single unmyelinated C-fibers that serve as nociceptors [3]. Dermatomal-evoked somatosensory potentials also have a high "false"-negative rate in correlations with symptoms [4]. Even with newer techniques of skin biopsies stained for nerve fibers, the correlation of symptoms and small fiber changes, the correlation with symptoms may be poor due to the influence of "fibromyalgia" affecting the patient's perception of pain [5].

The *differential diagnosis* of neuropathies found in SS patients includes those associated with diabetes or hypertension. A diagnostic dilemma is the patient with an *"idiopathic neuropathy" and a positive ANA/anti-SSA antibody*. Even though the patient may lack symptoms, signs, or biopsies characteristic of SS, these patients may be referred to rheumatologist with diagnosis of SS based on the positive anti-nuclear antibody (ANA) for consideration of systemic therapy.

Symptoms of dry mouth and neurological pain are frequent complaints in patients with depression unrelated to SS [6]. Again, the laboratory evaluation of these patients may reveal a low-titer ANA and raise the question of relationship of their depression and dryness to SS. This group probably includes the common complaint of "burning mouth syndrome" where no other etiology can be ascertained to explain the oral symptoms that appear out of proportion to examination of the oral mucosa or salivary flow measurements. The issue facing the rheumatologist is whether to initiate immunosuppressive therapy or simply pursue symptomatic relief.

Objective abnormalities of the central nervous system (CNS) manifestations include both white matter and cerebral atrophy that have been noted in MRI studies and CSF studies of SS patients [7–10]. SS patients with transverse myelitis may include relatively distinct subsets that involve the gray and white matter involvement [11], similar to distinct subsets of SLE patients with myelitis

Table 22.1 Neurological manifestations of Sjögren's syndrome: peripheral neuropathy

• Has been reported in 10–20% of patients, mainly in the form of sensorimotor and sensory polyneuropathies.
• Subclinical manifestations may be much more frequent and present in up to 50% of SS patients.
• The severity of symptoms as perceived by the patient may be significantly influenced by "central sensitization," i.e., "fibromyalgia."
• Motor involvement should suggest the presence of vasculitis or mononeuritis multiplex.
Central nervous system (CNS) manifestations of Sjögren's syndrome are diverse, with an array of clinical features including the following:
• Cognitive disorder and neuropsychiatric manifestations.
• Transient ischemic attack (TIA) and stroke.
• Thrombotic manifestations of the brain are more common than large or medium-sized vasculitic processes, particularly in association with anti-cardiolipin and anti-coagulants.
• Severe migraine headaches that may mimic TIA with focal weakness after the migraine.
• Myelopathy including transverse myelitis and demyelinating disease.
• Ganglionopathy.
• Seizures.
• Toxic-metabolic encephalopathy.
• Vasculitis and cranial neuropathies.
• Parkinson's disease.
The spectrum of CNS manifestations in SS is generally similar to systemic lupus erythematosus (SLE) patients with the caveat that SS patients have a higher frequency of lymphoproliferative manifestations and the associated neurologic sequelae.
SS patients may also have CNS manifestations caused by *secondary factors*, including infections associated with immunosuppressive therapy, side effects from corticosteroids, and occult nutritional deficiencies (resulting from altered eating habits due to mouth/dental problems or malabsorption from associated celiac sprue or pernicious anemia).
Treatment: Sensory peripheral neuropathies may respond to *pentagabalin* or *pregabalin*.
• *Traditional therapies* for peripheral sensory neuropathies, such as *tricyclic agents, amitriptyline* or *nortriptyline*, may not be tolerated at therapeutic doses due to their anti-cholinergic side effects.
• *The major dose-limiting side effect of anti-epileptics—which may lead to premature continuation of these medications—is aggravation of fatigue, which can be a major cause of subjective morbidity in Sjögren's patients. Such premature discontinuation can be mitigated by slower titration than is normally employed in other patients with neuropathic pain.*
• Newer agents such as *duloxetine* or *milnacipran* may be useful, particularly in combination with other agents.
• *Other causes of neuropathic pain or myelopathy including infections* with viruses (i.e., Herpes zoster), immune reactions to viruses (i.e., hepatitis C) or spirochetes (including Borrelia species), and mycobacterial infections including tuberculosis must be excluded.
• *Other causes of neuropathy* including hypertension and diabetes must be carefully controlled and recognition of their exacerbation by corticosteroids, as well as steroid myopathy.
Corticosteroids are the first-line treatment for myelopathy and vasculitis.
When SS patients fail to improve or deteriorate on corticosteroids, *non-steroidal immunosuppressant(s)* should be used for treatment or to help taper the steroid dose:
• *Pulse intravenous cyclophosphamide or oral cyclophosphamide* is often used for acute vasculitis in SS patients, although controlled trials are lacking.
• *Azathioprine, leflunomide,* and *methotrexate* may be used to help taper corticosteroids, in a manner similar to systemic lupus or rheumatoid arthritis patients.
• *Biologic agents (anti-CD20, infliximab, and anti-CD22 antibodies)* have been reported beneficial in small case series of SS patients with neurological manifestations.
• *IV-Ig* has been used in axonal polyneuropathies and ganglionopathies that are resistant to corticosteroids and non-steroidal immunosuppressants.

[12]. The "distinction" of purely anatomic separation of white and gray matter is used here as a simplified way for the rheumatologist to approach this complex diagnostic problem.

Perhaps, the greatest source of debate in the past 20 years has been the incidence of "multiple sclerosis" (MS) in SS patients. Initial references reported a relatively high frequency of possible demyelinating lesions on MRI in SS patients with vague symptoms of chronic fatigue. The diagnosis of MS associated with SS led to a great deal of concern on the part of patients and a therapeutic dilemma for physicians. However, using newer MRI techniques (described below), the frequency of demyelinating lesions in SS and SLE patients has been reported at less than 5% [13, 14]. *With the current benefit of the revised MS McDonald criteria* [15]*—which provides surrogate evidence for dissemination of lesions in space—future studies should characterize the white matter lesions in Sjögren's patients, through the prism of updated MRI criteria (i.e., Barkhof criteria)* [16]. *Such a comparison would be useful in determining whether the white matter lesions in Sjögren's patients have the radiographic and morphological features of MS lesions.*

Studies in SS have suggested a role for *accelerated vasculopathy* (particularly in patients with circulating anti-coagulants, leukopenia, and elevated C-reactive protein (CRP) and *"atherosclerotic" changes in "precocious" carotid intimal thickening* [17]. In SLE, accelerated atherosclerosis has been reported on MRI of the brain and correlated with decreased performance on neuropsychiatric testing. It should be noted that one review study failed to find accelerated atherosclerosis in SS patients, in comparison to SLE patients [18]. However, as noted in other chapters, the criteria for inclusion of SS patients have varied tremendously over the past decade. Therefore, any "meta-analysis" of studies that assess "early" atherosclerotic CNS changes in SS patients will need to include only SS patients identified by strict current diagnostic criteria. The same factors that led to accelerated atherosclerosis in SLE are also found in SS patients [17]. Therefore, the authors predicted that similar processes leading to accelerated vasculopathy will be found to affect the SS patient. Further, attention to preventable factors such as "tight control" of blood pressure, lipids, and diabetes will be important as well as control of the underlying inflammatory process that also contributes to vasculopathy.

22.2 Clinical Evaluation of Neurological Findings in SS

It is critical for the rheumatologist to make the following mental notes to guide in the triage of neurological symptoms including

a. *Onset of symptoms and signs* (gradual or sudden);
b. *Severity and rate of progression* of either central or peripheral findings;
c. *Distribution* as symmetric, asymmetric, proximal, distal, focal, or diffuse of peripheral findings;
d. *Evidence for co-existence of peripheral vasculitis*; and
e. *Evidence for infection* associated with onset of central findings (brain or spinal cord).

Although there are exceptions, our experience at Scripps [19] *suggests that:*

- *Seizures and meningoencephalitis tend to present acutely and early in the course of disease in association with active vasculitis, similar to that reported in SLE* [20].
- *Cognitive features due to structural CNS damage tend to develop slowly and later in the course of disease; the contribution of chronic fatigue syndrome (i.e., central sensitization, fibromyalgia) makes evaluation of "clinical disability" difficult.*
- *CNS manifestations do not closely correlate with peripheral manifestations of active vasculitis or elevation of acute phase reactants such as* erythrocyte sedimentation rate (ESR) *or CRP.*
- *Thrombotic lesions in the CNS are more common than large or medium-sized vasculitis, particularly in patients with circulating anticoagulants.*
- *Weakness as an objective presenting sign early in the course of disease may be due to*

transverse myelitis or CIDP, while myopathy later in the course of disease may result from steroid myopathy.

22.3 Pathogenesis of Neurological Manifestations

22.3.1 Role of Cell-Mediated Immunity

Peripheral nervous system involvement in SS was initially thought to be predominantly due to necrotizing vasculitis, similar to that visualized on SLE kidney biopsies or leukocytoclastic skin biopsies [21]. However, subsequent studies on biopsies from patients with peripheral neuropathies have found that "true" necrotizing vasculitis of medium or large-sized blood vessels are uncommon. Instead, a "microvasculitis" that has features similar to the peripheral neuropathy of diabetes has [22] been noted in SS biopsies [21, 23]. These studies have suggested a critical role for lymphocytes and dendritic cells that release cytokines leading to "vasculopathy" that includes complement activation and coagulation pathways [24–26].

Sural nerve biopsies in a study by Mori et al. [22] in Japanese SS patients have demonstrated lymphocytes in the small vessels (including arterioles and high endothelial venules) in association with vascular occlusions suggestive of chronic endothelium damage. Among 55 biopsies from Japanese SS patients [22], predominantly large fiber loss was observed in sensory ataxic neuropathy, whereas predominantly small fiber loss occurred in painful sensory neuropathy. Angiitis and perivascular cell invasion were seen most frequently in multiple mononeuropathy, followed by sensory ataxic neuropathy. The autopsy findings of one patient with sensory ataxic neuropathy showed severe large sensory neuron loss paralleling to dorsal root and posterior column involvement of the spinal cord and severe sympathetic neuron loss. Degrees of neuron loss in the dorsal and sympathetic ganglia corresponded to segmental distribution of sensory and sweating impairments. Multifocal T-cell invasion was seen in the dorsal root and sympathetic ganglia, perineurial space, and vessel walls in the *nerve* trunks. Similar changes have been reported in sural nerve biopsies of Caucasian SS patients [27]. Biopsies of dorsal root ganglia and autopsy studies of SS patients with CNS manifestations have noted vasculopathy involving the choroid plexus and suggested that alteration of the vascular permeability to antibodies, cytokines, and adhesion/entry of either lymphocytes or other pro-inflammatory cells plays a role [28–30].

Additional studies on sural nerve biopsy of patients with painful sensory neuropathy show reduced density of small diameter myelinated and unmyelinated fibers [31, 32], in contrast to ataxic neuropathy where large axonal fiber loss is seen [22, 33–35]. Axonal degeneration is present in teased fiber preparations, without axonal sprouting suggesting dorsal root ganglion pathology.

Epidermal nerve fiber density, as measured by immunostained panaxonal marker protein gene product ("PGP 9.5") (see Chapter 11), is reduced in patients with burning feet—in many cases in a non-length-dependent distribution [27].

The number of reported dorsal root ganglion biopsies in sensory ataxic neuropathy is relatively limited [22, 33, 34] but significant, in terms of the understanding of the pathophysiology. These abnormalities are characterized by T-cell infiltration, neuronal cell, and fiber loss, with inflammatory cells around neurons and blood vessels [35, 36]. Electron microscopy showed "onion bulbs" in one case suggesting prior inflammation [35, 36].

Pathological material associated with *motor neuropathies* in Sjögren's syndrome is restricted to sural nerve and muscle. Sural nerve biopsies show varying degrees of vasculitis of small vessels with decreased fiber density of myelinated axons [22, 33, 34, 37–39]. Perivascular or vascular inflammation in small epineural vessels with necrosis may be seen. Nerve fiber loss may be diffuse or multifocal.

Terrier et al. [39] had 8 patients with lymphocytic vasculitis and 14 with necrotizing vasculitis in their 34 patients, noting that vasculitis was present in patients with multiple mononeuropathy and sensorimotor neuropathy, but never in patients with ganglionopathy, and reduced in patients with pronounced sensory symptoms. In the myopathies [40], varying degrees of inflammatory changes occur, in a perivascular, endomysial, or perimysial distribution. The majority of infiltrating lymphocytes are T cells, and inflammatory cells in the perimysium are often associated with a vasculitis [41, 51]. Non-specific abnormalities with degeneration, regeneration, muscle fiber size variation, split fibers, atrophic fibers, and ragged red fibers are seen as well [41, 42].

There appears to be a complex "vicious cycle" that involves humeral immunity described below (including anti-coagulants), innate immune factors such as CRP, complement activation and associated coagulopathy, and cytokine/chemokine release that perpetuates the small vessel damage and leukocyte adherence.

Vasculopathy in the periphery and the CNS is characterized by a small-to-moderate perivascular accumulation of mononuclear cells, without destruction (e.g., fibrinoid necrosis) of the blood vessel [43]. There may be small infarcts due to luminal occlusion. The pathogenic basis of vasculopathy remains largely unknown, but the pathologic findings have some similarities to the biopsies from diabetic patients [43]. Indeed, rheumatologists have a great deal to learn about the pathogenesis of SS from the glandular and extraglandular manifestations of diabetes [44].

The accessibility of the salivary gland to biopsy may provide a tissue model for understanding the underlying processes that originate with vascular changes and perivascular infiltrates of mononuclear cells and dendritic cells. As outlined in the chapters on salivary gland pathology and neuroendocrine factors, analysis of the earliest vasculopathy changes in the SS gland may permit understanding of the molecular events that result in vasculopathy. These events include continued activation of the innate immune system that is reflected in type I interferon and interleukin-1 gene signatures found in SS salivary gland tissue biopsies [45] and the later homing of inflammatory cells with resultant metalloproteinase and cytokine induction.

22.3.2 The Role of Antibodies Associated with Neurological Manifestations of SS

The "purest" example of humoral factors in neuropathogenesis involves anti-SSA antibodies in pregnant SS patients, where maternal antibodies cross the placenta to interfere with the developing fetal cardiac neural conducting system [46–48]. Another example of humoral-mediated neuropathic damage is the presence of anti-myelin-associated protein in SS patients with chronic inflammatory demyelinating polyneuropathy (CIDP). Anti-cardiolipin antibodies and lupus anti-coagulants predispose to thrombotic events including strokes and microvascular nephritis with hypertensive crises.

Among *differences between SS and SLE*, SS patients have a higher frequency than SLE patients of lymphoproliferative disorders including lymphoma. Accordingly, they have a higher frequency of antibodies associated with mixed cryoglobulinemia (i.e., monoclonal rheumatoid factors that participate in type II mixed cryoglobulin) and other paraneoplastic antibodies such as ANNA-1 or Ri [49, 50–53].

In these SS patients, the pathogenetic role of autoantibodies in neurological manifestations has been established.

Other autoantibodies have been associated with neurological symptoms but the association may not be causal.

SS patients, in comparison to SLE patients, have a higher frequency of autoantibodies to muscarinic receptors [54] *and to fodrin, a structural brain antigen that has been found in circulation after stroke in non-autoimmune patients* [55].

These latter antibodies have been proposed to contribute to autonomic and central neurological manifestations, although it is unclear whether the antibodies are pathogenetic or the consequence of neurological damage.

Antibodies from SS patients can be infused into mice to interfere with neural innervation of the glands and the function of bladder smooth muscle of guinea pigs or rabbits in vitro. However, the structure of muscarinic receptors in rodents (and their glycosylation) differs from humans. Also, the ability of SS sera to reproducibly react with human cells transfected with muscarinic receptor suggests that the reactivity detected in the bladder muscle assays is not easy to translate to in vivo activity. However, the pathogenetic importance of these anti-muscarinic antibodies is potentially very important, since it would change our conception of SS from an SLE-like illness and make it more similar to a myasthenia gravis syndrome, where antibodies against muscarinic receptor are pathogenetic.

22.4 Investigations

22.4.1 Neurophysiology

Sensory nerve action potentials are often normal, but may be reduced or absent in painful sensory neuropathies and ataxic neuropathy. *The presence of preserved sensory nerve action potentials (SNAPs), in a patient with isolated examination findings of impaired "small fiber modalities" (i.e., pinprick and temperature), should immediately suggest the diagnosis of small fiber neuropathies in SS* [56, 57]. *Because the small fiber neuropathies often affect only the unmyelinated nociceptive nerves, the sensitivity of detection of abnormality is relatively low on routine electrodiagnostic studies.*

Motor nerve conduction abnormalities on EMG/nerve conduction velocity (NCV) among 28% of patients were reported in a large cohort study of SS patients from Johns Hopkins University [58]; the EMG/NCV most frequently demonstrated predominantly symmetric axonal sensorimotor polyneuropathy, although the patient's symptoms reflected a predominance of sensory symptoms, followed by cranial nerve involvement affecting trigeminal, facial, or cochlear nerves. Multiple mononeuropathy, myositis, and polyradiculoneuropathy were also reported by these patients. Often, the symptoms preceded the diagnosis of SS. These studies [58] indicated a relatively poor correlation of motor symptoms and abnormal EMG findings. Similarly, Andonopoulos et al. [59] performed EMG/NCV studies on 63 consecutive Greek SS patients with complaints of mild sensory neuropathy. One had pure *motor* neuropathy and another eight had EMG findings of mixed *sensory/motor* neuropathy. None volunteered neurological motor complaints. Also, similar results were found in neurological evaluation and EMG/NCV studies on consecutive Japanese SS patients [57] and European SS patients [60].

Sensory-evoked potentials are often abnormal in ataxic neuropathies [57, 61, 62]. In neuropathies with weakness, compound muscle action potentials are reduced in involved nerves, and sensory nerve action potentials may be affected as well. Motor conduction velocities may be slowed and F-wave latencies prolonged with root involvement [31, 33, 60, 63].

Neurogenic abnormalities are frequently present on needle electrode examination [37, 38]. In the myopathies, needle electrode abnormalities are characterized by fibrillation potentials, myopathic motor units, and increased recruitment of motor units with muscle activation.

22.4.2 Autonomic Studies

Heart rate and blood pressure homeostasis in SS patients are often abnormal with tilt table study [64, 65]. Heart rate and blood pressure variability measurements may be evaluated by several other different methods to evaluate spontaneous baroreflex sensitivity and cardiovascular reflex [66]. Segmental anhidrosis may also be noted in SS patients [67].

Abnormal reflex vasoconstrictor responses to contralateral cooling can be demonstrated with laser Doppler imaging [68, 69]. Marked decreases in ^{123}I-MIBG uptake, cardiac uptake indicating sympathetic innervation abnormalities, occur in patients with either sensory ataxic neuropathy or painful sensory neuropathy [57].

Thermoregulatory testing [70] may demonstrate abnormalities.

22.4.3 MR Imaging of the Spinal Cord

Spinal cord magnetic resonance imaging may be abnormal in patients with sensory ataxic neuropathy with T2-weighted hyperintensities in the fasciculus cuneatus and gracilis [57, 71, 72]. In one study [62], MRI abnormalities on T2* of the posterior columns correlated with the distribution and severity of the neuropathy. A review of imaging techniques for ganglionopathies in SS patients was recently reported [73].

22.5 Peripheral Clinical Manifestations

Frequencies of the reported prevalence of neuropathy associated with Sjögren's syndrome vary greatly in different centers, with incidence ranging between 4.5 and 60% depending on methods of patient selection, population, and criteria used for defining Sjögren's syndrome [33, 58, 74–77].

The clinical expression of the neuropathy associated with Sjögren's syndrome at Scripps [19] is similar to that reported at Johns Hopkins [58] and several other medical centers [22, 33].

There are several presentations of peripheral *neuropathy* associated with Sjögren's syndrome:

- *Sensory neuropathies* are a common presentation, dominated by either painful dysesthesia or by ataxia.
- *Motor neuropathy or neuromuscular weakness* is the outstanding part of the presentation in other patients, occurring less frequently according to patient's symptoms, but invariably associated with sensory findings.
- *Muscle weakness and pain* occur on the basis of direct muscle involvement.
- *The autonomic system is frequently involved,* often in combination with the other forms, and may be the presenting form as described above including anhidrosis on a neuropathic basis [78].
- *Ganglionopathies:* An *asymmetrical onset can be seen in the ganglionopathies—with initial clinical manifestations including ataxia and dysesthesia—or with the small fiber neuropathies, in which the distribution of pain can be asymmetrical and multifocal. These neuropathies may involve any distribution—even in a pattern not easily conforming to a dermatomal or neuropathic pattern—involving the trunk, proximal limb, or face.*
- *Pseudo-athetosis* is a continuous stream of slow, sinuous, writhing movements, typically of the hands and feet. This movement, usually of the fingers, occurs when the eyes are closed, caused by a failure of joint position sense (proprioception), for example, in peripheral neuropathy. The term is used to distinguish the movements from *athetosis,* which are caused by damage to the corpus striatum of the brain—specifically to the putamen—or caused by a lesion of the motor thalamus.
- *Finally, cranial nerves* and especially the *trigeminal nerve* may be affected.

  Anhidrosis can present similarly.

In these neuropathies with a multifocal or asymmetric onset, the neuropathy may evolve into a generalized form, enter a chronic phase, remit, or relapse. A *gradual onset* is more often the case, and the course is frequently mild, but may be particularly severe or disabling, and response to therapy is unpredictable.

22.6 Painful Sensory Neuropathies

Early case reports describe an asymmetric onset of painful neuropathic symptoms in patients with Sjögren's syndrome [60, 79, 80]. *In general, women in their mid-fifties are predominantly affected* [34, 57, 81] often with *burning feet* being the main complaint. The neuropathy may have a length-dependent onset and progress, but *early involvement of thigh, hands, trunk, or face* is not infrequent. *Paresthesia* may accompany the pain [37, 38].

A *unilateral presentation* with painful *dysesthesias spreading to trunk and face* chronically over months to years was found in 18 patients (20%) without ataxia in 1 study [34]. In this study, seven patients could not walk because of severe pain. In another study, Kaplan and Schaumburg [82] described a 21-year-old woman with painful left-sided numbness and dysesthesias beginning on the left side of her face, thumb, and fore-finger of the left hand, spreading in a week to involve the left arm, mid-forearm, and left foot. The neurological abnormalities were confined to the left side with profound *loss of vibration and position sense*, *pseudo-athetosis*, and *areflexia*.

Neuropathic symptoms are usually chronic, may gradually extend, and may be severe.

22.6.1 Differential Diagnosis

Potential causes of painful small fiber neuropathies include hypertension, diabetes and "impaired glucose tolerance," alcohol, paraproteins, hyperlipidemia, amyloidosis, Fabry's disease, hereditary sensory neuropathies, and drug toxicity including vincristine, paclitaxel, and other pharmacological toxins [83–87].

In a study of 124 patients with sensory neuropathy, Devigili et al. [87] diagnosed small fiber neuropathy in 67 patients, 5 of whom had Sjögren's syndrome and a sixth developed Sjögren's in the 2-year follow-up period.

22.7 Sensory Ataxic Neuropathy

Sensory ataxic neuropathies occur as a result of pathological involvement of dorsal root ganglia or their axons [71, 88].

Malinow et al. [36] described a patient with a subacute ataxic sensory neuropathy and Sjögren's syndrome. This patient developed a band-like tightness around the neck and thorax with pain, dysesthesia, and numbness in the left hand, face, and tongue, followed by progressive loss of dexterity in both hands, dysarthria, and labial anesthesia.

The examination showed facial numbness, profound loss of position and vibratory sensation in both upper extremities, and moderate loss in the lower extremities. Muscle strength was normal, and deep tendon reflexes were absent. There were pseudo-athetoid movements in both hands and the fingers were hyperextended. Gait was mildly ataxic. Bilateral somatosensory median-evoked, radial-evoked, and ulnar-evoked potentials were absent, but those from the peroneals were present. A thoracic dorsal root ganglion biopsy showed infiltration with mononuclear cells and neuronal degeneration.

The reported frequency of *ataxic neuropathy* is variable [33, 35, 76] and was the most commonly occurring presentation in one study [57] with 40% of patients affected, usually middle-aged women.

The *onset* may be abrupt, slowly progress over years, stabilize, or relapse [57, 89]. A unilateral presentation is frequent with a variable distribution with loss of proprioception and kinesthetic sensibility and pseudo-athetosis. Autonomic involvement is common [22].

22.7.1 Differential Diagnosis

Vasculitis, thrombotic (especially cardiolipin syndrome), embolic, malignant inflammatory sensory polyganglionopathy (associated with antibody to ANNA-1 and ANNA-2), idiopathic non-malignant inflammatory sensory polyganglionopathy [22], toxic-sensory polyganglionopathy (pyridoxine, cisplatin, paclitaxel), sensory variant of acute and chronic inflammatory demyelinating neuropathies, and IgM paraproteinemic neuropathy are all considerations in the differential diagnosis [89].

22.8 Neuromuscular Weakness

From a clinical perspective, one may recognize neuropathies to be characterized primarily by neuromuscular weakness and categorized as mononeuropathy, multiple mononeuropathy, polyradiculoneuropathy, or sensorimotor neuropathy based on electrophysiological studies.

The distribution of weakness may be segmental, multifocal, proximal or distal, and asymmetric. These forms may be associated with varying degrees of sensory involvement and as a general observation occur less frequently than the primarily sensory neuropathies. Frequencies and definitions of various types differ [32, 38, 39, 74, 76].

There is often an acute onset of weakness together with tingling or dysesthesias in a limb distally, extending to a multiple mononeuropathy pattern.

22.8.1 Differential Diagnosis

Acute inflammatory demyelinating polyneuropathy, chronic inflammatory demyelinating polyneuropathy, non-systemic vasculitic neuropathy, diabetic and non-diabetic radiculoplexus neuropathy, and the vasculitides associated with neuropathy are in the differential diagnosis [89, 90].

The latter includes classic polyarteritis nodosa, mixed connective disease, SLE, overlap syndrome, rheumatoid arthritis, and cryoglobulinemic vasculitis. *Cryoglobulinemic vasculitis may rarely occur in Sjogren's patients; isolated C4 hypocomplementemia (with normal C3) may be a clue to the presence of a cryoglobulin* [91, 92].

22.9 Neuromuscular Pain

Muscle pain occurs in about one-third [93] *of patients with Sjögren's syndrome*, and half of these patients fulfill criteria for fibromyalgia [94].

Pain affects shoulders, back, thighs, and calves and is usually symmetric and may be associated with weakness. The latter may occur in the absence of pain and is generally proximal and symmetric in distribution.

Sjögren's syndrome may be associated with polymyositis, dermatomyositis, and inclusion body myositis [95–97]. However, the inflammatory changes in muscle do not correlate closely with weakness or pain [41].

22.9.1 Differential Diagnosis

The main considerations are the inflammatory myopathies including polymyositis, dermatomyositis, inclusion body myopathy, rheumatoid arthritis, mixed connective disease, and scleroderma [40].

22.10 Autonomic Neuropathy

Sjögren's syndrome may present with generalized autonomic failure in the absence of other neurological abnormalities.

Sakakibara et al. [64] described a 64-year-old woman presenting with Raynaud's phenomenon followed by painful dry eyes, dry mouth, and parotid pain. Three years later, she was constipated; by 8 years had postural dizziness; and in 10 years presented to the hospital with decreased perspiration, urinary urgency, and decreased frequency of defecation to every fifth day.

Autonomic function tests showed supersensitivity of the pupils to noradrenaline, postural hypotension, and anhidrosis with provocative testing. Urinary flow decreased, anal resting pressure was low, and colonic transit time was 144 h. Motor and sensory nerve conduction studies were normal. There was cardiac supersensitivity to diluted noradrenaline infusion and cardiac denervation on [^{123}I]-MIBG scintigraphy.

Autonomic symptoms may be severe [22, 33] with hypotension and syncope as well as widespread anhidrosis, which may be segmental and asymmetric [67]. Milder involvement of the autonomic nervous system occurs more frequently (50% [98], 66% of those screened) [33] and may affect multiple autonomically controlled organs. Orthostatic intolerance, bladder symptoms, constipation, pupillomotor disorder, secretomotor dysfunction, male sexual dysfunction, gastroparesis, diarrhea, sleep dysfunction, and reflex syncope are common problems [33, 68–70, 99].

Parasympathetic nerve dysfunction may be mediated by a deficiency in neural transmission. Bacman and co-workers [100, 101] initially demonstrated the ability of antibodies from SS patients to inhibit lacrimal glandular function on transfer into rodents. Wang et al. [102] extended these studies by demonstrating that M3 muscarinic receptor-mediated bladder contractions in mice or guinea pig could be blocked in vitro with purified IgG from patients with Sjögren's syndrome.

22.10.1 Differential Diagnosis

The differential diagnosis includes *acute, subacute, and chronic autonomic neuropathies* [103, 104]. Post-infectious autoimmune autonomic neuropathy, paraneoplastic neuropathy, diabetes, amyloid neuropathy in its various forms including sporadic amyloid and genetically determined amyloidosis, drug-induced autonomic neuropathy (*cis*-platinum, vinca alkaloids, and amiodarone), and toxic-autonomic neuropathies (heavy metals, hexacarbon compounds, and acrylamide) are part of the differential diagnosis. Unusual disorders include hereditary and autonomic neuropathies, porphyria, and distal small fiber neuropathy [104].

22.11 Trigeminal Neuropathy and Other Cranial Neuropathies

Cranial nerve involvement occurs during the course of Sjögren's syndrome, *most frequently involving the trigeminal nerve. Numbness, paresthesia, dysesthesia, and altered taste perception* are presenting symptoms and *motor function is usually spared* [38, 57, 105]. Reported prevalence varies [33, 58] and may be higher in Japanese patients [74]. Other cranial nerve manifestations include *hearing loss, vestibular symptoms, facial nerve involvement, and loss of olfaction.*

Mori et al. reported five patients with multiple cranial neuropathies, one with involvement of cranial nerves III, V, VI, VII, IX, and X, one with bilateral involvement of VII, and recurrent III and VI involvement in one patient [57, 106].

22.12 Central Nervous System Manifestations

There is no unique central nervous system presentation of Sjögren's syndrome. A broad spectrum of abnormalities have been described, with reported prevalence ranging from 1 to 46% [74, 107–110].

Presentations include *mild cognitive impairment, subcortical dementia, encephalopathy, recurrent aseptic meningitis, seizures, movement disorders, myelitis (including pain, weakness, and sphincteric defects), and optic neuropathy with relapsing and remitting features similar to multiple sclerosis* [74, 107–110].

While given episodes can be transient and self-limited, there is generally progressive disease with cumulative neurological impairment [107].

Central nervous system inflammatory disease, cognitive disorders, movement disorders, and meningoencephalitis are described in more detail.

22.12.1 Central Nervous System Inflammatory Disease

Myelitis is a devastating inflammatory syndrome of the spinal cord causing weakness, numbness, and sphincteric deficits. It has *frequency* of approximately 5% in SS patients in the Johns Hopkin's cohort, which is more than a 1,000-fold greater than idiopathic myelitis in the general population [111]. The frequency and features appear similar to those recently reported in a cohort of SLE patients with myelitis from the same institution, in which two distinct syndromes could be distinguished clinically by involvement of the central gray or the outer white matter neural tracts [111]. It is recognized that the Johns Hopkin's experience (and other reported series referenced below) represents the referral bias of much sicker patients to a tertiary institution.

Patients with *gray matter dysfunction* (i.e., spasticity and hyperreflexia) were more likely to present with fever and urinary retention. These patients were more likely to present with high systemic activity of their underlying

SLE [111]. Their *CSF profile was similar to bacterial meningitis* and they were more likely to have *irreversible paraplegia*. Patients with white matter dysfunction were also more likely to meet criteria for *neuromyelitis optica* (*NMO, Devic's syndrome*) and were more likely to have *anti-phospholipid antibodies* [111]. The actual "anatomic distinctions" between gray matter and white matter involvement are actually much more intricate, but this simplification is provided to help rheumatologists recognize and categorize clinical patterns in SS patients.

Optic neuritis was seen in about 50% of the NMO patients and they had a characteristic *anti-NMO antibody*, which predicted an increased chance of relapse. A paradoxical finding was that spinal cord MRI showing post-gadolinium enhancement was seen more frequently in patients with white matter myelitis, despite the tendency of white matter myelitis to occur with less severe inflammatory and CSF findings. This was attributed to the swelling of the spinal cord and progressive venous hypertension that decreased perfusion between the spinal radicular arteries and the pial venous plexus. Thus, the same compromised blood flow to the gray matter tracts also limited efflux of the gadolinium [111].

Multiple sclerosis is an inflammatory disease of the nervous system for which no test is pathognomonic [15]. There has been debate over the past two decades over the frequency of this complication in SS patients.

Histopathological studies of demyelinated lesions show considerable heterogeneity at the cellular and molecular level thought to be related to the diversity of the clinical presentation [112].

In 1986, Alexander et al. described 20 patients with primary Sjögren's syndrome, with features indistinguishable from multiple sclerosis [107]. Ataxia, visual loss, hypesthesia, and hemiparesis were frequent occurrences, and the course was relapsing and remitting or progressive, with frequent spinal cord involvement.

Important differences from the usual presentation of multiple sclerosis were vasculitis on biopsy of skin or muscle with a predominantly mononuclear vasculopathy and reduced number of oligoclonal bands in cerebrospinal fluid that decreased sequentially with corticosteroid therapy. It was thought that CNS Sjögren's syndrome was an autoimmune inflammatory ischemic small vessel cerebral vasculopathy affecting subcortical and periventricular white matter.

Based on these findings, a higher prevalence of Sjögren's syndrome-associated nervous system inflammatory disease would be expected [113–115], but has not been confirmed, with the exception of Asia, where MS is rare [116].

In primary progressive multiple sclerosis-like syndromes with myelopathy, the association with Sjögren's syndrome is stronger [117]. However, the association of MS and SS is controversial, particularly in patients lacking antibodies to ANA [118].

A case described by Tsai et al. [119] summarizes the problem of distinguishing Sjögren's syndrome associated with CNS inflammatory disease from multiple sclerosis.

A 27-year-old woman developed diplopia and ataxia, which subsided after 10 days. Over the next 15 months, she had six discreet neurological episodes associated with T2-weighted hyperintensities on MRI of the brain. These included left optic neuritis, lower extremity numbness, leg numbness and neurogenic bladder, right optic neuritis, left leg weakness, and left facial palsy. Betaseron was started after the third episode. Each episode responded to high-dose steroids with the exception of the sixth episode that left her with paraparesis.

A month after the sixth attack, she developed diplopia, exacerbation of leg weakness, dry eyes, and dry mouth.

Sjögren's syndrome was diagnosed on the basis of a positive Schirmer's test, Grade IV changes on labial salivary gland biopsy, and xerostomia on sialoscintigraphy.

She was again treated with pulse therapy, this time followed by 60 mg daily of prednisone, which was tapered to 30 mg per day, with no relapse in 12 months.

The pathological basis for inflammatory central nervous system disease in Sjögren's syndrome has not been established. The underlying abnormality is thought to be intracranial vasculitis or vasculopathy [105].

Moore and Lisak long ago thought that alternative diagnoses should be considered in multiple sclerosis until tests to unequivocally define multiple sclerosis and Sjögren's syndrome become available.

22.12.2 Cognitive Impairment

Cognitive impairment—characterized by *inattention, poor concentration, memory impairment, and loss of verbal fluency*— is frequently reported by patients with Sjögren's syndrome or demonstrated with neuropsychological testing [109, 120]. Psychometric studies may show *impairments of visual memory, reduced perceptual speed, and loss of fluid intelligence* [110].

The clinical presentation may be characteristic of subcortical dementia [58] and Alzheimer-type dementia, and a frontal lobe syndrome has been described [121].

Two case descriptions illustrate the range and chronicity of the dementia in Sjögren's syndrome.

Kawashima described a patient with subcortical dementia [122]. This 48-year-old male schoolteacher developed lassitude, forgetfulness, and withdrawal over 6 months. The first symptom was a poorly delivered speech.

On examination he was oriented, inactive, irritable, slow, hostile, and circumferential. An MRI demonstrated ventricular dilatation and T2 periventricular hyperintensities. His verbal IQ was 82 and performance IQ was 66.

After treatment with prednisone, he became active, reasonable, and co-operative. His neurological condition worsened with tapering steroids, but improved with resumption of therapy.

Caselli et al. described a case of reversible dementia in a 56-year-old woman with a 16-year history of Sjögren's syndrome, who lost the ability to program her computer [123]. There was spontaneous improvement after 6 months, and 18 months later, she developed visual hallucinations and started hiding her medications.

Magnetic resonance imaging, cerebral angiography, and spinal fluid examinations were all normal. Alzheimer's disease was diagnosed and she continued to deteriorate. Fifteen months later, she was readmitted to the hospital with perseveration, phonemic errors, and memory impairment.

MRI of the brain and carotid angiography were again normal, but cerebrospinal fluid showed an elevated protein with one oligoclonal band. A right pre-frontal brain biopsy revealed lymphocytic perivascular leptomeningeal and rare intraparenchymal infiltration. Gliosis was seen in superficial cortical layers, but there were no areas of microinfarction, viral inclusions, and neurofibrillary tangles or amyloid plaques. Focal vascular wall infiltration was present, but no transmural vasculitis.

She was initially treated with 120 mg oral prednisone per day (tapered in 3 months to 25 mg daily) and made a dramatic clinical improvement returning to nearly normal, according to family.

An *abnormality of brain muscarinic acetylcholine receptor function and regulation* may be responsible for the cognitive abnormalities seen in Sjögren's syndrome. Orman et al. purified IgG from 15 patients with primary Sjögren's disease who were positive for anti-M1 and anti-M3 activities [124].

All patients had a frontal lobe disorder on neuropsychological testing. They showed that pSS IgG evoked nitric oxide synthase and prostaglandin E2 production from rat cerebral cortex. NOS in other systems has been associated with cell death [125, 126].

22.12.3 Movement Disorders

Parkinsonism and other movement disorders are generally degenerative or genetically determined, but there is evidence [127–132] that when associated with Sjögren's syndrome, the movement disorder may be driven by an immune mechanism.

Distinguishing features are lack of response to dopaminergic drugs, improvement with steroids, and diffuse periventricular T2-weighted hyperintensities on brain MRI.

Nishimura et al. described a 74-year-old woman with a 10-year history of primary Sjögren's syndrome who developed parkinsonism that was responsive to steroids [130].

The initial presentation was with a *short steppage gait* non-responsive to dopaminergic therapy. The gait deteriorated over the next 7 years with *hesitation, festination, freezing, akinesia, and rigidity*. MRI showed T2-weighted hyperintensities in deep white matter and basal ganglia.

Following the administration of 30 mg of prednisone daily, there was a brisk improvement in gait and bradykinesia, the sedimentation rate dropped from 106 to 20 mm/h, and MRI abnormalities decreased in size.

Other movement disorders associated with Sjögren's syndrome respond to steroids, although not invariably [133, 134].

Papageorgiou et al. reported a 57-year-old woman with a 2-year history of Sjögren's syndrome, who had involuntary muscle contractions around the mouth and eyes, progressing to face and neck that was diagnosed with orofacial dystonia [134].

She was non-responsive to dopamine, clonazepam, and levetiracetam, but after 1 g of methylprednisolone IV for 3 days followed by prednisone, the patient experienced a dramatic improvement and was virtually symptom-free in 2 months.

Similarly, Venegas Fanchke et al. described a 43-year-old woman with Sjögren's syndrome presenting with generalized *choreic movements* of the axial skeleton and face followed by depression and cognitive impairment that improved with steroids and azathioprine [133].

Elevated titers of anti-β2-glycoprotein I IgG [127] have been found in three patients with Sjögren's syndrome and Parkinson's disease. Purified α,β2 glycoprotein antibodies bind to cerebral endothelial cells, suggesting an immune-mediated vascular etiology.

22.12.4 Aseptic meningitis and Meningoencephalitis

Aseptic meningitis and meningoencephalitis have been described in patients with Sjögren's syndrome, often characterized by *pleocytosis, protein elevation , and increased IgG synthesis rate in spinal fluid.*

In some instances there is *vasculitis on biopsy of muscle and skin*. These disorders may be recurrent, associated with *other neurological abnormalities including seizures, cranial nerve palsies, and coma, and respond to steroids* [135–140].

A fatal case of meningoencephalitis, upon autopsy, was described by Gerraty et al. on an 18-year-old patient who initially presented with fever, somnolence, and seizures [141]. Findings had included positive sialography, anti-SSA and SSB antibodies, 62 lymphocytes on CSF examination with protein 0.34 g/dL, and the patient was treated with prednisone 0.5 mg daily followed by Cytoxan with no improvement.

She had responded markedly to plasmapheresis. A brain CT scan showed several small infarctions in the temporal and parietal lobes. She had memory impairment and frequent focal and generalized seizures.

The illness was protracted, but after 3 months, she had developed increased drowsiness that did not respond to plasmapheresis, and she expired 6 months after that initial hospital admission. Laminar necrosis of the frontal and parietal cortex was seen on autopsy together with small infarcts but no vasculitis.

22.12.5 Other Neurological Disorders

Various other unusual neurological syndromes occur during the course of Sjögren's syndrome. Syndromes include *epilepsy* [142], *acute cerebellar ataxia* [143], *cerebral venous thrombosis* [106], and progressive multifocal leukoencephalopathy [144].

Li et al. described a case of hypertrophic cranial pachymeningitis and lymphocytic hypophysitis in a 74-year-old with Sjögren's syndrome [145]. The original presentation was headache, dizziness, and general malaise with polydipsia and polyuria. CSF was negative, and MRI showed thickened meninges with gadolinium enhancement, mildly enlarged pituitary gland, and thickening of the pituitary stalk with extension along the basal hypothalamus.

Hypopituitarism was evident on endocrine study. MRI thickening of the dura was reduced with steroid therapy. Biopsy of dura mater 4 months later showed an inflammatory response characterized by patchy infiltration of small lymphocytes, plasma cells, and fibrosis hyalinized collagen tissue. There was no vasculitis. The cells were predominantly $CD3^+$ lymphocytes.

Niemela et al. described a 24-year-old with primary Sjögren's syndrome and grand mal seizures [142]. This patient had a past history of arthralgia, fever, and Raynaud's phenomenon and developed a confusional state and grand mal seizures. The cerebrospinal fluid had a protein of 5,000 mg/L, with 5 WBC.

Initial treatment with prednisone was ineffective, and the patient deteriorated, became somnolent, but responded to pain with eye opening. Cyclophosphamide (15 mg/kg) on days 0, 8, 29, and 50 resulted in improvement. The patient became oriented, walked in 3 weeks, and was normal cognitively in a year.

22.13 Investigations of Central Nervous System Manifestations

22.13.1 Serology

Serum anti-SSA and less frequently anti-SSB antibodies are present in patients with CNS disease and SS, more so with focal disease and when angiographic abnormalities are present [58, 146]. The patient's sera should also be tested for circulating anti-coagulants (anti-cardiolipin and/or anti-phospholipid antibody, lupus anti-coagulant) and rapid plasma reagin/fluorescent treponemal antibody (RPR/FTA). There have been some reports of association with antibody to ribosomal P protein [147, 148, 149] and to neuronal antigens [150–152] associated with neuropsychiatric manifestations. However, these assays have not been sufficiently replicated to advocate their use at present time. More recently, α-fodrin antibodies have been proposed to distinguish primary progressive multiple sclerosis from Sjögren's syndrome [97]. Again, confirmatory studies will be required.

Additional serologic abnormalities have been associated, including a higher prevalence of

- *C-reactive protein* (68% vs. 6%)
- *RF* (76% vs. 35%)
- hypocomplemententemia (56% vs. 19%)
- monoclonal gammopathy (36% vs. 6%)
- SSA/Ro (77% vs. 50%)
- SSB/La (55% vs. 28%)
- increased serum β2-microglobulin

in patients with vasculitis has been observed in some presentations [Terrier, 2007 #112].

22.13.2 Spinal Fluid

Spinal fluid examination, when performed, has shown protein elevation in a small proportion of cases of painful neuropathy and ataxic neuropathy, and pleocytosis may occur in ataxic neuropathy [33]. Albumin-cytological dissociation on spinal fluid examination has been described [33].

Pleocytosis, elevated protein, increased IgG synthesis rate, and oligoclonal bands occur during the course of central nervous system disease in Sjögren's syndrome [153, 154]. Anti-SSA and anti-SSB antibodies have also been found in the CSF in some cases with evidence of increased intrathecal synthesis of anti-SSA autoantibody [155].

22.13.3 MRI

Both white matter and cerebral atrophy have been noted in MRI studies of SS patients. Recent technological advances in MRI using diffusion tensor imaging (DTI) may make possible more detailed imaging to correlate *brain tissue integrity and volume loss* in SS patients and SLE patients [13, 14]. The higher resolution MRIs indicated that the previous studies were identifying vascular lacuni rather than demyelinating lesions [9]. These studies have shown an incidence of demyelinating lesions less than 5%, in contrast to the characteristic alterations found in well-characterized multiple sclerosis patients.

T2-weighted hyperintensities on brain MRI abnormalities are seen in SS affecting white and gray matter in periventricular or subcortical regions [8]. Frontal and parietal lobes are commonly involved and abnormalities in general may correlate with focal neurological signs [156].

MRI abnormalities are non-specific and T2-weighted hyperintensities may represent edema, gliosis, demyelination, or axonal loss [157]. The prevalence of cerebral MRI abnormalities varies in primary Sjögren's syndrome populations and is higher in patients with neurological impairment [157].

22.13.4 Nuclear Brain Imaging Studies

Cerebral blood flow measured with Technetium-99m-HMPAO SPECT and glucose metabolism measured with FDG-PET in patients with Sjögren's syndrome with neuropsychiatric symptoms including cognitive and memory impairment are frequently abnormal [120].

MRI brain scans may be normal in these cases. Researchers have found multiple areas of hypoperfusion, usually bilateral, in cortex and basal ganglia [158–160].

22.13.5 Cerebral Angiography

There are limited reports of cerebral angiography in Sjögren's syndrome. Alexander et al. reported on 45 patients with Sjögren's syndrome who had cerebral angiography for clinical reasons [146]. Twenty patients had abnormal studies, of which 18 had radiographic findings of stenosis, dilatation or occlusion of small cerebral blood vessels consistent, with small vessel angiitis. Small arteries of the anterior and posterior circulation were involved; four patients had involvement of medium size or larger vessels; five patients had one or more aneurysms.

22.14 The Puzzling Neurological Manifestations of Fibromyalgia

Perhaps, the most common clinical problem in the SS patient is *vague cognitive dysfunction* and *diffuse myalgia* (fibromyalgia). These problems are more difficult to assess as a consequence of the immune process as there are few clinically available objective tests. However, the frequency of fibromyalgia in SS patients is higher than the general population, and these complaints often overwhelm other aspects of the patient's (or physician's) global assessment of quality of life and the patient's disability (see chapter on fibromyalgia).

However, the problem of fibromyalgia (i.e., central pain sensitization) often has less obvious consequences than simply unexplained fatigue. The severity of pain or weakness reported is often out of proportion to observed clinical, EMG/NCV, or biopsy findings. It is difficult to know if these "amplifications" of pain result at the level of the dorsal root ganglia, the ascending/descending channels of the spinal cord, or in particular regions of the brain. It is not known if they result from an inflammatory process or a vasculopathy.

The high frequency of "fibromyalgia" symptoms in the SS patient is the "elephant in our diagnostic exam room," as these patients frequently complain of disabling pain or fatigue.

Among primary care physicians, there is little recognition of the lack of specificity of low-titer ANA and the relatively high frequency of "false-positive" results [161, 162]. This leads many primary care physicians to refer fibromyalgia patients with a low-titer ANA to a rheumatologist to "rule out" autoimmune disorders such as SS.

On the other hand, a neurologist may perform an extensive workup of peripheral neuropathy including nerve biopsy while evaluating an "idiopathic" neuropathy. If a positive ANA is noted, the patient often is termed SS even if the patient lacks dry eyes/mouth or other criteria for SS.

22.15 Interpretation of ANA in the Patient with Neurological Symptoms

Another area of diagnostic confusion is ANA. *There is a misconception that a positive ANA (singularly) "makes" the diagnosis of SLE or SS.*

The ANA is used to *confirm* the diagnosis, and the test done by immunofluorescence assay (IFA) is more sensitive than it is specific [162]. The test shows variability in different laboratories and the ELISA test has *many more false negatives* [163] than the IFA and may lead to missed or incorrect diagnosis as illustrated in a recent clinical pathologic conference published in *New England Journal of Medicine* [164].

The frequency of patients with a low-titer ANA increases with age [165]. Patients with Alzheimer's disease frequently have increased oral and ocular dryness complaints due to impairment of cortical white matter outflow, autonomic neuropathy, and changes in nerve growth factor as well as the normal atrophy of secretory glands that occurs with age [70]. Indeed, the basis of several approved drugs for Alzheimer's disease such as rivastatin is based on their cholinergic stimulatory activity [166]. Thus, the presence of a low-titer ANA in an older patient may lead to a clinical diagnosis of SS, even when the salivary gland biopsies are normal or show expected age-related atrophy.

22.16 Treatment

22.16.1 Peripheral Nervous System Treatment: Overview

There are no controlled clinical trials of treatment for the neuropathy of Sjögren's syndrome. Multiple immune-based therapies have been shown to be effective in many isolated cases based on individual case reports and several series of patients.

Our approach to therapy is largely based on our experience with treatment in SLE patients with central and peripheral neuropathies. Treatment has included corticosteroids, cyclophosphamide, intravenous gammaglobulin, plasma exchange, D-penicillamine, chlorambucil, rituximab, and infliximab [56, 167–174].

Few treatments of acute neurological syndromes are "controlled trials." Symptomatic treatment of painful neuropathies generally follows the guidelines used for treatment of diabetic neuropathies. However, the anti-cholinergic side effects of tricyclic agents make these agents poorly tolerated in SS patients.

Immune mechanisms are not necessarily the same in the various forms of neuropathy [116], and there may be marked differences in rates of favorable responses between the various neuropathic forms [9].

22.16.2 Painful Sensory Neuropathies

Kizawa et al. report a favorable response to IV-Ig in a patient with Sjögren's syndrome with severe sensory symptoms such that he could not open his hands and walk, with a recurrent episode 6 months later responding to the same treatment [175].

Caroyer et al. described a 68-year-old woman with Sjögren's syndrome who developed distal tingling and burning in both hands who responded to a course of infliximab [167].

Grant and Dyck reported treating sensory neuropathy with steroids, IV-Ig, and plasmapheresis and found the response to treatment to be equivocal and recommended controlled clinical trials to establish effective therapy [175].

22.16.3 Ataxic Neuropathy

Chen et al. described four patients with Sjögren's syndrome (one of whom had SLE) and ataxic sensory neuropathy treated with 5–9 plasma exchanges [171]. The two patients who had acute onset of symptoms responded to this therapy.

Takahashi et al. and others have shown a functional benefit of IV-Ig in long-standing severe ataxic neuropathy, where prior steroids and plasmapheresis had failed, and noted the rapid improvement and long-lasting effect in spite of long-standing chronic disability [109]. In IV-Ig-dependent neuropathy, rituximab may be effective [169]. Cyclophosphamide [56] and D-penicillamine [173] have also been reported as beneficial in this neuropathy.

22.16.4 Motor and Sensory Neuropathies

Mori et al. thought that corticosteroid therapy was likely to be effective for multiple mononeuropathy [22].

Terrier et al. [39] treated 40 highly selected patients with Sjögren's syndrome where neuromuscular biopsy was one of the inclusion criteria, with corticosteroids (38 patients), azathioprine (8 patients), cyclophosphamide (10 patients), hydroxychloroquine (3 patients), rituximab plus cyclophosphamide (1 patient), methotrexate (1 patient), CHOP (1 patient), and plasma exchange (4 patients). They found a good response in 12 of 40 patients, moderate response in 9 of 40, stabilization in 17 of 40, worsening in 2 of 40, and relapse in 19 of 40.

22.16.5 Central Nervous System Treatment

As with peripheral nervous system involvement in Sjögren's syndrome randomized blinded placebo-controlled studies are not available. In addition there is a lack of precise knowledge regarding the underlying pathogenesis [175].

Treatment is based on case reports and several case studies. Steroids are frequently effective in CNS Sjögren's syndrome [36, 176]. In progressive focal CNS destruction, monthly intravenous cyclophosphamide for 12 months until stabilization or improvement seen has been recommended [177]. Cyclophosphamide has also been recommended in treatment of myelopathy [178, 179].

Combination therapy with steroids and cyclophosphamide improved expanded disability status scale (EDSS) and ambulation in some patients with myelopathy [117]. Steroids and chlorambucil were effective in another instance [180].

There is one case report for each of the use of rituximab, IV-Ig, and plasma exchange.

Yamout et al. described a 47-year-old woman with recurrent weakness of the lower extremities due to an extensive demyelinating lesion T7–T10 that improved with rituximab after steroids and cyclophosphamide failed [181]. She had become bedridden, but returned to daily activities in 8 months.

Canhao et al. described a 67-year-old woman diagnosed at age 50 with Sjögren's syndrome, who developed recurrent ataxia and dysmetria, controlled with prednisone and cyclophosphamide for 3 years, at which point she worsened with confusion dysarthria and ataxia [182]. IV-Ig 400 mg/kg/day for 5 days resulted in a dramatic response of neurological symptoms, and recurrent relapses have remained responsive to this therapy.

Konttinen et al. described a 54-year-old woman with a 2-year history of Sjögren's syndrome, who developed myalgias followed by internuclear ophthalmoplegia, acute transverse myelitis at T6 with complete paraparesis, urinary retention, and fecal incontinence [183]. Visual-evoked potentials and MRI of the brain were normal. Prednisone was started at the onset of paraparesis and plasma exchange 6 days later. The first signs of improvement were within a week. She could stand with a tilt table at 6 weeks, had normal urination at that point, and at about 3 months could walk with a 4-point cane.

22.16.6 Side Effects of Immunosuppressive Therapy

Relatively, little has been reported about the side effects of steroidal or non-steroidal complications in SS patients, in contrast to larger studies focusing on SLE. The side effects of traditional therapies including oral and pulse cyclophosphamide, azathioprine, and cyclosporin A in SS patients have been recently reviewed by Mavragani et al. [184], who also have updated this topic in another chapter of this textbook. The problems of immune suppression and bone marrow toxicity with cyclophosphamide are similar to SLE patients [184]. Also, pneumonitis may reflect opportunistic infections including pneumocystic or "drug pneumonitis" such as "alkylator lung." These findings may present diagnostic dilemmas due to the relatively high frequency of leukopenia and/or thrombocytopenia as a result of the SS pathogenesis. Similarly, the increase in chest X-ray infiltrates may be due to the SS pneumonitis or infections. The problem is particularly difficult in treating neurological problems, where side effects including progressive multifocal leukoencephalopathy (PML) may occur in SS patients in the absence of immunosuppressive therapy [144] and has been recently associated with certain biologic agents such as rituximab (although at very low rates). Corticosteroids may have the effect of acceleration of dental decay, in addition to the side effects of osteoporosis, avascular necrosis, glaucoma, diabetes, and steroid myopathy.

22.17 Summary of Special Points to Neurologists

22.17.1 Neuropathic Pain in Sjogren's Patients

The management of neuropathic pain in Sjogren's patients may be especially challenging. The normal therapeutic armamentarium, which may be useful in other subgroups of patients with neuropathic pain, may present unique iatrogenic difficulties in Sjogren's patients. However, by working with Sjogren's patients to modulate expectations and anticipating such side effects, neurologists can facilitate the symptomatic manifestations of neuropathic pain.

The use of tricylic anti-depressants (TCAs) remains first-line agents in the treatment of neuropathic pain. Because of the anti-cholinergic side effects, which may aggravate sicca symptoms, they are often regarded as contraindicative in Sjogren's patients. However, some Sjogren's patients with milder sicca manifestations may be able to tolerate nortriptyline. In contrast, to amitriptyline—which is a tertiary amine—nortriptyline causes less anti-cholinergic side effects. Therefore, slow titration of nortriptyline may be useful.

The institution of neuropathic agents such as Neurontin and/or Lyrica is often attempted and abandoned, because of the exacerbation of *fatigue*, which may be an especially prominent symptom in Sjogren's patients. As for the use of TCAs, patients should be counseled that often the sedative effects of these agents habituate with time. Again, slow titration of agents toward doses, which are effective in therapeutic trials, may be necessary.

Neurologists should also be aware that Sjogren's patients might employ an imaginative, varied, and graphic description of neuropathic pain, with a nosology, which is sharply different from traditional descriptors of neuropathic pain. For example, neuropathic pain may be described as occurring in distributions not conforming to dermatomes or the distributions of peripheral nerves. There are several reasons why pain may not crisply conform to such orthodox boundaries. First, in patients with small fiber neuropathies, more than 50% of Sjogren's patients may experience pain in proximal as opposed to distal regions, i.e., disproportionately affecting the thighs versus the toes. In other scenarios, pain may be described as exquisite sensitivity, in virtually all regions of the torso. Such diffuse tenderness to palpation—which is termed as *dynamic touch allodynia* in many neuropathic pain questionnaires—may be due to the "central" sensitization of neuropathic pain. The term "central" sensitization of neuropathic pain refers to the constellation of changes which may amplify neuropathic pain, due to hyperexcitability of ion channels in the dorsal root ganglia (DRG) and the spinal cord, morphologic changes of cellular elements, and cytokine changes which may render "gating" of somatosensory cues intractable to central, inhibitory pathways (i.e., the GABA pathway). Therefore, the experiential features of "central" sensitization of neuropathic pain can be indistinguishable from fibromyalgia.

Whether fibromyalgia should be regarded as "central" neuropathic pain is currently controversial. Nevertheless, when neurologists are confronted with touch allodynia, which may not crisply conform to traditional neuroanatomic boundaries, the selective noradrenaline re-uptake inhibitor (SNRI) medications (i.e., Cymbalta) may be useful.

In addition to recognizing the unorthodox and heterogeneous descriptors of neuropathic pain, there may be concomitant causes of pain which often go overlooked, but which may be amplifying the experience of neuropathic pain. Overweight patients who complain of fibromyalgia may have sleep apnea; therefore, screening by sleep studies is important. Other co-morbid conditions may include hypothyroidism, adrenal insufficiency, and depression.

22.17.2 Demyelinating Syndromes in Sjogren's Patients

The sinuous relationship of Multiple Sclerosis (MS) has been described above, with discrepant attributions reported by different authors. When demyelinating episodes occur in Sjogren's patients, there is often a dilemma about whether the operative diagnosis should be Multiple Sclerosis (MS) or a demyelinating syndrome due to Sjogren's syndrome. This dilemma is not only important as a ritualistic, nosological debate, *but also has dramatic therapeutic repercussions*. Specifically, the interferon-based medications, which are useful in reducing new clinical attacks and brain lesions in MS, have been amply reported as potentiating or aggravating systemic rheumatic diseases. Therefore, neurologists can play a crucial role in directing rheumatologists toward the appropriate diagnosis and treatment.

First, neurologists should alert rheumatologists that not all demyelinating episodes are due to MS. In the past 5 years, there is increasing recognition that the demyelinating episodes constitute a heterogeneous group of disorders, with distinguishing clinical, radiographic, and serological features. For example, neuromyelitis optica/NMO can occur in patients with systemic rheumatic syndromes, including systemic lupus erythematosus (SLE), and Sjogren's syndrome.

A common source of consternation—for both neurologists and rheumatologist—is that the radiologists' interpretation of white matter lesions in Sjogren's patients has an unwieldy cornucopia of causes, ranging from "vasculitis" to "MS," to the diathesis of Sjogren's syndrome. However, a few principles should apply. First, CNS vasculitis is the rarest of the vasculitides and will likely never be the cause of such lesions. Second, neurologists can now apply the Barkhof MRI criteria, which have been incorporated into the revised 2005 McDonald diagnostic criteria for MS. The McDonald criteria incorporate the Barkhof criteria to serve as a MRI surrogate for the clinical requirement of lesions which may be "disseminated in space." The neurologist's meticulous application of the Barkhof criteria may demonstrate to rheumatologists that the distribution and morphologic features of such white matter lesions are inconsistent with MS. It is highly likely that earlier reports in the 1980s, attesting to the frequency of "MS" in Sjogren's patients, did not have the benefit of utilizing such radiographic criteria.

The potential mechanisms of white matter lesions not satisfying the Barkhof criteria are uncertain and have been reviewed earlier in this chapter.

22.17.3 Relationship of Neurological Symptoms to Sicca Manifestations

Both the central nervous system (CNS) and peripheral nervous system (PNS) manifestations may antedate emergence of glandular symptoms in up to 50% of Sjogren's patients, sometimes by up to a decade. Even in the absence of prominent sicca symptoms, neurologists should be especially vigilant for potential emergence of Sjogren's symptoms, especially when encountering neuropsychiatric manifestations, which may be prototypical of Sjogren's patients. Examples of such prototypical *PNS* manifestations would be the larger fiber ganglionopathies/sensory neuronopathies or small fiber neuropathies not occurring in a length-dependent gradient. In some scenarios, there may be subtle symptoms of xerostomia and keratoconjunctivitis sicca, but such "glandular" manifestations may be overlooked in the context of devastating neuropsychiatric disease. Examples of prototypical *CNS* manifestations would include opticospinal manifestations occurring in the context of neuromyelitis optica/NMO (see below) or demyelinating episodes not satisfying diagnostic criteria for multiple sclerosis (MS).

Therefore, neurologists must ruthlessly query and pursue even the subtlest manifestations of sicca symptoms. It is not sufficient to merely ask patients, "Do you have dry eyes or dry mouth?". The symptomatic manifestations of keratoconjunctivitis sicca are protean: patients should be asked about sensitivity to light and about inability to wear contact lenses. Similarly, the manifestation of xerostomia may be unearthed by an increased burden of caries or by complaints of halitosis. In female patients, incipient sicca symptoms may be heralded by vaginal dryness: patients should be asked about recurrent candidiasis or dyspareunia.

In other scenarios, even a meticulous assessment for subtle sicca manifestations may not suggest the glandular manifestations of Sjogren's syndrome. Although such patients may be provisionally relegated as having "idiopathic" neuropsychiatric syndromes, there should be hypervigilant suspicion on longitudinal evaluation, for eventual emergence of any glandular manifestations.

Lastly, neurologists should be aware that the current American–European classification criteria allow for the diagnosis of Sjogren's syndrome—*even when patients lack symptoms of dry eyes or dry mouth*. In such scenarios, the diagnosis is facilitated by both demonstration of sialadenitis on lip biopsy and seropositivity to anti-Ro/SSA and/or anti-La/SSB autoantibodies, along with at least one "functional" test, which may corroborate subclinical sicca symptoms. Therefore, we recommend that when patients without sicca symptoms present with the above prototypical PNS or CNS manifestations, which are suggestive of Sjogren's syndrome, that lip biopsy be performed when there is seropositivity to anti-Ro/SSA or anti-La/SSB autoantibodies.

In summary, the neurologist may play a crucial and gratifying role in diagnosing Sjogren's syndrome, by limning the expertise to recognize neuropsychiatric manifestations, which may be the "footprint" of Sjogren's disease, even in the absence of sicca symptoms.

22.18 Summary for Rheumatologists

Sjögren's syndrome has a wide variety of neurological manifestations ranging from peripheral to central signs and symptoms. The neurological symptoms are a key reason for extraglandular morbidity in SS and patient's assessment of their "quality of life."

The symptoms of *peripheral neuropathy* are common and correlate poorly with EMG measurements due to involvement of unmyelinated nerves. Also, the severity of symptoms is affected by the presence of "fibromyalgia" that may amplify "pain" signals at the level of the spinal cord or CNS. Evidence for immune system involvement is more specific with respect to the dorsal root ganglia. Thus, the early finding of dorsal root ganglion involvement correlates well with the ataxic neuropathy, as does the proportionately reduced fiber densities in sural nerve biopsies in ataxic and painful sensory neuropathies.

Motor peripheral neuropathies also may occur due to vasculitis or antibody-mediated demyelination (CIPD).

Therapy of neuropathies may include *corticosteroids, IVIg, and immunosuppressant therapy including cyclophosphamide* and perhaps *biologic agents.*

Central nervous involvement may involve both white and gray matter. Vasculitis as well as thrombotic and atherosclerotic manifestations must be considered. Newer MRI techniques may help identify structural damage in the CNS and spinal cord. Recent studies have identified a much lower incidence of demyelinating disease (approximately 5% or less) than was reported in previous years.

Central sensitization (fibromyalgia) and chronic fatigue remain a challenge to diagnosis as assessment of therapy. Recent studies *in mice* demonstrate that changes in cytokines and adrenal axis stress hormones strongly influence behavior without detectable associated change in brain structure [14, 185–187]. This *"stress" effect on memory and multitasking* in mice also can be reproduced with effect of stress on healthy adults [188]. Thus, neurological symptoms in SS patients present a diagnostic and therapeutic challenge that bridges immune activity, thrombotic complications, and manifestations from local cytokine release or hypothalamic axis alterations that may play a role in fibromyalgia.

22.19 Speculations on the Relationship of Neurological and Lacrimal/Salivary Aspects of Sjogren's Syndrome

In summary, we have a variety of neurological manifestations resulting from microvasculitis due to T cell and dendritic cells, antibody-mediated mechanisms, hormonally related factors, and the complement/coagulation pathways. In each of these acquired and innate immune systems, the release of cytokines and chemokines is activated. Thus, SS appears to represent an intersection of immune, hormonal, endocrine, and exocrine function. Each of these "immune" systems will influence neural function and the action of neurotransmitter on the end organ.

Thus, we can look at the body of neurological data in the mirror of our knowledge about salivary/lacrimal gland biopsies and function presented in other chapters. The salivary and lacrimal glands develop embryologically from the same brachial cleft as the brain and neural system. Thus in a sense, the glands are "hard wired" to the neural system from the time of development. The degree of xerostomia in patients with Sjögren's syndrome does not correlate with degree of glandular destruction on biopsy [189]. Thus, the release of cytokines and other factors paralyzes the function of the residual glands. It is likely that the release of similar factors influence the function of peripheral nerves and those in the central nervous system. Thus, studies of nerve–gland function and biopsy presented in other chapters will need to be applied to our understanding of neurological manifestations of SS. In the past, we were limited to sural or other nerve biopsies for evaluation of neuropathic processes. The methods of skin biopsy stained for neural markers may be modified to include immune markers so that correlation with changes on minor salivary gland biopsies can be made. Thus, we now have two sites that can be safely biopsied (glandular and extraglandular) to obtain a better understanding of pathogenesis and to direct therapy.

References

1. Delalande S, de Seze J, Fauchais AL, Hachulla E, Stojkovic T, Ferriby D, et al. Neurologic manifestations in primary Sjogren syndrome: a study of 82 patients. Medicine (Baltimore) 2004;83(5): 280–91.
2. Goldenberg D. Fibromyalgia, chronic fatigue syndrome, and myofascial pain syndrome. Curr Opin Rheumatol. 1995;7(2):127.
3. Hanson P, Schumacker P, Clerin M. Evaluation of somatic and autonomic small fibers neuropathy in diabetes. Am J Phys Med Rehabil. 1992;71(1):44.
4. Rodriquez A, Kanis L, Lane D. Somatosensory evoked potentials from dermatomal stimulation as an indicator of L5 and S1 radiculopathy. Arch Phys Med Rehabil. 1987;68(6):366.
5. Elert J, Rantapää-Dahlqvist S, Henriksson-Larsen K, Lorentzon R, Gerdle B. Muscle performance, electromyography and fibre type composition in fibromyalgia and work-related myalgia. Scand J Rheumatol. 1992;21(1):28–34.
6. Bergdahl M, Bergdahl J, Johansson I. Depressive symptoms in individuals with idiopathic subjective dry mouth. J Oral Pathol Med. 1997;26(10):448–50.
7. Bronge L, Wahlund L, Brauner A, Basun H, Garlind A. White matter lesions and soluble interleukin-1 receptor type II in CSF from demented and non-demented subjects. Neurochem Int. 2002;41(4):217–22.
8. Coates T, Slavotinek J, Rischmueller M, Schultz D, Anderson C, Dellamelva M, et al. Cerebral white matter lesions in primary Sjögren's syndrome: a controlled study. J Rheumatol. 1999;26(6): 1301.

9. Pierot L, Sauve C, Leger J, Martin N, Koeger A, Wechsler B, et al. Asymptomatic cerebral involvement in Sjögren's syndrome: MRI findings of 15 cases. Neuroradiology 1993;35(5):378–80.
10. Ramos-Casals M, Tzioufas A, Font J. Primary Sjogren's syndrome: new clinical and therapeutic concepts. Br Med J. 2005;64(3):347.
11. Birnbaum J, Kirr D. Frequency of neurologic disease in Sjogren syndrome patients versus controls. Arth Rheum. 2009;60:506.
12. Birnbaum J, Petri M, Thompson R, Izbudak I, Kerr D. Distinct subtypes of myelitis in systemic lupus erythematosus. Arthritis Care Res. 2009;60(11):3378–87.
13. Harboe E, Beyer M, Greve O, Gränsson L, Tjensvoll A, Kvalÿ J, et al. Cerebral white matter hyperintensities are not increased in patients with primary Sjögren's syndrome. Eur J Neurol. 2009;16(5): 576–81.
14. Harboe E, Tjensvoll A, Maroni S, Goransson L, Greve O, Beyer M, et al. Neuropsychiatric syndromes in patients with systemic lupus erythematosus and primary Sjogren syndrome: a comparative population-based study. Br Med J. 2009;68(10):1541.
15. McDonald W, Compston A, Edan G, Goodkin D, Hartung H, Lublin F, et al. Recommended diagnostic criteria for multiple sclerosis: guidelines from the International Panel on the diagnosis of multiple sclerosis. Ann Neurol. 2001;50(1):121–7.
16. Filippi M, Bozzali M, Rovaris M, Gonen O, Kesavadas C, Ghezzi A, et al. Evidence for widespread axonal damage at the earliest clinical stage of multiple sclerosis. Brain 2003;126(2):433.
17. Vaudo G, Bocci E, Shoenfeld Y, Schillaci G, Wu R, Del Papa N, et al. Precocious intima–media thickening in patients with primary Sjögren's syndrome. Arthritis Care Res. 52(12):3890–7.
18. Shoenfeld Y, Gerli R, Doria A, Matsuura E, Cerinic M, Ronda N, et al. Accelerated atherosclerosis in autoimmune rheumatic diseases. Circulation 2005;112(21):3337.
19. Fox RI. Sjogren's syndrome. Lancet 2005; 366(9482):321–31.
20. Sanna G, Bertolaccini M, Cuadrado M, Laing H, Khamashta M, Mathieu A, et al. Neuropsychiatric manifestations in systemic lupus erythematosus: prevalence and association with antiphospholipid antibodies. J Rheumatol. 2003;30(5):985–92.
21. Gemignani F, Marbini A, Pavesi G, Di Vittorio S, Manganelli P, Cenacchi G, et al. Peripheral neuropathy associated with primary Sjogren's syndrome. J Neurol Neurosurg Psychiatry. 1994;57(8):983–6.
22. Mori K, Iijima M, Koike H, Hattori N, Tanaka F, Watanabe H, et al. The wide spectrum of clinical manifestations in Sjogren's syndrome-associated neuropathy. Brain 2005;128(11):2518–34.
23. Sghirlanzoni A, Pareyson D, Lauria G. Sensory neuron diseases. Lancet Neurol. 2005;4(6):349–61.
24. Lafitte C, Amoura Z, Cacoub P, Pradat-Diehl P, Picq C, Salachas F, et al. Neurological complications of primary Sjögren's syndrome. J Neurol. 2001;248(7):577–84.
25. Alexander EL, Provost TT, Stevens MB, Alexander GE. Neurologic complications of primary Sjogren's syndrome. Medicine 1982;61(4):247.
26. Govoni M, Bajocchi G, Rizzo N, Tola MR, Caniatti L, Tugnoli V, et al. Neurological involvement in primary Sjögren's syndrome: clinical and instrumental evaluation in a cohort of Italian patients. Clin Rheumatol. 1999;18(4):299–303.
27. Chai J, Herrmann DN, Stanton M, Barbano RL, Logigian EL. Painful small-fiber neuropathy in Sjogren syndrome. Neurology 2005;65(6):925–7.
28. Moore PM, Lisak RP. Systemic lupus erythematosus: immunopathogenesis of neurologic dysfunction. In: Springer; 1995. pp. 43–60.
29. Moore PM. Central nervous system vasculitis. Curr Opin Neurol. 1998;11(3):241.
30. McCombe PA. Neurological complications of connective tissue diseases and vasculitis. Autoimmune Neurol Dis. 1995:345.
31. Goransson L, Brun J, Harboe E, Mellgren S, Omdal R. Intraepidermal nerve fiber densities in chronic inflammatory autoimmune diseases. Arch Neurol. 2006;63(10):1410.
32. Goransson L, Herigstad A, Tjensvoll A, Harboe E, Mellgren S, Omdal R. Peripheral neuropathy in primary Sjogren syndrome: a population-based study. Arch Neurol. 2006;63(11):1612.
33. Grant I, Hunder G, Homburger H, Dyck P. Peripheral neuropathy associated with sicca complex. Neurology 1997;48(4):855.
34. Mori K, Iijima M, Sugiura M, Koike H, Hattori N, Ito H, et al. Sjogren's syndrome associated painful sensory neuropathy without sensory ataxia. Br Med J. 2003;74(9):1320.
35. Griffin J, Cornblath D, Alexander E, Campbell J, Low P, Bird S, et al. Ataxic sensory neuropathy and dorsal root ganglionitis associated with Sjogren's syndrome. Ann Neurol. 1990;27:304–15.
36. Malinow K, Yannakakis G, Glusman S, Edlow D, Griffin J, Pestronk A, et al. Subacute sensory neuronopathy secondary to dorsal root ganglionitis in primary Sjögren's syndrome. Ann Neurol. 1986;20(4):535–7.
37. Mellgren S, Conn D, Stevens J, Dyck P. Peripheral neuropathy in primary Sjogren's syndrome. Neurology 1989;39(3):390.
38. Mellgren S, Göransson L, Omdal R. Primary Sjögren's syndrome associated neuropathy. Can J Neurol Sci. 2007;34(3):280–7.
39. Terrier B, Lacroix C, Guillevin L, Hatron P, Dhote R, Maillot F, et al. Diagnostic and prognostic relevance of neuromuscular biopsy in primary Sjögren's syndrome-related neuropathy. Arthritis Rheum. 2007;57(8).

40. Engel A, Hohlfeld R, Banker B. The polymyositis and dermatomyositis syndromes. Myology 1994;2:1335–83.
41. Lindvall B, Bengtsson A, Ernerudh J, Eriksson P. Subclinical myositis is common in primary Sjogren's syndrome and is not related to muscle pain. J Rheumatol. 2002;29(4):717–25.
42. Chahin N, Engel AG. Correlation of muscle biopsy, clinical course, and outcome in PM and sporadic IBM. Neurology 2008;70(6):418–24.
43. Kissel J, Mendell J. Vasculitic neuropathy. Neurol Clin. 1992;10:761–6.
44. Stevens MJ, Feldman EL, Thomas TP, Greene DA. The pathogenesis of diabetic neuropathy. Clin Manag Diabetic Neuropathy 1998;9:13–21.
45. Hu S, Wang J, Meijer J, Ieong S, Xie Y, Yu T, et al. Salivary proteomic and genomic biomarkers for primary Sjogren's syndrome. Arthritis Rheum. 2007;56(11):3588–600.
46. Taylor PV, Taylor KF, Norman A, Griffiths S, Scott JS. Prevalence of maternal Ro (SS-A) and La (SS-B) autoantibodies in relation to congenital heart block. Rheumatology 1988;27(2):128.
47. Buyon JP, Ben-Chetrit E, Karp S, Roubey RA, Pompeo L, Reeves WH, et al. Acquired congenital heart block. Pattern of maternal antibody response to biochemically defined antigens of the SSA/Ro-SSB/La system in neonatal lupus. J Clin Invest. 1989;84(2):627.
48. Waltuck J, Buyon JP. Autoantibody-associated congenital heart block: outcome in mothers and children. Ann Intern Med. 1994;120(7):544.
49. Logothetis J, Kennedy WR, Ellington A, Williams RC. Cryoglobulinemic neuropathy: incidence and clinical characteristics. Arch Neurol. 1968;19(4):389–97.
50. Hughes RAC. Inflammatory and immune mediated sensory neuropathies. Sens Neuropathies. 1995;7:151–9.
51. Griffin JW, Cornblath DR. Ataxic neuropathies. Sens Neuropathies. 1995:105–25.
52. Donfrid M, Apostolski S, Suvajdzic N, Jankovic G, Cemerikic-Martinovic V, Atkinson HDE, et al. Monocytoid B cell lymphoma associated with antibodies to myelin-associated glycoprotein and sulphated glucuronyl paragloboside. Acta Haematol. 2000;106(3):130–32.
53. Voltz R. Paraneoplastic neurological syndromes: an update on diagnosis, pathogenesis, and therapy. Lancet Neurol. 2002;1(5):294–305.
54. Bacman S, Sterin-Borda L, Camusso JJ, Arana R, Hubscher O, Borda E. Circulating antibodies against rat parotid gland M3 muscarinic receptors in primary Sjogren's syndrome. Clin Exp Immunol. 1996;104(3):454–9.
55. Watanabe T, Tsuchida T, Kanda N, Mori K, Hayashi Y, Tamaki K. Anti-{alpha}-fodrin antibodies in Sjogren syndrome and lupus erythematosus. Arch Dermatol. 1999;135(5):535.
56. Kastrup O, Maschke M, Diener H. Pulse cyclophosphamide in the treatment of ataxic sensory and cranial nerve neuropathy associated with Sjogren's syndrome. Clin Neurol Neurosurg. 2005;107(5):440–1.
57. Mori K, Iijima M, Koike H, Hattori N, Tanaka F, Watanabe H, et al. The wide spectrum of clinical manifestations in Sjogren's syndrome-associated neuropathy. Brain 2005;128(11):2518.
58. Delalande S, De Seze J, Fauchais A, Hachulla E, Stojkovic T, Ferriby D, et al. Neurologic manifestations in primary Sjögren syndrome. Medicine 2004;83(5):280–91.
59. Andonopoulos AP, Lagos G, Drosos AA, Moutsopoulos HM. The spectrum of neurological involvement in Sjogren's syndrome. Rheumatology 1990;29(1):21–4.
60. Font J, Valls J, Cervera R, Pou A, Ingelmo M, Graus F. Pure sensory neuropathy in patients with primary Sjogren's syndrome: clinical, immunological, and electromyographic findings. Br Med J. 1990;49(10):775.
61. Mori A, Shimazaki J, Shimmura S, Fujishima H, Oguchi Y, Tsubota K. Disposable eyelid-warming device for the treatment of meibomian gland dysfunction. Jpn J Ophthalmol. 2003;47(6):578–86.
62. Mori K, Koike H, Misu K, Hattori N, Ichimura M, Sobue G. Spinal cord magnetic resonance imaging demonstrates sensory neuronal involvement and clinical severity in neuronopathy associated with Sjogren's syndrome. Br Med J. 2001;71(4):488.
63. Kachi T, Sobue G, Yamamoto M, Igata A. Sensory conduction study in chronic sensory ataxic neuropathy. Br Med J. 1994;57(8):941.
64. Sakakibara R, Hirano S, Asahina M, Sawai S, Nemoto Y, Hiraga A, et al. Primary Sjogren's syndrome presenting with generalized autonomic failure. Eur J Neurol. 2004;11(9):635–8.
65. Kovacs L, Paprika D, Takacs R, Kardos A, Varkonyi TT, Lengyel C, et al. Cardiovascular autonomic dysfunction in primary Sjogren's syndrome. Rheumatology 2004;43(1):95–9.
66. Straub R, Baerwald C, Wahle M, Jä nig W. Autonomic dysfunction in rheumatic diseases. Rheum Dis Clin N Am. 2005;31(1):61–75.
67. Kumazawa K, Sobue G, Yamamoto K, Mitsuma T. Segmental anhidrosis in the spinal dermatomes in Sjögren's syndrome-associated neuropathy. Neurology 1993;43(9):1820.
68. Mandl T, Bornmyr S, Castenfors J, Jacobsson L, Manthorpe R, Wollmer P. Sympathetic dysfunction in patients with primary Sjögren's syndrome. J Rheumatol. 2001;28(2):296–301.
69. Mandl T, Granberg V, Apelqvist J, Wollmer P, Manthorpe R, Jacobsson L. Autonomic nervous symptoms in primary Sjogren's syndrome. Rheumatology 2008;47:914.

70. Wright R, Grant I, Low P. Autonomic neuropathy associated with sicca complex. J Auton Nerv Syst. 1999;75(1):70–6.
71. Sobue G. Pathophysiology of sensory ataxic neuropathy. Rinsh Shinkeigaku Clin Neurol. 1996;36(12):1356.
72. Sobue G, Yasuda T, Kumazawa K, Yamamoto K, Mitsuma T. MRI demonstrates dorsal column involvement of the spinal cord in Sjögren's syndrome-associated neuropathy. Neurology 1995;45(3):592–3.
73. Lin C, Chiu M. Teaching neuroimage: cervical cord atrophy with dorsal root ganglionopathy in Sjogren syndrome. Neurology 2008;70(7):e27.
74. Tajima Y, Mito Y, Owada Y, Tsukishima E, Moriwaka F, Tashiro K. Neurological manifestations of primary Sjögren's syndrome in Japanese patients. Int Med. 1997;36(10):690–3.
75. Govoni M, Bajocchi G, Rizzo N, Tola M, Caniatti L, Tugnoli V, et al. Neurological involvement in primary Sjögren's syndrome: clinical and instrumental evaluation in a cohort of Italian patients. Clin Rheumatol. 1999;18(4):299–303.
76. Gemignani F, Marbini A, Pavesi G, Di Vittorio S, Manganelli P, Cenacchi G, et al. Peripheral neuropathy associated with primary Sjogren's syndrome. Br Med J. 1994;57(8):983.
77. Servioli L, PÈrez C, Consani S, Surez A, Sehabiaga G, Collazo C, et al. Prevalence and characteristics of immunomediated neuropathies in a group of patients with autoimmune diseases. J Clin Neuromuscular Dis. 2007;9(2):285.
78. Vetrugno R, Liguori R, Cortelli P, Montagna P. Sympathetic skin response. Clin Auton Res. 2003;13(4):256–70.
79. Kaplan J, Rosenberg R, Reinitz E, Buchbinder S, Schaumburg H. Invited review: peripheral neuropathy in Sjogren's syndrome. Muscle Nerve 1990;13(7):570–9.
80. Graus F, Pou A, Kanterewicz E, Anderson N. Sensory neuronopathy and Sjögren's syndrome: clinical and immunologic study of two patients. Neurology 1988;38(10):1637.
81. Chai J, Herrmann D, Stanton M, Barbano R, Logigian E. Painful small-fiber neuropathy in Sjogren syndrome. Neurology 2005;65(6):925.
82. Kaplan J, Schaumburg H. Predominantly unilateral sensory neuronopathy in Sjogren's syndrome. Neurology 1991;41(6):948–9.
83. Lacomis D. Small-fiber neuropathy. Muscle Nerve 2002;26(2):173–88.
84. Periquet M, Novak V, Collins M, Nagaraja H, Erdem S, Nash S, et al. Painful sensory neuropathy: prospective evaluation using skin biopsy. Neurology 1999;53(8):1641.
85. Koike H, Sobue G. Alcoholic neuropathy. Curr Opin Neurol. 2006;19(5):481.
86. Laaksonen S, Roytta M, Jaaskelainen SK, Kantola I, Penttinen M, Falck B. Neuropathic symptoms and findings in women with Fabry disease. Clin Neurophysiol. 2008;119(6):1365–72.
87. Devigili G, Tugnoli V, Penza P, Camozzi F, Lombardi R, Melli G, et al. The diagnostic criteria for small fibre neuropathy: from symptoms to neuropathology. Brain 2008;131(7):1912.
88. Smith B, Windebank A, Dyck P. Nonmalignant inflammatory sensory polyganglionopathy. Peripheral neuropathy. Philadelphia, PA: WB Saunders; 1993. pp. 1525–31.
89. Smith A, Bromberg M. A rational diagnostic approach to peripheral neuropathy. J Clin Neuromuscular Dis. 2003;4(4):190.
90. Collins M. Localized vasculitis and the peripheral nervous system. J Rheumatol. 2005;32:769–71.
91. Ramos-Casals M, Anaya J, Garcla-Carrasco M, Rosas J, Bové A, Claver G, et al. Cutaneous vasculitis in primary Sjogren syndrome: classification and clinical significance of 52 patients. Medicine 2004;83(2):96.
92. Ramos-Casals M, Nardi N, Brito-Zeron P, Aguilo S, Gil V, Delgado G, et al. Atypical autoantibodies in patients with primary Sjogren syndrome: clinical characteristics and follow-up of 82 cases. Semin Arthritis Rheum. 2006;35(5):312–21.
93. Vitali C, Tavoni A, Neri R, Castrogiovanni P, Pasero G, Bombardieri S. Fibromyalgia features in patients with primary Sjögren's syndrome: evidence of a relationship with psychological depression. Scand J Rheumatol. 1989;18(1):21–7.
94. Tishler M, Barak Y, Paran D, Yaron M. Sleep disturbances, fibromyalgia and primary Sjögren's syndrome. Clin Exp Rheumatol. 1997;15(1):71.
95. Ringel S, Forstot J, Tan E, Wehling C, Griggs R, Butcher D. Sjogren's syndrome and polymyositis or dermatomyositis. Arch Neurol. 1982;39(3):157.
96. Cody D, Davidson J. Juvenile dermatomyositis and Sjogren's syndrome occurring concurrently in an adolescent male. Rheumatology 2002;41(6):698.
97. Kanellopoulos P, Baltoyiannis C, Tzioufas A. Primary Sjogren's syndrome associated with inclusion body myositis. Rheumatology 2002;41(4):440.
98. {Akpek E-B, 1979 #9; French, 2003 #8; Graves, 2003 #10; Jacobs, 1988 #11; Khurrum Baig, 2004 #2; Kiang, 1998 #5; Perry, 1997 #6; Pucci, 2002 #4; Smith, 1981 #12; Tang-Liu, 2005 #1; Temprano, 2005 #7}. The American College of Rheumatology response criteria for proliferative and membranous renal disease in systemic lupus erythematosus clinical trials. Arthritis Rheum. 2006;54(2):421–32.
99. Hocevar A, Tomsic M, Praprotnik S, Hojnik M, Kveder T, Rozman B. Parasympathetic nervous system dysfunction in primary Sjogren's syndrome. Br Med J. 2003;62(8):702.
100. Bacman S, Perez Leiros C, Sterin-Borda L, Hubscher O, Arana R, Borda E. Autoantibodies against lacrimal gland M3 muscarinic acetylcholine receptors in patients with primary Sjogren's

syndrome. Invest Ophthalmol Vis Sci. 1998;39(1): 151–6.
101. Bacman S, Sterin-Borda L, Camusso JJ, Arana R, Hubscher O, Borda E. Circulating antibodies against rat parotid gland M3 muscarinic receptors in primary Sjogren's syndrome. Clin Exp Immunol. 1996;104(3):454–9.
102. Wang F, Jackson M, Maughan V, Cavill D, Smith A, Waterman S, et al. Passive transfer of Sjögren's syndrome IgG produces the pathophysiology of overactive bladder. Arthritis Rheum. 2004;50(11): 3637–45.
103. Mandl T, Granberg V, Apelqvist J, Wollmer P, Manthorpe R, Jacobsson LTH. Autonomic nervous symptoms in primary Sjogren's syndrome. Rheumatology 2008;47(6):914.
104. Low P, Vernino S, Suarez G. Autonomic dysfunction in peripheral nerve disease. Muscle Nerve 2003;27(6):646–61.
105. Alexander E. Neurologic disease in Sjögren's syndrome: mononuclear inflammatory vasculopathy affecting central/peripheral nervous system and muscle. A clinical review and update of immunopathogenesis. Rheum Dis Clin N Am. 1993;19(4):869–908.
106. Urban P, Keilmann A, Teichmann E, Hopf H. Sensory neuropathy of the trigeminal, glossopharyngeal, and vagal nerves in Sjögren's syndrome. J Neurol Sci. 2001;186(1–2):59–63.
107. Alexander E. Central nervous system (CNS) manifestations of primary Sjögren's syndrome: an overview. Scand J Rheumatol Suppl. 1986;61:161.
108. Garcia-Carrasco M, Ramos-Casals M, Rosas J, Pallares L, Calvo-Alen J, Cervera R, et al. Primary Sjogren syndrome: clinical and immunologic disease patterns in a cohort of 400 patients. Medicine 2002;81(4):270.
109. Anaya J, Villa L, Restrepo L, Molina J, Mantilla R, Vargas S. Central nervous system compromise in primary Sjogren's syndrome. JCR 2002;8(4): 189.
110. Mauch E, Volk C, Kratzsch G, Krapf H, Kornhuber H, Laufen H, et al. Neurological and neuropsychiatric dysfunction in primary Sjogren's syndrome. Acta Neurol Scand. 1994;89(1):31–5.
111. Birnbaum J, Petri M, Thompson R, Izbudak I, Kerr D. Distinct subtypes of myelitis in systemic lupus erythematosus. Arthritis Rheum. 2009;60(11):3378–87.
112. Zeis T, Graumann U, Reynolds R, Schaeren-Wiemers N. Normal-appearing white matter in multiple sclerosis is in a subtle balance between inflammation and neuroprotection. Brain 2007.
113. Noseworthy J, Bass B, Vandervoort M, Ebers G, Rice G, Weinshenker B, et al. The prevalence of primary Sjögren's syndrome in a multiple sclerosis population. Ann Neurol. 1989;25(1):95–8.
114. Sandberg-Wollheim M, Axellm T, Hansen B, Henricsson V, Ingesson E, Jacobsson L, et al. Primary Sjogren's syndrome in patients with multiple sclerosis. Neurology 1992;42(4):845.
115. Miro J, Peña-Sagredo J, Berciano J, InsuA S, Leno C, Velarde R. Prevalence of primary Sjögren's syndrome in patients with multiple sclerosis. Ann Neurol. 1990;27(5):582–4.
116. Wang Y, Tsai K, Fuh J, Tsai C, Wang S. High frequency of primary Sjögren's syndrome in Taiwanese patients presenting as relapsing–remitting multiple sclerosis. Eur Neurol. 2004; 51(1):21–5.
117. de Seze J, Delalande S, Fauchais A, Hachulla E, Stojkovic T, Ferriby D, et al. Myelopathies secondary to Sjögren's syndrome: treatment with monthly intravenous cyclophosphamide associated with corticosteroids. J Rheumatol. 2006;33(4): 709–11.
118. Pericot I, Brieva L, Tintore M, Rio J, Sastre-Garriga J, Nos C, et al. Myelopathy in seronegative Sjogren syndrome and/or primary progressive multiple sclerosis. Multiple Sclerosis 2003;9(3):256–9.
119. Tsai K, Tsai C, Liao N. Sjögren's syndrome with central nervous system involvement presenting as multiple sclerosis with failure response to beta-interferon. Eur Neurol. 2001;45(1):59–60.
120. Chang C, Shiau Y, Wang J, Ho S, Kao A. Abnormal regional cerebral blood flow on ^{99m}Tc ECD brain SPECT in patients with primary Sjogren's syndrome and normal findings on brain magnetic resonance imaging. Br Med J. 2002;61(9):774.
121. Belin C, Moroni C, Caillat-Vigneron N, Debray M, Baudin M, Dumas JL, Moretti JL, Delaporte P, Guillevin L. Central nervous system involvement in Sjögren's syndrome: evidence from neuropsychological testing and HMPAO-SPECT. Ann de Méd. 1999;150:598–604.
122. Kawashima N, Shindo R, Kohno M. Primary Sjögren's syndrome with subcortical dementia. Intern Med. 1993;32(7):561–4.
123. Caselli R, Scheithauer B, Bowles C, Trenerry M, Meyer F, Smigielski J, et al. The treatable dementia of Sjögren's syndrome. Ann Neurol. 1991;30(1):98–101.
124. Orman B, Sterin-Borda L, De Couto Pita A, Reina S, Borda E. Anti-brain cholinergic auto antibodies from primary Sjögren syndrome sera modify simultaneously cerebral nitric oxide and prostaglandin biosynthesis. Int Immunopharmacol. 2007;7(12):1535–43.
125. Liberatore G, Jackson-Lewis V, Vukosavic S, Mandir A, Vila M, McAuliffe W, et al. Inducible nitric oxide synthase stimulates dopaminergic neurodegeneration in the MPTP model of Parkinson disease. Nature Med. 1999;5(12):1403–9.
126. Kim E, Lee J, Kwon K, Lee S, Moon C, Baik E. Differential roles of cyclooxygenase isoforms after kainic acid-induced prostaglandin E2 production and neurodegeneration in cortical and hippocampal cell cultures. Brain Res. 2001;908(1):1–9.

127. Hassin-Baer S, Levy Y, Langevitz P, Nakar S, Ehrenfeld M. Anti-2-glycoprotein I in Sjogren's syndrome is associated with Parkinsonism. Clinical Rheumatol. 2007;26(5):743–7.
128. Visser L, Koudstaal P, Van de Merwe J. Hemiparkinsonism in a patient with primary Sjögren's syndrome. A case report and a review of the literature. Clin Neurol Neurosurg. 1993;95(2):141–5.
129. Hashimoto S, Sawada T, Inoue T, Yamamoto K, Iwata M. Cholinergic-drug induced sicca syndrome in Parkinson's disease: a case report and a review of the literature. Clin Neurol Neurosurg. 1999;101(4):268–70.
130. Nishimura H, Tachibana H, Makiura N, Okuda B, Sugita M. Corticosteroid-responsive Parkinsonism associated with primary Sjögren's syndrome. Clin Neurol Neurosurg. 1994;96(4):327–31.
131. Creange A, Sedel F, Brugieres P, Voisin M, Degos J. Primary Sjögren's syndrome presenting as progressive parkinsonian syndrome. Mov Disord. 1997;12(1):121–3.
132. Walker R, Spiera H, Brin M, Olanow C. Parkinsonism associated with Sjögren's syndrome: three cases and a review of the literature. Mov Disord. 1999;14(2):262–8.
133. Venegas Fanchke P, Sinning M, Miranda M. Primary Sjögren's syndrome presenting as a generalized chorea. Parkinsonism Rel Disord. 2005;11(3):193–4.
134. Papageorgiou S, Kontaxis T, Bonakis A, Kalfakis N. Orofacial dystonia related to Sjogren's syndrome. Clin Rheumatol. 2007;26(10):1779–81.
135. Alexander E, Alexander G. Aseptic meningoencephalitis in primary Sjogren's syndrome. Neurology 1983;33(5):593.
136. Hirohata M, Yasukawa Y, Ishida C, Komai K, Yamada M. Reversible cortical lesions in primary Sjögren's syndrome presenting with meningoencephalitis as an initial manifestation. J Neurol Sci. 2005;232(1–2):111–3.
137. Rossi R, Valeria Saddi M. Subacute aseptic meningitis as neurological manifestation of primary Sjögren's syndrome. Clin Neurol Neurosurg. 2006;108(7):688–91.
138. Ishida K, Uchihara T, Mizusawa H. Recurrent aseptic meningitis: a new CSF complication of Sjogren's syndrome. J Neurol. 2007;254(6): 806–7.
139. Hoshina T, Yamaguchi Y, Ohga S, Kira R, Ishimura M, Takada H, et al. Sjogren's syndrome-associated meningoencephalomyelitis: cerebrospinal fluid cytokine levels and therapeutic utility of tacrolimus. J Neurol Sci. 2007.
140. Caselli R, Scheithauer B, O'Duffy J, Peterson G, Westmoreland B, Davenport P. Chronic inflammatory meningoencephalitis should not be mistaken for Alzheimer's disease. Mayo Clin Proc. 1993;68:846–53.
141. Gerraty R, McKelvie P, Byrne E. Aseptic meningoencephalitis in primary Sjögren's syndrome. Acta Neurol Scand. 1993;88:309–11.
142. Niemela RK, Hakala M. Primary Sjögren's syndrome with severe central nervous system disease. Semin Arthritis Rheum. 1999;29:4–13.
143. Wong S, Pollock A, Burnham J, Sherry D, Dlugos D. Acute cerebellar ataxia due to Sjogren syndrome. Neurology 2004;62(12):2332.
144. Hayashi Y, Kimura A, Kato S, Koumura A, Sakurai T, Tanaka Y, et al. Progressive multifocal leukoencephalopathy and $CD4^+$ T-lymphocytopenia in a patient with Sjögren syndrome. J Neurol Sci. 2008;268(1–2):195–8.
145. Li J, Lai P, Lam H, Lu L, Cheng H, Lee J, et al. Hypertrophic cranial pachymeningitis and lymphocytic hypophysitis in Sjogren's syndrome. Neurology 1999;52(2):420.
146. Alexander E, Ranzenbach M, Kumar A, Kozachuk W, Rosenbaum A, Patronas N, et al. Anti-Ro (SS-A) autoantibodies in central nervous system disease associated with Sjogren's syndrome (CNS-SS): clinical, neuroimaging, and angiographic correlates. Neurology 1994;44(5):899.
147. Spezialetti R, Bluestein H, Peter J, Alexander E. Neuropsychiatric disease in Sjögren's syndrome: anti-ribosomal P and anti-neuronal antibodies* 1. Am J Med. 1993;95(2):153–60.
148. Arnett F, Reichlin M. Lupus hepatitis: an under-recognized disease feature associated with autoantibodies to ribosomal P. Am J Med. 1995;99(5): 465–72.
149. Ghirardello A, Doria A, Zampieri S, Gerli R, Rapizzi E, Gambari P. Anti-ribosomal P protein antibodies detected by immunoblotting in patients with connective tissue diseases: their specificity for SLE and association with IgG anticardiolipin antibodies. Br Med J. 2000;59: 975–80.
150. Moll J, Markusse H, Pijnenburg J, Vecht C, Henzen-Logmans S. Antineuronal antibodies in patients with neurologic complications of primary Sjogren's syndrome. Neurology 1993;43(12):2574.
151. Owada K, Uchihara T, Ishida K, Mizusawa H, Watabiki S, Tsuchiya K. Motor weakness and cerebellar ataxia in Sjögren syndrome—identification of antineuronal antibody: a case report. J Neurol Sci. 2002;197(1–2):79–84.
152. Shams' ili S, Grefkens J, de Leeuw B, van den Bent M, Hooijkaas H, van der Holt B, et al. Paraneoplastic cerebellar degeneration associated with antineuronal antibodies: analysis of 50 patients. Brain 2003;126(6):1409.
153. Bourahoui A, De Seze J, Guttierez R, Onraed B, Hennache B, Ferriby D, et al. CSF isoelectrofocusing in a large cohort of MS and other neurological diseases. Eur J Neurol. 2004;11(8):525–9.
154. Vrethem M, Ernerudh J, Lindstrm F, Skogh T. Immunoglobulins within the central nervous system

in primary Sjögren's syndrome. J Neurol Sci. 1990;100(1–2):186.
155. Cauli A, Yanni G, Pitzalis C, Challacombe S, Panayi G. Cytokine and adhesion molecule expression in the minor salivary glands of patients with Sjogren's syndrome and chronic sialoadenitis. Br Med J. 1995;54(3):209.
156. Alexander E, Beall S, Gordon B, Selnes O, Yannakakis G, Patronas N, et al. Magnetic resonance imaging of cerebral lesions in patients with the Sjogren syndrome. Ann Intern Med. 1988;108(6):815.
157. Morgen K, McFarland H, Pillemer S. Central nervous system disease in primary Sjögren's syndrome: the role of magnetic resonance imaging. Semin Arthritis Rheum. 2004;34:623–30.
158. Kao C, Ho Y, Lan J, ChangLai S, Chieng P. Regional cerebral blood flow and glucose metabolism in Sjogren's syndrome. J Nucl Med. 1998;39(8):1354.
159. Kao C, Lan J, ChangLai S, Chieng P. Technetium-99m-HMPAO SPECT and MRI of brain in patients with neuro-Behcet's syndrome. J Nucl Med. 1998;39(10):1707.
160. Lass P, Krajka-Lauer J, Homziuk M, Iwaszkiewicz-Bilikiewicz B, Koseda M, Hebanowski M, et al. Cerebral blood flow in Sjogren's syndrome using ^{99}Tcm-HMPAO brain SPET. Nucl Med Commun. 2000;21(1):31.
161. Tan EM. Antinuclear antibodies. Diagnostic markers for autoimmune diseases and probes for cell biology. Adv Immunol 1989;44:93–151.
162. Tan EM, Feltkamp TE, Smolen JS, Butcher B, Dawkins R, Fritzler MJ, et al. Range of antinuclear antibodies in "healthy" individuals. Arthritis Rheum. 1997;40(9):1601–11.
163. Tan EM, Smolen JS, McDougal JS, Butcher BT, Conn D, Dawkins R, et al. A critical evaluation of enzyme immunoassays for detection of antinuclear autoantibodies of defined specificities. I. Precision, sensitivity, and specificity. Arthritis Rheum. 1999;42(3):455–64.
164. Infirmary E, Stone J, Caruso P, Deshpande V. Case 24—2009: a 26-year-old woman with painful swelling of the neck. N Engl J Med. 2009;361: 511–8.
165. Craig W, Ledue T, Johnson A, Ritchie R. The distribution of antinuclear antibody titers in normal children and adults. J Rheumatol. 1999;26(4): 914–9.
166. Rosler M, Anand R, Cicin-Sain A, Gauthier S, Agid Y, Dal-Bianco P, et al. Efficacy and safety of rivastigmine in patients with Alzheimer's disease: international randomised controlled trial. Commentary: another piece of the Alzheimer's jigsaw. Br Med J. 1999;318(7184):633.
167. Caroyer J, Manto M, Steinfeld S. Severe sensory neuronopathy responsive to infliximab in primary Sjogren's syndrome. Neurology 2002;59(7):1113.
168. Kizawa M, Mori K, Iijima M, Koike H, Hattori N, Sobue G. Intravenous immunoglobulin treatment in painful sensory neuropathy without sensory ataxia associated with Sjogren's syndrome. Br Med J. 2006;77(8):967.
169. Takahashi Y, Takata T, Hoshino M, Sakurai M, Kanazawa I. Benefit of IVIG for long-standing ataxic sensory neuronopathy with Sjogren's syndrome. Neurology 2003;60(3):503.
170. Rajabally Y, Seow H, Abbott R. Immunoglobulin-responsive dysautonomia in Sjögren's syndrome. J Neurol. 2007;254(5):674–5.
171. Chen W, Yeh J, Chiu H. Plasmapheresis in the treatment of ataxic sensory neuropathy associated with Sjögren's syndrome. Eur Neurol. 2000;45(4): 270–4.
172. Gorson K, Natarajan N, Ropper A, Weinstein R. Rituximab treatment in patients with IVIg-dependent immune polyneuropathy: a prospective pilot trial. Muscle Nerve 2007;35(1):66–9.
173. Asahina M, Kuwabara S, Nakajima M, Hattori T. D-Penicillamine treatment for chronic sensory ataxic neuropathy associated with Sjögren's syndrome. Neurology 1998;51(5):1451–3.
174. Wyszynski A, Wyszynski B. Treatment of depression with fluoxetine in corticosteroid-dependent central nervous system Sjogren's syndrome. Psychosomatics 1993;34(2):173.
175. Pascual J, Cid C, Berciano J, Grant I, Dyck P. High-dose IV immunoglobulin for peripheral neuropathy associated with Sjogren's syndrome. Authors' reply. Neurology 1998;51(2):650–1.
176. Alexander E, Malinow K, Lejewski J, Jerdan M, Provost T, Alexander G. Primary Sjogren's syndrome with central nervous system disease mimicking multiple sclerosis. Ann Intern Med. 1986;104(3):323.
177. Ozgocmen S, Gur A. Treatment of central nervous system involvement associated with primary Sjogrens syndrome. Curr Pharm Des. 2008;14(13):1270–3.
178. Williams C, Butler E, Roman G. Treatment of myelopathy in Sjogren syndrome with a combination of prednisone and cyclophosphamide. Arch Neurol. 2001;58(5):815.
179. Rogers S, Williams C, Roman G. Myelopathy in Sjogren's syndrome: role of nonsteroidal immunosuppressants. Drugs 2004;64(2):123–32.
180. Wright R, O'Duffy J, Rodriguez M. Improvement of myelopathy in Sjögren's syndrome with chlorambucil and prednisone therapy. Neurology 1999;52(2):386.
181. Yamout B, El-Hajj T, Barada W, Uthman I. Successful treatment of refractory neuroSjogren with rituximab. Lupus 2007;16(7):521.
182. Canhao H, Fonseca J, Rosa A. Intravenous gammaglobulin in the treatment of central nervous system vasculitis associated with Sjögren's syndrome. J Rheumatol. 2000;27(4):1102.

183. Konttinen Y, Kinnunen E, Martin Von Bonsdorff M, Lillqvist P, Immonen I, Bergroth V, et al. Acute transverse myelopathy successfully treated with plasmapheresis and prednisone in a patient with primary Sjögren's syndrome. Arthritis Care Res. 30(3):339–44.
184. Mavragani C, Moutsopoulos H. Conventional therapy of Sjogren's syndrome. Clin Rev Allergy Immunol. 2007;32(3):284–91.
185. Szechtman H, Sakic B, Denburg J. Review: behaviour of MRL mice: an animal model of disturbed behaviour in systemic autoimmune disease. Lupus 1997;6(3):223.
186. Tomita M, Holman B, Williams L, Pang K, Santoro T. Cerebellar dysfunction is associated with overexpression of proinflammatory cytokine genes in lupus. J Neurosci Res. 2001;64(1): 26–33.
187. Arnsten A. Stress signalling pathways that impair prefrontal cortex structure and function. Nat Rev Neurosci. 2009;10(6):410–22.
188. Luethi M, Meier B, Sandi C. Stress effects on working memory, explicit memory, and implicit memory for neutral and emotional stimuli in healthy men. Front Behav Neurosci. 2008;2.
189. Waterman SA, Gordon TP, Rischmueller M. Inhibitory effects of muscarinic receptor autoantibodies on parasympathetic neurotransmission in Sjogren's syndrome. Arthritis Rheum. 2000;43(7):1647–54.

Part V

The Views from Japan, China, India, and Australia

New Approaches for the Management of Dry Mouth in Sjögren's Syndrome in Japan

23

Yoichi Nakagawa and Ichiro Saito

Abstract

The management of xerostomia (dry mouth) in Sjögren's syndrome includes rinsing of the mouth with water or mouthwash, the application of salivary substitutes and lubricants, and systemic secretagogues. There are three secretagogues suitable for alleviation of dry mouth in Sjögren's syndrome patients in Japan. Because cevimeline is the most prevalent secretagogue now, we describe the prediction of the effect of cevimeline in patients with Sjögren's syndrome. In addition, the usefulness of the mouth guard for prevention of hyperevaporation of saliva and immunological management are discussed in this chapter.

Keywords

Cevimeline • Minor salivary gland biopsy • Sialography • Sialometory • Bite guard

23.1 Introduction

Sjögren's syndrome (SS) is an autoimmune disease which shows exocrinopathies characterized by lymphocytic infiltration into the salivary and lacrimal glands, resulting in dry mouth and dry eyes [1]. The management of xerostomia (dry mouth) has included using air humidifiers, rinsing the mouth with water or mouthwash, and the application of a salivary substitute. Recently, the usefulness of a reservoir bite guard [2] and an intraoral lubricating device [3–5] was reported to deliver a saliva substitute to the oral cavity for the hyposalivation patients. Additionally, a large number of systemic agents have been proposed as secretagogues but only a few have shown consistent salivary-enhancing properties in well-designed, controlled trials [6]. There are three secretagogues (cevimeline hydrochloride hydrate (cevimeline), pilocarpine hydrochloride, and anetholtrithion) suitable for alleviation of dry mouth in Sjögren's syndrome patients in Japan. Cevimeline is the most prevalent secretagogue now.

Cevimeline, which is an agonist of muscarinic type 1 and 3 receptors [7], has shown clinical efficacy in increasing saliva production and improving the subjective perception of oral dryness in

I. Saito (✉)
Department of Pathology, Tsurumi University School of Dental Medicine, Yokohama, Japan
e-mail: saito-i@tsurumi-u.ac.jp

R.I. Fox, C.M. Fox (eds.), *Sjögren's Syndrome*, DOI 10.1007/978-1-60327-957-4_23,

Sjögren's syndrome patients [8, 9]. Sjögren's syndrome leads to the loss of salivary acinar cells and secretagogues are expected to enhance salivation from the remaining functional acinar cells. It can thus be hypothesized that the greater the salivary gland tissue damage, the less the cevimeline effect. However, to the best of our knowledge the correlation between the severity of Sjögren's syndrome and the effectiveness of cevimeline has not been reported. In addition, IgG from patients with primary Sjögren's syndrome reduced the carbachol-evoked increase in calcium ions (Ca^{2+}) in both mouse and human acinar cells showing that IgG from patients with primary Sjögren's syndrome contains autoantibodies capable of damaging saliva production [10]. The study suggests the involvement of autoantibodies to the receptors in the response to cevimeline in patients with Sjögren's syndrome. Therefore, the clinical effect of cevimeline to enhance salivary secretion would be influenced multifactorially and little is known as to which clinical or immunological factors can predict the effect. If the efficacy of cevimeline can be predicted from the findings of diagnostic clinical examinations before treatment, it would be useful in arriving at the prognosis in patients with Sjögren's syndrome. The relationship between the effect of cevimeline and clinical findings in combination with immunological features in patients with Sjögren's syndrome will be discussed as one of the topics in this chapter.

Xerostomia is defined as a subjective complaint of oral dryness [11] and is caused by the hyposalivation and/or hyperevaporation of saliva. Hyposalivation occurs due to various causes such as Sjögren's syndrome, radiation therapy to the head and neck, the use of medications, and diabetes mellitus [11]. Hyperevaporation is mainly caused by mouth opening or mouth breathing, which often occurs during the night without an apparent decrease in the salivary flow. Hyperevaporation occurs even in the Sjögren's syndrome patients. Recently, we applied a simple mouth guard for sleep-related xerostomia [12] and as the mouth guard is expected to alleviate xerostomia in patients with Sjögren's syndrome, we will also discuss this as another topic.

23.2 Japanese Criteria for Diagnosis of Sjögren's Syndrome

The Committee on Sjögren's Syndrome of the Ministry of Health and Welfare of Japan proposed the revised diagnostic criteria for Sjögren's syndrome in 1999. The criteria are composed of four examinations: histopathology, oral, ocular, and serological examinations [13] and do not include subjective evaluation of the symptoms (Table 23.1). Although the revised Japanese criterion is widely used in Japan as the diagnostic guideline, clinicians often refer to the Sjögren's syndrome criteria proposed by the American–European Consensus Group to make a diagnosis [14].

In 2002, Tsurumi University Dental Hospital opened a Dry Mouth Clinic. Of the 2,269 cases attended to at this clinic with the complaint of a dry mouth sensation, 159 (7.0%) were diagnosed with Sjögren's syndrome (Fig. 23.1). As for the distribution according to age of these Sjögren's syndrome patients, 59 patients were 60–69 years old and 33 patients were 50–59 years old. These results demonstrated that the causes of dry mouth were various, and that Sjogren's syndrome existed in only less than 10% of the dry mouth cases, thus the importance of examinations for the diagnosis was emphasized.

23.3 Efficacy Prediction of Cevimeline in Patients with Sjögren's Syndrome

Thirty consecutive Japanese female primary SS patients with a mean age of 62.3 ± 11.2 (range 22–78 years) treated with cevimeline for their dry mouth at the Tsurumi University Dental Hospital Dry Mouth Clinic were enrolled in this study. The diagnosis of SS was based on the revised diagnostic criteria for Sjögren's syndrome by the Committee on Sjögren's syndrome of the Ministry of Health and Welfare of Japan and the SS criteria proposed by the American–European Consensus Group [14].

Table 23.1 Revised Japanese criteria for Sjögren's syndrome (1999)

1. Histopathology
Definition: positive for at least 1 of A or B:
A. Focus score ≥1 (periductal lymphoid cell infiltration ≥50 in a 4-mm^2 minor salivary gland biopsy)
B. Focus score ≥1 (periductal lymphoid cell infiltration ≥50 in a 4-mm^2 lacrimal gland biopsy)
2. Oral examination
Definition: positive for at least 1 of A or B:
A. Abnormal findings in sialography ≥Stage I (diffuse punctate shadows of less than 1 mm)
B. Decreased salivary secretion (flow rate ≤10 mL/10 min according to chewing gum test or 2 g/2 min according to Saxon test) and decreased salivary function according to salivary scintigraphy
3. Ocular examination
Definition: positive for at least 1 of A or B:
A. Schirmer's test ≤5 mm/5 min and Rose Bengal test ≥3 according to van Bijsterveld score
B. Schirmer's test ≤5 mm/5 min and positive fluorescein staining test
4. Serological examination
Definition: positive for at least 1 of A or B:
A. Anti-Ro/SS-A antibody
B. Anti-La/SS-B antibody

Diagnostic criteria: a diagnosis of Sjögren's syndrome can be made when the patient meets at least two of the above four criteria.

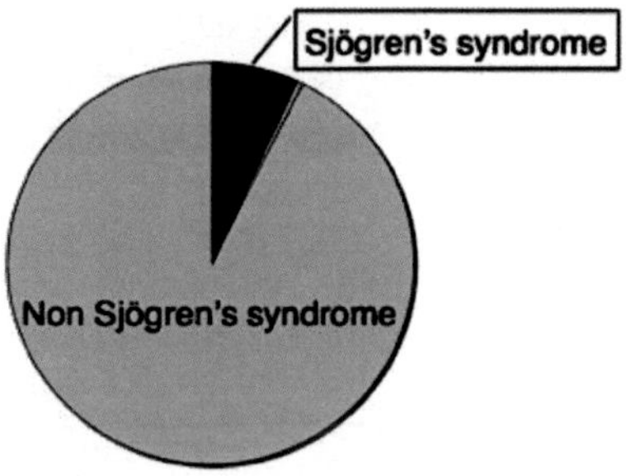

Fig. 23.1 Cause of dry mouth. Of the 2,269 cases seen at Tsurumi University Dental Hospital Dry Mouth Clinic during November 2002–April 2007, 159 (7.0%) were diagnosed with Sjögren's syndrome

Whole stimulated sialometry (WSS) was determined by measuring a volume of stimulated whole saliva, which was stimulated by chewing a piece of gum (Free zone gum, Lotte Co., Ltd, Tokyo, Japan). WSS was compared between the pre-treatment and post-treatment points (4 weeks after cevimeline administration).

Our study on parotid sialography showed that Sjögren's syndrome patients with sialectasis were less sensitive to cevimeline than those without sialectasis [15]. In addition, those patients with severe periductal lymphocyte infiltration in the minor salivary gland demonstrated a lower efficacy of cevimeline than those with slight lymphocyte infiltration.

List of products available in Japan

Product name		Manufacturer/sales agency
Viva-Jellwet	Gel	Tokyo Giken, Inc.
Denture Gel	Gel	Kamemizu Chemical Ind Co., Ltd
Biotene Oral Balance Liquid	Liquid	Laclede, Inc./T&K, Inc.
Biotene Oral Balance Gel	Gel	Laclede, Inc./T&K, Inc.
Biotene Mouthwash	Liquid	Laclede, Inc./T&K, Inc.
Biotene Toothpaste	Toothpaste	Laclede, Inc./T&K, Inc.

Product name		Manufacturer/sales agency
Bioxtra Alcohol-free Mouthrinse	Liquid	Weltec
Bioxtra Mild Toothpaste Jell	Toothpaste	Weltec
Bioxtra Aqua Mouth Jell	Gel	Weltec
Bioxtra Aqua Mouth Spray	Spray	Weltec
Oral Aqua Gel	Gel	GC Co
Dry Mouth Gel	Gel	GC Co
Saliveht®	artificial saliva	Teijin Pharma, Ltd
Kinusui® Spray	Spray	Seikagaku Co/Sunstar, Inc.
Dent Health Moisturizing Mouthwash	Liquid	Lion Co
Wet Care	Spray	Kissei Pharmaceutical Co., Ltd
Wet Care Lemon	Spray	Kissei Pharmaceutical Co., Ltd
Wet Care Plus (apple flavor)	Spray	Kissei Pharmaceutical Co., Ltd
Butler Dental Tablet	Tablet	Sunstar, Inc.
Oral Gelwetkeeping	Gel	Oralcare
Stoppers for	Spray	Sundental Co., Ltd
Honey Wet	Gel	Nippon Zettoc Co., Ltd
Oral Control Moistwash	Liquid	Nippon Zettoc Co., Ltd/ Daiichi Sankyo Healthcare Co., Ltd
Oral Control Moistliquid	Liquid	Nippon Zettoc Co., Ltd/ Daiichi Sankyo Healthcare Co., Ltd
Oral Control Moistgel	Gel	Nippon Zettoc Co., Ltd/Daiichi Sankyo Healthcare Co., Ltd
Oral Refre Jell	Gel	Toho Co., Ltd/Morita Co.
Aqua Mucus Gel	Gel	Life Co.
Aqua Mucus Liquid	Liquid	Life Co.

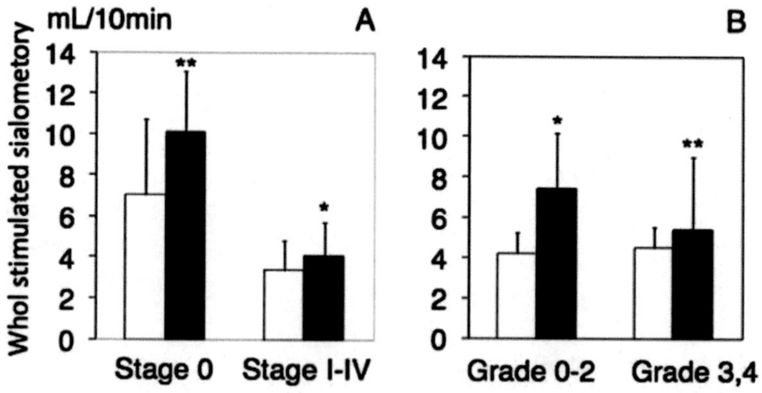

Fig. 23.2 Effect of cevimeline on whole stimulated sialometry. **a** Classification of sialography. **b** Classification of labial minor salivary gland biopsy. Data show mean ± s.d. (white bars: pre-WSS, black bars: post-WSS); $^{*}P < 0.05$, $^{**}P < 0.01$

Figure 23.2a shows the pre-treatment and post-treatment WSS in groups classified according to the sialography findings. In both the Stage 0 and the Stage I–IV groups, post-treatment WSS demonstrated a significant increase compared with the pre-treatment values (P = 0.008 and P = 0.015, respectively).

The magnitude of the increase in WSS after cevimeline treatment in the Stage 0 group was significantly higher than that in the Stage I–IV

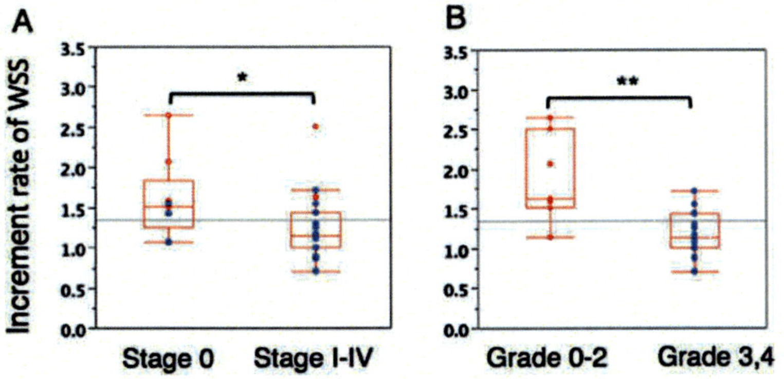

Fig. 23.3 Comparison of the increment rate of WSS after 4 weeks of cevimeline treatment. WSS was compared between the pre-treatment and post-treatment points (4 weeks after cevimeline administration) and the increment rate was also calculated by dividing the post-treatment value by the pre-treatment value. **a** Classification of the sialography. **b** Classification of the labial minor salivary gland biopsy; box plots represent the median (*line*), 25th and 75th percentiles (*box*), and *whiskers* indicate the tenth and ninetieth percentiles (*red dot*: Grade 0–2, *blue dot*: Grade 3 and4); $^{*}P < 0.05$, $^{**}P < 0.01$

group ($P < 0.001$). The increment rate of WSS after cevimeline treatment in the Stage 0 group was significantly higher than that in the Stage I–IV group ($P = 0.042$) (Fig. 23.3a).

23.3.1 Labial Minor Salivary Gland Biopsy

Biopsy specimens were obtained through normal-appearing lower labial mucosa. Three trained pathologists evaluated the focal lymphocytic sialadenitis in the minor salivary glands by hematoxylin and eosin (HE)-stained section according to Greenspan's criteria [16]: Grade 0, absent; Grade 1, slight infiltrate; Grade 2, moderate infiltrate or less than one focus per 4 mm^2; Grade 3, one focus per 4 mm^2; and Grade 4, more than one focus per 4 mm^2. Grades 3 and 4 were considered to be positive according to the SS criteria.

23.3.2 Sialography

Sialography of the unilateral parotid gland was performed once before treatment with cevimeline using the conventional hand-injection method. A lateral projection was taken immediately after injection of 1 mL of contrast medium (76% diatrizoate sodium) (Urografin: Nihon Schering Co., Ltd, Osaka, Japan) into the Stensen's duct. After an addition of 0.5 mL of contrast medium, a posterior–anterior radiograph was taken. Two trained examiners evaluated the sialography in all cases according to the classification of Rubin and Holt [17]: Stage 0, normal; Stage I, punctate; Stage II, globular; Stage III, cavitary; and Stage IV, destructive. Stages I–IV were considered to be positive according to the SS criteria.

Figure 23.2b shows the pre-treatment and post-treatment WSS in groups classified according to the findings of the labial minor salivary gland biopsy. In both the Grade 0–2 and the Grade 3 and 4 groups, post-treatment WSS demonstrated a significant increase compared to the pre-treatment values ($P = 0.018$ and $P = 0.006$, respectively). The magnitude of increase of WSS after cevimeline treatment in the Grade 0–2 group was significantly higher than that in the Grade 3 and 4 group ($P = 0.001$).

Patients with positive sialography findings (Stages I–IV) had a significantly lower pre-treatment WSS and response to cevimeline compared to those with negative findings. In contrast, positive findings of labial minor salivary gland biopsy were not related to pre-treatment WSS in patients with Sjögren's syndrome. As WSS is contributed principally by the parotid gland [18], this discrepancy might be due to the difference

Table 23.2 Results of multiple regression analysis to examine factors influencing the objective variable of post-treatment whole stimulated sialometry

	Coefficient (*b*)	SE	Standardized coefficient (*b*)	*P* Value
Intercept	5.784	1.126		<0.001
WSS before treatment	0.874	0.100	0.707	<0.001
Grade of lip biopsy	−0.869	0.269	−0.232	0.003
Stage of sialography	−0.867	0.269	−0.259	0.004
SS-B	−0.001	0.003	−0.014	0.847

WSS whole stimulated sialometry, *Lip biopsy* labial minor salivary gland biopsy, *SS-B* anti-La/SS-B antibodies.

of the evaluation site (parotid gland versus minor salivary gland). These results are congruent with those reported by Saito et al. [19].

The increment rate of WSS after cevimeline treatment in the Grade 0–2 group was significantly higher than that in the Grade 3 and 4 group ($P = 0.002$) (Fig. 23.3b).

Similar findings [20] were reported by the use of pilocarpine, a cholinergic parasympathomimetic agent, which has shown efficacy in treating dry mouth symptoms in Sjögren's syndrome patients [21, 22]. Rosas et al. [20] reported that Sjögren's syndrome patients with a pilocarpine-stimulated salivary flow less than 1.5 mL had a higher prevalence of positive anti-Ro/SS-A, anti-La/SS-B, parotid scintigraphy class III or IV, and positive salivary gland biopsy compared to those with a pilocarpine-stimulated flow over 1.5 mL. Our findings that the effect of cevimeline is influenced by the severity of SS concur with those reported by Rosas et al. [20].

Interestingly, the response to cevimeline was quite different between the Grade 0–2 and the Grade 3 and 4 groups. This implies the existence of soluble factors interfering with cevimeline in the Grade 3 and 4 group. When considering the higher prevalence of autoantibodies to La/SS-B in the Grade 3 and 4 group compared to the Grade 0–2 group, local production of autoantibodies or cytokines might lead to dysfunction of the residual glandular tissues. The prevalence of anti-La/SS-B antibodies in the Grade 3 and 4 group was significantly higher than that in the Grade 0–2 group ($P = 0.022$).

Multiple regression was employed to examine the relative contributions of sialography stage, grade of lip biopsy, and titer of anti-La/SS-B antibody to the post-treatment WSS. Results showed that post-treatment WSS was predicted by the model ($R^2 = 0.880$): Post-treatment WSS = 5.784 + (0.847 × pre-treatment WSS) – (0.869 × grade of lip biopsy) – (0.867 × stage of sialography) – (0.001 × anti-La/SS-B antibody), and that the stage classification of sialography ($P = 0.004$) and the histological grade of the labial minor salivary gland biopsy ($P = 0.003$) were significantly associated with the post-treatment WSS (Table 23.2).

Our preliminary results demonstrated the relationship between the effect of cevimeline on saliva secretion and the degree of salivary gland destruction evaluated by sialography and histopathological findings in the labial minor salivary glands. These diagnostic approaches could provide useful prognostic information on the efficacy of cevimeline in SS patients. However, this study is a preliminary open-label trial without placebo-treated patients from a practical standpoint, which is limited by its relatively small sample size and the lack of blinding of patients and outcome assessors. Therefore, to verify the results in the present study, a placebo-controlled, double-blind randomized trial should be done in the next step.

23.4 The Application of a Bite Guard

Sleep-related xerostomia is a sensation of dry mouth associated with a report of either mouth and/or throat discomfort that induces awakenings for water intake [23, 24]. The prevalence of

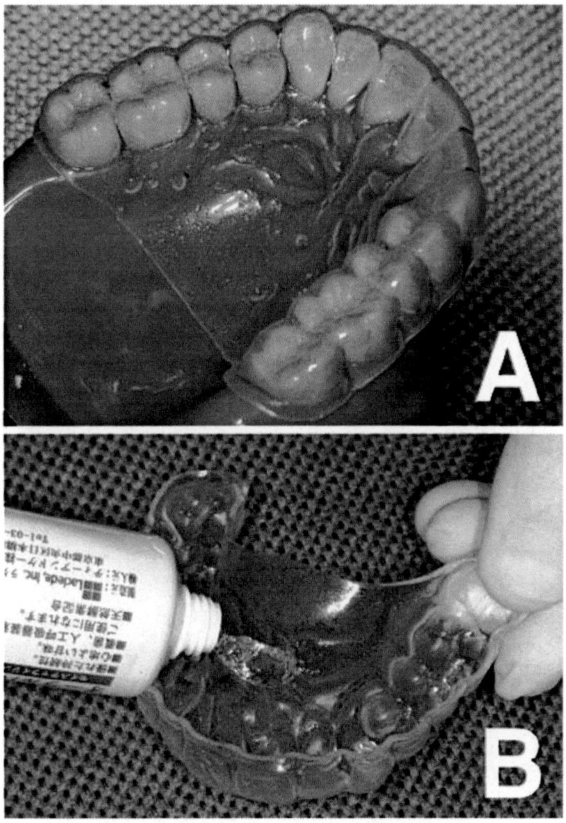

Fig. 23.4. The night guard was fabricated with soft material. **a** The night guard covered the dental arch and the hard palate and did not possess a reservoir for retaining a saliva substitute. **b** Patients can use the device to maintain the lubricants

self-reported dry mouth complaints during sleep in a survey of Swedish pensioners was estimated to be 13.7% for men and 24.1% for women [25]. However, the etiology of sleep-related xerostomia has not been revealed. The secretory response to mastication is associated with the stimulation of periodontal mechanoreceptors of the teeth and taste receptors, which usually occur during food intake in the daytime [26]. During the night, salivary secretion diminishes dramatically, even in healthy subjects [27, 28].

We applied a simple mouth guard for the sleep-related xerostomia [12]. The device, fabricated with a soft material, is often used as a sports mouth guard or as a night guard for the treatment of nighttime bruxism. The 1.5-mm-thick ethylene vinyl acetate sheet (Sof-Tray Sheets, Ultradent Products, Inc., South Jordan, UT, USA) was heated and aspirated to secure the model using a vacuum-forming system (Dental Sta-Vac Model; Buffalo Dental Manufacturing, Syosset, NY, USA). The night guard covered the dental arch and the hard palate and did not possess a reservoir for retaining the saliva substitute (Fig. 23.4a).

The participants in the preliminary study complained of nocturnal oral dryness, but they showed normal salivation during the examination at the clinic. No factors that cause nocturnal hyposalivation, such as medication side effects, could be identified. The patients did not show any signs in their oral cavity. Fourteen patients (7 males, 7 females; mean age 66.5 ± 9.2, ranging from 55 to 93 years) were allocated to the treatment group, while 14 patients (7 males, 7 females; mean age 73.1 ± 10.0, ranging from 54 to 78 years) were allocated to the control group. The control group used a mouth rinse three times daily (daytime and before going to bed). There were no significant differences between the groups in terms of age, WRS (whole resting saliva flow), and WSS by the Mann–Whitney test at the pre-treatment period.

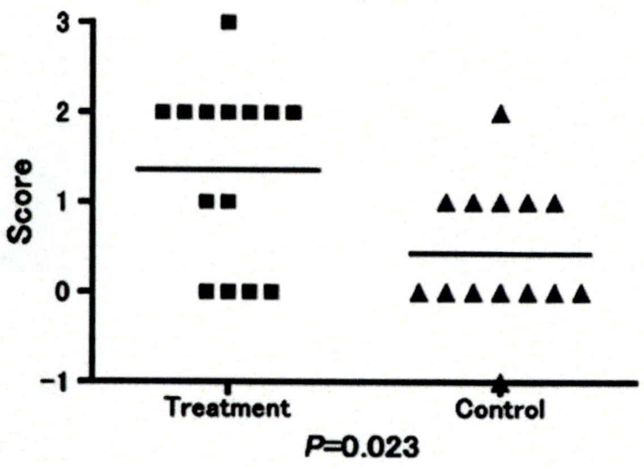

Fig. 23.5 Comparison of the improvement in general impression between treatment and control groups. The general impression was scaled using five levels: 3, extremely improved; 2, improved; 1, improved a little; 0, unchanged; −1, deteriorated (Mann–Whitney test)

Table 23.3 Comparison of VAS between the treatment and control groups

	P Value	
	Treatment group	Control group
Sensation of oral dryness	0.0295	0.0942
Thirstiness	0.0012	0.3013
Stickiness in oral cavity	0.0640	0.4961
Change of taste	0.2500	0.0547
Burning sensation of the tongue	0.0371	0.8501

The Wilcoxon signed-rank test was used to compare the visual analog scale (VAS) between pre-treatment and post-treatment periods.

Following completion of the 2-week treatment, substantial improvement was reported by the treatment group (Fig. 23.5). In the results of the general impression, the treatment group showed that 10 of the 14 patients (71%) showed improvement in their symptoms, but 4 expressed that their symptoms were unchanged. No patients experienced an aggravation or worsening of symptoms. As for the results of the visual analog scale (VAS), the sensation of dryness was improved in the treatment group except in two cases. The post-treatment VAS value significantly decreased compared with that of the pre-treatment period in sensation of oral dryness, thirstiness, and burning sensation of the tongue in the treatment group (Table 23.3).

A hypothesis was proposed that unconscious episodes of rhythmic masticatory muscle activity play an important role in lubricating the oral cavity [23, 24] and that the night guard could help to regulate appropriate rhythmic muscle activity. Alternatively, secretion was accelerated by mechanical stimulation to the oral mucosa. Stimulation of the fauces is known to lead to an increase in salivation [29], therefore the night guard possibly stimulates the oral mucosa mechanically, which may thus induce saliva secretion.

A second possible mechanism for nocturnal xerostomia improvement with the night guard is maintenance of saliva volume in the oral cavity. It was suggested that patients recognized the sensation of dryness when there was not enough saliva to cover the various oral surfaces, especially the palate [30]. In addition, the resting flow rates from the palatal salivary gland less than 6.0 L/cm^2 cause patients to suffer from a dry mouth [31]. Due to the ability of the night guard to cover the palate, enough saliva volume on the palate could be maintained between the palate and the night guard, resulting in a decreased sensation of dryness.

A third possible factor for symptom improvement could be that the night guard decreases vaporization of saliva from the oral cavity, which is dependent upon how long the mouth is open.

Mouth breathing occurs due to malocclusion, nasal congestion, and enlarged adenoids.

We concluded that the application of a night guard is therefore suggested to be a useful and simple method for the management of nocturnal xerostomia. If the mouth guard possesses the functions of an increase of salivary secretion, the maintenance of saliva volume in the oral cavity, and a decrease of saliva vaporization, the device could also be useful for Sjögren's syndrome patients. The device can be used not only during the night but also during the day time. Furthermore, patients can use the device to maintain the lubricants (Fig. 23.4b).

23.5 Immunological Treatment for Primary Sjögren's Syndrome

Immunological management will be one of the options for patients who could neither expect the effect of secretagogues nor moisturizing agents using the bite guard. However, no trial concerning immunological treatment of primary Sjögren's syndrome such as interferon-α [32, 33] and anti-CD20 antibody [34, 35] has been conducted so far. Even systemic administration of corticosteroid to the primary Sjögren's syndrome patients has not been accepted by all clinicians in Japan, and thus the corticosteroid irrigation of the parotid gland has been an alternative option [36].

References

1. Fox RI, Saito I. Criteria for diagnosis of Sjögren's syndrome. Rheum Dis Clin North Am. 1994;20(2):391–407.
2. Robinson PG, Pankhurst CL, Garrett EJ. Randomized-controlled trial: effect of a reservoir biteguard on quality of life in xerostomia. J Oral Pathol Med. 2005;34(4):193–7.
3. Frost PM, Gardner RM, Price AR, Sinclair GF. A preliminary assessment of intra-oral lubricating systems for dry mouth patients. Gerodontology 1997;14(1):54–8.
4. Frost PM, Shirlaw PJ, Challacombe SJ, Fernandes-Naglik L, Walter JD, Ide M. Impact of wearing an intra-oral lubricating device on oral health in dry mouth patients. Oral Dis. 2006;12(1):57–62.
5. Frost PM, Shirlaw PJ, Walter JD, Challacombe SJ. Patient preferences in a preliminary study comparing an intra-oral lubricating device with the usual dry mouth lubricating methods. Br Dent J. 2002;193(7):403–8.
6. Fox PC. Salivary enhancement therapies. Caries Res. 2004;38(3):241–6.
7. Iwabuchi Y, Katagiri M, Masuhara T. Salivary secretion and histopathological effects after single administration of the muscarinic agonist SNI-2011 in MRL/lpr mice. Arch Int Pharmacodyn Ther. 1994;328(3):315–25.
8. Fife RS, Chase WF, Dore RK, et al. Cevimeline for the treatment of xerostomia in patients with Sjogren syndrome: a randomized trial. Arch Intern Med. 2002;162(11):1293–300.
9. Petrone D, Condemi JJ, Fife R, Gluck O, Cohen S, Dalgin P. A double-blind, randomized, placebo-controlled study of cevimeline in Sjogren's syndrome patients with xerostomia and keratoconjunctivitis sicca. Arthritis Rheum. 2002;46(3):748–54.
10. Dawson LJ, Stanbury J, Venn N, Hasdimir B, Rogers SN, Smith PM. Antimuscarinic antibodies in primary Sjogren's syndrome reversibly inhibit the mechanism of fluid secretion by human submandibular salivary acinar cells. Arthritis Rheum. 2006;54(4):1165–73.
11. Guggenheimer J, Moore PA. Xerostomia: etiology, recognition and treatment. J Am Dent Assoc. 2003;134(1):61–9.
12. Yamamoto K, Nagashima H, Yamachika S, et al. The application of a night guard for sleep-related xerostomia. Oral Surg Oral Med Oral Pathol Oral Radiol Endod. 2008;106(3):e11–4.
13. Fujibayashi T, Sugai S, Miyasaka N, Hayashi Y, Tsubota K. Revised Japanese criteria for Sjögrens syndrome (1999): availability and validity. Mod Rheumatol. 2004;14:425–34.
14. Vitali C, Bombardieri S, Jonsson R, et al. Classification criteria for Sjogren's syndrome: a revised version of the European criteria proposed by the American-European Consensus Group. Ann Rheum Dis. 2002;61(6):554–8.
15. Yamada H, Nakagawa Y, Wakamatsu E, et al. Efficacy prediction of cevimeline in patients with Sjogren's syndrome. Clin Rheumatol. 2007;26(8):1320–27.
16. Greenspan JS, Daniels TE, Talal N, Sylvester RA. The histopathology of Sjogren's syndrome in labial salivary gland biopsies. Oral Surg Oral Med Oral Pathol. 1974;37(2):217–29.
17. Rubin P, Holt JF. Secretory sialography in diseases of the major salivary glands. Am J Roentgenol Radium Ther Nucl Med. 1957;77(4):575–98.
18. Edgar WM. Saliva: its secretion, composition and functions. Br Dent J. 1992;172(8):305–12.
19. Saito T, Fukuda H, Arisue M, et al. Relationship between sialographic findings of parotid glands

and histopathologic finding of labial glands in Sjogren's syndrome. Relation to clinical and immunologic findings. Oral Surg Oral Med Oral Pathol. 1991;72(6):675–80.
20. Rosas J, Ramos-Casals M, Ena J, et al. Usefulness of basal and pilocarpine-stimulated salivary flow in primary Sjogren's syndrome. Correlation with clinical, immunological and histological features. Rheumatology 2002;41(6):670–5.
21. Vivino FB, Al-Hashimi I, Khan Z, et al. Pilocarpine tablets for the treatment of dry mouth and dry eye symptoms in patients with Sjogren syndrome: a randomized, placebo-controlled, fixed-dose, multicenter trial. P92-01 Study Group. Arch Intern Med. 1999;159(2):174–81.
22. Papas AS, Sherrer YS, Charney M, et al. Successful treatment of dry mouth and dry eye symptoms in Sjogren's Syndrome patients with oral pilocarpine: a randomized, placebo-controlled, dose-adjustment study. J Clin Rheumatol. 2004;10(4): 169–77.
23. Thie NM, Kato T, Bader G, Montplaisir JY, Lavigne GJ. The significance of saliva during sleep and the relevance of oromotor movements. Sleep Med Rev. 2002;6(3):213–27.
24. Lavigne GJ, Goulet JP, Zuconni M, Morrison F, Lobbezoo F. Sleep disorders and the dental patient: an overview. Oral Surg Oral Med Oral Pathol Oral Radiol Endod. 1999;88(3):257–72.
25. Asplund R. Nocturia in the elderly in relation to thirst, dry mouth and dry eyes. Can J Urol. 2004;11(4):2322–6.
26. Anderson DJ, Hector MP. Periodontal mechanoreceptors and parotid secretion in animals and man. J Dent Res. 1987;66(2):518–3.
27. Dawes C, Ong BY. Circadian rhythms in the flow rate and proportional contribution of parotid to whole saliva volume in man. Arch Oral Biol. 1973;18(9):1145–53.
28. Ferguson DB, Fort A. Circadian variations in human resting submandibular saliva flow rate and composition. Arch Oral Biol. 1974;19(1):47–5.
29. Edgar WE, O'Mullane DM. Saliva and oral health. 2nd ed. London: British Dental Association; 1996.
30. Wolff M, Kleinberg I. Oral mucosal wetness in hypo- and normosalivators. Arch Oral Biol. 1998;43(6):455–62.
31. Niedermeier W, Huber M, Fischer D, et al. Significance of saliva for the denture-wearing population. Gerodontology 2000;17(2):104–18.
32. Ship JA, Fox PC, Michalek JE, Cummins MJ, Richards AB. Treatment of primary Sjogren's syndrome with low-dose natural human interferon-alpha administered by the oral mucosal route: a phase II clinical trial. IFN Protocol Study Group. J Interferon Cytokine Res. 1999;19(8):943–51.
33. Cummins MJ, Papas A, Kammer GM, Fox PC. Treatment of primary Sjogren's syndrome with low-dose human interferon alfa administered by the oromucosal route: combined phase III results. Arthritis Rheum. 2003;49(4):585–93.
34. Pijpe J, van Imhoff GW, Spijkervet FK, et al. Rituximab treatment in patients with primary Sjogren's syndrome: an open-label phase II study. Arthritis Rheum. 2005;52(9):2740–50.
35. Steinfeld SD, Tant L, Burmester GR, et al. Epratuzumab (humanised anti-CD22 antibody) in primary Sjogren's syndrome: an open-label phase I/II study. Arthritis Res Ther. 2006;8(4):R129.
36. Izumi M, Eguchi K, Nakamura H, Takagi Y, Kawabe Y, Nakamura T. Corticosteroid irrigation of parotid gland for treatment of xerostomia in patients with Sjogren's syndrome. Ann Rheum Dis. 1998;57(8):464–9.

New Approaches for the Management of Dry Mouth and Dry Eye in Sjogren's Syndrome in Japan

24

Dry Eye Part

Kazuo Tsubota

Abstract

The first-line of treatment in the management of dry eye Sjogren's syndrome patients is using artificial tears without preservatives and hyaluronic acid, which brings moisture to the ocular surface, preventing desiccation. However, recent findings suggest that dry eye is caused not only by the desiccation, but also by the lack of tear components. The second treatment regimen should include the supply of the tear components such as vitamin A and EGF to the ocular surface. The punctum plug is one choice of treatment when the patient has a minimal level of tear production. However, those patients who do not even produce even the smallest amount of tears, treatment by autologous serum eye drops becomes necessary. Serum has many components that exist in tears, so the 20% diluted autologous serum can be a good source of tear components for the ocular surface. In this chapter we focus on this tear component supply treatment.

Keywords

Autologous serum • Hyaluronic acid • Punctal plug • Dry eye • Tear

24.1 Introduction

Sjogren's syndrome (SS) is an organ-specific autoimmune disorder characterized by lymphocytic infiltration and destruction of the exocrine glands such as lacrimal and salivary glands. The pathology is accompanied by systemic production of autoantibodies to ribonucleoprotein particles SS-A/Ro and SS-B/La [1]. The disease is not fatal, however, the dysfunctions of the exocrine glands cause hyposecretion of tears and saliva, resulting in decreased quality of life due to the dry eyes and dry mouth. These are common complaints among the elderly, and living with dry eye and/or dry mouth syndrome can be a devastating experience for the sufferer, where living with the symptoms is more severe than would non-sufferers realize.

K. Tsubota (✉)
Department of Ophthalmology, Keio University School of Medicine, Tokyo, Japan
e-mail: tsubota@z3.keio.jp

R.I. Fox, C.M. Fox (eds.), *Sjögren's Syndrome*, DOI 10.1007/978-1-60327-957-4_24,

The fundamental problem is the lack of tear, resulting in the desiccation itself. The naming of dry eye suggests that dryness itself is the major problem of sicca syndrome. In some aspects, it is right especially in the evaporative type of dry eye [2, 3]. However, the dry eye in Sjogren's syndrome is often severer than the evaporative dry eye or simple tear-deficient dry eye [4]. We have previously hypothesized that the severity of dry eye in Sjogren's syndrome is due to the lack of the tear component supply to the ocular surface, because Sjogren's syndrome-type dry eye do not only have basic tearing but also reflex tearing, resulting in the deficiency of the tear components [4]. Thus the treatment options include not only the prevention of desiccation but also the supply of essential tear components.

24.2 How to Provide the Essential Tear Components to the Ocular Surface

Available artificial tears are known to improve symptoms of dry eye such as irritation, they do not include the essential tear components, thus we have had to seek an alternative way. There are several options for this purpose.

(1) Punctal plug
(2) Secretagogues
(3) Autologous serum eye drops

Punctal plug is often used for the treatment of severe dry eye [5]. The occlusion of the punctum increases the volume of tears on the ocular surface, providing the tear components to the ocular surface, because SS patients still have minimal lacrimal secretion even in the late stage. This treatment is popular in the United States, estimating that 400,000 plugs are used every year. The second option is the use of secretagogues such as cevimeline or pilocarpine to stimulate muscarinic receptors. Those drugs are effective for the salivation, but the efficacy to the recovery of lacrimal function is somehow limited [6] and not widely used by ophthalmologists. I believe there are patients with certain types of dry eye who respond well to these secretagogues but the efficacy and dosage of these drugs have not been fully elucidated, and future study is expected to be ongoing.

The third option, the use of autologous serum eye drops, has been gaining in popularity by Japanese dry eye specialists. The first several cases using autologous serum were originally described by Fox et al. [7]. The theory and further development have been mainly followed by our dry eye team and now is a widely accepted therapy [8–10]. The Dry Eye Society of Japan compiles a list of ophthalmologists who are preparing and administering autologous serum for the treatment of severe dry eye (http://www.dryeye.ne.jp/). Patients looking for relief are able to find ophthalmologists who can provide such treatment. In this review, I would like to focus on the treatment for Sjogren's syndrome with autologous serum eye drops.

24.3 Use of Autologous Serum Eye Drops for the Treatment of Dry Eye

Sjogren's syndrome patients exhibit more severe ocular surface changes than those seen in non-Sjogren dry eye patients due to insufficient basic and reflex tearing. This is caused by infiltrating lymphocytes that destroy the lacrimal gland [11–13]. Basal tears and serum share many similar components (Table 24.1) such as epidermal growth factor (EGF) and vitamin A and are important for maintaining the health of the ocular surface epithelium [14–17]. In addition, transforming growth factor (TGF)-β concentration in human serum, which is five times higher than in tear, is believed to control epithelial proliferation and maintain cells in an undifferentiated state such as the induction of basic keratins in epidermal cells [18]. Fibronectin, insulin-like growth factors, and substance P, all present in serum, have been reported to be essential for wound healing, especially for patients with dry eye [19–21]. Since artificial tears do not contain these components, it became important to find a tear substitute, and the use of autologous serum is appealing for this reason [22].

Table 24.1 Comparison of tears and autologous serum

Components	Basal tears	Serum
Growth factors		
EGF	1.66 ng/mL	0.72 ng/mL
TGF-α (males)	247 pg/mL	147 pg/mL
TGF-α (females)	180 pg/mL	147 pg/mL
Vitamins		
Vitamin A	16 ng/mL	883 ng/mL
Vitamin C	117 μg/mL	7–20 μg/mL
Proteins		
Lysozyme	2.39 g/L	4.0–15 mg/L
Lactoferrin	1.51 g/L	ND
Albumin	5.4 mg/dL	3.5–5.5 g/dL
IgA	41.1 mg/dL	90–450 mg/dL
Electrolytes		
Na^+	145 mEq/L	135–146 mEq/L
K^+	24.1 mEq/L	3.5–5.0 mEq/L
Ca^{2+}	1.5 mEq/L	5 mEq/L
Cl^-	128 mEq/L	96–108 mEq/L
HCO_3^-	26 mEq/L	21–29 mEq/L

ND, not detected.

24.4 Ongoing Research with Autologous Serum Eye Drops

Our study of Sjogren's syndrome patients showed the advantage of using autologous serum eye drops for the treatment of dry eye by measuring EGF, vitamin A, and TGF-β concentrations in serum and tears. We demonstrated that autologous serum application provided these components to the ocular surface [23]. Autologous serum is preservative-free so patients were instructed to diligently take precautions to avoid contamination. The concentration of essential serum components remained stable after 1 month of refrigeration and 3 months of being frozen. Serum contains proteins such as albumin or globulin, which can protect the deterioration of key cytokines. Clinical application of autologous serum is possible through the extended preservation offered by these components. Ohashi et al. reported that the concentration of EGF was 0.7–8.1 ng/mL in reflex tears and 1.9–9.7 ng/mL in non-reflex tears [15], which is higher than EGF found in serum, which is approximately 0.5 ng/mL [23]. In contrast, the amount of retinol in human tear fluid was reported by Speek et al. to be 0.4–10.6 ng/mL [24]. Retinol in serum is 55 ng/mL, which contains over 1000 times the amount in tears. Squamous metaplasia tends to occur when the epithelium lacks enough vitamin A [23–25]. The application of autologous serum may provide appropriate levels of retinol for ocular health.

TGF-β in serum is five times higher than in tears so in high concentrations it remains controversial due to its anti-proliferative effects and possible suppression of wound healing of the ocular surface epithelium [23]. In order to maintain TGF-β levels similar to tears, the serum was diluted, which also enabled the preparation of serum eye drops from a small blood sample.

24.5 Preparation of Autologous Serum Eye Drops

First, informed consent should be obtained after explanation to the patient of the autologous serum preparation and use, including effects of the treatment. The patient should test negative for HIV and hepatitis B and C infections. Next, 40 mL of venous blood is obtained and centrifuged (Fig. 24.1). This provides 20 mL of serum, which is then diluted with saline in a sterile manner to 20%. The 40-mL sample provides 100 mL of serum and is adequate for a 3-month supply. Figure 24.2 shows the graphic preparation of autologous serum eye drops.

One 100-mL supply yields about 2,000 eye drops of 5 μL each. Sjogren's syndrome dry eye patients use a maximum of 20 drops a day (up to 10 drops per eye), thus 2,000 drops are enough for more than 100 days. The autologous serum eye drops are divided into 20 5-mL bottles, and patients are advised to store bottles in the freezer until use [23]. The patients are encouraged to keep the bottle currently being used in the refrigerator.

Fig. 24.1 Preparation of venous blood for centrifugation

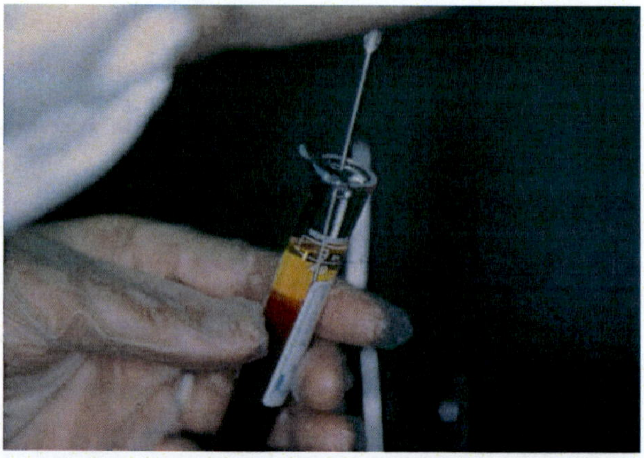

Fig. 24.2 Preparation of autologous serum eye drops

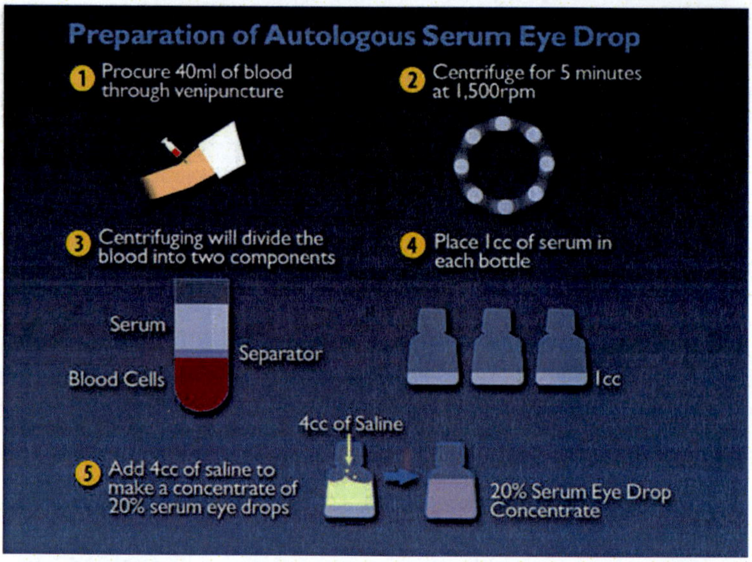

24.6 Autologous Serum Eye Drops for Sjogren's and Non-Sjogren's Syndrome

Studies have shown the beneficial effects of autologous serum eye drops for both Sjogren's syndrome and non-Sjogren's syndrome dry eye patients, with striking improvements seen in Rose Bengal (Fig. 24.3a, b) and fluorescein staining scores, which may be multifactorial. Additionally, increased mucin (MUC)-1 expression of the cultured conjunctival epithelium suggested a direct effect of the serum on the ocular surface epithelium [23].

The study by Nobel et al. evaluated the efficacy of autologous serum for the treatment of severe ocular surface disorders, including Sjogren's syndrome patients in a prospective randomized controlled crossover study comparing 50% autologous serum eye drops and conventional treatment. When the treatment was reversed to conventional therapy from autologous serum eye drops, the cytological improvements and ocular surface vital staining scores were reversed [26].

We performed a randomized prospective controlled clinical trial by evaluating the solitary effects of autologous treatment by assigning patients into two groups using only autologous

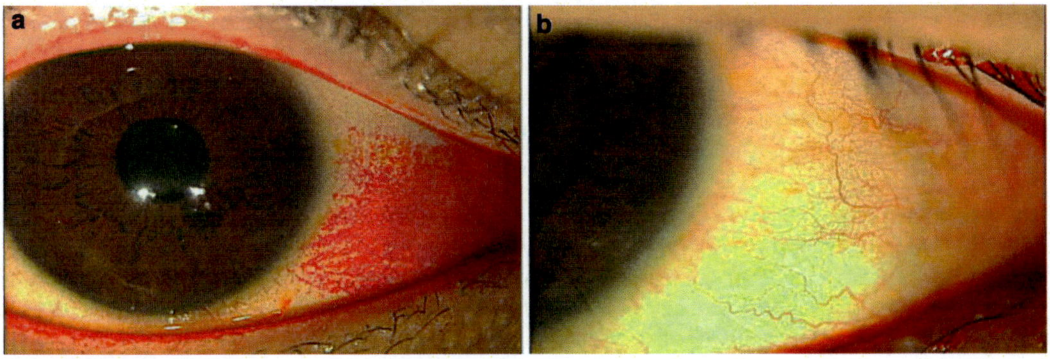

Fig. 24.3 Sjogren's syndrome—43-year-old male patient. **a** Rose Bengal staining before autologous serum treatment. **b** Rose Bengal staining after treatment by autologous serum

Fig. 24.4 Comparison of Rose Bengal score between patients using artificial tears and patients using autologous serum. Rose Bengal score was significantly lower in the group using artificial tears compared to the group using autologous serum after treatment ($P < 0.05$). Reprinted from Kojima et al. [9], with permission from Elsevier, Inc

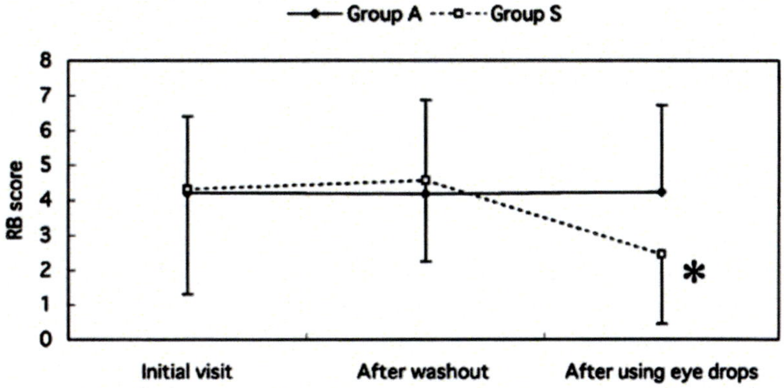

serum eye drops or artificial tear drops after a washout period of 2 weeks. After 2 weeks of treatment, tear stability, ocular surface vital staining scores, and pain symptom scores in patients treated with autologous serum eye drops showed significant improvement compared to those assigned to preservative-free artificial tears (Fig. 24.4) [9].

24.7 Future Studies of Autologous Serum Treatment

Future studies may shed light on the exact mechanism of the use of serum on the ocular surface epithelium, which still remains unexplained. However, several studies have shown the positive benefits of serum as a likely tear substitute for the maintenance of ocular surface health since many of the essential components in tears are also present in serum. The primary disadvantage of autologous serum treatment is the necessity of obtaining blood from the patients and contraindication in cases with HIV or hepatitis B or C infection. Cultured conjunctival cells by autologous serum increased MUC-1 expression, which suggests a direct effect of the serum on the ocular surface epithelia, but it remains unknown if serum upregulates other ocular surface mucins. Hyaluronate eye drops are popular artificial tears, so a comparative prospective study in combination with serum would prove interesting, especially in consideration of the longer exposure hyaluronate would provide the essential components of serum to the ocular surface. Additionally, combining other conventional treatments with serum would also be highly valuable. Refinement of an artificial tear substitute containing all essential tear components would be ideal. Long-term studies showing the efficacy and safety of prolonged use of autologous serum eye drops at various concentrations should also be included in future investigations. As tear components are fully elucidated, we believe artificial tear substitutes that include all essential tear components will eventually replace autologous serum eye drops in the future.

24.8 Conclusion

This review has described the unique treatment of Sjogren's syndrome dry eye by autologous serum eye drops. As I have described in the introduction, autologous serum treatment can be replaced by the punctal plug or secretagogues in certain types of patients. Punctal plug insertion is more convenient for most of the patients and may be the method of first choice to supply essential tear components. However, autologous serum is most beneficial and necessary for patients who do not have enough tearing even with a punctal plug or when there has been no response to the secretagogues. It was been my pleasure to report to you, the reader, this unique treatment initially described by Fox, who is the editor of this book.

24.9 Late-Breaking Update

Recently, P2Y2 receptor agonist (Diquafosol tetrasodium, Santen Pharmaceutical Co., Ltd.) was approved as the first drug for the treatment of dry eye in the world. We are expecting the improvement of dry eye symptoms in the management of Sjogren's syndrome with this drug.

References

1. Fox R. Sjögren's syndrome: primer on the rheumatic diseases. Atlanta: Arthritis Foundation; 1998. pp. 283–286.
2. Tsubota K, Nakamori K. Dry eyes and video display terminals. N Engl J Med. 1993 Feb 25;328(8):584.
3. Xu KP, Yagi Y, Toda I, Tsubota K. Tear function index. A new measure of dry eye. Arch Ophthalmol. 1995 Jan;113(1):84–8.
4. Tsubota K, Xu KP, Fujihara T, Katagiri S, Takeuchi T. Decreased reflex tearing is associated with lymphocytic infiltration in lacrimal glands. J Rheumatol. 1996 Feb;23(2):313–20.
5. Kaido M, Goto E, Dogru M, Tsubota K. Punctal occlusion in the management of chronic Stevens–Johnson syndrome. Ophthalmology 2004 May;111(5):895–900.
6. Ono M, Takamura E, Shinozaki K, Tsumura T, Hamano T, Yagi Y, Tsubota K. Therapeutic effect of cevimeline on dry eye in patients with Sjögren's syndrome: a randomized, double-blind clinical study. Am J Ophthalmol 2004 Jul;138(1):6–17.
7. Fox RI, Chan R, Michelson JB, Belmont JB, Michelson PE. Beneficial effect of artificial tears made with autologous serum in patients with keratoconjunctivitis sicca. Arthritis Rheum. 1984 Apr;27(4):459–61.
8. Matsumoto Y, Dogru M, Goto E, Ohashi Y, Kojima T, Ishida R, Tsubota K. Autologous serum application in the treatment of neurotrophic keratopathy. Ophthalmology 2004 Jun;111(6):1115–20.
9. Kojima T, Ishida R, Dogru M, Goto E, Matsumoto Y, Kaido M, Tsubota K. The effect of autologous serum eyedrops in the treatment of severe dry eye disease: a prospective randomized case–control study. Am J Ophthalmol. 2005 Feb;139(2):242–6.
10. Kojima T, Higuchi A, Goto E, Matsumoto Y, Dogru M, Tsubota K. Autologous serum eye drops for the treatment of dry eye diseases. Cornea 2008;27: S25–30.
11. Tsubota K, Kaido M, Yagi Y, Fujihara T, Shimmura S. Diseases associated with ocular surface abnormalities: the importance of reflex tearing. Br J Ophthalmol. 1999 Jan;83(1):89–91.
12. Tsubota K. Reflex tearing in dry eye not associated with Sjogren's syndrome. In: Sullivan D, et al., editors. Lacrimal gland, tear film and dry eye syndromes. 2nd ed. New York, NY: Plenum Press; 1998. pp. 903–907.
13. Tsubota K, Toda I, Yagi Y, Ogawa Y, Ono M, Yoshino K. Three different types of dry eye syndrome. Cornea 1994 May;13(3):202–9.
14. Ubels JL, Foley KM, Rismondo V. Retinol secretion by the lacrimal gland. Invest Ophthalmol Vis Sci. 1986 Aug;27(8):1261–8.
15. Ohashi Y, Motokura M, Kinoshita Y, Mano T, Watanabe H, Kinoshita S, Manabe R, Oshiden K, Yanaihara C. Presence of epidermal growth factor in human tears. Invest Ophthalmol Vis Sci. 1989 Aug;30(8):1879–82.
16. van Setten G, Viinikka L, Tervo T. EGF is a constant component of normal human tear fluid. Graefes Arch Clin Exp Ophthalmol. 1989:22:184–7.
17. van Setten GB, Tervo T, Tervo K, Tarkkanen A. Epidermal growth factor (EGF) in ocular fluids: presence, origin and therapeutical considerations. Acta Ophthalmol Suppl. 1992;(202):54–9.

18. Gupta A, Monroy D, Ji Z, Yoshino K, Huang A, Pflugfelder SC. Transforming growth factor beta-1 and beta-2 in human tear fluid. Curr Eye Res. 1996 Jun;15(6):605–14.
19. Nishida T, Ohashi Y, Awata T, Manabe R. Fibronectin. A new therapy for corneal trophic ulcer. Arch Ophthalmol. 1983 Jul;101(7):1046–8.
20. Nishida T, Nakamura M, Ofuji K, Reid TW, Mannis MJ, Murphy CJ. Synergistic effects of substance P with insulin-like growth factor-1 on epithelial migration of the cornea. J Cell Physiol. 1996 Oct;169(1):159–66.
21. Nishida T, Nakagawa S, Awata T, Tani Y, Manabe R. Fibronectin eye drops for traumatic recurrent corneal lesion. Lancet 1983 Aug 27;2(8348):521–2.
22. Tsubota K. New approaches in dry eye management: supplying missing tear components to the ocular surface epithelium. 1st Annual Meeting of the Kyoto Cornea Club. Amsterdam: Kugler. 1997; 1. pp. 27–32.
23. Tsubota K, Goto E, Fujita H, Ono M, Inoue H, Saito I, Shimmura S. Treatment of dry eye by autologous serum application in Sjögren's syndrome. Br J Ophthalmol. 1999 Apr;83(4):390–5.
24. Speek AJ, van Agtmaal EJ, Saowakontha S, Schreurs WH, van Haeringen NJ. Fluorometric determination of retinol in human tear fluid using high-performance liquid chromatography. Curr Eye Res. 1986 Nov;5(11):841–5.
25. el-Ghorab M, Capone A Jr, Underwood BA, Hatchell D, Friend J, Thoft RA. Response of ocular surface epithelium to corneal wounding in retinol-deficient rabbits. Invest Ophthalmol Vis Sci. 1988 Nov;29(11):1671–6.
26. Noble BA, Loh RS, MacLennan S, Pesudovs K, Reynolds A, Bridges LR, Burr J, Stewart O, Quereshi S. Comparison of autologous serum eye drops with conventional therapy in a randomised controlled crossover trial for ocular surface disease. Br J Ophthalmol. 2004 May;88(5):647–52.

Sjögren's Syndrome in Australia: Clinical Practice and Research

25

Tom Gordon and Maureen Rischmueller

Abstract

Sjögren's syndrome is commonly encountered in clinical practice in Australia. Management is conservative and biological therapies have yet to be approved for use. Intravenous immunoglobulins have improved autonomic symptoms in some patients. Research has focused on the molecular and genetic analysis of anti-Ro/La antibodies; characterization of muscarinic receptor autoantibodies; immunohistology of salivary gland biopsies; and the role of BAFF/BLyS.

Keywords

Sjögren's syndrome • Australia • Research

There have been no formal studies on the incidence and prevalence of primary and secondary Sjögren's syndrome in Australia. Notwithstanding this, Sjögren's syndrome is encountered commonly in clinical practice; indeed most rheumatologists and clinical immunologists would see more patients with primary Sjögren's syndrome than with systemic lupus erythematosus. Patients treated for rheumatoid arthritis and systemic sclerosis frequently have sicca symptoms. A recent South Australian study reported a 50% prevalence of secondary Sjögren's syndrome in patients with systemic sclerosis [1].

T. Gordon (✉)
Department of Immunology, Flinders Medical Center, Flinders, Australia
e-mail: t.gordon@flinders.edu.au

The clinical features observed in Australian patients with primary Sjögren's syndrome are comparable to reports from North America and Europe. As expected, the dominant symptoms are dry eyes and xerostomia with signs relating to salivary and lacrimal gland involvement. In our experience with a cohort of more than 200 patients, 50% or more have Raynaud's phenomenon and about one-third of patients have extraglandular complications involving the skin, lungs, kidneys, muscles, peripheral sensory nerves, or central nervous system. A small number of patients (2–3%) have developed non-Hodgkin's lymphomas of the salivary/lacrimal glands and/or gastrointestinal tract that have generally responded well to conventional chemotherapy. Overall, the clinical patterns seen in Australia are similar to the overseas experience. A particular area of interest has been the study of autonomic complications involving

R.I. Fox, C.M. Fox (eds.), *Sjögren's Syndrome*, DOI 10.1007/978-1-60327-957-4_25,

the bladder, bowel, and cardiovascular system in patients with primary Sjögren's syndrome, with a recent controlled study confirming the presence of mild autonomic dysfunction, as measured by both self-reported symptoms and objective assessment. Most treating physicians have observed cases of primary Sjögren's syndrome with monoclonal rheumatoid factors and mixed cryoglobulinemia requiring high dose steroids.

The treatment of patients with primary Sjögren's syndrome in Australia remains conservative, and no biological therapies have been approved for use in this condition as yet. Topical lubricants are baseline therapy, with occasional punctual occlusion of the nasolacrimal ducts. Systemic pilocarpine is used as a secretagogue by a minority of patients, due to minor drug intolerances. Topical ocular cyclosporin A is not approved for Sjögren's syndrome in Australia, but is used by a few patients via a special access scheme. Hydroxychloroquine is often prescribed for cutaneous manifestations, myalgias, and arthralgias and short courses of steroids often employed for lymphocytic infiltrations of the lungs (lymphatic pneumonia) or kidneys (interstitial nephritis). Sodium bicarbonate is employed for renal tubular acidosis. Low dose methotrexate is the drug of choice for patients who develop an inflammatory arthritis despite hydroxychloroquine therapy and has also been successfully used as a steroid-sparing agent for patients with inflammatory myositis. Some patients with central nervous system involvement or vasculitic neuropathy have required pulse steroids and cyclophosphamide, and one patient with cyclic fever responded to off-label use of rituximab. Therapeutic courses of intravenous immunoglobulins have improved autonomic symptoms in some patients, apparently by neutralizing autoantibodies directed against muscarinic receptors [2].

Sjögren's syndrome research in Australia has centered on the characterization of the fine specificity and genetic control of anti-Ro-La responses [3]; detection of anti-muscarinic receptor antibodies by physiological assays [4]; analysis of chemokine expression, cellular adhesion molecules, and dendritic cells in salivary gland biopsy specimens [5, 6]; and the role of BAFF/BLyS in patients and experimental models [7]. Australia has a strong tradition of translational research in the autoimmune diseases, and Sjögren's syndrome, as a prototypic systemic autoimmune disorder, will continue to remain a key focus of research. The aims will be to discover new biomarkers and improve our understanding of pathogenesis with the hope of developing new therapeutic strategies.

References

1. Swaminathan S, Goldblatt F, Dugar M, Gordon TP, Roberts-Thomson PJ. Prevalence of sicca symptoms in a South Australian cohort with systemic sclerosis. Intern Med J. Epub 2008;38:897–903.
2. Smith AJ, Jackson MW, Wong F, Cavill D, Rischmueller M, Gordon TP. Neutralisation of muscarinic receptor autoantibodies by intravenous immunoglobulin in Sjögren's syndrome. Hum Immunol. 2005;66:411–6.
3. McCluskey J, Farris AD, Keech CL, et al. Determinant spreading: lessons from animal models and human disease. Immunol Rev. 1998;164:209–29.
4. Waterman SA, Gordon TP, Rischmueller M. Inhibitory effects of muscarinic receptor autoantibodies on parasympathetic neurotransmission in Sjögren's syndrome. Arthritis Rheum. 2000;43:1647–1654.
5. Azis KE, McCluskey PJ, Wakefield D. Characterisation of follicular dendritic cells in labial salivary glands of patients with primary Sjögren's syndrome. Ann Rheum Dis. 1997;56:140–143.
6. Cuello C, Palladinetti P, Tedla N, DiGirolamo N, Lloyd AR, McCluskey PJ, Wakefield D. Chemokine expression and leucocyte infiltration in Sjögren's syndrome. Br J Rheumatol. 1998;37:779–83.
7. Groom J, Kalled SL, Cutler AH, et al. Association of BAFF/BLyS over-expression and altered B cell differentiation with Sjögren's syndrome. J Clin Invest. 2002;109:59–68.

Primary Sjögren's Syndrome: Report from India

26

Ramnath Misra, Sapan Pandya, and Debashish Danda

Abstract

A decade ago primary Sjögren's syndrome (SS) had been rarely reported from India. Contrary to Western data, the reported occurrence of disease has been low. Even in dedicated clinics for rheumatic diseases, only about 0.5% of all patients seen are diagnosed to have SS. However, in recent years larger dataset of SS has been presented. One of the notable differences was the earlier age at presentation, almost a decade earlier than reported. The occurrence of dry eyes, dry mouth, arthritis, skin manifestations, systemic features and presence of antibodies to Ro and La are similar to published series. Patients have been diagnosed when they present with delayed complications like renal tubular acidosis. It is recommended to go for biopsy of the minor salivary gland. It provides definitive proof while excluding diseases like tuberculosis, lymphoma, and sarcoidosis, which can mimic SS.

Keywords

India • SS • Younger age • Diagnosis

A decade earlier, primary Sjögren's syndrome (SS) had been rarely reported from India. Even a population-based study [1] of rheumatic diseases in India, by a rheumatology center, makes no mention of this disease. Contrary to Western data, the reported occurrence of disease has been low. Even in dedicated clinics for rheumatic diseases, only about 0.5% of all patients seen are diagnosed to have SS. We had reported a series of 26 North Indian patients with SS [2]. Subsequently, two series of patients were presented in the annual national rheumatology meeting from the Western and the Southern regions of India. The California criteria were used for diagnosis in our series whereas the latter two used the American–European Consensus criteria for diagnosis. There is thus an increasing awareness to diagnose SS at rheumatology centers. This brief write up will attempt to summarize the clinical picture of the disease and similarities and dissimilarities with patients reported from Western countries.

One of the striking features is the younger age at the time of diagnosis. The mean age of our

R. Misra (✉)
Department of Immunology, Sanjay Gandhi Post Graduate Institute of Medical Sciences, Lucknow, India
e-mail: rnmisra2000@gmail.com

R.I. Fox, C.M. Fox (eds.), *Sjögren's Syndrome*, DOI 10.1007/978-1-60327-957-4_26,

patients is 10 years younger than that reported from Europe. Though we cannot explain this earlier occurrence, we have observed this "shift to the left" phenomenon in other diseases such as multiple myeloma, which normally has been described in the sixth decade. Due to lack of awareness and availability of appropriate diagnostic facility, there is a delay in diagnosis by an average of 4 years. There was some variation in the sex ratio among the three series, but the female predominance was similar to that reported elsewhere. The series from North India has less number of females, which is a referral bias and could reflect that less number of females do seek specialist's attention for apparently milder and innocuous symptoms like dry eyes and dry mouth. The occurrence of xerostomia, dry eyes, parotid gland enlargement, purpura, hypergammaglobulinemia, and presence of autoantibodies are comparable to that seen in Western countries (Table 26.1) [7]. Some delayed complications of the disease such as renal tubular acidosis and even glomerulonephritis was observed by us. The retrospective series from South India had a biopsy done in all patients who had dry mouth along with polyarthralgia/arthritis or chronic fibromyalgia-like pain. Hence, the number of patients with arthritis was higher. Besides, it observed dental problem (193, 83.5%), neurological features (25, 11%), respiratory (26, 11%), and lymphoma (2, 0.01%).

Diagnosis was based on both the presence of antibodies to Ro and antibodies to La and/or the biopsy of minor salivary gland. The prevalence of various autoantibodies in present series is similar to that reported in other series.

Many of the patients with SS are labeled as rheumatoid arthritis or systemic lupus erythematosus (SLE) due to overlapping features and it is only after extensive investigations for the dry eyes and dry mouth that proper diagnosis is reached. Documenting a reduction or absolute lack in salivation by objective tests is an issue as investigational facilities like salivary scintigraphy, parotid sialography, and measurement of salivary flow are not available at all centers. Antibodies to Ro and La are still not widely available. Though minor salivary gland biopsy remains a simple and definitive diagnostic test, there are reservations in getting their biopsies done by both patients and physicians. It also helps in excluding diagnosis like tuberculosis, sarcoidosis, and lymphoma, which may mimic the clinic picture of SS. We encountered

Table 26.1 Frequency of various manifestations of patients with primary Sjögren's syndrome as reported in three cohort of Indian patients from different regions of the country. The figures in parenthesis are percentages

N	Misra et al. ($n = 26$)[3]	Pandya ($n = 68$)[+]	Danda ($n = 231$)[+]
Region	North India	West India	South India
Period	1990–2000	2004–2009	1997–2005
Mean age in years	42.9	42.9	45
Duration prior to diagnosis	3.93	5.9	5.9
Sex	4:1	9:1	8:1
Dry eyes	22 (85)	68 (100)	231 (100)
Dry mouth	23 (88)	68 (100)	231 (100)
Arthritis/arthralgia	20 (77)	42 (62)	231 (100)
Purpura	4 (15)	26 (42)	14 (6)
Parotid gland enlargement	6 (23)	30 (44)	43 (19)
Renal tubular acidosis	1 (4)	12 (17)	27 (12)
Biopsy proven	16/26 (60)	44/45 (98)	231 (100)
Antibodies to ANA	18/26 (69)	57/62 (92)	203 (84)
Antibodies to Ro and La	16	52 (85)	16/40 (40)

[+]Personal communication, 2010.

one patient each with tuberculosis and sarcoidosis, which was revealed on labial salivary gland biopsy.

Symptomatic treatment included artificial tears, frequent use of sips of water, and care of teeth. Corticosteroids (1 mg/kg/day to start with and later tapered over a period of 6 months) were used only in patients with glomerulonephritis and vasculitis. Immunosuppressive drugs like azathioprine or cyclophosphamide or biological agents were rarely used. Arthritis was managed with NSAIDs and low dose methotrexate (7.5–15 mg/week) or hydroxychloroquine (3–5 mg/kg/day).

Thus, in conclusion, primary SS is an underdiagnosed entity in India. Many cases are not diagnosed due to lack of awareness among physicians, ophthalmologists, or dentists who would be looking after patients with dryness of eyes or mouth. These patients receive scant attention and a prompt rheumatologist referral may help to diagnose them at an early stage. Definitive primary SS with classical history of sicca syndrome is less often seen than probable cases. It is worth considering a lip biopsy and antinuclear antibody (ANA) on all patients presenting with features of sicca syndrome with systemic features like arthritis/arthralgia or fibromyalgic pain. Hepatitis C and HIV infection need to be ruled out.

References

1. Chandrasekaran AN, Venugopal B, Thenmozhivilli PR, Partibhan M. Spectrum of clinical and immunological features of systemic rheumatic disorders in a referral hospital in South India—Sjögren's syndrome. J Indian Rheum Assoc. 1994;2:71–5.
2. Malaviya AN, Singh RR, Kapoor SK, Sharma A, Kumar A, Singh YN. Prevalence of rheumatic diseases in India. Results of a population survey. J Indian Rheum Assoc. 1994;2:13–7.
3. Misra R, Hissaria P, Tandon V, Aggarwal A, Krishnani N, Dabadghao S. Primary Sjögren's syndrome: rarity in India. J Assoc Phys India. 2003;51:859–62.
4. Dabadghao S, Aggarwal A, Arora P, Pandey R, Misra R. Glomerulonephritis leading to end stage renal disease in a patient with primary Sjögren syndrome. Clin Expl Rheumatol. 1995;13:509–11.
5. Fox RI, Saito I. Criteria for diagnosis of Sjögrens's syndrome. Rheum Clin North Am. 1994;20:391–407.
6. Vitali C, Bombardieri S, Jonsson R, et al. Classification criteria for Sjögren's syndrome: a revised version of the European criteria proposed by the American–European Consensus Group. Ann Rheum Dis. 2002:61:554.
7. Skopouli FN, Dafni U, Ioannidis JP, Moutsopoulos HM. Clinical evolution, and morbidity and mortality of primary Sjögren's syndrome. Semin Arthritis Rheum. 2000;29:296–304.

Sjögren's Syndrome in China

27

Jing He and Zhan-Guo Li

Abstract

Primary Sjögren's syndrome (SS) is a debilitating systemic autoimmune disorder. In this chapter, SS in China was introduced. The prevalence of SS was 0.77% by Copenhagen criterion, and more than 62% of the patients were delayed or misdiagnosed in this country. The novel autoantibodies were used routinely in diagnosis of SS in some hospitals, such as anti-a(alpha)-fodrin and anti-M3 receptor (M3R). Treatment of SS is much the same as that in Western countries, including corticosteroid and immunosuppressant. Herbs are also applied by rheumatologists practicing traditional Chinese medicine (TCM).

Keywords

Sjögren's syndrome • Anti-α(alpha)-fodrin • Anti-M3 receptor (M3R) • Herbs • Traditional Chinese medicine

27.1 A Disease of Antiquity in Ancient China

Historically a condition of severe dry eyes and dry mouth with glandular swelling was originally described as "燥痹" (Zao Bi) in ancient China at around 500 BC in the medical book called *Huang Di Nei Jing*. It is very difficult to compare the clinical features of patients in antiquity with modern SS patients due to the profound differences in diagnosis and treatment in traditional Chinese and Western medicine. For over a thousand years, symptoms of SS have been treated by a variety of different herbal medicines provided by Traditional Chinese Practitioners (TCPs). Chinese history records the use of acupuncture and herbal mixtures such as Tea of Increased Tears in detailed records of treatments given to the emperor and his household a thousand years ago. It is likely that these herbal remedies contain a variety of cholinergic agonists and anti-inflammatory properties, similar to the use of the herbal agents including pilocarpine, quinine, and salicylates in the West.

The approach to diagnosis and treatment of SS has changed dramatically in China over the

J. He (✉)
Department of Rheumatology and Immunology, People's Hospital, Peking University Medical School, Beijing, China
e-mail: hejing_1105@yahoo.com

R.I. Fox, C.M. Fox (eds.), *Sjögren's Syndrome*, DOI 10.1007/978-1-60327-957-4_27,

past generation. These changes reflect the enormous changes in the health care system of China, the availability of economic resources, and increased introduction of Western diagnostic and therapeutic methods in China. These changes are the result of Chinese physicians having the opportunity to study in the West as well as the availability of Western medical literature translated into Chinese. There are also several key changes in China that have contributed to this change in clinical features and treatment of SS: (1) a generation ago, virtually all patients were seen and treated predominantly by traditional Chinese medicine practitioners with little access to Western medicine; (2) sanitation changes have altered the frequency of infections including hepatitis B, hepatitis C, tuberculosis, and EBV-related diseases (such as nasopharyngeal carcinoma that mimicked SS); (3) Western style hospitals in academic centers were previously accessible to only a very small number of patients and the clinical presentation of patients to these centers was limited to patients with life-threatening manifestations such as periodic paralysis due to renal tubular acidosis or vasculitis. This bias toward very sick patients skewed the initial distribution of patient clinical associations.

Pioneers in the evaluation of SS in China include Prof. Nai-Zheng Zang and his protégé Prof. Dong Yi in Beijing and Prof. Cheng Shun-li in Shanghai who had training in Western-oriented medicine [1]. It soon became clear that the clinical manifestations in Chinese mainland SS patients were not the same as those seen among Chinese of similar genetic background who were living in the United States, Europe, or Australia; it was deduced that environmental co-factors (such as the ubiquitous use of herbs) played a role in manifestations such as renal tubular acidosis or infections such as TBC or hepatitis viruses biased the presentations; and symptoms such as dry eyes and dry mouth were "quality of living issues" that were largely ignored a generation ago against the background of providing treatment for life-threatening manifestations even when patients were seen in Western style academic institutions. As showed in studies by Doctors Nai-Zheng Zhang and Yi Dong and Chen Shun-li in early 1980s, the prevalence of SS was 0.77% by Copenhagen criterion and 0.33% by Fox criterion, respectively [2].

Even today outside large urban medical centers in China, SS is not a well-recognized disease and traditional medicine remains the mainstay of health care in the rural regions of China and for many patients in large urban centers. As demonstrated in a survey carried out recently by our group, only 37.9% of SS patients attended rheumatology clinic at their first visit to hospital. Most of the SS patients tended to consult with hematologists, stomatologists, gastroenterologists, or doctors practicing traditional Chinese medicine. It is not surprising that Sjögren's syndrome is often diagnosed with delay or misdiagnosed, which is largely due to unawareness of the disease by public as well as the atypical clinical features [3].

As shown by a survey including 224 Chinese SS patients, there are many different manifestations and patients are seen by multiple specialties (Tables 27.1 and 27.2) [3, 11]. The

Table 27.1 The specialties attended by Sjögren's syndrome patients at their first visit to hospital

Specialties	Patient no.	%	Specialties	Patient no.	%
Rheumatology	85	37.9	Ophthalmology	13	5.8
Hematology	26	11.6	Orthopedics	10	4.5
Gastroenterology	22	9.8	ENT	10	4.5
Stomatology	19	8.5	Dermatology	3	1.3
Pneumology	17	7.5	Nephrology	2	0.9
TCM	15	6.7	Neurology	2	0.9

ENT ear–nose–throat department, *TCM* traditional Chinese medicine

Table 27.2. Complications of 224 Sjögren's syndrome patients

Complications	No.	%
Leukopenia	74	33.0
Arthritis	56	25.0
Raynaud's syndrome	37	16.5
Aminotransferase ↑	35	15.6
Purpura	26	11.6
Anemia	18	8.0
Thrombocytopenia	13	5.8
Renal tubular acidosis	8	3.6

most common symptoms include leukopenia (33%), arthritis (25%), and Raynaud's phenomena (16.5%). Interestingly, it appears that SS-associated leukopenia is more common in Chinese patients than that in Western countries. In contrast, there is less Raynaud's phenomena in Chinese patients. In addition, thyroid dysfunction is one of the major complications in Chinese SS patients. The prevalence is up to 44.4% in a large-scale study, including hyperthyroidism, hypothyroidism, and thyroxin abnormality [4].

Another recent study by An et al. in our group focusing on SS in youth has shown that parotid gland swelling, hematological involvement, and hyperglobulinemia were much more common in early-onset Sjögren's syndrome [5].

It has been shown that a portion of patients developed lupus shortly after SS (SS-onset lupus), while others might suffer from SS and lupus almost at the same time. In 2006, Jia et al. from our group studied the clinical and serologic features of 22 SS patients associated with systemic lupus erythematosus (SLE) [6]. It was found that 36% (8/22) of patients were SS-onset SLE, 32% (7/22) of patients developed SS and SLE simultaneously, while the other 32% (7/22) were lupus-onset SS. The ages at onset of SLE–SS were older than SLE and younger than SS. Another study in China showed that SS–SLE patients with distinctive clinical manifestations and favorable prognosis require less glucocorticoids and immunosuppressants [7].

27.2 "A Light in Darkness"—Value of Novel Autoantibodies in Diagnosis of SS

It has been a long time that rheumatologists puzzled in the diagnosis of SS, the "unclear" and "misleading" syndromes. This is partially owing to patients' reluctance to have a labial gland biopsy and low specificity and lack of ready availability of anti-SSB and anti-SSA antibody tests. In recent years, the role of anti-α(alpha)-fodrin antibody in diagnosing SS has been studied extensively by our group and others have been explored in China [3, 11].

In addition, several studies in China have suggested the diagnostic value of a novel anti-M3 receptor (M3R) antibody in Sjögren's syndrome. Fang et al. from our group have shown that anti-M3R is probably a serologic biomarker in SS with a sensitivity of 91.3% and a specificity of 84.6%. Our recent study showed that antibodies against a peptide derived from the second loop of M3 receptor are valuable in the diagnosis of SS with sensitivity at 62.2% and specificity at 95.1%, respectively. The anti-M3R antibodies were detected in most of the SS patients lacking anti-SSB or anti-SSA. These data indicated that anti-M3R might be of significance in diagnosis of SS. However, our studies are limited by the absence of salivary gland biopsies that serve as the "gold standard."

27.3 "Pearls" of Chinese Medicine

Treatment of SS in China is much the same as that in Western countries [8]. Most patients with mild disease are treated symptomatically with eye drops, mouth syrup, and nose syrup, while patients with systemic involvement might be put on with corticosteroid or immunosuppressant, such as cyclophosphamide, azathioprine, or leflunomide. Biological agents including rituximab are occasionally used under certain restricted conditions, e.g., severe thrombocytopenia.

Traditional Chinese medicine (TCM) has been applied by a number of practitioners in China. There is substantial evidence that TCM improved symptoms and even laboratory parameters of SS patients. It was shown by Guo et al. that herbs such as *Pueraria lobota*, *Tripterygium wilfordii* Hook. f. (TWH), *Dendrobium*, *Fructus lycii*, and *Adenophora* are efficacious in improving dryness of mouth and eyes [9]. TWH has been used for many years to treat autoimmune diseases as anti-inflammatory and immunosuppressive agent. A number of studies have suggested that TCM might regulate immune responses by raising CD4(+)CD25(+) T cells and by promoting the Foxp3 mRNA expression [10]. Increased evidence over the last three decades indicates that TCM can be used clinically based on the symptoms and severity of the diseases [11]. Collectively, TCM is potentially therapeutic in Sjögren's syndrome and more studies should be carried out to evaluate its clinical value and underlying mechanism.

References

1. Bowman SJ, Ibrahim GH, Holmes G, et al. Estimating the prevalence among Caucasian women of primary Sjögren syndrome in two general practices in Birmingham, UK. Scand J Rheumatol. 2004;33:39–43.
2. Zhang NZ, Shi QS, Yao QP, et al. Epidemiological studies on primary Sjögren syndrome. Chin J Intern Med. 1993;32(8):522–3.
3. He J, Liu X, Jia Y. Survey of clinical patterns of Sjögren syndrome in China. Chin J Misdiagnos. 2009;9(20):4799–4780.
4. Huang JM, Zhang XW, Jia Y, Mu R, Li ZG. Thyroid disease in primary Sjögren syndrome. Chin J Rheumatol. 2002;6(6):4780–99.
5. An Y, Zhang XW, Li ZG. Clinical features of primary Sjögren syndrome in youth. J Peking Univ. 2009;41(3):324–7.
6. Jia Y, Liu X, Liu CH, Li ZG. The clinical and laboratory features of patients with Sjögren syndrome associated with systemic lupus erythematosus. Chin J Rheumatol. 2006;10(1):23–6.
7. Xu D, Tian X, Zhang W, et al. Sjögren syndrome-onset lupus patients have distinctive clinical manifestations and benign prognosis: a case–control study. Lupus 2009;18:1–4.
8. Fox RI. Sjögren syndrome. Lancet 2005;366:321–31.
9. Guo FQ. The progress of Chinese medicine treatment in Sjögren syndrome. J Modem Stomatol. 2003;17(4):359–61.
10. Li S, Xu KL, Li ZY. Effects of *Triptergium hypoglaucun* Hutch extraction on regulatory T cells in mice after allogeneic bone marrow transplantation. Zhongguo Zhong Xi Yi Jie He Za Zhi. 2009;29(10):910–14.
11. Liu F, Liu H, Wang CL. Sjögren syndrome. J Practical Traditional Chin Int Med. 2009;23(4):18–9.

Sjögren's Syndrome in China

28

Chak-sing Lau

Abstract

Primary Sjögren's syndrome (pSS) is as commonly seen in Chinese as in people of other ethnic origins. Previous studies have suggested that Chinese pSS patients may have more severe disease and a higher frequency of major organ involvement, including the cardiac, pulmonary, and neurological diseases. Protein-losing enteropathy, in particular, appears to be a characteristic variant of gastrointestinal disease seen in Chinese patients. As with all patients, keratoconjunctivitis sicca and xerostomia have a major impact in Chinese patients with pSS. This is particularly important for patients from China and other Asian countries because of the lack of a comprehensive dental health service and habitual smoking among patients.

Keywords

Primary Sjögren's syndrome • Ethnic differences • Geographic variations • Protein-losing enteropathy

Sjögren's syndrome (SS) is probably one of the commonest systemic autoimmune rheumatic disorders seen in Chinese. However, it has attracted disproportionately less academic interest compared with conditions such as systemic lupus erythematosus (SLE). Most of the studies on SS carried out in Chinese have been observational. The prevalence of primary SS (pSS) has been estimated to be between 0.45 and 0.77% in Chinese [1, 2], with the peak age of onset between 40 and 50 years of age. As with patients of other ethnic origins, there is a female predominance with a female to male patient ratio of 9:1. A large number of patients suffering from rheumatoid arthritis, SLE, and other connective tissue disorders may also be complicated by secondary SS. The frequency of secondary SS has not been reported previously but an early study showed that extra-articular manifestations, including sicca symptoms, are uncommon in southern Chinese with rheumatoid arthritis [3].

The spectrum of clinical manifestations of pSS in Chinese is probably similar to that reported in other ethnic groups. For example, the 2002 International Classification Criteria for pSS [4] have been shown to be sensitive and specific for

C.-s. Lau (✉)
Division of Rheumatology and Clinical Immunology, Li Ka Shing Faculty of Medicine, The University of Hong Kong, Hong Kong, China
e-mail: cslau@hku.hk

R.I. Fox, C.M. Fox (eds.), *Sjögren's Syndrome*, DOI 10.1007/978-1-60327-957-4_28,

the diagnosis of this condition in Chinese in routine clinical practice [5]. Serologically, 70 and 40% of patients are positive for anti-SSA and anti-SSB antibodies, respectively. Rheumatoid factor (RF) is reported to be positive in 70–90% of patients and cryoglobulin is said to be positive in 25% of patients. Patients who are anti-nuclear antibodies (ANAs) and/or RF positive appear to be younger, have more severe keratoconjunctivitis complex, and other organ involvement [6].

No previous studies have been carried out comparing the clinical manifestations, treatment responses, and outcome of primary SS in Chinese and patients of other ethnic origins. Clinical observation and previous descriptive studies tend to suggest that Chinese patients with pSS probably develop more severe organ disease. For example, in a retrospective study that involved 522 patients with pSS, 221 (42.3%) were reported to have developed some form of pulmonary complications after a median follow up of 48 months from disease onset. Of these patients, 23.3% had interstitial lung involvement, 12.5% pulmonary hypertension, 9.2% pulmonary bullae, 6.0% pleural effusion, and 5.6% pulmonary nodules. Patients with pulmonary disease were older, had more severe sicca symptoms, Raynaud's phenomenon and articular complaints, and higher levels of serum γ(gamma)-globulin. The mortality rate was 5.5 times higher in patients with pulmonary complications than those without lung disease [7]. A recent computed tomographic and histopathologic study of patients with interstitial lung disease showed features of non-specific interstitial pneumonia with organizing pneumonia, non-caseating granulomas, chronic bronchiolitis, and lymphocytic interstitial pneumonia [8]. It therefore appears that regular monitoring with careful clinical assessment, pulmonary function tests, and radiological examination are warranted when following up on Chinese patients with pSS.

Cardiac disease is also thought to be common in Chinese patients with pSS, though many patients are asymptomatic [9]. In the retrospective study by Ye et al. [9], of the 124 patients examined, pericardial effusion, left ventricular diastolic dysfunction, and pulmonary arterial hypertension were found in 20.2, 13.7, and 12.9% of patients, respectively.

Besides pulmonary and cardiac involvement, neurological manifestations have also been suggested to be commonly seen in Chinese patients with pSS. Peripheral neuropathy is commonly reported and up to 5% of patients may present with major central nervous disease including tonic–clonic seizures, psychosis, and organic brain syndromes. Cerebrospinal fluid examination may reveal increased white cell count and protein levels, while CT scan of the brain may show plague-like lesions. Similarly, renal diseases, including renal tubular acidosis, interstitial nephritis, and glomerulonephritis, are said to be commonly seen in Chinese SS patients. However, it is not sure whether the patients with glomerulonephritis may indeed have SLE and secondary SS rather than pSS.

Of the various organs involved in pSS, Chinese or oriental pSS patients may present with a characteristic variant of gastrointestinal disease—protein-losing enteropathy [10, 11]. These patients often present with periorbital and peripheral edema and hypoalbuminemia without marked features of keratoconjunctivitis complex. Serologically, there is hypergammaglobulinemia and positive RF, ANA, and anti-SSA and anti-SSB antibodies. Excessive intestinal protein loss may be confirmed by albumin-labeled scan or stool α(alpha)-1 anti-trypsin clearance measurement. Treatment with systemic corticosteroid often results in an improvement and the prognosis is generally good with maintenance immunosuppressive therapy such as azathioprine.

As with all patients with pSS, xerostomia presents a major challenge in the management of this condition in Chinese. Few studies have evaluated the extent of xerostomia and its impact on patients' health-related quality of life (HR-QOL) and oral health in Chinese because of a lack of appropriate and culturally validated measurement tools. Recently, however, questionnaires that measure general health-related QOL [12, 13] and oral health-related QOL in southern Chinese have been validated [14]. Using a Chinese version of the SF-36 questionnaire [12], both pSS and secondary SS patients from Hong

Kong were found to have poorer QOL in the physical functioning, role physical, and general health domains [15]. Interestingly, fibromyalgia, which is commonly described as a co-morbidity in pSS patients in the West, is uncommonly seen in Chinese.

Salivary flow and saliva pH and buffering capacity were found to be reduced in patients with SS. In addition, xerostomia had a negative impact on oral health-related QOL, which correlated with the number of missing, filled, and decayed teeth [16]. Dental caries is a major problem in patients with SS in China, probably because of the lack of a comprehensive national dental service and habitual smoking among patients. Anecdotal evidence suggests that half of all these patients have severe dental caries, with many of them losing all of their teeth. Interestingly, patients with secondary SS had poorer dry mouth measures than pSS. Treatment with muscarinic receptor agonist was well tolerated with improvement in oral health-related QOL but not salivary flow [17].

References

1. Zeng QY, Chen R, Darmawan J, et al. Rheumatic diseases in China. Arthritis Res Ther. 2008;10:R17. Epub 2008 Jan 31.
2. Xiang YJ, Dai SM. Prevalence of rheumatic diseases and disability in China. Rheumatol Int. 2009;29(5):481–90.
3. Cohen MG, Li EK, Ng PY, Chan KL. Extra-articular manifestations are uncommon in southern Chinese with rheumatoid arthritis. Brit J Rheumatol. 1993;32:209–11.
4. Vitali C, Bombardieri S, Jonsson R, et al. Classification criteria for Sjögren's syndrome: a revised version of the European criteria proposed by the American–European Consensus Group. Ann Rheum Dis. 2002;61:554–8.
5. Zhao Y, Kang J, Zheng WJ, et al. Evaluation of International Classification Criteria (2002) for primary Sjögren's syndrome in Chinese patients. Chin Med Sci J. 2005;20:190–3.
6. AP Huo, KC Lin, CT Chou. Predictive and prognostic value of antibodies and rheumatoid factor in primary Sjögren's syndrome. Int J Rheum Dis. 2010;13(1):39–47.
7. Yan SM, Zhao Y, Zeng XF, Zhang FC, Dong Y. Lung involvement of primary Sjögren's syndrome. Zhonghua Jie He He Hu Xi Za Zhi. 2008;31:513–6.
8. Shi JH, Liu HR, Xu WB, et al. Pulmonary manifestations of Sjögren's syndrome. Respiration 2009;78:377–86.
9. Ye YC, Zeng Y, Zhu WL, et al. Cardiac manifestations in Sjögren's syndrome. Zhonghua Xin Xue Buan Bing Za Zhi. 2008;36:327–31.
10. Mok MY, Lau CS. Protein losing enteropathy and primary Sjögren's syndrome. Clin Exp Rheumatol. 1997;15:705.
11. Nagashima T, Hoshino M, Shimoji S, et al. Protein-losing gastroenteropahy associated with primary Sjögren's syndrome: a characteristic oriental variant. Rheumatol Int. 2009;29:817–20.
12. Lam CLK, Gandek B, Ren SZ, Chan MS. Tests of scaling assumptions and construct validity of the Chinese (HK) version of the SF-36 health survey. J Clin Epidemiol. 1998;51:1139–47.
13. Lam CLK, Launder IJ, Lam TP, Gandek B. Population based norming of the Chinese (HK) version of the SF-36 health survey. HK Pract. 1999;21:460–70.
14. Wong MCM, Lo ECM, McMillan AS. Validation of a Chinese version of the oral health impact profile (OHIP). Comm Dent Oral Epidemiol. 2002;30: 423–30.
15. McMillan AS, Leung KCM, Leung WK, Wong MCM, Lau CS, Mok TMY. Impact of Sjögren's syndrome on oral health related quality of life in southern Chinese. J Oral Rehab. 2004;31:653–9.
16. Leung KCM, McMillan AS, Leung WK, Wong MCM, Lau CS, Mok TMY. Oral condition and saliva flow in southern Chinese with Sjögren's syndrome. Int Dent J. 2004;54:159–65.
17. Leung KCM, McMillan AS, Wong MCM, Leung WK, Mok MY, Lau CS. The efficacy of cevimeline hydrochloride in the treatment of xerostomia in Sjögren's syndrome in southern Chinese patients: a randomized double-blind, placebo crossover study. Clin Rheumatol. 2008;27:429–36.

Sjögren's Syndrome in Israel: A Scientific Point of View

29

Moshe Tishler and Yehuda Shoenfeld

Abstract

The knowledge about primary and secondary Sjögren's syndrome in Israel is well established by physicians of all specialties. Studies from Israel have dealt with both clinical and scientific patterns of the disease. Many studies have been published exploring the various inflammatory markers both in the saliva and in the tear fluid trying to assess disease activity. Studies on the prevalence of various autoantibodies in this disease and their similarity to other autoimmune disorders shed more light on the concept of "the mosaic of autoimmunity."

Keywords

Autoantibodies • Salivary proinflammatory markers • Clinical disease spectrum

Primary and secondary Sjögren's syndrome (SS) are common diseases in Israel, but their precise prevalence has not been investigated. The knowledge about the disease and its manifestation is well established by physicians of all specialties. The local SS patients' association is also very active by promoting local patients' conferences and editing a local quarterly newsletter. SS has been investigated in depth by Israeli physicians, thus leading to better understanding of the clinical and pathophysiological aspects of this complex disease. Israeli rheumatologists have been involved in the European study group, which has determined the European diagnostic criteria for SS that were used for more than a decade until replaced later on by the American–European Consensus Group classification criteria [1, 2]. A study assessing the clinical and laboratory data of 60 SS patients, done by Tishler et al. revealed that despite the different genetic background the clinical features and immunological specificities were the same as those of many European centers [3].

Some important clinical findings have been reported by this group concerning allergy, sleep disorders, and fibromyalgia in SS patient. We have detected that moderate-to-severe sleep disturbances have been reported by 49 out of 65 SS patient (75%) and that fibromyalgia was also common in this group (55%) and was associated with the sleep disturbances that were detected [4].

M. Tishler (✉)
Department of Medicine "B", Asaf Harofe Medical Center, Zerifin, Israel 70300
e-mail: tishlerm@netvision.net.il

R.I. Fox, C.M. Fox (eds.), *Sjögren's Syndrome*, DOI 10.1007/978-1-60327-957-4_29,

In another study, allergic manifestations were reported frequently by this group of SS patients (65%) and were significantly higher than that reported in other rheumatic disorders. These allergic manifestations and especially contact dermatitis and drug eruptions were closely related to the existence of anti-ρ(rho) antibodies [5].

In order to try and have better markers of local inflammation that could be of value in the diagnosis of SS, Tishler's group examined several markers in the saliva and tears of SS patients. They have found increased concentrations of salivary eicosanoids (thromboxane B_2 and prostaglandin E_2) in SS patients as compared to a control group of patient with dry mouth [6]. Similar data were found while examining hyaluronic acid concentrations that were elevated in the saliva but not in the sera of SS patient [7].

In order to define the role of several proinflammatory cytokines in the pathophysiology of SS patients, we examined some of them in various fluids. Elevated levels of IL-6 and soluble IL-2 receptor were found in the saliva of patients suffering from Sjögren's syndrome as well as elevation of IL-6 in their tears.

The fact that no parallel elevation in the concentration of these cytokines was found in the sera of these patients points to the fact that these increases are the result of local inflammation [8–10].

An important work in the field of basic research concerning SS was done by the group of Shoenfeld et al. by defining experimental and induced animal models in this disease as well in SLE [11].

Yehuda Shoenfeld's group concentrated on the specific anti-ρ(rho) and anti-λ(lambda) antibodies and found high incidence of these antibodies' activities in patients with monoclonal gammopathies. They found also that patients with SS had a predominance of IgG1 subclass of anti-ρ(rho) (SSA) antibodies while IgG2 and IgG3 anti-λ(lambda) (SSB) antibodies were more frequent in patients with an extraglandular disease [12].

The important role of IgA in SS was also widely investigated and published by Shoenfeld's group [13]. A mutual work of Shoenfeld and Tishler investigated the whole spectrum of autoantibodies in SS patients. In this work the frequencies of various antibodies were compared between SS patients and patients suffering from primary biliary cirrhosis [14]. The data that yielded similarities in different autoantibodies between the two diseases with different clinical presentations shed more light on the concept of the "mosaic of autoimmunity," suggested by Yehuda Shoenfeld [15–16].

Concerning the treatment issue of SS patients, therapy in Israel is much the same as in other Western countries and mainly involves symptomatic medications aimed at alleviation of mouth and ocular dryness. In an open label study done by Tischler et al., they tried to evaluate treatment with hydroxychloroquine (HCQ) 200 mg/d for 12 months on a group of SS patients. The results of this study showed that HCQ treatment reduced both salivary and serum IL-6 levels with almost no clinical effect on disease symptomatology [17].

Although much progress has been made in Israel in understanding the pathophysiological mechanisms underlying this disease the way to treatment is still obscure.

References

1. Vitali C, Bombardieri S, Moutsopoulos HM, et al. Assessment of the European classification criteria for Sjögren's syndrome in a series of clinically defined cases: results of a prospective multicentre study. The European Study Group on Diagnostic Criteria for Sjögren's Syndrome. Ann Rheum Dis. 1996;55(2):116–21.
2. Vitali C, Bombardieri S, Moutsopoulos HM, et al. Preliminary criteria for the classification of Sjögren's syndrome. Results of a prospective concerted action supported by the European Community. Arthritis Rheum. 1993;36:340–7.
3. Tishler M, Alosachie I, Barka N, et al. Primary Sjögren's syndrome and primary biliary cirrhosis: differences and similarities in the autoantibody profile. Clin Exp Rheumatol. 1995;(4): 497–500.
4. Tishler M, Barak Y, Paran D, Yaron M. Sleep disturbances, fibromyalgia and primary Sjögren's syndrome. Clin Exp Rheumatol. 1997;5(1): 71–4.

5. Tishler M, Paran D, Yaron M. Allergic disorders in primary Sjögren's syndrome. Scand J Rheumatol. 1998;27(3):166–9.
6. Tishler M, Yaron I, Raz A, Meyer FA, Yaron M. Salivary eicosanoid concentration in patients with Sjögren's syndrome. Ann Rheum Dis. 1996;55(3):202–4.
7. Tishler M, Yaron I, Shirazi I, Yaron M. Salivary and serum hyaluronic acid concentrations in patients with Sjögren's syndrome. Ann Rheum Dis. 1998;57(8):506–508.
8. Tishler M, Yaron I, Geyer O, Shirazi I, Naftaliev E, Yaron M. Elevated tear interleukin-6 levels in patients with Sjögren syndrome. Ophthalmology 1998;105(12):2327–29.
9. Tishler M, Yaron I, Shirazi I, Yossipov Y, Yaron M. Increased salivary interleukin-6 levels in patients with primary Sjögren's syndrome. Rheumatol Int. 1999;18(4):125–7.
10. Tishler M, Yaron I, Shirazi I, Levartovsky D, Yaron M. Salivary and serum soluble interleukin-2 receptor in primary Sjögren's syndrome. Arch Oral Biol. 1999;44(4):305–8.
11. Shoenfeld Y. Experimental and induced animal models of SLE and Sjögren's syndrome. Curr Opin Rheumatol. 1989;1:360–8.
12. Maran R, Dueymes M, Pennec YL, Casburn-Budd R, Shoenfeld Y, Youinou P. Predominance of IgG subclass of anti-λ(rho)/SS-A, but not anti-λ(lambda)/S-B antibodies in primary Sjögren's syndrome. J Autoimmunity. 1993;6:379–87.
13. Levy Y, Dueymes M, Pennec YL, Shoenfeld Y, Youinou P. IgA in Sjögren's syndrome. Clin Exp Rheumatol. 1994;12:543–51.
14. Tishler M, Alosachie I, Barak N, et al. Primary Sjögren's syndrome and primary biliary cirrhosis: differences and similarities in the autoantibody profile. Clin Exp Rheumatol. 1995;13:497–500.
15. Shoenfeld Y, Zandman-Goddard G, Stojanovich L, et al. The mosaic of autoimmunity: hormonal and environmental factors involved in autoimmune diseases—2008. IMAJ 2008;10:8–12.
16. Shoenfeld Y, Blank M, Abu-Shakra M, et al. The mosaic of autoimmunity: prediction, autoantibodies, and therapy in autoimmune diseases—2008. IMAJ 2008;10:13–9.
17. Tishler M, Yaron I, Shirazi I, Yaron M. Hydroxychloroquine treatment for primary Sjögren's syndrome: its effect on salivary and serum inflammatory markers. Ann Rheum Dis. 1999;58(4):253–6.

Part VI

Future Perspectives

30 Looking into the Future—The EULAR Disease Activity Scores: Toward a Consensual Evaluation of Primary Sjogren's Syndrome

Raphaèle Seror, Philippe Ravaud, Claudio Vitali, Simon J. Bowman, and Xavier Mariette

Abstract

In primary Sjögren's syndrome (SS), clinical features can be divided into two facets: the benign subjective but disabling manifestations such as dryness, articular and muscular pain, and fatigue, and the systemic manifestations such as synovitis, vasculitis, skin, lung, renal and neurological involvement, or lymphoma. Great efforts have been made to develop valid activity indexes needed to assess the effectiveness of new therapies. First, for evaluation of patients' symptoms: the Profile of Fatigue and Discomfort (PROFAD) and Sicca Symptoms Inventory (SSI) then for systemic features: the SS Disease Activity Index (SSDAI) and Sjögren's Systemic Clinical Activity Index (SCAI). The development of these indexes served as bases of an international collaborative project promoted by European League Against Rheumatism (EULAR). Thirty-nine primary SS experts were involved in the development of these two consensus disease activity indexes: the EULAR Sjögren's Syndrome Patients Reported Index (ESSPRI), a patient-administered questionnaire to assess subjective features, and the EULAR Sjögren's Syndrome Disease Activity Index (ESSDAI), a systemic activity index to assess systemic complications. Both indexes have good correlations with existing scores and also global evaluation of disease activity by physician for ESSDAI and by patient for ESSPRI. In addition, ESSDAI had a good sensitivity to change and detects changes more accurately, when compared to other scores. These both indexes are simple and aimed to be used for both clinical trials and clinical practice. They are currently being validated for that purpose.

Keywords

Primary Sjögren's syndrome • Disease activity index • Patient-reported outcome • Outcome assessment • Systemic activity

R. Seror (✉)
Assistance Publique-Hopitaux de Paris, Hôpital Bicêtre, Department of Rheumatology, Institut Pour la Santé et la Recherche Médicale (INSERM) U 802, Université Paris-Sud 11, Le Kremlin Bicêtre, France
e-mail: raphaele.se@gmail.com

30.1 Introduction

Primary Sjögren's syndrome (SS) is a systemic disorder characterized by lymphocytic infiltration of exocrine glands resulting in their progressive

R.I. Fox, C.M. Fox (eds.), *Sjögren's Syndrome*, DOI 10.1007/978-1-60327-957-4_30,

destruction. Apart from its tropism for exocrine glands, the inflammatory process can, however, affect any organ. As a result, clinical features can be divided into two facets: (i) benign subjective but disabling manifestations such as dryness, articular and muscular pain, and fatigue, affecting almost all patients and (ii) systemic manifestations such as synovitis, vasculitis, skin, lung, renal and neurological involvement, or lymphoma. Systemic involvement of the disease, which refers to active inflammatory disease with potential severity, affects 20–40% of patients.

Until recently, evidence-based therapy for Sjögren's syndrome was largely limited to treatments that may improve sicca features [1]. Consequently, for decades, the evaluation of primary SS in clinical trials has been primarily based on the assessment of glandular features, either with objective or subjective parameter [2–4]. Moreover, all these studies used a different measurement tool, which makes comparisons impossible. Outcome criteria using composite criteria have also been proposed in the most recent clinical trials [5, 6]. But, none of these measures was able to capture the activity of systemic features of the disease, and, until now, therapeutic evaluation of primary SS has never focused on systemic features, despite their potential severity.

Over the past few years, evidence-based evaluation of therapies has become important, with an increasing number of large clinical trials conducted in this disease [1–6]. Valid activity indexes were needed [7–9] to assess the effectiveness of new targeted therapies, such as B-cell-targeted therapies that have shown promising results for both severe systemic [10, 11] and glandular features [12–16]. Therefore, in the past decade, great efforts have been made to determine a core set of outcome measure [7, 8]. The primary SS core set includes sicca features (oral and ocular, subjective and objective), fatigue, health-related quality of life, composite activity score, and laboratory measures. However, assessing the benefit of therapies for primary SS lacks consensual outcome measures.

Different disease-specific indexes have then been developed, first, for evaluation of patients' symptoms (subjective features), such as Profile of Fatigue and Discomfort (PROFAD) and Sicca Symptoms Inventory (SSI) [17, 18], and, more recently, for systemic features, such as Ss Disease Activity Index (SSDAI) [19] and Sjögren's Systemic Clinical Activity Index (SCAI) [20]. The development of these indexes was based on exploratory studies conducted in a single country, but served as bases of the present collaborative project. Thus, EULAR has promoted an international collaboration between primary SS experts to develop consensus disease activity indexes. Two indexes have been developed: (i) a patient-administered questionnaire to assess subjective features, the EULAR Sjögren's Syndrome Patients Reported Index (ESSPRI), and (ii) a systemic activity index to assess systemic complications, the EULAR Sjögren's Syndrome Disease Activity Index (ESSDAI).

30.2 Evaluation of Systemic Features of Primary SS

As previously mentioned, three disease activity scores have been recently developed to assess activity in patients with systemic complication of primary SS. Table 30.1 compared these three scores.

30.2.1 The SSDAI: Sjögren's Syndrome Disease Activity Index

The SSDAI [19] is a disease activity index that includes 11 items grouped in 8 domains. The weights of each item were obtained with multivariate model using PhGA as gold standard, in a cohort of 206 patients. The relative weightings of each domain are indicated in brackets: pleuropulmonary (4), articular (2), change in vasculitis (3), lymph node/spleen enlargement (2), active renal (2), constitutional (3), change in salivary gland swelling (3), recent onset peripheral neuropathy (1), and leukopenia (1). The final score, the sum of all items, varies from 0 to 21.

Table 30.1 Description of disease activity indexes for primary Sjogren's syndrome

Score	ESSDAI [25] EULAR Sjögren's Syndrome Disease Activity Index	SSDAI [19] Sjögren's Syndrome Disease Activity Index	SCAI* [20, 26] Sjögren's Systemic Clinical Activity Index
Year of publication	2009	2007	2007
Setting of development	Multicenter Worldwide	Multicenter Italy	Multicenter UK
Definition of items	By expert consensus	By expert consensus	By expert consensus, derived from BILAG
Method for determining weights	Multiple regression modeling	Multiple regression modeling	No weighting
Gold standard	Physician global assessment	Physician global assessment	Intention to treat
Number of patients	702 clinical vignettes based on 96 real patients	206 patients	104 patients
Number of domains	12	8	8
Number of items	44 (3–4 by domain ranked by level of activity)	11	42
Scoring of items - Present/absent - New/worse	 Yes No	 Yes (8/15) Yes (7/15)	 No Yes
Domains and weights	Constitutional (3)	Constitutional (3 × 1)	Fatigue
	Lymphadenopathy (4)	Lymph node/spleen enlargement (2)	Constitutional
	Articular (2)	Articular (2)	Musculoskeletal
	Muscular (6)		
	Cutaneous (3)	Change in vasculitis (3)	Skin/vasculitis
	Glandular (2)	Change in salivary gland swelling (3)	Salivary gland
	Pulmonary (5)	Pleuropulmonary (4)	Respiratory

Table 30.1 (continued)

Score	ESSDAI [25] EULAR Sjögren's Syndrome Disease Activity Index	SSDAI [19] Sjögren's Syndrome Disease Activity Index	SCAI* [20, 26] Sjögren's Systemic Clinical Activity Index
	Renal (5)	Active renal (2)	Renal
	Peripheral nervous system (5)	Recent onset peripheral neuropathy (1)	Neurological
	Central nervous system (5)		
	Hematological (2)		Hematological
	Biological (1)	Leukopenia (1)	
Final score	Numerical	Numerical	Intention to treat alphabetical scoring for each domain Possible numerical conversion
Scoring	– Final score = sum of the score of each domain – Score of each domain = activity level × weight of the domain	– Final score = sum of the score of each item	Alphabetical scoring by domain A = requiring prednisolone >20 mg and/or immunosuppressants B = requiring prednisolone <20 mg and/or anti-malarials and/or NSAIDs C = stable, mild disease D = previously affected but inactive E = never involved
			Numerical conversion: A = 9; B = 3; C = 1; D or E = 0
Range of theoretical values	0–123	0–21	E–A Numerical conversion: 0–72
Range of observed values	0–49	0–7	0–31

BILAG: British Isles Lupus Activity Group; NSAIDs: non-steroidal anti-inflammatory drugs.
*A modified SCAI excludes subjective features such as fatigue, myalgias, arthralgias, Raynaud's phenomenon, shortness of breath, and pleuropericardial pain.

30.2.2 The SCAI: Sjögren's Systemic Clinical Activity Index

The SCAI is an ordinal transition scale, derived from the British Isles Lupus Activity Group (BILAG) scoring system, developed in a cohort of 104 patients [20, 21]. It reflects changes in clinical symptoms during the 4-week period prior to evaluation or compared to the previous visit. SCAI includes 42 items that are clearly defined and grouped into the 8 following domains: constitutional, musculoskeletal, skin/vasculitis, respiratory, neurological, renal, salivary gland, and hematological. Each item is scored as absent, improving, the same, worse, or new. This scoring is used to score each domain with an "intention to treat" alphabetical scoring system. Category A denotes disease that requires prednisolone >20 mg and/or immunosuppressants for treatment. Category B denotes disease requires prednisolone <20 mg and/or anti-malarials and/or NSAIDs. Category C indicates stable, mild disease. Category D is assigned to a domain that was previously affected, but where disease is currently inactive. Category E indicates an organ system that has never been involved. Categories were derived from the BILAG index for systemic lupus (created by nominal consensus techniques). This scoring could be converted into a numeric variable according to the author recommendation a A score = 9, a B score = 3, a C score = 1, and a D or E score = 0. Therefore the maximum theoretical SCAI score is 72. This numerical conversion has never been evaluated.

30.2.3 The ESSDAI: EULAR Sjögren's Syndrome Disease Activity Index

The ESSDAI (Table 30.2) is a disease activity index that was generated in 2009, by consensus of a large group of worldwide experts from European and North American countries. The ESSDAI is a systemic disease activity index and includes 12 domains (i.e., organ systems). Each domain is divided in three to four levels depending on their degree of activity. The weights of each domain were obtained with multiple regression modeling using the physician global assessment of disease activity (PhGA) as gold standard, in a cohort of 702 clinical vignettes based on 96 real patients. The relative weightings of each domain are indicated in brackets: constitutional (3), articular (2), cutaneous (3), glandular (2), lymphadenopathy (4), pulmonary (5), renal (5), muscular (6), peripheral nervous system (5), central nervous system (5), hematological (2), and biological (1). Before rating the score, experts are asked to rate only manifestations related to the disease and to avoid rating long-lasting clinical features. No item is rated as new or worse. The final score, the sum of all weighted scores, falls between 0 and, theoretically, 123, with 0 being the less disease activity.

30.2.4 Comparisons of Systemic Disease Activity Scores

In a recent study, we evaluated and compared sensitivity to change of disease activity indexes for primary SS [22]. In this study we included 96 profiles, were abstracted from real pSS patients' medical charts. Patient profiles were scored according the 3 scoring systems at 3 consecutive visits by 39 experts. In addition, experts also assessed profiles according to whether disease activity had improved, worsened, or remained stable at follow-up visits. In this study we showed that, compared to SCAI and SSDAI, the ESSDAI was the most correlated with PhGA of disease activity. Also, when assessing sensitivity to change we found that for patients whose disease activity had improved, all disease activity scores showed a similar large sensitivity to change. But, the ESSDAI adequately varied according to the degree and the direction of change in disease activity, and therefore detects changes more accurately than did the SSDAI and SCAI. Notably, for patients with stable disease activity, the ESSDAI scores did not show erroneous improvement contrarily on SSDAI and SCAI.

Table 30.2 The EULAR Sjögren's Syndrome Disease Activity Index (ESSDAI): domain and item definitions and weights

Domain (Weight)	Activity level	Description
Constitutional (3)	No = 0	Absence of the following symptoms
Exclusion of fever of infectious origin and voluntary weight loss	Low = 1	Mild or intermittent fever (37.5–38.5°C)/night sweats and/or involuntary weight loss of 5–10% of body weight
	Moderate = 2	Severe fever (>38.5°C)/night sweats and/or involuntary weight loss of >10% of body weight
Lymphadenopathy (4)	No = 0	Absence of the following features
Exclusion of infection	Low = 1	Lymphadenopathy ≥ 1 cm in any nodal region or ≥ 2 cm in inguinal region
	Moderate = 2	Lymphadenopathy ≥ 2 cm in any nodal region or ≥ 3 cm in inguinal region and/or splenomegaly (clinically palpable or assessed by imaging)
	High = 3	Current malignant B-cell proliferative disorder
Glandular (2)	No = 0	Absence of glandular swelling
Exclusion of stone or infection	Low = 1	Small glandular swelling with enlarged parotid (≤3 cm) or limited submandibular or lacrimal swelling
	Moderate = 2	Major glandular swelling with enlarged parotid (>3 cm) or important submandibular or lacrimal swelling
Articular (2)	No = 0	Absence of currently active articular involvement
Exclusion of osteoarthritis	Low = 1	Arthralgias in hands, wrists, ankles, and feet accompanied by morning stiffness (>30 min)
	Moderate = 2	1–5 (of 28 total count) synovitis
	High = 3	≥6 (of 28 total count) synovitis
Cutaneous (3)	No = 0	Absence of currently active cutaneous involvement
Rate as "No activity" stable long-lasting features related to damage	Low =1	Erythema multiforma
	Moderate = 2	Limited cutaneous vasculitis, including urticarial vasculitis, or purpura limited to feet and ankle, or subacute cutaneous lupus
	High = 3	Diffuse cutaneous vasculitis, including urticarial vasculitis, or diffuse purpura, or ulcers related to vasculitis
Pulmonary (5)	No = 0	Absence of currently active pulmonary involvement
Rate as "No activity" stable long-lasting features related to damage or respiratory involvement not related to the disease (tobacco use, etc.)	Low = 1	Persistent cough or bronchial involvement with no radiographic abnormalities on radiography Or radiological or HRCT evidence of interstitial lung disease with: No breathlessness and normal lung function test.
	Moderate = 2	Moderately active pulmonary involvement, such as interstitial lung disease shown by HRCT with shortness of breath on exercise (NHYA II) or abnormal lung function tests restricted to 70% > DL_{CO} ≥ 40% or 80% > FVC ≥ 60%
	High = 3	Highly active pulmonary involvement, such as interstitial lung disease shown by HRCT with shortness of breath at rest (NHYA III, IV) or with abnormal lung function tests: DL_{CO} < 40% or FVC < 60%

Table 30.2 (continued)

Domain (Weight)	Activity level	Description
Renal (5) *Rate as "No activity" stable long-lasting features related to damage and renal involvement not related to the disease.* *If biopsy has been performed, please rate activity based on histological features first*	No = 0	Absence of currently active renal involvement with proteinuria <0.5 g/d, no hematuria, no leukocyturia, no acidosis, or long-lasting stable proteinuria due to damage
	Low = 1	Evidence of mild active renal involvement, limited to tubular acidosis without renal failure or glomerular involvement with proteinuria (between 0.5 and 1 g/d) and without hematuria or renal failure (GFR $\geq$ 60 mL/min)
	Moderate = 2	Moderately active renal involvement, such as tubular acidosis with renal failure (GFR < 60 mL/min) or glomerular involvement with proteinuria between 1 and 1.5 g/d and without hematuria or renal failure (GFR $\geq$ 60 mL/min) or histological evidence of extramembranous glomerulonephritis or important interstitial lymphoid infiltrate
	High = 3	Highly active renal involvement, such as glomerular involvement with proteinuria > 1.5 g/d or hematuria, or renal failure (GFR < 60 mL/min), or histological evidence of proliferative glomerulonephritis or cryoglobulinemia related renal involvement
Muscular (6) *Exclusion of weakness due to corticosteroids*	No = 0	Absence of currently active muscular involvement
	Low = 1	Mild active myositis shown by abnormal EMG or biopsy with no weakness and creatine kinase (N <CK $\leq$ 2N)
	Moderate = 2	Moderately active myositis proven by abnormal EMG or biopsy with weakness (maximal deficit of 4/5) or elevated creatine kinase (2N <CK $\leq$4N)
	High = 3	Highly active myositis shown by abnormal EMG or biopsy with weakness (deficit $\leq$ 3/5) or elevated creatine kinase (>4N)
PNS (5) *Rate as "No activity" stable long-lasting features related to damage or PNS involvement not related to the disease*	No = 0	Absence of currently active PNS involvement
	Low = 1	Mild active peripheral nervous system involvement, such as pure sensory axonal polyneuropathy shown by NCS or trigeminal (V) neuralgia
	Moderate = 2	Moderately active peripheral nervous system involvement shown by NCS, such as axonal sensory-motor neuropathy with maximal motor deficit of 4/5, pure sensory neuropathy with presence of cryoglobulinemic vasculitis, ganglionopathy with symptoms restricted to mild/moderate ataxia, chronic inflammatory demyelinating polyneuropathy (CIDP) with mild functional impairment (maximal motor deficit of 4/5 or mild ataxia) Or cranial nerve involvement of peripheral origin (except trigeminal (V) neuralgia)
	High = 3	Highly active PNS involvement shown by NCS, such as axonal sensory motor neuropathy with motor deficit $\leq$ 3/5, peripheral nerve involvement due to vasculitis (mononeuritis multiplex, etc.), severe ataxia due to ganglionopathy, chronic inflammatory demyelinating polyneuropathy (CIDP) with severe functional impairment: motor deficit $\leq$ 3/5 or severe ataxia

Table 30.2 (continued)

Domain (Weight)	Activity level	Description
CNS (5) *Rate as "No activity" stable long-lasting features related to damage or CNS involvement not related to the disease*	No = 0	Absence of currently active CNS involvement
	Moderate = 2	Moderately active CNS features, such as cranial nerve involvement of central origin, optic neuritis, or multiple sclerosis-like syndrome with symptoms restricted to pure sensory impairment or proven cognitive impairment
	High = 3	Highly active CNS features, such as cerebral vasculitis with cerebrovascular accident or transient ischemic attack, seizures, transverse myelitis, lymphocytic meningitis, and multiple sclerosis-like syndrome with motor deficit
Hematological (2) *For anemia, neutropenia, and thrombopenia, only autoimmune cytopenia must be considered* *Exclusion of vitamin or iron deficiency, drug-induced cytopenia*	No = 0	Absence of autoimmune cytopenia
	Low = 1	Cytopenia of autoimmune origin with neutropenia (1,000 < neutrophils < 1,500/mm^3), and/or anemia (10 < hemoglobin < 12 g/dL), and /or thrombocytopenia (100,000 < platelets < 150,000/mm^3) Or lymphopenia (500 < lymphocytes < 1,000/mm^3)
	Moderate = 2	Cytopenia of autoimmune origin with neutropenia (500 ≤ neutrophils ≤ 1,000/mm^3), and/or anemia (8 ≤ hemoglobin ≤ 10 g/dL), and/or thrombocytopenia (50,000 ≤ platelets ≤ 100,000/mm^3) Or lymphopenia (≤500/mm^3)
	High = 3	Cytopenia of autoimmune origin with neutropenia (neutrophils < 500/mm^3), and/or or anemia (hemoglobin < 8 g/dL), and/or thrombocytopenia (platelets < 50,000/mm^3)
Biological (1)	No = 0	Absence of any of the following biological feature
	Low = 1	Clonal component, and/or hypocomplementemia (low C4 or C3 or CH50), and/or hypergammaglobulinemia or high IgG level between 16 and 20 g/L
	Moderate = 2	Presence of cryoglobulinemia, and/or hypergammaglobulinemia or high IgG level > 20 g/L, and/or recent onset hypogammaglobulinemia or recent decrease of IgG level (<5 g/L)

CIDP= chronic inflammatory demyelinating polyneuropathy; CK = creatine kinase; CNS = central nervous system; DLCO= diffusing CO capacity; EMG= electromyogram; FVC= forced vital capacity; GFR = glomerular filtration rate; Hb = hemoglobin; HRCT = high-resolution computed tomography; IgG = immunoglobulin G; NCS = nerve conduction studies; NHYA = New York heart association classification; Plt = platelet; PNS = peripheral nervous system.

30.3 Evaluation of Primary SS Patients' Symptoms

Since correlation between objective measures of dryness and symptoms is poor [18, 23], the evaluation of symptoms, along the measure of objective tests, such as Schirmer's test and salivary flow, is necessary. For these reasons, three disease-specific scores are now available for evaluation of patients' symptoms (Table 30.3). The first two scores were the SSI for evaluation of dryness features [18] and the PROFAD for evaluation of fatigue and discomfort [17]. More recently, we developed a simple global score the ESSPRI that encompasses these both components [24].

30.3.1 The SSI: Sicca Symptoms Inventory

The SSI was the first disease-specific score developed in a multicenter cohort of 112 UK primary SS patients in 2002 [18]. The definition of each item was based on phrases elicited by patients. Among a large number of initial phrases, items were selected based on the symptom frequencies. Severity of each item is assessed by a 0–7 numerical scale. A principal component analysis was then used to gather the ten items into four domains: ocular, oral, vaginal, and cutaneous dryness. Oral and ocular domains include, respectively, five and three items, but have the same weight on the final score than cutaneous and vaginal dryness. The final score is the sum of the four domains and varied from 0 to 28.

30.3.2 The PROFAD: Profile of Fatigue and Discomfort

The PROFAD was developed in 2004 using the same methodology as SSI. It includes nine items gathered into four domains: somatic fatigue, mental fatigue, arthralgias and Raynaud's phenomenon. Even if somatic fatigue is the predominant domain and includes four items, like for the SSI, in the PROFAD all domains have the same weight on the final score. The final score is the sum of the four domains and varied from 0 to 28.

30.3.3 The ESSPRI: EULAR Sjögren's Syndrome Patients Reported Index

The ESSPRI has been recently developed in a multicenter international cohort of 230 patients (Table 30.4). The domains were selected based on previous data from development of SSI and PROFAD. Selection of domains and determination of their weights were determined from the patients' perspective, using multiple linear regression with patient global assessment as gold standard. The ESSPRI uses 0–10 numerical scales, one for assessment of each of the three domains: dryness, fatigue, and pain (articular and/or muscular). The weights of the domains were identical, and the final score is the mean of the score of each domain.

30.3.4 Comparisons of Scores for Evaluation of Patients' Symptoms

Table 30.3 compared the methodology used to develop the three scores. Until development of ESSPRI, the SSI assessed dryness features and the PROFAD fatigue and discomfort; these both scores are not supposed to be combined, and no global score was available. Therefore, having a global score, such as the ESSPRI, able to capture all important symptoms of the disease, may be a consistent help to design and conduct clinical trials in primary SS. Compared to ESSPRI, which evaluated all dryness features and also all fatigue component with only one scale for each, the SSI evaluates separately each dryness feature and separate fatigue in two components (somatic and mental). Even if the number of items is higher for the most relevant components (oral and ocular dryness in SSI, and somatic fatigue in PROFAD), these domains have the same weight

Table 30.3 Comparisons of the three patients' indexes for primary Sjogren's syndrome

Score	ESSPRI [24]	SSI [18]	PROFAD [17]
	EULAR Sjögren's Syndrome Patients Reported Index	Sicca Symptoms Inventory	Profile of Fatigue and Discomfort
Year of publication	2010	2002	2004
Setting of development	Multicenter Worldwide	Multicenter (12 centers) UK	Multicenter UK
Items definition	Based on previous studies and literature review	Elicited by patients	Elicited by patients
Method for items/domains selection	Based on patient's opinion using multiple regression modeling	Symptom frequency	Symptom frequency
Method for determining weights and domain gathering	Multiple regression modeling Each question is a domain (no gathering)	No weighting Principal component analysis to gather items from domains	No weighting Principal component analysis to gather items from domains
Gold standard	Patient global assessment	None	None
Number of patients	240 patients	112 patients	137 patients
Number of domains	3	4	4
Number of items	3	10	9
Scoring of items	0–10 numerical scale	0–7 numerical scale	0–7 numerical scale
Domains	Dryness (1 item) Pain (1 item) Fatigue (1 item)	Oral dryness (5 items) Ocular dryness (3 items) Vaginal dryness (1 item) Cutaneous dryness (1 item)	Somatic fatigue (4 items) Mental fatigue (2 items) Arthralgias (2 items) Vascular dysfunction (1 item)
Scoring	– Final score = mean of the score of each domain	– Final score = sum of the score of each domain – Domain score = mean of the score of each item of the domain	– Final score = sum of the score of each domain – Domain score = mean of the score of each item of the domain
Range of theoretical values	0–10	0–28	0–28

Table 30.4 The EULAR Sjögren's syndrome patients reported index (ESSPRI)

1) How severe has your *dryness* been during the last 2 weeks?

No dryness	0	1	2	3	4	5	6	7	8	9	10	Maximal imaginable dryness

2) How severe has your *fatigue* been during the last 2 weeks?

No fatigue	0	1	2	3	4	5	6	7	8	9	10	Maximal imaginable fatigue

3) How severe has your *pain* (joint or muscular pains in your arms or legs) been during the last 2 weeks?

No pain	0	1	2	3	4	5	6	7	8	9	10	Maximal imaginable pain

on the final score than other less important domains (vaginal or cutaneous dryness in the SSI or mental fatigue and vascular dysfunction in the PROFAD). This might dilute the effect of the most relevant domains in the SSI and PROFAD compared to ESSPRI. Effectively, in the development of ESSPRI, there was specific questions for all types of dryness and fatigue (mental or somatic); but with the patient global assessment as gold standard, we found that they did not add anything compared with the generic question. In addition, the ESSPRI was modeled on judgment of a worldwide panel of patients which ensured a good content validity by inclusion of different *trans*-cultural patients' views. Compared with PROFAD, SSI, the ESSPRI, including only three questions, offers the advantage of simplicity. But, the ESSPRI should now be validated.

30.4 Conclusion

The ESSDAI and ESSPRI seemed to be promising tools for outcome assessment of patient with primary SS. Their content validity was ensured by participation of a large worldwide panel of primary SS experts for the ESSDAI and patients for the ESSPRI. Compared to previous and recently developed tools, these both indexes are simple, particularly the ESSPRI. Also, both indexes have good construct validity when physician global assessment or patient global assessment is considered as the gold standard. ESSDAI and ESSPRI are currently being validated and evaluated for sensitivity to change in a large cohort of patients all around the world, independent from the target population. In future clinical trials, depending of the therapeutic objectives of the new drugs to evaluate, it will be possible to use ESSDAI, ESSPRI, and objective measures of dryness, alone or a combination of these outcome measures.

References

1. Vivino FB, Al-Hashimi I, Khan Z, LeVeque FG, Salisbury PL, 3rd, Tran-Johnson TK, et al. Pilocarpine tablets for the treatment of dry mouth and dry eye symptoms in patients with Sjogren syndrome: a randomized, placebo-controlled, fixed-dose, multicenter trial. P92-01 Study Group. Arch Intern Med. 1999;159(2):174–81.
2. Drosos AA, Skopouli FN, Costopoulos JS, Papadimitriou CS, Moutsopoulos HM. Cyclosporin A (CyA) in primary Sjogren's syndrome: a double blind study. Ann Rheum Dis. 1986;45(9): 732–5.
3. Kruize AA, Hene RJ, Kallenberg CG, van Bijsterveld OP, van der Heide A, Kater L, et al. Hydroxychloroquine treatment for primary Sjogren's syndrome: a two year double blind crossover trial. Ann Rheum Dis. 1993;52(5):360–4.

4. Price EJ, Rigby SP, Clancy U, Venables PJ. A double blind placebo controlled trial of azathioprine in the treatment of primary Sjogren's syndrome. J Rheumatol. 1998;25(5):896–9.
5. Mariette X, Ravaud P, Steinfeld S, Baron G, Goetz J, Hachulla E, et al. Inefficacy of infliximab in primary Sjogren's syndrome: results of the randomized, controlled Trial of Remicade In Primary Sjogren's Syndrome (TRIPSS). Arthritis Rheum. 2004;50(4):1270–6.
6. Sankar V, Brennan MT, Kok MR, Leakan RA, Smith JA, Manny J, et al. Etanercept in Sjogren's syndrome: a twelve-week randomized, double-blind, placebo-controlled pilot clinical trial. Arthritis Rheum. 2004;50(7):2240–5.
7. Pillemer SR, Smith J, Fox PC, Bowman SJ. Outcome measures for Sjogren's syndrome, April 10–11, 2003, Bethesda, Maryland, USA. J Rheumatol. 2005;32(1):143–9.
8. Bowman SJ, Pillemer S, Jonsson R, Asmussen K, Vitali C, Manthorpe R, et al. Revisiting Sjogren's syndrome in the new millennium: perspectives on assessment and outcome measures. Report of a workshop held on 23 March 2000 at Oxford, UK. Rheumatology (Oxford) 2001;40(10):1180–8.
9. Asmussen KH, Bowman SJ. Outcome measures in Sjogren's syndrome. Rheumatology (Oxford) 2001;40(10):1085–8.
10. Pijpe J, van Imhoff GW, Spijkervet FK, Roodenburg JL, Wolbink GJ, Mansour K, et al. Rituximab treatment in patients with primary Sjogren's syndrome: an open-label phase II study. Arthritis Rheum. 2005;52(9):2740–50.
11. Seror R, Sordet C, Guillevin L, Hachulla E, Masson C, Ittah M, et al. Tolerance and efficacy of rituximab and changes in serum B cell biomarkers in patients with systemic complications of primary Sjogren's syndrome. Ann Rheum Dis. 2007;66(3): 351–7.
12. Dass S, Bowman SJ, Vital EM, Ikeda K, Pease CT, Hamburger J, et al. Reduction of fatigue in Sjogren syndrome with rituximab: results of a randomised, double-blind, placebo-controlled pilot study. Ann Rheum Dis. 2008;67(11):1541–4.
13. Devauchelle-Pensec V, Pennec Y, Morvan J, Pers JO, Daridon C, Jousse-Joulin S, et al. Improvement of Sjogren's syndrome after two infusions of rituximab (anti-CD20). Arthritis Rheum. 2007;57(2): 310–7.
14. Pijpe J, van Imhoff GW, Vissink A, van der Wal JE, Kluin PM, Spijkervet FK, et al. Changes in salivary gland immunohistology and function after rituximab monotherapy in a patient with Sjogren's syndrome and associated MALT lymphoma. Ann Rheum Dis. 2005;64(6):958–60.
15. Meijer JM, Vissink A, Meiners PM, Spijkervet FK, Kallenberg CG, Boostma H. Rituximab treatment in primary Sjögren's syndrome: a double-blind controlled trial. Arthritis Rheum. 2008;58(9 Suppl):S430–1.
16. Meijer J, Meiners P, Vissink A, Spijkervet F, Abdulahad W, Kamminga N, et al. Effective rituximab treatment in primary Sjogren's syndrome: a randomised, double-blind, placebo-controlled trial. Arthritis Rheum. 2010;62(4):960–8.
17. Bowman SJ, Booth DA, Platts RG. Measurement of fatigue and discomfort in primary Sjogren's syndrome using a new questionnaire tool. Rheumatology (Oxford) 2004;43(6):758–64.
18. Bowman SJ, Booth DA, Platts RG, Field A, Rostron J. Validation of the Sicca Symptoms Inventory for clinical studies of Sjogren's syndrome. J Rheumatol. 2003;30(6):1259–66.
19. Vitali C, Palombi G, Baldini C, Benucci M, Bombardieri S, Covelli M, et al. Sjogren's syndrome disease damage index and disease activity index: scoring systems for the assessment of disease damage and disease activity in Sjogren's syndrome, derived from an analysis of a cohort of Italian patients. Arthritis Rheum. 2007;56(7):2223–31.
20. Bowman SJ, Sutcliffe N, Isenberg DA, Goldblatt F, Adler M, Price E, et al. Sjogren's systemic clinical activity index (SCAI)—a systemic disease activity measure for use in clinical trials in primary Sjogren's syndrome. Rheumatology (Oxford) 2007;46(12):1845–51.
21. Hay EM, Bacon PA, Gordon C, Isenberg DA, Maddison P, Snaith ML, et al. The BILAG index: a reliable and valid instrument for measuring clinical disease activity in systemic lupus erythematosus. Q J Med. 1993;86(7):447–58.
22. Seror R, Mariette X, Bowman S, Baron G, Gottenberg JE, Boostma H, et al. Accurate detection of changes in disease activity in primary Sjogren's syndrome by the European League Against Rheumatism Sjogren's Syndrome Disease Activity Index. Arthritis Care Res (Hoboken). 2010;62(4):551–8.
23. Hay EM, Thomas E, Pal B, Hajeer A, Chambers H, Silman AJ. Weak association between subjective symptoms or and objective testing for dry eyes and dry mouth: results from a population based study. Ann Rheum Dis. 1998;57(1):20–4.
24. Seror R, Ravaud P, Mariette X, Bootsma H, Theander E, Hansen A, et al. EULAR Sjogren's Syndrome Patient Reported Index (ESSPRI): development of a consensus patient index for primary Sjogren's syndrome. Ann Rheum Dis. 2011;70(6):968–92.
25. Seror R, Ravaud P, Bowman S, Baron G, Tzioufas A, Theander E, et al. EULAR Sjogren's Syndrome Disease Activity Index (ESSDAI): development of a consensus systemic disease activity index in primary Sjogren's syndrome. Ann Rheum Dis. 2009;69(6):1103–9.
26. Barry RJ, Sutcliffe N, Isenberg DA, Price E, Goldblatt F, Adler M, et al. The Sjogren's syndrome damage index—a damage index for use in clinical trials and observational studies in primary Sjogren's syndrome. Rheumatology (Oxford) 2008;47(8):1193–8.

Looking into the Crystal Ball: Initiatives from the Sjögren's Syndrome Foundation That Will Impact Patient Care

31

Elaine Alexander, Frederick B. Vivino, Steven E. Carsons, and Katherine Morland Hammitt

Abstract

The Sjögren's Syndrome Foundation (SSF) has developed and implemented programs critical to the health and well-being of Sjögren's syndrome (SS) patients worldwide and that will have a profound impact on patients as well as on the diverse range of physicians who care for them. Some of the most recent initiatives include the development of Clinical Practice Guidelines, a Clinical Trials Consortium, and broad-reaching projects to increase professional education and awareness of SS. The development of Clinical Practice Guidelines will delineate, for the first time, guidelines which will lead to better decision-making in treating SS patients. Standardization of care across practices will decrease disease-related morbidity and improve patient quality of life. The launching of a Clinical Trials Consortium in SS will accelerate the availability and accessibility of drugs/biologics/over-the-counter products for treatment of SS. The implementation of numerous professional educational programs will enhance knowledge and awareness of SS on the part of health care providers. The SSF remains committed to expanding and solidifying its leadership role worldwide to improve the lives of SS patients and arm the clinician with the latest and best tools and resources for treating their patients.

Keywords

Sjogren's syndrome • Sjogren's Syndrome Foundation • Autoimmune • Clinical guidelines • Clinical trials • Biologics • Medical education

The Sjögren's Syndrome Foundation (SSF) has launched several major initiatives that will have a profound impact on SS patients and the diverse range of physicians who care for them. These initiatives include the development of Clinical Practice Guidelines, the creation of a Clinical Trials Consortium, as well as the pursuit of broad-reaching projects to increase professional education and awareness of SS as an important autoimmune disorder with exocrine gland dysfunction and multiple, often serious systemic (extra-glandular) manifestations.

E. Alexander (✉)
Sjögren's Syndrome Foundation Medical and Scientific Advisory Board, San Diego, CA, USA
e-mail: elaine@easandiego.com

R.I. Fox, C.M. Fox (eds.), *Sjögren's Syndrome*, DOI 10.1007/978-1-60327-957-4_31,

31.1 Clinical Practice Guidelines

The development of Clinical Practice Guidelines will delineate, for the first time, guidelines that will lead to improvement of quality of care and decision-making in treating SS patients. This dynamic and evolving process will develop guidelines for assessment and management of the glandular (dry eye and dry mouth) as well as the systemic manifestations of SS. The initial focus of this initiative is with US clinicians, but it will have broader international implications. By creating a document delineating SS Clinical Practice Guidelines, the Foundation aims to define standards of care, educate health care providers, increase acceptance of standard practices for insurance reimbursement, and obtain broad acceptance of the guidelines by key professional and government organizations. Finally, the initiative will identify gaps in our scientific knowledge and encourage future research and clinical studies.

The process employed by the leading medical SS experts in establishing Clinical Practice Guidelines begins with the determination of management areas and potential clinical scenarios that need to be addressed. Additional stakeholders including patients and allied health professionals also will have input. Following this initial step an extensive review of published peer-reviewed literature will establish existing evidence for treatment decisions in SS and grade the strength of evidence. When definitive evidence does not exist or is not strong, expert opinion will be determined using a method such as a Delphi panel approach.

All working groups for key areas of clinical coverage will convene to present their findings and engage in a consensus conference. Once the guidelines are finalized, articles on the different specialty aspects will be submitted for peer-reviewed publication in leading journals for the specialty areas covered, presented at professional meetings, and reproduced in toto on the SSF website.

While diagnosis is not a feature of the Clinical Practice Guidelines, choice of therapy depends on assessment, so management decisions will be based on clearly delineated assessment factors. The guidelines will also discuss risk/benefit ratios and prioritize the importance of specific interventions.

SS Clinical Practice Guidelines will remain a work in progress as our knowledge of SS continuously evolves. As we learn more about the etiopathogenesis of SS and identify the multiple genetic and biologic targets in the complex effector cascade, new therapeutic targets should emerge for clinical drug/biologic development. In the interim, physicians and other health care professionals will have recommended state-of-the-art standards of care for management of SS. Standardization of care across practices will undoubtedly decrease disease-related morbidity and improve patient quality of life.

31.2 Clinical Trials Consortium

The SSF recently launched a Clinical Trials Consortium designed to increase the availability and accessibility of drugs/biologics/over-the-counter products for treatment of SS. The Foundation has been building the framework for the consortium via several initiatives:

- Fostering interest in research within the scientific and medical community
- Convening workshops to catalyze ideas and develop collaborations
- Launching efforts to support clinical trial criteria and outcome measures

These efforts have led to the development of the American–European Consensus Group classification criteria and validated internationally accepted European League Against Rheumatism (EULAR) clinical outcome measures and the establishment of partnerships with biotech and pharmaceutical companies. These initiatives have raised industry awareness of the market value of SS and initiated a dialogue with the US Food and Drug Administration (FDA) to develop guidelines for new drug/biologic registration. SSF leaders have also developed collaborative relationships with the National Institutes of Health (NIH), served on numerous NIH committees, and advocated for and advised on an National Institute of Dental and Craniofacial Research (NIDCR) sponsored international registry in SS (SICCA) at the University of California, San Francisco (UCSF). The NIDCR-funded SICCA registry marks the largest SS research grant awarded by the NIH.

Over the last decade, the first-ever FDA-approved drugs for SS came to market: Salagen and Evoxac for dry mouth and Restasis for dry eye. More recently, additional drugs have been approved for marketing: Numoisyn, Neutrasal, and CalphoVess for dry mouth and FreshKote for dry eye. All of these drugs, however, target specific symptoms and signs of SS and do not treat the underlying immunological basis for the disease or its many systemic manifestations. The Foundation believes that the consortium will serve to accelerate the discovery and clinical development of novel agents that will treat the underlying disease process and thus systemic complications. More than two dozen candidate drugs/biologics either in development or already approved for use in other closely related autoimmune diseases have been identified and targeted for review and discussions with the companies that manufacture or market them.

As we enter an era characterized by an ever-expanding repertoire of effective biologic therapies for multiple autoimmune disorders, it is anticipated that a number of these therapies will also have the potential for clinical efficacy in SS. For example, the successful clinical development of Benlysta for the treatment of systemic lupus erythematosus (SLE) will soon result in an FDA regulatory submission for approval (NDA). Such a targeted B-cell therapy and others in development are ideal candidates for clinical trials in SS. A number of early stage clinical trials already have been or are being conducted with B-cell therapies in SS. The SSF has worked closely with the companies sponsoring these clinical trials to expand the potential clinical indications to SS. The SSF Clinical Trials Consortium will continue to interface with biotechnology/pharmaceutical companies to facilitate the development of new therapies and provide guidance in the conduct, design, and execution of clinical trials.

31.3 Professional Education and Awareness

Efforts to improve education and awareness about SS among various health care professionals who treat this complex, multifaceted disorder are a major focus of the SSF. The SSF has developed a number of approaches to attain these goals. The first-ever publication for professionals, the *Sjögren's Quarterly*, was launched in 2006, providing a unique educational resource for clinicians and researchers. By early 2010, about 4,000 US professionals were receiving the newsletter as well as another 500 international recipients. Annual meetings organized by the SSF at the American College of Rheumatology (ACR) address the latest topics of interest to rheumatologists such as the promise of new therapeutics in SS. Additionally, SSF leaders have partnered with the ACR to increase the number of Sjögren's-related workshops and symposia presented at its national and regional meetings. A Nursing Education Committee was also formed to provide updated presentations on SS as a women's health issue to the nursing community. A basic guide on all aspects of Sjögren's syndrome, *The Sjögren's Syndrome Handbook*, is published by Oxford University Press as an official publication of the SSF and is regularly updated.

In order to increase our knowledge about disease morbidity in SS patients and provide this information to educate physicians, the SSF in 2007 worked with Harris Interactive and a company sponsor to compile a major survey of SS patients. The study on Burden of Illness and General Health-Related Quality of Life in a US Sjögren's Syndrome Population has led to numerous publications in professional journals and presentations at professional conferences.

The Foundation also provides educational materials for physicians to distribute to their patients, including brochures, booklets on self-help tips, and products for symptoms of SS. Medical professionals are encouraged to join the SSF and invite their patients also to become members and receive "The Moisture Seekers," a newsletter geared toward patient education and support; discounts on regional and national patient conferences, books, and CDs; and the latest information on SS. Visit the SSF at www.sjogrens.org.

The SSF continues to work closely with several institutes of the National Institutes of Health (NIDCR, NEI, NIAMS, NIAID, NCI, and the Office of Woman's Health) and with the US Congress (Senate and House of Representatives) to foster education and awareness of SS, promote increased research funding for autoimmune disorders (including SS), and sponsor scientific and educational workshops and symposia.

In conclusion, over the last 10 years, and under the leadership of CEO Steven Taylor, the SSF has emerged as a major non-profit organization with a substantial multifaceted impact on numerous areas crucial to the health and well-being of SS patients worldwide. The SSF remains committed to expanding and solidifying this important role in the future.

31.4 SSF Clinical Practice Guidelines

Guidelines Chair
Frederick Vivino, MD

31.4.1 Rheumatology Working Group

Co-Chairs
Steve Carsons, MD, and Ann Parke, MD
Elaine Alexander, MD, PhD
Julius Birnbaum, MD
Nancy Carteron, MD
Robert Fox, MD, PhD
Hal Scofield, MD
Barbara Segal, MD
Frederick Vivino, MD

31.4.2 Ocular Working Group

Co-Chairs
Gary Foulks, MD, and Lance Forstot, MD
Peter Donshik, MD
Michael Goldstein, MD
Michael Lemp, MD
J. Daniel Nelson, MD
Kelly Nichols, OD, PhD
Stephen Pflugfelder, MD

31.4.3 Oral Working Group

Co-Chairs
Troy Daniels, DDS, MS, and Philip C. Fox, DDS
Ibtisam Al-Hashimi, BDS, MS, PhD
Mike Brennan, DDS, MHS
Mahvash Navazesh, DMD
Athena Papas, DMD, PhD, FACD
Dorothy Perry, RDH, PhD
Andres Pinto, DMD
Nelson Rhodus, DMD, MPH, FACD
James Sciubba, DMD, PhD
Carol M. Stewart, DDS
Ava Wu, DDS
Domenick Zero, DDS, MS

31.4.4 SSF Clinical Trials Consortium

Consortium Chair
Elaine Alexander, MD, PhD
Steering Committee Members
Philip L. Cohen, MD
Philip C. Fox, DDS
Ann Parke, MD
Frederick Vivino, MD
Claudio Vitali, MD

31.4.5 Facilitator for Both Initiatives

Katherine Morland Hammitt, MA, Vice President of Research, Sjögren's Syndrome Foundation

Biological Treatment for Sjögren's Syndrome

32

Philip L. Cohen and Pamela Traisak

Abstract

The diffuse lymphocyte infiltration of target organs in Sjögren's syndrome seems potentially amenable to therapies which might alter specific lymphocyte populations or their migration to tissues. Especially because this illness responds unsatisfactorily to conventional immunosuppression, efforts are underway to ameliorate disease using monoclonal antibodies, cytokines, and gene therapy. Promising data have been obtained using B-cell depletion with monoclonal antibodies, although further trials are necessary. Because B-cell homeostasis depends to a large degree on the cytokine BAFF/Blys, blocking of these molecules or their receptors may be a valuable approach in some patients. In Sjögren's syndrome, the activation of interferon type I genes has opened the possibility that blocking antibodies to interferon-α or interferon-β may interrupt the disease process and reduce lymphocytic tissue infiltration. Monoclonal antibodies to adhesion molecules and other structures affecting lymphocyte homing may be particularly useful in this illness as well as antibodies to cytokines and their receptors, such as IL-6. Co-stimulation blockade using CTLA-4 is worthy of consideration for Sjögren's syndrome treatment, in light of the important role for T cells in this illness. Finally, while far from clinical use, the delivery of cytokines such as IL-10 by viral vectors or other forms of gene therapy is also an appealing approach. The next few years should bear witness to important new, rational biological approaches to Sjögren's syndrome which should increase our understanding of its basis and provide welcome relief for patients with severe illness.

Keywords

B cells • Sjögren's syndrome • Biological therapies • Monoclonal antibodies • Immunosuppression • Rituximab • BAFF

P.L. Cohen (✉)
Section of Rheumatology, Department of Medicine,
Temple University School of Medicine, Philadelphia,
PA, USA
e-mail: philco@temple.edu

R.I. Fox, C.M. Fox (eds.), *Sjögren's Syndrome*, DOI 10.1007/978-1-60327-957-4_32,

32.1 Introduction

We are in an era of potent biological treatments for rheumatic diseases. Specific cytokines and cytokine receptors can be efficiently blocked, interactions between T and B lymphocytes can be targeted, co-stimulatory receptors on T cells can be blocked, and B-cell or T-cell populations can be drastically reduced or eliminated through the administration of monoclonal antibodies. Primary Sjögren's syndrome seems ripe for intervention with biologicals. The central abnormality is abnormal accumulation of lymphocytes in exocrine organs. Strategies to destroy these unwelcome lymphocytes, to neutralize the harmful cytokines they secrete, or to interfere with their trafficking are attractive solutions to the problem of ectopic lymphocyte accumulation. Somewhat less attractive approaches are to inhibit the global reactivity of T or B cells with monoclonal antibodies or to inhibit cellular interactions.

Given the lack of any specific therapy for Sjögren's syndrome (SS), physicians have begun to administer various biological agents in the hope of intervening in a beneficial way to reduce the cellular infiltrate so characteristic of SS and, more importantly, to reverse or ameliorate functional changes wrought by SS autoimmunity. In this chapter, we will discuss the rationale for therapy, review the published experience with biological agents, and outline promising future directions in this area.

32.2 For Which Patients Should Biological Therapy Be Considered?

Sjögren's syndrome manifestations are highly variable, ranging from localized sicca symptoms to serious complications of central nervous system disease, vasculitis, and cytopenias. Given the cost and risk of present biological therapy, it seems reasonable that patients with severe systemic manifestations of SS, particularly those refractory to conventional therapy, are the candidates for biological therapy. These would include patients with severe vasculitis, cryoglobulinemia, neurological manifestations (both CNS and peripheral), cytopenias, and severe and active interstitial lung disease. Patients with severe parotid enlargement and intractable ophthalmological problems related to sicca have been considered candidates in some trials. Less clear is the use of biological agents in patients with disabling fatigue. The development of validated clinical assessment tools for SS disease severity should help clarify just which patients have disease sufficiently active or severe to merit biological treatment.

Should biological therapy be given early in the course of disease or should it be reserved for patients with advanced pathology? Late in the course of disease, much of the architecture of exocrine glands becomes obliterated due to scarring and fibrosis. It seems sensible that candidates for therapies aimed at intervening in active immunological processes should have evidence of ongoing destruction of tissue. As biological markers of Sjögren's syndrome activity are not readily available, clinical assessment is needed. In a B-cell depletion study cited below, patients with salivary flow rates less than 0.15 mL/min were excluded in an effort to select those with the most potential to benefit.

32.3 Scientific Rationale for Biological Treatment

Any biological intervention to ameliorate SS must consider the mechanisms of lymphocytic infiltration in the illness; the trafficking and turnover of infiltrating cells; the mechanism of epithelial injury; and the potential degree of reversibility of pathology.

Lymphocytes in SS lesions must enter glandular tissue from the circulation and then must localize in tissue through the action of adhesion molecules and chemokines. In particular, CXCL13 and CCL21 [1] seem of special importance in T-cell trafficking to exocrine glands. As will be discussed later, intervention at the level of lymphocyte migration is an exciting approach that has not yet been tried.

Once lymphocytes are in glandular tissue, their activation and their generation of local immune responses provide opportunities for intervention. Both T and B lymphocytes are present in inflammatory infiltrates, and both show evidence of activation as assessed by acquisition of co-stimulatory molecules, other activation molecules, and class II MHC molecules [2]. Whether T-cell activation precedes and causes B-cell activation, or vice versa, is still a matter of controversy and therapeutic trials of biologics may help to resolve this question. T cells may cause tissue injury through cytokine production, through cognate interactions with B cells mediated by CD40–CD40L, and via secretion of cytokines [3]. This injury may take the form of induction of apoptosis in glandular epithelial tissue, with consequent destruction and loss of secretory function, as well as the injury and interruption of autonomic nervous system pathways, leading to impaired glandular innervation and decreased tear or saliva production [4]. Targeting of T cells, and in particular of T-cell subsets in affected tissues, might lead to decreased glandular infiltration and damage.

T cells may enhance activation of B cells or may act to attract them to glands. Alternatively, SS pathology may predominantly be due to glandular attraction and accumulation of B cells. Once within tissues, B cells may mediate injury by cytokine production, by presentation of antigens, and by secretion of antibodies with potential functional consequences.

32.4 TNF-α(alpha) Inhibition

Tumor necrosis factor-α (TNF-α) is expressed in salivary gland duct cells in patients with Sjögren's syndrome. TNF-α initiates the release of matrix metalloproteinases from glandular epithelial cells, triggers the expression of endothelial adhesion molecules, and promotes the influx of mononuclear cells into the salivary glands and other epithelia such as lung and kidney. The administration of pegylated recombinant methionyl human soluble TNF receptor type I in animal models of Sjögren's syndrome prevented lymphocytic infiltration into lacrimal and salivary glands and blocked the development of autoimmunity [5]. These findings provided the basis for investigating TNF-α inhibition. The three primary biologic agents targeting tumor necrosis factor-α are the chimeric monoclonal IgG1 antibody infliximab, the receptor fusion protein etanercept, and the fully humanized monoclonal antibody adalimumab. The initial studies of anti-TNF-α therapy for Sjögren's syndrome appeared promising, however, subsequent studies failed to demonstrate efficacy of TNF-α inhibitors.

A pilot study and a 1-year follow-up trial with infliximab showed improvement in objective and subjective parameters of Sjögren's syndrome tested. In the pilot study, 16 patients with primary Sjögren's syndrome received 3 infusions (3 mg/kg) at weeks 0, 2, and 6, which yielded significant improvement in global assessments, erythrocyte sedimentation rate, whole salivary flow rate, tear secretion, tender joint count, fatigue score, and sensation of dry eyes and dry mouth [5]. In the follow-up study, a maintenance regimen of 1 infusion every 12 weeks was evaluated in 10 of the original 16 patients. Retreatment led to sustained improvement of primary Sjögren's syndrome that was comparable with the effects from the initial three loading infusions [6]. However, a subsequent large randomized, double-blind, placebo-controlled study, the Trial of Remicade In Primary Sjögren's Syndrome (TRIPSS) failed to confirm any benefit of infliximab monotherapy. In this multicenter trial, 103 patients with active primary Sjögren's syndrome were randomly assigned to either receive treatment with infliximab infusions (5 mg/kg) or placebo at weeks 0, 2, and 6 and had follow-up over a 22-week period. There were no significant differences found in improvement from baseline of pain, fatigue, or sicca symptoms or in objective measures of salivary flow, swollen joints, tender joints, erythrocyte sedimentation rate, or C-reactive protein [7].

Etanercept has also been evaluated in a small prospective uncontrolled study and a randomized placebo controlled pilot study. The first study evaluated 15 patients with primary Sjögren's syndrome treated with 25 mg of etanercept given subcutaneously twice a week for 12 weeks along with repeated treatments for up to 26 weeks. There was no reduction in sicca symptoms or signs; however, there was a decrease in fatigue in a subset of four patients as well as a reduction in erythrocyte sedimentation rate [8]. The second study evaluated subcutaneous administration of etanercept versus placebo in 28 patients for 12 weeks and also showed no significant clinical efficacy [9]. No trials of adalimumab treatment in primary Sjögren's syndrome have been reported.

TNF-α may not have the critical role in Sjögren's syndrome as previously thought given the results of the above studies. The failure of TNF-α blockade to protect BAFF-transgenic mice against autoimmunity may also provide insight for the observed lack of efficacy of TNF-α blockers in humans. BAFF-transgenic mice developed Sjögren's syndrome-like features and inhibition of TNF-α in these mice did not alter secretion of autoantibodies and salivary lesions [10]. Additionally, in human SS, TNF-α inhibition with etanercept was associated with increased levels of interferon-α and BAFF [11]. Another potential explanation for the inefficacy of TNF-α blockers may be that TNF-α blockers administered systemically did not achieve therapeutic levels in the target glands [12]. None of the above studies evaluated tissue levels of the drugs or local TNF-α activity before or after treatment. Local gene transfer of a TNF-α blocker to salivary and lacrimal glands was successful in preventing and in some cases reversing the damage in animal studies [13].

32.5 B-cell Depletion

The presence of hypergammaglobulinemia and various autoantibodies such as rheumatoid factor and anti-SSA/SSB antibodies in Sjögren's syndrome provide evidence of B-cell hyperactivity. B-cell infiltrates, largely consisting of memory B cells, have been found in salivary gland biopsy specimens [14]. Five percent of patients with Sjögren's syndrome develop malignant B-cell lymphoma, usually the mucosa-associated lymphoid tissue (MALT) type [15]. Rituximab is a chimeric humanized monoclonal antibody directed against the B-cell surface molecule CD20, which is expressed on the surface of normal and malignant pre-B and mature B lymphocytes. Rituximab leads to peripheral blood B-cell depletion for a period of 6–12 months. Rituximab was first developed for the treatment of B-cell lymphoma and subsequently has been applied to various autoimmune disorders [16].

Several case series demonstrate the potential of rituximab as a therapeutic agent in Sjögren's syndrome. One phase II study evaluated 15 patients with primary Sjögren's syndrome treated with 4 infusions of rituximab (375 mg/m^2) once weekly and observed over a 3-month period. Eight of the patients had primary Sjögren's syndrome for less than 4 years and seven patients had MALT-type lymphomas. There was favorable improvement of subjective symptoms and an increase in salivary gland function. All patients showed a rapid depletion of peripheral B cells within a few weeks accompanied by a decrease in IgM-RF levels. Three of the seven patients with MALT-type lymphoma had a complete remission, three remained stable, and one progressed. Additionally, a high incidence of human anti-chimeric antibodies (HACA) and associated side effects such as serum sickness were observed [17]. In one patient who underwent biopsy before and after treatment, there was improvement in salivary gland histological appearance with apparent regeneration of ductal tissue, along with an increased salivary flow [18].

In a retrospective study, six patients with primary Sjögren's syndrome treated with four infusions of rituximab (375 mg/m^2) once weekly were evaluated. Five of the six patients had regression of parotid gland swelling and improvement of arthralgias. Two of the six patients had major improvement in cryoglobulinemia-related vasculitis [19]. A third study examined 16 patients with primary Sjögren's syndrome who received rituximab for lymphoma and systemic manifestations. Four of 5 patients with lymphoma obtained complete remission and efficacy was observed in 9 out of 11 patients with systemic involvement. Rituximab use also allowed a significant reduction in corticosteroid use and decreased serum B-cell biomarker levels [20]. In another study, 16 patients with primary Sjögren's syndrome received 2 infusions of rituximab (375 mg/m^2) at weeks 0 and 2 without corticosteroids and had follow-up over 36 weeks. Visual analog scale (VAS) scores for fatigue and dryness, tender point count, and quality of life evaluated by the Short Form 36 questionnaire (SF-36) at week 12 were significantly improved. At week 36, significant improvement continued with both tender point count and tender joint count [21].

One double-blind randomized pilot study investigated 2 infusions of rituximab (1 g) versus placebo in 17 patients with primary Sjögren's syndrome with follow-up over 6 months. Significant improvement from baseline in VAS scores for fatigue in the rituximab group as compared to the placebo group was noted. There was also a significant difference between the groups at 6 months in the social functioning score of SF-36 and the mental health score of SF-36 [13]. This study was the first double-blind study of rituximab in primary Sjögren's syndrome to demonstrate benefit but outcome measures were somewhat limited.

Another double-blind placebo study of rituximab in primary Sjögren's syndrome was recently presented. Thirty patients—selected to have salivary flow rates above 0.15 mL/min—were randomized to rituximab treatment (20 patients) or placebo. All patients received IV methylprednisolone before infusion and a tapering course of oral prednisolone afterward. There was significant improvement in salivary secretion rates in the rituximab-treated group, with a decrease observed in the placebo group. Rheumatoid factor levels fell substantially in the B-cell depleted patients and were slightly increased in the placebo group. There was a significant improvement in the visual analog scale score for oral dryness in the rituximab group. Interestingly, both placebo and actively treated groups reported an improvement in generalized fatigue, but those rituximab-treated patients whose disease duration was less than 4 years showed the greatest degree of improvement. Only one patient developed serum sickness, which was judged to be mild. This study is encouraging and suggests that patients with earlier and more active disease are more likely to benefit from B-cell depletion therapy than are patients with long-standing illness [22].

An open trial of rituximab in 12 patients with primary SS showed significant improvement in physicians' and patients VAS, yet no significant change in saliva production [23]. All patients underwent nearly complete B-cell depletion, and at the time of reconstitution peripheral B cells showed a transitional phenotype (CD19$^+$, CD38hi, IgM$^+$, IgD$^+$, CD5$^+$, CD10$^+$, CD23$^+$, CD27$^+$). There was also an increase in the percentage and absolute numbers of peripheral blood B cells with a plasmablast phenotype (CD19$^+$, CD20$^-$, CD38hi, IgD$^-$, CD27^{++}) prior to the increase in transitional B cells [24]. Patients showed low levels of peripheral blood CD27$^+$ memory cells after reconstitution, suggesting that this feature of the Sjögren's phenotype may have been corrected, at least temporarily. There were no changes in CD4, CD8, NK, or T regulatory cells. Levels of IgG autoantibodies were unchanged, but there was a decrease in IgA autoantibodies against Ro and M3 muscarinic receptors [25].

32.6 Monoclonal Antibody Modulation of B-cell Function

An alternative target for B-cell depletion is the B-cell-specific transmembrane protein CD22, co-receptor of the B-cell receptor (BCR) that functions as a negative regulator of BCR signaling. Epratuzumab is a fully humanized monoclonal antibody to CD22 that has been investigated in primary Sjögren's syndrome. Compared with rituximab, epratuzumab provokes a modest decrease in B-cell numbers and acts as an immunomodulator. Epratuzumab is also less immunogenic with reduced potential for human anti-human antibody (HAHA) development and therefore suitable for repeated dosing in patients with chronic autoimmune diseases [26].

Sixteen patients in an open-label phase I/II study received four infusions of epratuzumab (360 mg/m^2) at weeks 0, 2, 4, and 6 and were followed over a 6-month period. A composite endpoint involving the Schirmer-I test, unstimulated whole salivary flow, fatigue VAS, and the laboratory parameters (erythrocyte sedimentation rate and IgG) was used to define clinical response. Twenty percent improvement or more in at least two of the parameters constituted a clinical response. Of all the patients who received at least one dose of epratuzumab, 53% achieved a clinical response at 6 weeks, 53% at 10 weeks, 47% at 18 weeks, and 67% at 32 weeks. Peripheral B-cell levels were decreased by 54% at 6 weeks and 39% at 18 weeks. T-cell levels, immunoglobulins, and routine safety parameters did not change significantly [27]. Epratuzumab is a promising therapy, however, randomized, placebo-controlled trials are needed to confirm therapeutic efficacy.

32.7 BAFF Inhibition

BAFF (B-cell-activating factor or B-lymphocyte stimulator, BLys) is a cytokine necessary for B-cell survival and maturation. BAFF may have a major role in Sjögren's syndrome pathogenesis by regulating B-cell activation and autoantibody activation [28]. BAFF-transgenic mice develop severe sialadenitis, decreased saliva production, and destruction of submaxillary glands. Agents that inhibit BAFF and a related molecule (APRIL) could be an effective in Sjögren's syndrome. Monoclonal antibody blockade of BAFF (belimumab, Lymphostat B) has shown activity in RA and lupus and is worthy of further consideration in SS, as are soluble receptor antagonists BAFF-R3 Ig and TACI Ig.

32.8 Interferon Inhibition

Interferons are proteins with anti-viral activity and strong immunomodulating properties. Patients with Sjögren's syndrome have an activated type I interferon system that includes IFN-α among other interferons. IFN-α improves phagocytic antigen processing and immunoregulatory activity of macrophages and specific cytotoxicity of lymphocytes for target cells and natural killer cell activity [29]. It has been postulated that viral infection may initiate the production of IFN-α, however, continued IFN-α synthesis may be caused by nucleic acid-containing immune complexes that activate plasmacytoid dendritic cells to produce IFN-α at the tissue level [30]. Much recent work has underscored the importance of a type I interferon "signature" in SLE, with many patients exhibiting increased transcription of type I IFNs and of genes regulated by these cytokines [31]. In SLE, disease activity parallels the activation of these genes. Patients with primary Sjögren's syndrome also show increased IFN-related gene activation [32]. It is reasonable to propose that agents that inhibit the action or production of interferon-α may have a therapeutic role in SLE or Sjögren's syndrome. Receptor antagonists that prevent uptake of immune complexes by dendritic cells, inhibitory oligonucleotides that block binding of internalized DNA or RNA to Toll-like receptors, soluble IFN-α receptor, anti-IFN-α antibodies, or agents that block the signal transduction downstream of IFN-α receptors are potential targets of therapy.

Two monoclonal antibodies to type I interferon are in clinical trials in SLE. Preliminary reports have emphasized the apparent safety of this approach and have hinted at its efficacy in SLE [33]. Further studies are required to determine whether this approach will be of value in Sjögren's syndrome.

It is of interest that there have been reports that low doses of IFN-α administered via the oromucosal route increase unstimulated salivary output. A phase II study showed that administration of low doses of IFN-α by dissolving lozenges was safe and improved salivary output as well as decreased complaints of xerostomia [34]. These results prompted a randomized, double-blinded, placebo-controlled clinical trial with 497 patients. The patients in the treatment arm received a 24-week daily treatment of 450 IU IFN-α via the oromucosal route. The study failed to demonstrate a significant effect on VAS score for oral dryness and stimulated whole salivary flow. However, there was a significant increase in unstimulated whole saliva in the patients treated with IFN-α [34].

These results seem contradictory to the postulated role of IFN-α in Sjögren's syndrome. A potential explanation is that oral IFN-α treatment increases saliva secretion via up regulation of transcription of aquaporin 5, a membrane water channel, without influencing the underlying autoimmune process that could still be maintained by IFN-α. Further research is needed to fully understand the effect of IFN-α on salivary gland tissue and in Sjögren's syndrome.

32.9 Gene Therapy

Biologic agents generally have short half-lives and patients require frequent injections or infusions, which can be inconvenient and uncomfortable. Gene therapy offers the opportunity for stable and regulated expression of a therapeutic protein. There have been gene transfer studies conducted on animal models of Sjögren's syndrome; however, no gene transfer studies have been conducted in human patients with Sjögren's syndrome. Several gene delivery systems are available. They include recombinant viral vectors such as adeno-associated virus (AAV) and non-viral methods such as plasmid–cationic liposome mixtures, DNA–protein conjugates, and naked DNA. The recombinant serotype 2 adeno-associated virus vector (rAAV2) has been successfully used in animal models of Sjögren's syndrome [29]. Several successful examples of gene therapy in animals exist.

Local human IL-10 gene delivery to the submandibular glands in female non-obese diabetic (NOD) mice with Sjögren's syndrome resulted in increased salivary flow rate and less focal infiltration in the submandibular glands. Prophylactic adenovirus-mediated viral IL-10 delivery to the lacrimal gland partially suppressed the appearance of Sjögren's syndrome-like features, such as reduced tear production, accelerated tear breakup time, and ocular surface disease [35]. An adenovirus encoding a human TNF receptor was used in a dacryoadenitis rabbit model. Prophylactic administration to the lacrimal glands with concurrent induction of dacryoadenitis led to a partial suppression of Sjögren's syndrome-like features [36]. Administration of a rAAV2 vector encoding TNF receptor to the submandibular glands of the NOD mice increased salivary flow and reduced local infiltration [16]. Delivery of vasoactive intestinal peptide (VIP) via a rAAV2 vector to the submandibular glands of NOD mice increased salivary flow rate, reduced levels of IL-2, IL-10, IL-12, and TNF-α in the submandibular glands and decreased serum levels of the chemokine RANTES [37].

Although localized salivary and lacrimal gland gene transfers have been encouraging in animal models of Sjögren's syndrome, the clinical application of gene therapy in humans with Sjögren's syndrome is uncertain and still needs extensive research. However, gene therapy studies have been useful in providing additional insight into the pathogenesis of Sjögren's syndrome.

32.10 Other Targets for Biologic Therapy

Abatacept (CTLA-4 Ig) inhibits T-cell activation by binding to CD80 and CD86 on B cells, dendritic cells, and other antigen-presenting cells; it has been shown to be effective in rheumatoid arthritis [38]. The rationale for use of this agent in Sjögren's syndrome derives from the observation of activated T cells within glandular tissue and from the presence of co-stimulatory-like molecules within Sjögren's lesions [39]. Blocking of T-cell co-stimulation might reduce lymphocyte accumulation by interrupting T-cell production of chemoattractive cytokines and chemokines and by reducing the degree of interactions between T cells and B cells or antigen-presenting cells. There are also conflicting reports regarding whether Sjögren's disease patients have a genetic polymorphism in the CTLA-4 gene itself [40].

A potentially very interesting approach to Sjögren's therapy is natalizumab (Tysabri), a monoclonal antibody to α4 integrin. This agent is believed to inhibit migration of lymphocytes from lymph nodes to active sites of inflammation by blocking intracellular adhesion. It has been used with success in multiple sclerosis [41] and in Crohn's disease [41] and seems especially well suited to Sjögren's syndrome and other disorders of inappropriate lymphocytic infiltration. While it is generally well-tolerated, enthusiasm for its use is tempered by rare cases of progressive multifocal leukoencephalopathy, a severe and often fatal neurological disease [41].

While not a biological therapy, FTY-720 (fingolimod) has a similar mechanism of action, but acts by blocking binding to sphingosine receptors [42]. It is under evaluation for multiple sclerosis and other autoimmune diseases and may be worth considering for Sjögren's syndrome.

Efalizumab (Raptiva) blocks the binding of leukocyte function-associated antigen-1 (LFA-1) to intercellular adhesion molecules (ICAM-1) [43]. It has a potent effect on lymphocyte trafficking and was approved for the treatment of psoriasis. An National Institute of Dental and Craniofacial Research (NIDCR) study of its effectiveness in primary Sjögren's syndrome is underway. In April, 2009, Genentech voluntarily withdrew Raptiva from the market because of concerns about progressive multifocal leukoencephalopathy. Three confirmed and one possible case of this illness were reported in patients receiving this treatment. Further safety evaluation is underway for this agent.

Alefacept is a monoclonal antibody that blocks the interaction between LFA-3 and CD2, an accessory activation molecule on T cells [44]. Despite its potent effect on T cells and its in vivo depletion of $CD4^+$ T cells, opportunistic infections are not common and the agent is effective in psoriasis. Its use in Sjögren's syndrome has not yet been evaluated.

Tocilizumab, currently approved for treatment of rheumatoid arthritis in some countries, is a monoclonal antibody which blocks binding of IL-6 to its receptor [45]. As IL-6 may contribute to Sjögren's syndrome inflammation [46], it is possible that this agent will prove to be of value in Sjögren's syndrome therapy.

32.11 Conclusions and Future Directions

Though data are still preliminary, it seems that B-cell depletion therapy of Sjögren's syndrome is the most promising biological therapy. Blocking of TNF-α, at least using agents effective for other illnesses, seems ineffective. There is much to be done in the evaluation of other biological interventions for this illness, particularly in the area of therapies that interfere with lymphocyte migration and with the action of interferon. The next decade should see significant advances in the treatment of moderate-to-severe Sjögren's syndrome with biological agents.

References

1. Barone F, Bombardieri M, Manzo A, Blades MC, et al. Association of CXCL13 and CCL21 expression with the progressive organization of lymphoid-like structures in Sjögren's syndrome. Arthritis Rheum. 2005;52:1773–184.
2. Fox RI, Adamson TC 3rd, Fong S, Young C, Howell FV. Characterization of the phenotype and function of lymphocytes infiltrating the salivary gland in patients with primary Sjögren syndrome. Diagn Immunol. 1983;1:233–9.
3. Soliotis FC, Moutsopoulos HM. Sjögren's syndrome. Autoimmunity 2004;37:305–7.
4. Manganelli P, Fietta P. Apoptosis and Sjögren syndrome. Semin Arthritis Rheum. 2003;33:49–65.
5. Steinfeld SD, Demols P, Salmon I, Kiss R, Appelboom T. Infliximab in patients with primary Sjögren's syndrome: a pilot study. Arthritis Rheum. 2001;44:2371–5.
6. Steinfeld SD, Demols P, Appelboom T. Infliximab in primary Sjögren's syndrome: one-year follow up. Arthritis Rheum. 2002;46:3301–3.

7. Mariette X, Ravaud P, Steinfeld S, et al. Inefficacy of infliximab in primary Sjögren's syndrome: results of the randomized, controlled Trial of Remicade in Primary Sjögren's Syndrome (TRIPSS). Arthritis Rheum. 2004;50:1270–6.
8. Zandbelt MM, de Wilde P, van Damme P, Hoyng CB, van de Putte L, van den Hoogen F. Etanercept in the treatment of patients with primary Sjögren's syndrome: a pilot study. J Rheumatol. 2004;31:96–101.
9. Sankar V, Brennan MT, Kok MR, et al. Etanercept in Sjögren's syndrome: a twelve-week randomized, double-blind, placebo-controlled pilot clinical trial. Arthritis Rheum. 2004;50:2240–5.
10. Batten M, Fletcher C, Ng LG, et al. TNF deficiency fails to protect BAFF transgenic mice against autoimmunity and reveals a predisposition to B cell lymphoma. J Immunol. 2004;172:812–22.
11. Mavragani CP, Niewold TB, Moutsopoulos N, Pillemer SR, Wahl SM, Crow MK. Augmented interferon-alpha pathway activation in patients with Sjögren's syndrome treated with etanercept. Arthritis Rheum. 2007;56:3995–4004.
12. Moutsopoulos NM, Katsifis GE, Angelov N, et al. Lack of efficacy of etanercept in Sjögren syndrome correlates with failed suppression of tumour necrosis factor alpha and systemic immune activation. Ann Rheum Dis. 2008;67:1437–43.
13. Thanou-Stavraki A, James JA. Primary Sjögren's syndrome: current and prospective therapies. Semin Arthritis Rheum. 2008;37:273–92.
14. Le Pottier L, Devauchelle V, Pers JO, Jamin C, Youinou P. The mosaic of B-cell subsets (with special emphasis on primary Sjögren's syndrome). Autoimmun Rev. 2007;6:149–54.
15. Jonsson V, Wiik A, Hou-Jensen K, et al. Autoimmunity and extranodal lymphocytic infiltrates in lymphoproliferative disorders. J Intern Med. 1999;245:277–86.
16. Looney RJ, Anolik J, Sanz I. B cells as therapeutic targets for rheumatic diseases. Curr Opin Rheumatol. 2004;16:180–5.
17. Pijpe J, van Imhoff GW, Spijkervet FK, et al. Rituximab treatment in patients with primary Sjögren's syndrome: an open-label phase II study. Arthritis Rheum. 2005;52:2740–50.
18. Pijpe JG. van Imhoff W, Vissink A, et al. Changes in salivary gland immunohistology and function after rituximab monotherapy in a patient with Sjögren's syndrome and associated MALT lymphoma. Ann Rheum Dis. 2005;64:958–60.
19. Gottenberg JE, Guillevin L, Lambotte O, et al. Tolerance and short term efficacy of rituximab in 43 patients with systemic autoimmune diseases. Ann Rheum Dis. 2005;64:913–20.
20. Seror R, Sordet C, Guillevin L, et al. Tolerance and efficacy of rituximab and changes in serum B cell biomarkers in patients with systemic complications of primary Sjögren's syndrome. Ann Rheum Dis. 2007;66:351–7.
21. Devauchelle-Pensec V, PennecY, Morvan J, et al. Improvement of Sjögren's syndrome after two infusions of rituximab (anti-CD20). Arthritis Rheum. 2007;57:310–7.
22. Meijer JM, Meiners PM, Vissink A, et al. Effectiveness of rituximab treatment in primary Sjögren's syndrome: a randomized, double-blind, placebo-controlled trial. Arthritis Rheum. 2010.62(4):960–8.
23. St. Clair E, Levesque MC, Luning Prak N, Vivino FB, AlapattC, Wallace D, Cohen P. Rituximab therapy for primary Sjögren's syndrome (pSS): an open-label trial. Arthritis Rheum. 2007;56(Suppl 9):S449 (abst).
24. Levesque M, Luning Prak N, St. Clair EW, et al. Longitudinal analysis of lymphocyte subsets in patients with primary Sjögren's syndrome (pSS) treated with rituximab: results from an open-label clinical trial. Arthritis Rheum. 2007;56(Suppl 9):S445.
25. Cohen P, Silverman G, Peck AB, Cornelius JG, Luning Prak N, Levesque MC, Vivino F, Srikishnan R, St. Clair EW. IgA autoantibodies fall selectively in B-cell depleted Sjogren patients. Ann Rheum Dis. 2008;67:214 (abst).
26. Carnahan J, Stein R, Qu Z, Hess K, Cesano A, Hansen HJ, Goldenberg DM. Epratuzumab, a CD22-targeting recombinant humanized antibody with a different mode of action from rituximab. Mol Immunol. 2007;44:1331–41.
27. Steinfeld SD, Tant L, Burmester GR, Teoh NK, Wegener WA, Goldenberg DM, Pradier O. Epratuzumab (humanised anti-CD22 antibody) in primary Sjögren's syndrome: an open-label phase I/II study. Arthritis Res Ther. 2006;8:R129.
28. Groom J, Kalled SL, Cutler AH, Olson C, Woodcock SA, Schneider P, Tschopp J, Cachero TG, Batten M, Wheway J, Mauri D, Cavill D, Gordon TP, Mackay CR, Mackay F. Association of BAFF/BLyS overexpression and altered B cell differentiation with Sjögren's syndrome. J Clin Invest. 2002;109:59–68.
29. Lodde BM, Baum BJ, Tak PP, Illei G. Experience with experimental biological treatment and local gene therapy in Sjögren's syndrome: implications for exocrine pathogenesis and treatment. Ann Rheum Dis. 2006;65:1406–13.
30. Ueno H, Klechevsky E, Morita R, Aspord C, Cao T, Matsui T, Di Pucchio T, Connolly J, Fay JW, Pascual V, Palucka AK, Banchereau J. Dendritic cell subsets in health and disease. Immunol Rev. 2007;219: 118–42.
31. Ronnblom L, Pascual V. The innate immune system in SLE: type I interferons and dendritic cells. Lupus 2008;17:394–9.
32. Nordmark G, Alm GV, Ronnblom L. Mechanisms of disease: primary Sjögren's syndrome and the type I interferon system. Nat Clin Pract Rheumatol. 2006;2:262–9.
33. Wallace D, Petri M, Olsen N, et al. MEDI-545, an anti-interferon alpha monoclonal antibody, shows

evidence of clinical activity in systemic lupus erythematosus. Arthritis Rheum. 2007;56(Suppl 9):S526.
34. Ship JA, Fox PC, Michalek JE, Cummins MJ, Richards AB. Treatment of primary Sjögren's syndrome with low-dose natural human interferon-alpha administered by the oral mucosal route: a phase II clinical trial. IFN Protocol Study Group. J Interferon Cytokine Res. 1999;19:943–51.
35. Kok MR, Yamano S, Lodde BM, Wang J, Couwenhoven RI, Yakar S, Voutetakis A, Leroith D, Schmidt M, Afione S, Pillemer SR, Tsutsui MT, Tak PP, Chiorini JA, Baum BJ. Local adeno-associated virus-mediated interleukin 10 gene transfer has disease-modifying effects in a murine model of Sjögren's syndrome. Hum Gene Ther. 2003;14:1605–18.
36. Zhu Z, Stevenson D, Ritter T, Schechter JE, Mircheff AK, Kaslow HR, Trousdale MD. Expression of IL-10 and TNF-inhibitor genes in lacrimal gland epithelial cells suppresses their ability to activate lymphocytes. Cornea 2002;21:210–4.
37. Lodde BM, Mineshiba F, Wang J, Cotrim AP, Afione S, Tak PP, Baum BJ. Effect of human vasoactive intestinal peptide gene transfer in a murine model of Sjögren's syndrome. Ann Rheum Dis. 2006;65:195–200.
38. Kremer JM, Genant HK, Moreland LW, Russell AS, Emery P, Abud-Mendoza C, Szechinski J, Li T, Teng J, Becker JC, Westhovens R. Results of a two-year follow up study of patients with rheumatoid arthritis who received a combination of abatacept and methotrexate. Arthritis Rheum. 2008;58:953–63.
39. Fox RI. Clinical features, pathogenesis, and treatment of Sjögren's syndrome. Curr Opin Rheumatol. 1996;8:438–45.
40. Gottenberg JE, Loiseau P, Azarian M, Chen C, Cagnard N, Hachulla E, Puechal X, Sibilia J, Charron D, Mariette X, Miceli-Richard C. CTLA-4 + 49A/G and *CT60* gene polymorphisms in primary Sjogren syndrome. Arthritis Res Ther. 2007;9:R24.
41. Meyer MA. Natalizumab for relapsing multiple sclerosis. N Engl J Med. 2006;354:2387–9; author reply 87–9.
42. Weissert R. The curtain is drawn for both natalizumab and fingolimod (FTY720): a new era of multiple sclerosis therapy has arrived. Expert Rev Neurother. 2006;6:1587–90.
43. Marecki S, Kirkpatrick P. Efalizumab. Nat Rev Drug Discov. 2004;3:473–4.
44. Chamian F, Lowes MA, Lin SL, Lee E, Kikuchi T, Gilleaudeau P, Sullivan-Whalen M, Cardinale I, Khatcherian A, Novitskaya I, Wittkowski KM, Krueger JG. Alefacept reduces infiltrating T cells, activated dendritic cells, and inflammatory genes in psoriasis vulgaris. Proc Natl Acad Sci USA. 2005;102:2075–80.
45. Ohsugi Y, Kishimoto T. The recombinant humanized anti-IL-6 receptor antibody tocilizumab, an innovative drug for the treatment of rheumatoid arthritis. Expert Opin Biol Ther. 2008;8:669–81.
46. Tishler M, Yaron I, Geyer O, Shirazi I, Naftaliev E, Yaron M. Elevated tear interleukin-6 levels in patients with Sjogren syndrome. Ophthalmology 1998;105:2327–9.

Further Reading

1. Abdulahad WH, Meijer JM, Kroese FG, Meiners PM, Vissink A, Spijkervet FK, Kallenberg CG, Bootsma H. B-cell reconstitution and T-helper-cell balance after rituximab treatment of active primary Sjögren's syndrome. Arthritis Rheum. 2011 Jan; 10. [Epub ahead of print]
2. Meijer JM, Pijpe J, Vissink A, Kallenberg CG, Bootsma H. Treatment of primary Sjogren syndrome with rituximab: extended follow-up, safety and efficacy of retreatment. Ann Rheum Dis. 2009 Feb;68(2):284–5.

33 Looking into the Future—Emerging Therapies Based on Pathogenesis

Jacques-Eric Gottenberg and Xavier Mariette

Abstract

Previously in this textbook, improvement in the knowledge on the pathogenesis of primary Sjögren's syndrome (pSS) has already been emphasized as well as the absence of any specific drug for treatment of this disease. In this section, we will try to reconcile pathogenesis and treatment by focusing on the crucial pathogenic steps that could be targeted by emerging therapies. The main new insights into the pathogenesis of the disease are represented by the accumulating data on the involvement of type I interferon and the triggers of B-lymphocyte activation in pSS. First, we will summarize the pathogenic involvement of type I interferon (IFN) and B-cell-activating factor of the TNF family (BAFF) in B-cell activation. Interestingly, these recent genetic and pathogenic studies evidenced number of similarities between pSS and lupus, and pSS could be considered as a sort of lupus of mucosa. We will subsequently discuss the different therapeutics that could target such an IFN–BAFF–B-lymphocyte axis.

Keywords

Interferon • BAFF • TLRs • Rituximab • Anti-CD22

33.1 Overview of the Pathogenesis of pSS

33.1.1 Initial Steps

The initial steps in the pathogenesis of pSS involve the interaction between environmental/genetic factors and epithelial cells. Infectious triggering factors or other "danger signals" may have different consequences.

33.1.1.1 Breach of Self-tolerance

Environmental factors, like viruses, might contribute to the triggering of the disease by enhancing autoantigen presentation through molecular mimicry or surface exposure of endogenous ribonucleoproteins like SS-A, SS-B, normally hidden from the immune system, in apoptotic blebs, or exosomes. The breach of tolerance might be of central or peripheral origin. Regarding the peripheral origin of the breach of

X. Mariette (✉)
Assistance Publique-Hôpitaux de Paris (AP-HP), Hôpital Bicêtre, Institut Pour la Santé et la Recherche Médicale (INSERM) U 1012, Université Paris-Sud 11, Le Kremlin Bicêtre, France
e-mail: xavier.mariette@bct.aphp.fr

R.I. Fox, C.M. Fox (eds.), *Sjögren's Syndrome*, DOI 10.1007/978-1-60327-957-4_33,

tolerance, some studies have investigated the role of blood or salivary regulatory T cells, without any consistent evidence of decrease or functional defect in pSS [1, 2]. Thus, to date, there is no rationale for potential cell therapy based on the induction of regulatory T cells in pSS.

33.1.1.2 Activation of Innate Immunity and Interferon Pathways

Recently, the presence of interferon-producing cells and of IFN-α has been shown exclusively in salivary glands of patients with pSS. Likewise, three different gene expression studies (two studies in salivary glands [3, 4] and one in peripheral blood mononuclear cells (PBMCs) [5]) demonstrated the activation of interferon pathways in pSS. The type I interferon response is, at least partly, genetically determined. Gene polymorphisms of *IRF5*, a pivotal transcription in IFN pathways, are associated with pSS [6]. In addition to the role of genetic factors, immune complexes are the key drivers of the persistent activation of IFN pathways.

One of the main pathogenic consequences of the activation of IFN pathways is the induction of BAFF (B-cell-activating factor of the TNF family, also termed BLyS). BAFF promotes B-cell survival and antibody secretion. Autoreactive B cells are more dependent on BAFF for their survival than alloreactive B cells. The BAFF/APRIL "system" has five members: BAFF and APRIL (a proliferation-inducing ligand), present on monocytes, dendritic cells, and activated T cells, and their receptors. BAFF, which has membrane-bound and soluble forms, is recognized by three receptors: BAFF receptor (BR3), TACI on B and T cells, and BCMA on B cells (Fig. 33.1). BAFF-transgenic mice develop polyarthritis and clinical features of lupus and SS [7]. In patients with pSS, serum BAFF levels correlate with levels of autoantibodies (anti-SS-A/SS-B, rheumatoid factor) [8].

BAFF expression is also increased in salivary glands of patients with pSS compared with controls. Interestingly, Sellam et al. recently found a decrease of BAFF-R expression on B cells of patients with pSS and with systemic lupus erythematosus (SLE) [9]. This decrease of BAFF-R was

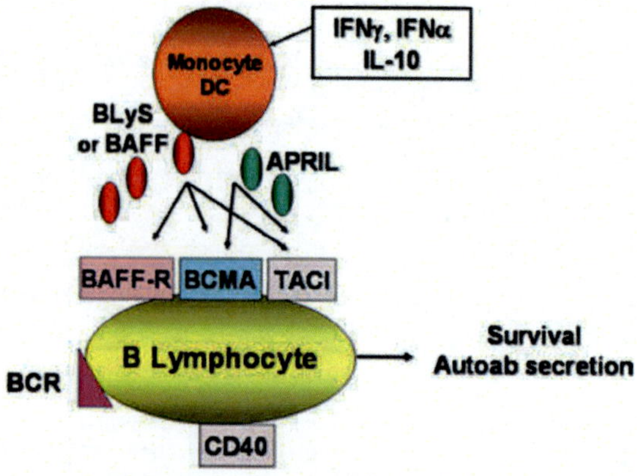

Fig. 33.1 The BAFF(BLyS)/BAFF receptor system: a crucial role for B-cell activation in autoimmune diseases, notably in pSS

correlated with disease activity in both diseases. There was a negative correlation between BAFF-R expression on B cells and serum BAFF level, suggesting that high serum BAFF level negatively regulates BAFF-R expression on B cells, either by internalization of the receptor or by shedding out of the membrane.

The role of APRIL in autoimmunity is less clear than that of BAFF. Indeed, APRIL-transgenic mice do not develop either B-cell abnormalities, serological, or clinical signs of autoimmunity [10].

Interestingly, through TACI targeting, APRIL could have a dual effect:

- A B-cell stimulatory effect mainly on immunoglobulin isotype switch. Indeed, TACI signaling is involved in immunoglobulin switch. TACI mutations are found in 10% of patients with common variable immunodeficiency [11].
- A negative signal on B cells explaining hyperactivation of B cells in TACI$^{-/-}$ mice [12]. Accordingly, APRIL could serve as a homeostatic down-modulator of B-cell hyperactivation induced by BAFF.

33.1.1.3 Multiple Cellular Origins of BAFF in pSS

In pSS, BAFF is not only expressed by the usual "professional" secreting cells (monocytes and dendritic cells), but also by

- *resident cells of target organs of autoimmunity.* Salivary epithelial cells may express and secrete BAFF, both in patients with SS and healthy subjects [13]. Interestingly, this expression is largely increased by stimulation with type I or type II interferon (IFN). Patients with SS seem to be more sensible to the effect of type I interferon for inducing BAFF expression and secretion by salivary epithelial cells. Thus, resident cells of target organs of autoimmunity are not only passive victims, but also play an active role by secreting BAFF after innate immune stimulation, resulting in activation of autoreactive B lymphocytes. The active contribution of epithelial cells to the pathogenesis of pSS, for which the term of "autoimmune epithelitis" [14] has been proposed, is also illustrated by their expression of HLA class II molecules, co-stimulatory molecules (CD80 or B7-1, CD86 or B7-2, CD40), adhesion molecules (ICAM-1) [14], and some innate immune receptors, like Toll-like receptors (TLRs).
- *T cells.* The first report from Groom et al. in 2002 showed the presence of BAFF within the salivary lymphoid infiltrate characteristic of this disease. Later, Lavie et al. demonstrated that both T cells of the infiltrate and epithelial cells could express BAFF [15]. In autoimmune conditions, BAFF can also be expressed and secreted by circulating blood T cells and by monocytes. In some pathologic conditions, T cells could also express BAFF [16, 17].
- *B cells.* Recently, Deridon et al. suggested that the B cells of the infiltrate, which are the target of BAFF and express the different receptors of BAFF, could also express the ligand (BAFF itself), leading to an autocrine pathway for BAFF secretion and activation of B cells [18].

33.1.1.4 Regulation of BAFF Secretion

IFNs are the main cytokines which stimulate BAFF secretion. Firstly, it was shown that type II γ-IFN was able to induce BAFF in monocytes and dendritic cells. Then, Litinskiy et al. demonstrated that type I IFN could induce BAFF secretion by monocytes [19]. Type I IFN is also able to induce BAFF secretion by salivary epithelial cells [14]. Viruses, or *double-stranded RNAs*, are capable of inducing directly and strongly BAFF secretion by salivary epithelial cells or bronchial epithelial cells, using pathways dependent or not on TLRs and IFN [20]. Other cytoplasmic RNA sensors, such as PKR, could be involved [21]. Thus, immune complexes might contribute to the persistence of BAFF overexpression in pSS. *BAFF* gene polymorphism is not associated with the disease but might also regulate BAFF secretion [22].

33.1.1.5 BAFF Overexpression Results in Polyclonal B-cell Activation Inside Target Organs and Might Contribute to the Development of Lymphoma

BAFF, along with other cytokines and chemokines, creates a microenvironment supportive of B-cell aggregation and differentiation, and production in target organs of the disease of anti-SS-A/SS-B antibodies, with structural features remarkably similar to germinal centers, observed in lymph nodes [23]. The co-expression of BAFF and BAFF receptor (BR-3) in some B lymphocytes might contribute to BAFF-mediated autocrine loop of B-cell activation in salivary glands [18]. Persistent polyclonal B-cell activation by BAFF overexpression and by immune complexes stimulating the RF-bearing activity of some B-cell receptors might result in the development of lymphomas in 5% of patients with pSS (16–18-fold increase compared with the general population) [24, 25]. Interestingly, increase in serum BAFF is associated with a poor survival in patients with lymphoma [26]. BAFF might thus represent not only one of the bridges joining innate immunity and autoimmune B-cell activation, but also between autoimmunity and lymphoma in pSS.

33.1.1.6 Other Cytokines, Chemokines, and Adhesion Molecules Are Involved in the Pathogenesis of the Disease

A predominant local Th1 response is observed in salivary glands of patients with pSS, with

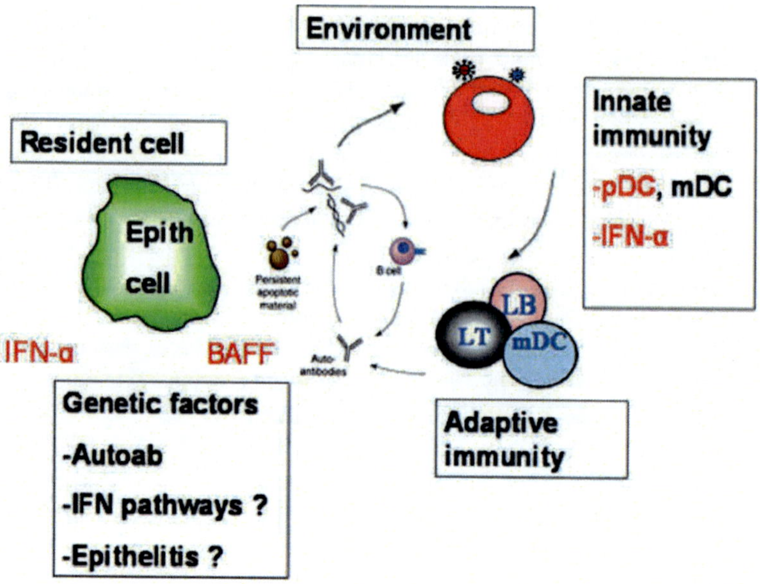

Fig. 33.2 Contribution of genetic and environmental factors and innate and adaptive immunity to the pathogenesis of pSS. pDC: plasmacytoid dendritic cell, mDC: myeloid dendritic cell

increased levels of not only IL-2 and IFN-γ, but also of other pro-inflammatory cytokines, like IL-1 and TNF-α. However, Th2 cytokines are also secreted, with high peripheral blood levels of IL-6 and IL-10, cytokines which promote antibody secretion. A decrease of TGF-β, though controversial, and IL-4 expression in salivary glands of pSS patients has been reported. T-cell-attracting chemokines, such as CXCL-9 (Mig) and CXCL-10 (IP-10), are involved in the migration of T cells in the salivary glands. B-cell-attracting chemokines (CXCL-12 or SDF-1, CXCL-13 or BCA-1) are expressed by epithelial cells, endothelial cells (CXCL-13), contributing to the recruitment of B cells, and activated T cells [27, 28]. An increase of IL-17 was also reported [29].

33.1.2 Autoantibody Secretion Is Pivotal for the Persistence of Autoimmunity

Anti-SS-A/SS-B antibodies might complex with double-stranded RNAs (Y-RNA) or single-stranded RNA and drive the continuous stimulation of interferon-producing cells through their Fc and Toll-like receptors. The persistent activation of the interferon pathways might thus be related to a vicious circle, in which the environment interacts with genetic factors (HLA-DRB1*15 and DRB1*03 associated with production of autoantibodies [30] and subsequent formation of immune complexes with self-RNA; increased secretion of IFN in patients with predisposing IRF5 haplotypes [31, 6]) to drive the mutually co-stimulatory innate and adaptive immune responses (Fig. 33.2). Immune complexes might not only stimulate BAFF secretion indirectly, by promoting the activation of IFN, but also directly, as shown by the induction of BAFF by epithelial expression after double-stranded RNA stimulation [20]. Thus, immune complexes lead to the enhancement of IFN activation and of BAFF secretion, mediating the characteristic B-cell hyperactivation observed in pSS.

33.1.3 Glandular Hypofunction Rather Than Glandular Destruction

Recent data suggest that the glandular dysfunction in SS could result from immune-mediated inhibition of secretory processes rather than

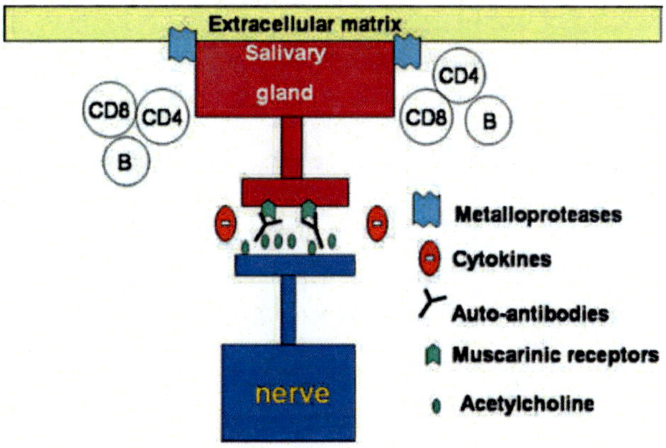

Fig. 33.3 Dysfunction of the neuroexocrine synapse in pSS, due to metalloproteinases, autoantibodies, cytokines, and T-lymphocyte-mediated cytotoxicity

from glandular destruction [32] (Fig. 33.3). First, apoptosis of the salivary gland epithelial cells has been shown to be a rare event [33]. Secondly, many patients with pSS with disabling objective dryness retain large amounts (30–50%) of histological normal salivary glands. Last, this residual tissue is functional in vitro and can be stimulated in vivo in patients with pSS using systemic sialogogues.

Salivary and lacrimal secretion is controlled by the binding of acetylcholine on type-3 muscarinic acetylcholine (M3) receptors on the surface of the acinar cells (Fig. 33.3). Many interactions between the immune system and the secretory process could inhibit this neuroexocrine junction:

- inhibition of neurotransmitter release by cytokines (IL-1, TNF-α) [34]
- enhanced breakdown of acetylcholine by increased levels of cholinesterase in pSS [35]
- blockade of M3 receptors by anti-muscarinic autoantibodies [36]
- altered NO production and intracellular calcium mobilization
- altered fluid movement due to abnormal distribution of aquaporins (AQP). Salivary acinar cells express AQP5 on the apical cell membrane and AQP1 on the basolateral membrane. Some data indicated that the expression of AQP5 could be reduced at the luminal membrane of salivary acinar cells in pSS but a recent study showed that the distribution of AQP5 in SS was unaltered [37].

33.2 Emerging Therapies

33.2.1 Prerequisite for the Development of New Drugs in pSS

33.2.1.1 Disease Activity Score

It is mandatory to validate a consensual disease activity score. After the very interesting preliminary works of Vitali et al. [38] and Bowman et al. [39], an international consensus Sjögren's activity score is being set up on behalf of EUropean Ligue Against Rheumatism (EULAR) [40].

33.2.1.2 Selection of Patients

For each drug evaluated, the target population should be defined: patients with glandular symptoms only (which must have residual salivary flow, so that a possible improvement can be assessed) or with associated systemic features, patients with recent onset or long-standing disease. Depending on the mechanism of action of the drug evaluated, specific inclusion criteria might be necessary. Likewise, for B-cell inhibitors, controlled trials should first focus on patients with systemic involvement and/or increase in B-cell biomarkers.

33.2.2 New Insights into the Pathogenesis of pSS Explain the Inefficacy of TNF Antagonists

33.2.2.1 Increase of BAFF Could Explain the Lack of Efficacy of Anti-TNF in SS

Two randomized controlled trials, one with infliximab [41] and one with etanercept [42], demonstrated absence of efficacy of TNF blockers in SS. A recent work showed the reason of the failure of anti-TNF. On etanercept and not on placebo, pSS patients experienced an increase in type I interferon and BAFF secretion which could explain the absence of improvement [43].

33.2.3 Blockade of the IFN–BAFF–B-lymphocyte Axis

33.2.3.1 Inhibition of the Triggering Factors of IFN Activation

The main potential therapeutic targets leading to IFN activation are immune complexes, Fcγ receptors, and innate immune receptors including TLR and other RNA sensors. Indeed, immune complexes have to be internalized by dendritic cells and B lymphocytes through Fcγ receptors. Then immune complexes activate TLRs in late, acidified, endosomes and might also stimulate other cytoplasmic RNA sensors, such as RIG-I, MDA-5, or PKR. Various strategies could be envisioned to inhibit subsequent IFN activation and BAFF secretion:

- Inhibition of immune complexes uptake by inhibitors of Fcγ receptors
- Increase in expression of "inhibitory" Fcγ receptors (Fcγ RII-B)
- Antagonists of TLRs involved in the recognition of immune complexes (TLR3, TLR7, TLR8, and TLR9)
- Inhibition of the activation of endosomes using hydroxychloroquine
- This "old" drug has shown some interesting effects, notably on the decrease of gammaglobulin levels, in open studies, which might result from the inhibition of TLRs. Thus, the therapeutic interest of hydroxychloroquine should be reassessed in controlled trials (a French multicenter controlled trial is ongoing)
- Inhibition of other RNA sensors, such as PKR

33.2.3.2 IFN Blockade

Recently it was presented the first phase I study with an anti-type I IFN monoclonal antibody in SLE with good safety and promising efficacy [44]. Safety and efficacy have to be confirmed in controlled phase II–III studies.

However, inhibiting type I IFN could lead to adverse side effect. In diseases for which an interferon signature has been demonstrated, BAFF-targeted therapy could be safer and maybe as efficient.

33.2.3.3 Antagonists of BAFF and APRIL

BAFF could be a possible bridge between innate and adaptive immunity, and between autoimmunity and lymphoma in pSS, which makes it a particularly interesting therapeutic target.

To date, three different drugs have been designed (Fig. 33.4):

- Belimumab is a monoclonal anti-BAFF antibody which targets only BAFF [45],
- Atacicept is a TACI-Fc molecule which targets both BAFF and APRIL, and
- BR3-Fc targets only BAFF.

To date, two large phase II studies (400–500 patients each) have been presented with belimumab. In rheumatoid arthritis (RA), the results are rather disappointing with around 30% of ACR 20 response in all belimumab groups versus 15% in the placebo group [46]. This may be explained by the fact that B-cell activation in RA may not be driven only by BAFF. In SLE, the results are more encouraging. Although the primary endpoint (decrease of SLEDAI of more than three points) was not achieved in the whole study including 449 patients, the analysis restricted to 70% of patients with anti-nuclear antibodies or anti-DNA antibodies showed a significant effect of belimumab on the decrease of disease activity measured by Systemic Lupus Erytjhematosus Disease Activity Index (SLEDAI) and anti-DNA antibody level. Phase III studies have confirmed efficacy of belimumab in SLE (Navarra et al.,

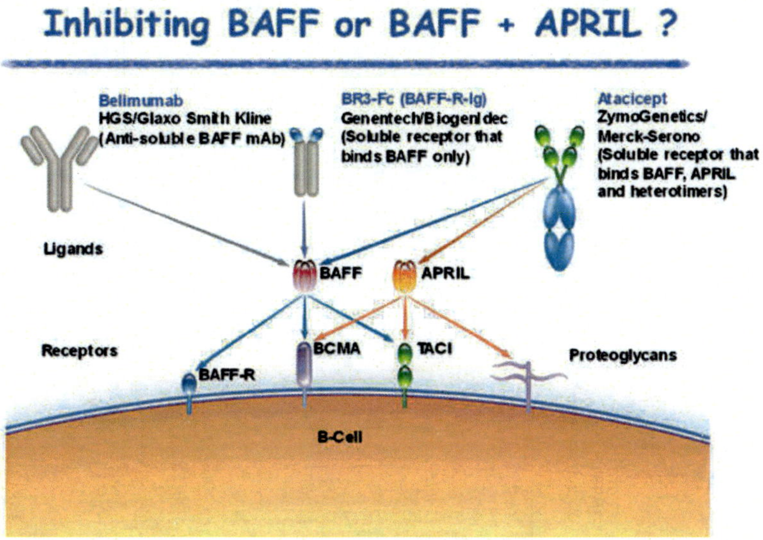

Fig. 33.4 The three treatments on development inhibiting BAFF or BAFF + APRIL

Lancet 2011;377:721–31) and the drug has been approved for SLE in 2011. Phase II studies in SS have began. Phase II studies with atacicept are ongoing in SLE.

Another possible interest of anti-BAFF therapy is its use just after rituximab treatment. Indeed, in all autoimmune diseases treated with rituximab, an increase in serum BAFF after rituximab therapy was observed [47–50]. This increase is not exclusively related to the disappearance of BAFF-binding B cells in peripheral blood. Thus, two studies showed a true homeostatic feedback characterized by the increase in BAFF mRNA expression in monocytes after rituximab [48, 50]. This increase in BAFF after rituximab could favor the stimulation of new autoimmune B cells. Using BAFF-targeted therapy after rituximab to avoid this BAFF increase could therefore be of interest.

33.2.3.4 B-cell Depletion

Rituximab in SS

Rituximab, a monoclonal anti-CD20 antibody, has been approved in the treatment of anti-TNF refractory rheumatoid arthritis. Three randomized controlled studies demonstrated its efficacy in this pathology.

Targeting B cells seems also very promising in SS. To date, rituximab has been used in three open studies that included 15–16 patients [51, 52] and in case reports of lymphomas complicating SS [53, 54] (Table 33.1). In two of these open studies [51, 52], efficacy on dryness was restricted to patients with early diseases. The third open study included patients with systemic complications since B-cell hyperactivity is higher in this category of patients [55]. There was a clear effect of rituximab on systemic complications: parotidomegaly, synovitis, and cryoglobulinemia-associated vasculitis. Individual cases with lung or renal infiltrate also improved. However, in this study, there was no change in subjective or objective dryness.

In a first randomized control trial of rituximab in SS [56], 17 patients without any systemic complications were included. Due to the low number of patients, there was no statistically significant difference on the primary endpoint (fatigue assessed by visual analog scale (VAS)) between the two groups, but the decrease of fatigue was statistically significant only in the rituximab group (decrease of around 50% vs. 20% in the placebo group).

In a second controlled study [57], 30 patients—selected to have salivary flow rates above 0.15 mL/min—were randomized to rituximab treatment ($n = 20$) or placebo ($n = 10$). There was a significant improvement in the visual analog scale score for oral and mouth dryness and in salivary secretion rates in the rituximab-treated group.

Table 33.1 Efficacy and indications of RTX (rituximab) in patients with pSS

Authors, years	Number of patients	Indications of RTX	Efficacy for lymphoma	Efficacy for systemic features	Efficacy for objective dryness	Efficacy for subjective dryness	Adverse events
Somer, 2003 [53]	1	Lymphoma	Yes	NR	Yes	Yes	No
Voulgarelis, 2004 [54]	4	Lymphoma (4/4)	4/4 (100%)	3/3 (100%)	NM	NM	2/4 (50%) 2 IRR
Harner, 2004 [62]	1	Lymphoma	Yes	NR	NM	Yes	NM
Ramos-Casals, 2004 [63]	2	Lymphoma (2/2)	Yes	NR	NM	NM	NM
Pijpe, 2005 [51]	1	Lymphoma	Yes	NR	Yes	Yes	No
Gottenberg, 2005 [64]	6	Lymphoma (2/6) Systemic features (4/6)	1/2 (50%) NR	NR 4/4 (100%)	N (0/2)	3/6 (50%)	2/6 (33%) 1 SSR, 1 IRR
Ahmadi-Simab, 2005 [65]	1	Scleritis	NR	Yes	NM	NM	NM
Pijpe, 2005 [51]	15	Lymphoma (7/15) Early pSS (8/15)	3/7 (43%)	NM	28.6% (2/7) 100% (7/7)	Yes	6/14 (43%) 3 SSR, 2 IRR
Ring, 2005 [66]	1	Renal tubular acidosis	NR	No	Yes	Yes	No
Seror, 2006 [55]	16	Lymphoma (5/16) Systemic features (11/16)	4/5 (80%) NR	NR 9/119 (82%)	2/16 (18%)	5/16 (36%)	4/16 (25%) 2 SSR, 2 IRR
Meijer, 2008 [57]	30	Mainly glandular symptoms	NR	Yes	Yes	Yes	1 SSR, 2 IRR
Devauchelle, 2007 [52]	16	Mainly glandular symptoms	NR	Yes	No	Yes	1 SSR, 2 IRR
Saint-Clair, 2007 [67]	12	Glandular symptoms	NR	NR	No	No	4 IRR
Dass, 2008 [56]	17	Glandular symptoms	NR	NR	No	No	1 SSR, 2 IRR

IRR infusion-related reaction; NR: not relevant; NM: not mentioned; SSR: serum sickness-like reaction

Of note, approximately 10% of treated patients of the different studies (case reports, open, and controlled studies) presented serum sickness-like disease 3–7 days after rituximab infusion (fever, arthralgia, and purpura). This complication, usually benign, must be differentiated from immediate infusion reactions which are probably due to cytokines release and which will not recur after the next infusions. Serum sickness disease may occur after treatment with chimeric antibodies. Curiously, it is exceptional after treatment of lymphoma with rituximab and has not been described in the randomized control trials of rituximab in RA. Cases of serum sickness diseases have also been described in open studies of rituximab in lupus. The higher frequency of serum sickness disease in SS may be due to hypergammaglobulinemia, which is much more common in SS and SLE than in RA.

33.2.3.5 Other B-cell-Targeted Therapy: Other Anti-CD20 and Anti-CD22

With the development of humanized or human anti-CD20 monoclonal antibodies or small oral molecules against CD20, the interest of B-cell inhibition using other agents might be further evaluated in pSS.

An open study including 15 patients has been performed with epratuzumab, an anti-CD22 monoclonal antibody [58]. This anti-B-cell antibody leads to only partial B-cell depletion (50% in blood). The results of this open study are interesting with improvement of dryness, fatigue, and pain VAS. Moreover, salivary flow seems to be improved in patients with early disease. A controlled trial is now necessary to confirm these data.

33.3 Other Therapeutic Perspectives

33.3.1 Inhibition of Other Cytokines and Chemokines

Inhibition of IL-6, which has a demonstrated efficacy in RA, or IL-21, other pivotal cytokines for B-cell activation, might be of interest in pSS. Inhibition of lymphotoxin-β, which allows, along with BAFF, the formation of germinal center-like structures in salivary glands, also deserves to be evaluated. Indeed, baminercept, a lymphotoxin-β receptor immunoglobulin fusion protein, has a dramatic effect in reducing salivary B-cell infiltrates of NOD mice. Moreover, salivary flow was partially restored in the treated mice [59].

33.3.2 Inhibition of T-cell Co-stimulation

Abatacept (CTLA-Ig), which has demonstrated its efficacy in RA, could be of therapeutic interest in pSS. Abatacept could also interact with the antigen-presenting cell properties of epithelial cells, which express CD80 and CD86.

33.3.3 Gene Therapy

For patients with glandular symptoms only, it could be speculated that progress in designing harmless vectors might make gene therapy become a true possibility in pSS [60, 61]. The good candidate genes for gene therapy remain to be determined. Of interest is the ongoing evaluation of the possibility of aquaporin 1 gene local livery in the salivary glands, currently evaluated in the NIH for radiotherapy-related dryness (phase I).

33.4 Conclusion

Looking into the future for therapies of pSS, we can feel rather optimistic. pSS is a wonderful model of autoimmunity for translational research, with an easy access to target organs of autoimmunity. Interestingly, recent genetic and pathogenic studies evidenced number of similarities between pSS and lupus, and pSS could be considered as a sort of lupus of mucosa. In pSS like in lupus, new pathogenic pathways have been and will be unraveled, resulting in the definition of new targets. To convert our optimism into the improvement of patients in daily care, a consensual disease activity score must be validated and clinicians and pharmaceutical companies have to design new trials with adequate inclusion criteria. Indeed, pSS is not a lost battle for the development of efficient biotherapies!

References

1. Christodoulou MI, Kapsogeorgou EK, Moutsopoulos NM, Moutsopoulos HM. Foxp3+ T-regulatory cells in Sjogren's syndrome: correlation with the grade of the autoimmune lesion and certain adverse prognostic factors. Am J Pathol. 2008;173:1389–96.
2. Gottenberg JE, Lavie F, Abbed K, Gasnault J, Le Nevot E, Delfraissy JF, Taoufik Y, Mariette X. CD4 CD25high regulatory T cells are not impaired in patients with primary Sjogren's syndrome. J Autoimmun. 2005;24:235–42.
3. Hjelmervik TO, Petersen K, Jonassen I, Jonsson R, Bolstad AI. Gene expression profiling of minor salivary glands clearly distinguishes primary Sjögren's syndrome patients from healthy controls. Arthritis Rheum. 2005;52:1534–44.
4. Gottenberg JE, Cagnard N, Lucchesi C, Letourneur F, Mistou S, Lazure T, Jacques S, Ba N, Ittah M, Lepajolec C, Labetoulle M, Ardizzone M, Sibilia J, Fournier C, Chiocchia G, Mariette X. Activation of IFN pathways and plasmacytoid dendritic cell recruitment in target organs of primary Sjogren's syndrome. Proc Natl Acad Sci USA. 2006;103:2770–5.
5. Emamian ES, Leon JM, Lessard CJ, Grandits M, Baechler EC, Gaffney PM, Segal B, Rhodus NL, Moser KL. Peripheral blood gene expression profiling in Sjögren's syndrome. Genes Immun. 2009;10:285–96. Epub 2009 Apr 30.
6. Miceli-Richard C, Comets E, Loiseau P, Puechal X, Hachulla E, Mariette X. Association of an *IRF5* gene functional polymorphism with Sjogren's syndrome. Arthritis Rheum. 2007;56:3989–94.
7. Gross JA, Johnston J, Mudri S, Enselman R, Dillon SR, Madden K, Xu W, Parrish-Novak J, Foster D, Lofton-Day C, Moore M, Littau A, Grossman A, Haugen H, Foley K, Blumberg H, Harrison K, Kindsvogel W, Clegg CH. TACI and BCMA are receptors for a TNF homologue implicated in B-cell autoimmune disease. Nature 2000;404:995–9.
8. Mariette X, Roux S, Zhang J, Bengoufa D, Lavie F, Zhou T, Kimberly R. The level of BLyS (BAFF) correlates with the titre of autoantibodies in human Sjogren's syndrome. Ann Rheum Dis. 2003;62: 168–71.
9. Sellam J, Miceli-Richard C, Gottenberg JE, Ittah M, Lavie F, Lacabaratz C, Gestermann N, Proust A, Lambotte O, Mariette X. Decreased BAFF-R on peripheral lymphocytes associated with increased disease activity in primary Sjogren's syndrome and systemic lupus erythematosus. Ann Rheum Dis. 2007 Jun;66:790–7.
10. Stein JV, López-Fraga M, Elustondo FA, Carvalho-Pinto CE, Rodríguez D, Gómez-Caro R, De Jong J, Martínez-A C, Medema JP, Hahne M. APRIL modulates B and T cell immunity. J Clin Invest. 2002;109:1587–98.
11. Castigli E, Wilson SA, Garibyan L, Rachid R, Bonilla F, Schneider L, Geha RS. TACI is mutant in common variable immunodeficiency and IgA deficiency. Nat Genet. 2005;37:829–34.
12. Yan M, Wang H, Chan B, Roose-Girma M, Erickson S, Baker T, Tumas D, Grewal IS, Dixit VM. Activation and accumulation of B cells in TACI-deficient mice. Nat Immunol. 2001;2: 638–43.
13. Ittah M, Miceli-Richard C, Eric Gottenberg J, Lavie F, Lazure T, Ba N, Sellam J, Lepajolec C, Mariette X. B-cell activating factor of the TNF family (BAFF) is expressed under stimulation by interferon in salivary gland epithelial cells in primary Sjögren's syndrome. Arthritis Res Ther. 2006 8;R51
14. Kapsogeorgou E, Manoussakis MN, The central role of epithelial cells in Sjogren's syndrome or autoimmune epithelitis. Autoimmun Rev. 2004;3(Suppl 1): S61–3.
15. Lavie F, Miceli-Richard C, Quillard J, Roux S, Leclerc P, Mariette X. Overexpression of BAFF in T cells infiltrating labial salivary glands from patients with Sjögren's syndrome. J Pathol. 2004;202: 496–502.
16. Morimoto S, Nakano S, Watanabe T, Tamayama Y, Mitsuo A, Nakiri Y, Suzuki J, Nozawa K, Amano H, Tokano Y, Kobata T, Takasaki Y. Expression of B-cell activating factor of the tumour necrosis factor family (BAFF) in T cells in active systemic lupus erythematosus: the role of BAFF in T cell-dependent B cell pathogenic autoantibody production. Rheumatology (Oxford) 2007;46:1083–6.
17. Lavie F, Miceli-Richard C, Ittah M, Sellam J, Gottenberg JE, Mariette X. B-cell activating factor of the tumour necrosis factor family expression in blood monocytes and T cells from patients with primary Sjögren's syndrome. Scand J Immunol. 2008;67:185–92.
18. Daridon C, Devauchelle V, Hutin P, Le Berre R, Martins-Carvalho C, Bendaoud B, Dueymes M, Saraux A, Youinou P, Pers JO. Aberrant expression of BAFF by B lymphocytes infiltrating the salivary glands of patients with primary Sjögren's syndrome. Arthritis Rheum. 2007 ;56:1134–44.
19. Litinskiy MB, Nardelli B, Hilbert DM, He B, Schaffer A, Casali P, Cerutti A. DCs induce CD40-independent immunoglobulin class switching through BLyS and APRIL. Nat Immunol. 2002;3:822–829.
20. Ittah M, Miceli-Richard C, Gottenberg JE, Sellam J, Eid P, Lebon P, Pallier C, Lepajolec C, Mariette X. Viruses induce high expression of B cell-activating factor by salivary gland epithelial cells through Toll-like receptor- and type-I interferon-dependent

and -independent pathways. Eur J Immunol. 2008 Apr;38:1058–64.
21. Ittah M, Miceli-Richard C, Gottenberg JE, Sellam J, Lepajolec C, Mariette X. B-cell-activating factor expressions in salivary epithelial cells after dsRNA virus infection depends on RNA-activated protein kinase activation. Eur J Immunol. 2009;39:1271–9.
22. Gottenberg JE, Sellam J, Ittah M, Lavie F, Proust A, Zouali H, Sordet C, Sibilia J, Kimberly RP, Mariette X, Miceli-Richard C. No evidence for an association between the −871 T/C promoter polymorphism in the B-cell-activating factor gene and primary Sjögren's syndrome. Arthritis Res Ther. 2006;8:R30. Epub 2006 Jan 9. PubMed PMID: 16507129.
23. Salomonsson S, Jonsson MV, Skarstein K, Brokstad KA, Hjelmström P, Wahren-Herlenius M, Jonsson R. Cellular basis of ectopic germinal center formation and autoantibody production in the target organ of patients with Sjögren's syndrome. Arthritis Rheum. 2003;48:3187–3201.
24. Theander E, Henriksson G, Ljungberg O, Mandl T, Manthorpe R, Jacobsson LT. Lymphoma and other malignancies in primary Sjogren's syndrome. A cohort study on cancer incidence and lymphoma predictors. Ann Rheum Dis. 2006;65:796–803.
25. Zintzaras E, Voulgarelis M, Moutsopoulos HM. The risk of lymphoma development in autoimmune diseases: a meta-analysis. Arch Intern Med. 2005;165:2337–2344.
26. Novak AJ, Grote DM, Stenson M, Ziesmer SC, Witzig TE, Habermann TM, Harder B, Ristow KM, Bram RJ, Jelinek DF, Gross JA, Ansell SM. Expression of BLyS and its receptors in B-cell non-Hodgkin lymphoma: correlation with disease activity and patient outcome. Blood 2004;104: 2247–53.
27. Ogawa N, Ping L, Zhenjun L, Takada Y, Sugai S. Involvement of the interferon-gamma-induced T cell-attracting chemokines, interferon-gamma-inducible 10-kd protein (CXCL10) and monokine induced by interferon-gamma (CXCL9), in the salivary gland lesions of patients with Sjogren's syndrome. Arthritis Rheum. 2002;46:2730–41.
28. Barone F, Bombardieri M, Manzo A, Blades MC, Morgan PR, Challacombe SJ, Valesini G, Pitzalis C. Association of CXCL13 and CCL21 expression with the progressive organization of lymphoid-like structures in Sjogren's syndrome. Arthritis Rheum. 2005;52:1773–84.
29. Nguyen CQ, Hu MH, Li Y, Stewart C, Peck AB. Salivary gland tissue expression of interleukin-23 and interleukin-17 in Sjögren's syndrome: findings in humans and mice. Arthritis Rheum. 2008;58: 734–43.
30. Gottenberg JE, Busson M, Loiseau P, Cohen-Solal J, Lepage V, Charron D, Sibilia J, Mariette X. In primary Sjogren's syndrome, HLA class II is associated exclusively with autoantibody production and spreading of the autoimmune response. Arthritis Rheum. 2003;48:2240–5.
31. Kariuki SN, Kirou KA, MacDermott EJ, Barillas-Arias L, Crow MK, Niewold TB. Cutting edge: autoimmune disease risk variant of STAT4 confers increased sensitivity to IFN-alpha in lupus patients in vivo. J Immunol. 2009 Jan 1;182:34–8.
32. Dawson LJ, Fox PC, Smith PM. Sjogrens syndrome—the non-apoptotic model of glandular hypofunction. Rheumatology (Oxford) 2006;45:792–8.
33. Ohlsson M, Skarstein K, Bolstad AI, Johannessen AC, Jonsson R. Fas-induced apoptosis is a rare event in Sjogren's syndrome. Lab Invest. 2001;81:95–105.
34. Zoukhri D, Kublin CL. Impaired neurotransmitter release from lacrimal and salivary gland nerves of a murine model of Sjogren's syndrome. Invest Ophthalmol Vis Sci. 2001;42:925–32.
35. Dawson LJ, Caulfield VL, Stanbury JB, Field AE, Christmas SE, Smith PM. Hydroxychloroquine therapy in patients with primary Sjogren's syndrome may improve salivary gland hypofunction by inhibition of glandular cholinesterase. Rheumatology (Oxford) 2005;44:449–55.
36. Waterman SA, Gordon TP, Rischmueller M. Inhibitory effects of muscarinic receptor autoantibodies on parasympathetic neurotransmission in Sjogren's syndrome. Arthritis Rheum. 2000;43:1647–54.
37. Beroukas D, Hiscock J, Jonsson R, Waterman SA, Gordon TP. Subcellular distribution of aquaporin 5 in salivary glands in primary Sjögren's syndrome. Lancet 2001;358:1875–76.
38. Vitali C, Palombi G, Baldini C, Benucci M, Bombardieri S, Covelli M, Del Papa N, De Vita S, Epis O, Franceschini F, Gerli R, Govoni M, Bongi SM, Maglione W, Migliaresi S, Montecucco C, Orefice M, Priori R, Tavoni A, Valesini G. Sjögren's syndrome disease damage index and disease activity index: scoring systems for the assessment of disease damage and disease activity in Sjögren's syndrome, derived from an analysis of a cohort of Italian patients. Arthritis Rheum. 2007;56:2223–31.
39. Bowman SJ, Sutcliffe N, Isenberg DA, Goldblatt F, Adler M, Price E, Canavan A, Hamburger J, Richards A, Rauz S, Regan M, Gadsby K, Rigby S, Jones A, Mathew R, Mulherin D, Stevenson A, Nightingale P. Sjögren's systemic clinical activity index (SCAI)—a systemic disease activity measure for use in clinical trials in primary Sjögren's syndrome. Rheumatology (Oxford) 2007;46:1845–51.
40. Seror R, Ravaud P, Bowman S, Baron G, Tzioufas A, Theander E, Gottenberg JE, Bootsma H, Mariette X, Vitali C. EULAR Sjogren's syndrome disease activity index (ESSDAI): development of a consensus systemic disease activity index in primary Sjogren's syndrome. Ann Rheum Dis. 2009 Jun 28; Epub ahead of print.
41. Mariette X, Ravaud P, Steinfeld S, Baron G, Goetz J, Hachulla E, Combe B, Puéchal X, Pennec Y, Sauvezie B, Perdriger A, Hayem G, Janin A, Sibilia

J. Inefficacy of infliximab in primary Sjögren's syndrome. Results of the randomized controlled Trial of Remicade In Primary Sjögren's Syndrome (TRIPSS). Arthritis Rheum. 2004;50:1270–6.
42. Sankar V, Brennan MT, Kok MR, Leakan RA, Smith JA, Manny J, Baum BJ, Pillemer SR. Etanercept in Sjogren's syndrome: a twelve-week randomized, double-blind, placebo-controlled pilot clinical trial. Arthritis Rheum. 2004;50:2240–5.
43. Mavragani CP, Niewold TB, Moutsopoulos NM, Pillemer SR, Wahl SM, Crow MK. Augmented interferon-alpha pathway activation in patients with Sjögren's syndrome treated with etanercept. Arthritis Rheum. 2007;56:3995–4004.
44. Wallace DJ, Petri M, Olsen N, et al. MEDI-545, an anti-interferon alpha monoclonal antibody, shows evidence of clinical activity in systemic lupus erythematosus. Arthritis Rheum. 2007;56:S526.
45. Stohl W, Chatham W, Weisman M, et al. Belimumab (BmAb), a novel fully human monoclonal antibody to B-lymphocyte stimulator (BLyS), selectively modulates B-cell sub-populations and immunoglobulins in a heterogeneous rheumatoid arthritis subject population. Arthritis Rheum. 2005;52:S444
46. Petri M, Furie R, Ginzler E, et al. Novel combined response endpoint and systemic lupus erythematosus (SLE) flare index (SFI) demonstrate belimumab (fully human monoclonal antibody to BLyS) improves or stabilizes SLE disease activity and reduces flare rate over 2.5 years of therapy. Arthritis Rheum. 2007;56:S527 (abstract 316).
47. Toubi E, Kessel A, Slobodin G, Boulman N, Pavlotzky E, Zisman D, Rozenbaum M, Rosner I. Changes in macrophage function after rituximab treatment in patients with rheumatoid arthritis. Ann Rheum Dis. 2007;66:818–20. Epub 2006 Dec 5.
48. Cambridge G, Stohl W, Leandro MJ, Migone TS, Hilbert DM, Edwards JC. Circulating levels of B lymphocyte stimulator in patients with rheumatoid arthritis following rituximab treatment: relationships with B cell depletion, circulating antibodies, and clinical relapse. Arthritis Rheum. 2006;54: 723–32.
49. Pers JO, Devauchelle V, Daridon C, Bendaoud B, Le Berre R, Bordron A, Hutin P, Renaudineau Y, Dueymes M, Loisel S, Berthou C, Saraux A, Youinou P. BAFF-modulated repopulation of B lymphocytes in the blood and salivary glands of rituximab-treated patients with Sjögren's syndrome. Arthritis Rheum. 2007;56:1464–77.
50. Lavie F, Miceli-Richard C, Ittah M, Sellam J, Gottenberg JE, Mariette X. Increase of B-cell activating factor of the TNF family (BAFF) after rituximab: insights into a new regulating system of BAFF production. Ann Rheum Dis. 2007;66:700–3.
51. Pijpe J, van Imhoff GW, Spijkervet FK, et al. Rituximab treatment in patients with primary Sjogren's syndrome: an open-label phase II study. Arthritis Rheum. 2005;52:2740–50.
52. Devauchelle-Pensec V, Pennec Y, Morvan J, et al. Improvement of Sjögren's syndrome after two infusions of rituximab (anti-CD20). Arthritis Rheum. 2007;57:310–7.
53. Somer BG, Tsai DE, Downs L, et al. Improvement in Sjogren's syndrome following therapy with rituximab for marginal zone lymphoma. Arthritis Rheum. 2003;49:394–8.
54. Voulgarelis M, Giannouli S, Tzioufas AG, et al. Long term remission of Sjogren's syndrome associated aggressive B cell non-Hodgkin's lymphomas following combined B cell depletion therapy and CHOP (cyclophosphamide, doxorubicin, vincristine, prednisone). Ann Rheum Dis. 2006;65: 1033–7.
55. Seror R, Sordet C, Guillevin L, Hachulla E, Masson C, Ittah M, Candon S, Le Guern V, Aouba A, Sibilia J, Gottenberg JE, Mariette X. Tolerance and efficacy of rituximab and changes in serum B cell biomarkers in patients with systemic complications of primary Sjogren's syndrome. Ann Rheum Dis. 2007;66: 351–7.
56. Dass S, Bowman SJ, Vital EM, Ikeda K, Pease CT, Hamburger J, Richards A, Rauz S, Emery P. Reduction of fatigue in Sjogren's syndrome with rituximab: results of a randomised, double-blind, placebo controlled pilot study. Ann Rheum Dis. 2008 Nov;67:1541–4.
57. Meijer J, Vissink A, Meiners PM, Spijkervet FKL, Kallenberg CGM, Bootsma H. Rituximab treatment in primary Sjögren's syndrome: a double-blind placebo controlled trial. Arthritis Rheum. 2008;56:S430 (abstract 713).
58. Steinfeld SD, Tant L, Burmester GR, et al. Epratuzumab (humanised anti-CD22 antibody) in primary Sjögren's syndrome: an open-label phase I/II study. Arthritis Res Ther. 2006;8(4):R129.
59. Gatumu MK, Skarstein K, Papandile A, Browning JL, Fava RA, Bolstad AI. Blockade of lymphotoxin-beta receptor signaling reduces aspects of Sjögren's syndrome in salivary glands of non-obese diabetic mice. Arthritis Res Ther. 2009;11:R24. Epub 2009 Feb 18.
60. Kok MR, Yamano S, Lodde BM, Wang J, Couwenhoven RI, Yakar S, Voutetakis A, Leroith D, Schmidt M, Afione S, Pillemer SR, Tsutsui MT, Tak PP, Chiorini JA, Baum BJ. Local adeno-associated virus-mediated interleukin 10 gene transfer has disease-modifying effects in a murine model of Sjögren's syndrome. Hum Gene Ther. 2003;14: 1605–18.
61. Lodde BM, Mineshiba F, Wang J, Cotrim AP, Afione S, Tak PP, Baum BJ. Effect of human vasoactive intestinal peptide gene transfer in a murine model of Sjogren's syndrome. Ann Rheum Dis. 2006 Feb;65:195–200.
62. Harner KC, Jackson LW, Drabick JJ. Normalization of anticardiolipin antibodies following rituximab therapy for marginal zone lymphoma in a patient

with Sjogren's syndrome. Rheumatology. 2004;43: 1309–10.
63. Ramos-Casals M, López-Guillermo A, Brito-Zerón P, Cervera R, Font J, SS-HCV Study Group. Treatment of B-cell lymphoma with rituximab in two patients with Sjögren's syndrome associated with hepatitis C virus infection. Lupus 2004;13:969–71.
64. Gottenberg JE, Guillevin L, Lambotte O, Combe B, Allanore Y, Cantagrel A, Larroche C, Soubrier M, Bouillet L, Dougados M, Fain O, Farge D, Kyndt X, Lortholary O, Masson C, Moura B, Remy P, Thomas T, Wendling D, Anaya JM, Sibilia J, Mariette X, Club Rheumatismes et Inflammation (CRI). Tolerance and short term efficacy of rituximab in 43 patients with systemic autoimmune diseases. Ann Rheum Dis. 2005;64:913–20.
65. Ahmadi-Simab K, Lamprecht P, Nölle B, Ai M, Gross WL. Successful treatment of refractory anterior scleritis in primary Sjogren's syndrome with rituximab. Ann Rheum Dis. 2005;64: 1087–8.
66. Ring T, Kallenbach M, Praetorius J, Nielsen S, Melgaard B. Successful treatment of a patient with primary Sjögren's syndrome with rituximab. Clin Rheumatol. 2006 Nov;25(6):891–4. Epub 2005 Nov 8.
67. St. Clair E, Levesque MC, Luning Prak N, Vivino FB, Alappatt C, Wallace D, Wedgwood J, Cohen P. Rituximab therapy for primary Sjögren's syndrome (pSS): an open-label trial. Arthritis Rheum. 2007;56:S449 (abstract 1102).

34 Into the Future: Autonomic Neuropathy, MicroRNAs, and Gene Therapy

Ilias Alevizos, John A. Chiorini,
and Nikolay P. Nikolov

Abstract

Understanding the pathogenesis of Sjögren's syndrome (SS) has proved to be challenging. Both immune-mediated and non-immune-mediated mechanisms have been implicated, which adds to the complexity of the problem. However, recent developments in science and technology have given researchers new opportunities for exploring this fascinating disease. In this chapter we provide a synopsis of the progress in our understanding of the role of the autonomic nervous system in SS pathogenesis, the role of microRNAs as novel tools in advancing research in this field, and gene therapy as potential therapeutic avenue.

Keywords

Autonomic nervous system • Dysautonomia • microRNA • Gene therapy

34.1 Introduction

Sjögren's syndrome (SS) is an enigmatic disease of unknown etiology and elusive pathogenesis. The current understanding of the complex immune and non-immune mechanisms driving SS is covered in detail by Gottenberg and Meriette earlier in this textbook. Recognition that glandular dysfunction without overt inflammation in a significant number of patients has led to the hypothesis that glandular dryness may be caused by mechanisms independent of or in addition to immune-mediated glandular destruction, atrophy, or fibrosis. Autonomic nervous system (ANS) dysfunction has emerged as one plausible mechanism underlying the sicca manifestations. In addition, advancements in our understanding of microRNAs (miRNAs) as gene expression regulators have highlighted the importance of exploring miRNAs as potential biomarkers and therapeutic targets for SS. The need for new and effective therapies for SS has led researchers to explore new approaches such as gene therapy, which could provide a local delivery mechanism of key molecules directly to the gland. Using targeted gene delivery in animal models may also be a powerful tool to investigate critical pathways in the pathogenesis of SS.

N.P. Nikolov (✉)
Sjögren's Syndrome Clinic, National Institute of Dental and Craniofacial Research, Bethesda, MD, USA
e-mail: nikolovn@mail.nih.gov

R.I. Fox, C.M. Fox (eds.), *Sjögren's Syndrome*, DOI 10.1007/978-1-60327-957-4_34,

34.2 Autonomic Neuropathy in Sjögren's Syndrome

Current understanding about the etiopathogenesis of SS stems from the assumption that the immune-mediated destruction of the exocrine glands leads to their hypofunction and subsequently symptoms of dryness. However, multiple examples raise concerns with this view: (1) the degree of glandular inflammation or destruction correlates only poorly with the degree of dysfunction or symptoms of dryness; (2) many patients do not show evidence of systemic autoimmunity or inflammation; (3) traditional immunosuppressive and anti-rheumatic medications have not proven to be beneficial, unlike the symptomatic sialogogues, to the sicca manifestations. Thus, the existing evidence does not fully support this assumption and cannot explain the underlying pathogenic mechanisms of SS.

Exocrine glands are innervated by the autonomic nervous system (ANS), and, interestingly, dysautonomia can mimic many of the features of SS, particularly cardinal manifestations, such as xerostomia and xerophthalmia. The ANS regulates homeostasis via effects on the smooth muscles, glands, and cardiovascular system. Recent studies have focused on the fact that regulation of tear and salivary flow involves an entire functional system that includes the mucosal surfaces, glands, afferent nerve signals sent to the midbrain (lacrimal and salivary response region), and efferent neural signals from the brain to the acinar/ductal epithelial structures in the gland. Saliva-secreting glands have both sympathetic and parasympathetic innervations with the latter being predominant. Postganglionic parasympathetic stimulation results in postsynaptic release of the neurotransmitter acetylcholine responsible for activation of G-protein-coupled muscarinic receptors on acinar cells leading to saliva secretion, while sympathetic glandular innervation is responsible for secretion of salivary proteins and glandular vascular responses.

Several systematic studies in patients with SS have found multiple clinical and subclinical abnormalities in parasympathetic and sympathetic cholinergic, sympathetic noradrenergic, enteric, and adrenomedullary hormonal ANS components, underscoring the role of the autonomic neuropathy in the pathogenesis of the syndrome [1–3]. Identifying the patterns of abnormalities in the different ANS domains will help us to better understand the mechanisms involved in the initiation and tenacity of the disease. The importance of salivary gland innervation in the pathogenesis of SS is further supported by the positive results of a study utilizing a local salivary reflex (lingual nerve) electrostimulator to relieve severe xerostomia [4].

In addition, recent recognition of the "cholinergic anti-inflammatory pathway" [5] indicates the existence of a critical crosstalk between the immune and the nervous systems, supporting the need for an interdisciplinary approach to understand the mechanisms underlying dryness in SS.

34.3 MicroRNAs in Sjögren's Syndrome

Over the past decade, microRNAs (miRNAs) have become a "hot" area of interest in the research community to identify mechanism of disease, biomarkers, and therapeutic targets. MiRNAs are endogenous, small (approximately 22 nucleotides in length) non-coding RNAs that regulate gene expression posttranscriptionally [6]. MiRNAs have been shown to play important roles in numerous physiological as well as pathological processes. Their discovery dates to 1993 when *lin-4*, the first described miRNA was shown to downregulate LIN-14 protein levels in *Caenorhabditis elegans*. It was only in 2001 that the term miRNA was used in the concurrent publication of three articles [7–9]. The number of publications related to miRNAs has since been exponentially increasing and their role is being explored in both functional and biomarker discovery studies.

MiRNA biogenesis has been extensively studied [10]. In mammalian cells, the first step involves the transcription of the pri-microRNAs by RNA polymerase II. Pri-microRNAs are usually thousands of nucleotides (nt) long. The second step in biogenesis involves the processing of pri-miRNAs to pre-microRNAs in the nucleus by Drosha, an RNase III enzyme. The pre-microRNAs form a hairpin duplex structure and typically have a length of 70–100 nt. Pre-microRNAs are subsequently actively transported from the nucleus to the cytoplasm where they are processed by Dicer, a cytoplasmic endonuclease, and other RNA-binding proteins into double-stranded RNAs, 19–24 nt long. Those double-stranded RNAs are then dissociated and get loaded to a ribonucleoprotein complex called RISC, so that they can exert their effect by binding on the target mRNAs and either degrading them or blocking their translation. The target selectivity of the miRNAs depends on the complementarities of their sequences with the sequences of the mRNA. Initially it was believed that miRNA–mRNA binding occurs only on the 3′-UTR, but it has been shown since that binding can also occur on the 5′-UTR and the coding sequence of the mRNA [11].

Some of the specific physiological functions that miRNAs have been implicated with include lymphocytic differentiation, embryonic stem cell fate, tissue morphogenesis, and organ development. Non-malignant pathologies in which miRNAs have been implicated include hepatitis infections [12], rheumatoid arthritis [13], neuropsychiatric disorders [14], and Alzheimer's disease [15]. Moreover, miRNA expression alterations have been identified in almost all major malignancies [16–22].

One of the most important characteristics of miRNAs is that a single miRNA can regulate the expression of hundreds of mRNAs simultaneously, potentially exerting a much greater effect on a cellular phenotype than a single mRNA [11, 23]. This is the reason why miRNAs are also called master regulators of gene expression. For autoimmune diseases such as Sjögren's syndrome, the functional importance of miRNAs is currently being explored. Their roles in Sjögren's syndrome should be investigated in two major directions. First, miRNA alterations might be associated with the autoimmune characteristics of lymphocytes, i.e., increased immune activation or loss of immune regulation. Second, miRNAs might be playing a role in the altered salivary gland function, especially in cases where inflammatory cells do not constitute the majority of the cells within the glands and there is functional salivary tissue remaining.

The use of miRNAs as biomarkers for diagnosis, prognosis, and disease activity in autoimmune diseases is currently unexplored. MiRNAs possess some characteristics that make them excellent candidates for biomarker studies. First, one miRNA can potentially capture a lot of information about the physiological status of a cell or tissue, since one miRNA controls the expression of a large number of genes. Clinically this translates into using a more limited number of miRNAs in biomarker assays reducing the complexity of measurements. Second, miRNAs can be isolated readily and reproducibly from easily obtained biological fluids such as saliva [24], urine [25], and plasma [26] and from formalin-fixed paraffin-embedded tissues [27]. The use of existing paraffin-embedded samples with their associated clinical information can greatly accelerate biomarker discovery. Third, in complex diseases such as cancer, miRNAs have been shown to have the specificity and sensitivity required for clinical applications. Fourth, miRNAs have a long half-life in vivo [23] and are remarkably stable and resistant to degradation by nucleases in vitro [28], thus allowing for detection in clinical specimens in which mRNA isolation is hindered by quick degradation.

In summary, miRNAs appear to be a promising tool to dissect critical mechanisms of disease, identify biomarkers for diagnosis, prognosis, and disease activity. MiRNAs also have the potential for identifying new therapeutic targets in SS and other disorders.

34.4 Gene Therapy in Sjögren's Syndrome

Current treatment strategies for SS are focused on symptomatic relief and the rationale for using available immunosuppressive and immunomodulatory therapies draws analogy from treatments

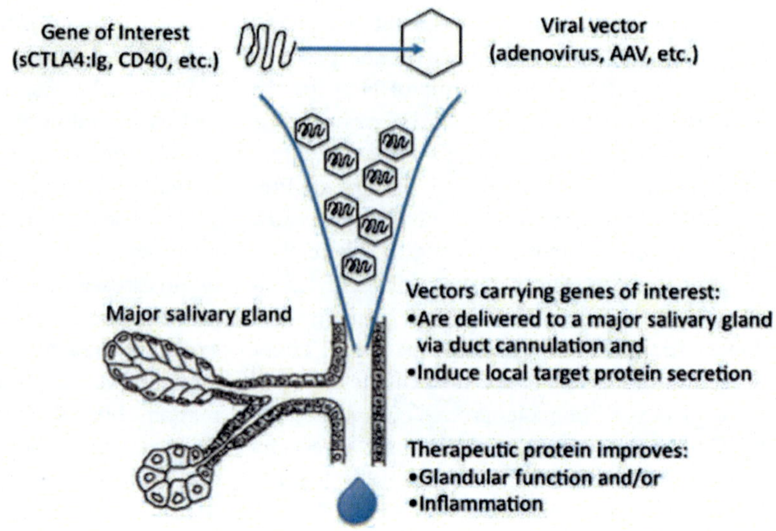

Fig. 34.1 Schema of local gene therapy for Sjögren's syndrome

of other rheumatic diseases. This approach, however, has not been very productive and indicates the need for development of new therapies based on better understanding of the disease itself. Identifying appropriate therapeutic targets is an active area of research and one aspect of successfully targeting the identified molecule(s) is the delivery method. Major salivary glands are considered a "prime suspect" in the initiation and perpetuation of sicca manifestations and perhaps the extraglandular features of SS. Therefore, local delivery of key immunomodulatory proteins or other potential therapeutic molecules directly to the gland using gene therapy is a sensible treatment approach. Advantages of this approach include ease of access via retrograde cannulation of the entire salivary gland (Fig. 34.1). Depending on the choice of vector, both long-term and short-term expressions are possible and systemic complication of the drugs can be limited by treating only the salivary glands. Although several viral vectors tested in pre-clinical studies appear to be safe vehicles for gene transfer, further work will be required to develop vectors with improved transduction activity in both ductal and acinar cells with limited immune response. Incorporation of regulated expression systems and the addition of tissue-specific promoters would further improve the safety profile of the vectors.

Despite the lack of correlation between local infiltrate scores and salivary gland activity, several proof of concept studies with immunomodulatory proteins delivered by gene therapy in animal models have been completed and demonstrated the feasibility of this approach. One of the first studies to test the local application of gene therapy to the salivary gland used a viral vector encoding the anti-inflammatory cytokine IL-10 [29]. IL-10 was administered locally to the salivary glands of NOD mice by retrograde cannulation of the salivary gland ducts or intramuscular injection in the quadriceps muscle using a recombinant adeno-associated viral type 2 (AAV2) vector. In contrast to the control or IM-treated groups, the mice treated with IL-10 locally in the salivary gland showed significantly higher salivary flow and lower infiltrate scores.

Similarly, positive results have also been observed using viral vectors encoding the neuropeptide vasoactive intestinal peptide (VIP) [30]. Although IL-10 has clear anti-inflammatory activity, it can promote B-cell proliferation, a concern in Sjögren's patients in which 5% of the patients develop lymphomas. Similarly, while VIP did restore salivary gland activity following local expression in the salivary glands of mice, it did not reduce the focal inflammation associated with this model. These findings suggest that immunomodulation can have a significant role in the treatment of SS. Other pro-inflammatory molecules such as IL-17, IFN-γ(gamma), and IL-12 as well as several chemokines have been associated with this disease and inhibitors of these molecules could be expressed locally in the gland [31]. Molecules that block costimulation such as sCTLA4, CD40, and sICAM are reported to be beneficial in the treatment of other autoimmune disease and should be explored in SS.

At present the primary treatment of SS and other autoimmune disorders is immune suppression or modulation. However, markers of immune activation do not always correlate with glandular dysfunction suggesting that other non-immunomodulatory approaches may be useful in preventing the sicca symptoms and restoring gland activity. In addition to therapies that enhance the sensitivity of salivary and lacrimal glands to neurostimulatory signals, approaches that reengineer the gland could be used to restore salivary gland activity. The altered expression and distribution of the water channel, AQP5, have been proposed as a mechanism for xerostomia [32]. Gene transfer technology offers the possibility to reengineer the glands by expressing other water channels such as AQP1 that could aid in fluid movement from the ductal structure still intact in the gland [33]. A similar approach was taken in developing a treatment for radiation-induced xerostomia and is currently in a Phase 1 study to assess the safety and efficacy of adenoviral vector delivery of the *AQP1* gene to parotid glands to restore fluid movement [34].

MiRNA profiling in minor glands presents not only a new window into the transcriptome of the salivary gland but also the potential for identifying new therapeutic targets. Short hairpin RNAs (shRNAs) which can have the same gene regulatory activity as miRNAs have been incorporated into gene therapy vectors for the treatment of hepatitis B virus as well as local expression in the eye for treatment of age-related macular degeneration [35–36]. Similarly as we gain clarity about the role of miRNAs in salivary gland function, those miRNAs differentially expressed in Sjögren's patients or that regulate key pathways in salivary gland function can be studied using current gene transfer vectors. Furthermore, these miRNAs may offer a new avenue for therapeutic intervention.

34.5 Conclusion

Thinking "outside the box" allowed SS researchers to focus on dissecting not only immune-mediated but also non-inflammatory disease mechanisms including autonomic neuropathy. Recent developments in science and technology have opened new and unorthodox avenues for studying the complex mechanisms underlying SS and other rheumatic diseases. Exploring miRNAs presents enormous opportunities to reveal critical pathways in the pathogenesis of SS and many other disorders. In the quest for new therapies, gene delivery may have its role as targeted therapeutic strategy for SS and potentially other local and systemic diseases.

References

1. Mandl T, Granberg V, Apelqvist J, Wollmer P, Manthorpe R, Jacobsson LT. Autonomic nervous symptoms in primary Sjogren's syndrome. Rheumatology 2008;47:914–9.
2. Cai FZ, Lester S, Lu T, et al. Mild autonomic dysfunction in primary Sjogren's syndrome: a controlled study. Arthritis Res Ther. 2008;10:R31.
3. Kovacs L, Papos M, Takacs R, et al. Autonomic nervous system dysfunction involving the gastrointestinal and the urinary tracts in primary Sjogren's syndrome. Clin Exp Rheumatol. 2003;21:697–703.
4. Strietzel FP, Lafaurie GI, Bautista Mendoza GR, et al. Efficacy and safety of an intraoral electrostimulation device for xerostomia relief: a multicenter randomized trial. Arthritis Rheum. 2011;63(1):180–90.
5. Tracey KJ. Reflex control of immunity. Nat Rev Immunol. 2009;9:418–28.
6. Chua JH, Armugam A, Jeyaseelan K. MicroRNAs: biogenesis, function and applications. Curr Opin Mol Ther. 2009;11:189–99.
7. Lagos-Quintana M, Rauhut R, Lendeckel W, Tuschl T. Identification of novel genes coding for small expressed RNAs. Science 2001;294:853–8.
8. Lau NC, Lim LP, Weinstein EG, Bartel DP. An abundant class of tiny RNAs with probable regulatory roles in *Caenorhabditis elegans*. Science 2001;294:858–62.
9. Lee RC, Ambros V. An extensive class of small RNAs in *Caenorhabditis elegans*. Science 2001;294:862–4.

10. Lee Y, Kim M, Han J, et al. MicroRNA genes are transcribed by RNA polymerase II. EMBO J. 2004;23:4051–60.
11. Miranda KC, Huynh T, Tay Y, et al. A pattern-based method for the identification of microRNA binding sites and their corresponding heteroduplexes. Cell 2006;126:1203–17.
12. Sarasin-Filipowicz M, Krol J, Markiewicz I, Heim MH, Filipowicz W. Decreased levels of microRNA miR-122 in individuals with hepatitis C responding poorly to interferon therapy. Nat Med. 2009;15:31–3.
13. Nakamachi Y, Kawano S, Takenokuchi M, et al. MicroRNA-124a is a key regulator of proliferation and monocyte chemoattractant protein 1 secretion in fibroblast-like synoviocytes from patients with rheumatoid arthritis. Arthritis Rheum. 2009;60:1294–304.
14. Zhu Y, Kalbfleisch T, Brennan MD, Li Y. A microRNA gene is hosted in an intron of a schizophrenia-susceptibility gene. Schizophrenia Res. 2009;109:86–9.
15. Niwa R, Zhou F, Li C, Slack FJ. The expression of the Alzheimer's amyloid precursor protein-like gene is regulated by developmental timing microRNAs and their targets in *Caenorhabditis elegans*. Dev Biol. 2008;315:418–25.
16. Spizzo R, Nicoloso MS, Croce CM, Calin GA. SnapShot: microRNAs in cancer. Cell 2009;137: 586–6.
17. Szafranska AE, Doleshal M, Edmunds HS, et al. Analysis of microRNAs in pancreatic fine-needle aspirates can classify benign and malignant tissues. Clin Chem. 2008;54:1716–24.
18. Visone R, Croce CM. MiRNAs and cancer. Am J Pathol. 2009;174:1131–8.
19. Yanaihara N, Caplen N, Bowman E, et al. Unique microRNA molecular profiles in lung cancer diagnosis and prognosis. Cancer Cell 2006;9:189–98.
20. Liston A, Lu LF, O'Carroll D, Tarakhovsky A, Rudensky AY. Dicer-dependent microRNA pathway safeguards regulatory T cell function. J Exp Med. 2008;205:1993–2004.
21. Marcucci G, Radmacher MD, Maharry K, et al. MicroRNA expression in cytogenetically normal acute myeloid leukemia. N Engl J Med. 2008;358:1919–28.
22. Schetter AJ, Leung SY, Sohn JJ, et al. MicroRNA expression profiles associated with prognosis and therapeutic outcome in colon adenocarcinoma. JAMA 2008;299:425–36.
23. Lim LP, Lau NC, Garrett-Engele P, et al. Microarray analysis shows that some microRNAs downregulate large numbers of target mRNAs. Nature 2005;433:769–73.
24. Michael A, Bajracharya SD, Yuen PS, et al. Exosomes from human saliva as a source of microRNA biomarkers. Oral Dis. 2010;16:34–8.
25. Hanke M, Hoefig K, Merz H, et al. A robust methodology to study urine microRNA as tumor marker: microRNA-126 and microRNA-182 are related to urinary bladder cancer. Urol Oncol. 2009. (Epub ahead of print).
26. Huang Z, Huang D, Ni S, Peng Z, Sheng W, Du X. Plasma microRNAs are promising novel biomarkers for early detection of colorectal cancer. Int J Cancer 2010;127:118–26.
27. Hasemeier B, Christgen M, Kreipe H, Lehmann U. Reliable microRNA profiling in routinely processed formalin-fixed paraffin-embedded breast cancer specimens using fluorescence labelled bead technology. BMC Biotechnol. 2008;8:90.
28. Chen X, Ba Y, Ma L, et al. Characterization of microRNAs in serum: a novel class of biomarkers for diagnosis of cancer and other diseases. Cell Res. 2008;18:997–1006.
29. Kok MR, Yamano S, Lodde BM, et al. Local adeno-associated virus-mediated interleukin 10 gene transfer has disease-modifying effects in a murine model of Sjogren's syndrome. Hum Gene Ther. 2003;14:1605–18.
30. Lodde BM, Mineshiba F, Wang J, et al. Effect of human vasoactive intestinal peptide gene transfer in a murine model of Sjogren's syndrome. Ann Rheum Dis. 2006;65:195–200.
31. Roescher N, Tak PP, Illei GG. Cytokines in Sjogren's syndrome. Oral Dis. 2009;15:519–26.
32. Soyfoo MS, De Vriese C, Debaix H, et al. Modified aquaporin 5 expression and distribution in submandibular glands from NOD mice displaying autoimmune exocrinopathy. Arthritis Rheum. 2007;56:2566–74.
33. Zheng C, Goldsmith CM, Mineshiba F, et al. Toxicity and biodistribution of a first-generation recombinant adenoviral vector, encoding aquaporin-1, after retroductal delivery to a single rat submandibular gland. Hum Gene Ther. 2006;17:1122–33.
34. Baum BJ, Zheng C, Alevizos I, et al. Development of a gene transfer-based treatment for radiation-induced salivary hypofunction. Oral Oncol. 2010;46: 4–8.
35. Chen Y, Du D, Wu J, et al. Inhibition of hepatitis B virus replication by stably expressed shRNA. Biochem Biophys Res Commun. 2003;311: 398–404.
36. Hadj-Slimane R, Lepelletier Y, Lopez N, Garbay C, Raynaud F. Short interfering RNA (siRNA), a novel therapeutic tool acting on angiogenesis. Biochimie 2007;89:1234–44.

Index

Note: The letters 'f' and 't' following the locators refer to figures and tables respectively.

R.I. Fox, C.M. Fox (eds.), *Sjögren's Syndrome*, DOI 10.1007/978-1-60327-957-4,

M

U

V

W

X